AF829080

Pearls and Pitfalls in CARDIOVASCULAR IMAGING

Pseudolesions, Artifacts and Other Difficult Diagnoses

Pearls and Pitfalls in CARDIOVASCULAR IMAGING

Pseudolesions, Artifacts and Other Difficult Diagnoses

Edited by

Stefan L. Zimmerman

Assistant Professor of Radiology and Radiological Sciences, Johns Hopkins University School of Medicine, Baltimore, MD, USA

Elliot K. Fishman

Professor of Radiology and Radiological Sciences, Johns Hopkins University School of Medicine, Baltimore, MD, USA

CAMBRIDGE UNIVERSITY PRESS

CAMBRIDGE
UNIVERSITY PRESS

University Printing House, Cambridge CB2 8BS, United Kingdom

Cambridge University Press is part of the University of Cambridge.

It furthers the University's mission by disseminating knowledge in the pursuit of education, learning and research at the highest international levels of excellence.

www.cambridge.org
Information on this title: www.cambridge.org/9781107023727

© Cambridge University Press 2015

This publication is in copyright. Subject to statutory exception and to the provisions of relevant collective licencing agreements, no reproduction of any part may take place without the written permission of Cambridge University Press.

First published 2015

Printed in the United Kingdom by Bell and Bain Ltd

A catalog record for this publication is available from the British Library

Library of Congress Cataloging in Publication data
Pearls and pitfalls in cardiovascular imaging : variants and other difficult diagnoses / [edited by] Stefan L. Zimmerman, Elliot K. Fishman.
p. ; cm.
Includes bibliographical references and index.
ISBN 978-1-107-02372-7 (Hardback)
I. Zimmerman, Stefan L., editor. II. Fishman, Elliot K., editor.
[DNLM: 1. Cardiovascular Diseases–diagnosis. 2. Diagnostic Imaging. 3. Diagnostic Techniques, Cardiovascular. WG 141]
RC683.5.I42
616.1′0754–dc23 2014039489

ISBN 978-1-107-02372-7 Hardback

DAMAGED

Cambridge University Press has no responsibility for the persistence or accuracy of URLs for external or third-party internet websites referred to in this publication, and does not guarantee that any content on such websites is, or will remain, accurate or appropriate.

Every effort has been made in preparing this book to provide accurate and up-to-date information which is in accord with accepted standards and practice at the time of publication. Although case histories are drawn from actual cases, every effort has been made to disguise the identities of the individuals involved. Nevertheless, the authors, editors and publishers can make no warranties that the information contained herein is totally free from error, not least because clinical standards are constantly changing through research and regulation. The authors, editors and publishers therefore disclaim all liability for direct or consequential damages resulting from the use of material contained in this book. Readers are strongly advised to pay careful attention to information provided by the manufacturer of any drugs or equipment that they plan to use.

Contents

Section 9. Mesenteric vascular

Section 10. Peripheral vascular

Section 11. Veins

Contributors

Sumera Ali, MD
Post-doctoral Fellow, Department of Radiology and Radiological Sciences, Johns Hopkins University School of Medicine, Baltimore, MD, USA

David Bonekamp, MD
Attending Radiologist, Department of Neuroradiology, University Hospital Heidelberg, Heidelberg, Germany

Tessa S. Cook, MD, PhD (senior contributor)
Assistant Professor of Radiology, Hospital of the University of Pennsylvania, PA, USA

Celia P. Corona-Villalobos, MD
Researcher, Department of Radiology, Division of Body MRI, Johns Hopkins Hospital, Baltimore, MD, USA

Benoit Desjardins, MD, PhD
Associate Professor of Radiology, Hospital of the University of Pennsylvania, Philadelphia, PA, USA

Maera Haider, MD
Post-doctoral Fellow, Department of Radiology and Radiological Sciences, Johns Hopkins University School of Medicine, Baltimore, MD, USA

Vivek Halappa, MD
Post-doctoral Fellow, Department of Radiology and Radiological Sciences, Johns Hopkins University School of Medicine, Baltimore, MD, USA

Saurabh Jha, MBBS (senior contributor)
Assistant Professor of Radiology, Hospital of the University of Pennsylvania, Philadelphia, PA, USA

Nathan Johnson, MD
Diagnostic Radiologist, United Imaging Consultants, Mission, KS, USA

Pamela T. Johnson, MD (senior contributor)
Associate Professor of Radiology and Radiological Sciences, Johns Hopkins University School of Medicine, Baltimore, MD, USA

Satomi Kawamoto, MD (senior contributor)
Associate Professor of Radiology and Radiological Sciences, Johns Hopkins University School of Medicine, Baltimore, MD, USA

Spencer T. Lake, MD
Radiology Resident, University of California at San Francisco, San Francisco, CA, USA

Pejman Motarjem, MD
Diagnostic Radiologist, Desert Radiologists, Las Vegas, NV, USA

Koteswara Pothineni, MD
Third-year Cardiology Fellow, Louisiana State University School of Medicine, Section of Cardiology, New Orleans, LA, USA

Siva P. Raman, MD
Assistant Professor of Radiology and Radiological Sciences, Department of Radiology, Johns Hopkins University School of Medicine, Baltimore, MD, USA

Mark Stellingworth, MD
Assistant Professor, Section of Cardiology, University of South Carolina Medical School, Columbia, SC, USA

Atif Zaheer, MD (senior contributor)
Associate Professor of Radiology and Radiological Sciences, Johns Hopkins University School of Medicine, Baltimore, MD, USA

Stefan L. Zimmerman, MD
Assistant Professor of Radiology and Radiological Sciences, Johns Hopkins University School of Medicine, Baltimore, MD, USA

Preface

As with other titles in the *Pearls and Pitfalls* series, this book is a reference for those uncommon clinical diagnoses, artifacts, and other confusing or strange entities that are not typically covered in standard textbooks. This is not a collection of the classic cases that are so often encountered during board review or in continuing education materials. Rather, this title focuses on challenging scenarios and entities that we often encounter in day-to-day clinical practice but are not widely described or discussed in the broader radiology literature.

This collection of cardiovascular pearls and pitfalls is intended for imagers from the trainee level to the senior clinician in practice. It is intended to help one who encounters a cardiovascular finding that just doesn't seem right, but can't exactly put his or her finger on it. These are not your typical "Aunt Minnie" cases, but rather true-to-life cases that can result in real interpretive problems for the radiologist. In this book, we have tried to include cases that we think are clinically relevant and likely to be encountered by the practicing imager, rather than focusing on the rare zebra that may never be encountered within the career of most imagers.

Within, we have included examples of uncommon appearances of common diseases, benign lesions that can be misinterpreted as something more sinister, and pseudolesions due to technical artifacts. We have focused on the modalities of cardiovascular MRI and CT. While there is certainly a wealth of potential pitfalls in cardiac echocardiography, we thought this was beyond the scope of the current publication.

The cases are organized broadly into a mix of anatomic groups, categories of pseudolesions, and types of artifacts. Each case features one or several clinical examples collected by the authors as well as a short explanatory text focusing on the typical imaging findings, clinical relevance, and differential diagnosis.

We have greatly appreciated the opportunity to share our broad clinical experiences through compiling this quite heterogeneous but highly informative group of cases. We hope that our readers will enjoy reading this text as much as we have putting it together.

Stefan L. Zimmerman,
on behalf of the co-authors.

To my wife, Ginny, whose love and support make everything possible, and to my children, Owen, Joey, and Olivia, who make it all worthwhile.

Stefan L. Zimmerman

CASE 1

Right atrial pseudotumor due to crista terminalis

Stefan L. Zimmerman

Imaging description

The crista terminalis is a smooth, vertically oriented, muscular ridge within the posterior wall of the right atrium (Figure 1.1). It is located at the site of embryonic fusion of the trabeculated and smooth-walled portions of the right atrium. The smooth-walled portion is also known as the sinus venosus. The crista terminalis is a critical structure for the cardiac conduction system, containing the sinoatrial node superiorly, and a frequent location of atrial tachyarrhythmias.[1] Most often the crista terminalis has low attenuation on computed tomography (CT) and is isointense to the right atrial wall on magnetic resonance imaging (MRI) (Figure 1.1).[2] In patients with lipomatous hypertrophy of the interatrial septum, the crista terminalis may also be enlarged and will include fat,[3] which will be low attenuation on CT (Figure 1.2) and high signal on bright blood and T1-weighted MRI images. In these cases, an etching artifact may also be recognized on bright blood steady-state free precession images, due to the interface of crista terminalis fat and the right atrial wall (Figure 1.3). The fat within an enlarged crista terminalis is contiguous with periatrial fat.

Importance

A prominent crista terminalis can be mistaken for a right atrial mass.[4] This could lead to inappropriate therapy and the associated risks of that therapy; for example, increased bleeding risk if anticoagulation is used in cases of suspected thrombus, or unnecessary open heart surgery if mistaken for myxoma.

Typical clinical scenario

The size of the crista terminalis has an average thickness of 4.5 mm; however, it is highly variable in size and can range from almost imperceptible to prominent and polypoid, projecting into the lumen of the right atrium.[1,4] It is often enlarged in patients with increased periatrial fat and lipomatous hypertrophy of the interatrial septum.

Differential diagnosis

A prominent crista terminalis should be distinguished from right atrial masses. In particular, right atrial thrombus or right atrial myxoma should be considered when an intraluminal polypoid mass is visualized attached to the right atrial wall. The crista terminalis can be distinguished by its characteristic location extending from the superior vena cava (SVC) to the inferior vena cava (IVC), smooth borders, and vertical orientation on coronal reformatted images. When present, fat within an enlarged crista terminalis will also exclude other entities. An atrial myxoma will demonstrate heterogenous enhancement, whereas crista terminalis will show mild enhancement identical to the adjacent atrial wall. Right atrial thrombus will often be found in the setting of a central venous catheter and will not have the characteristic shape or enhancement of the crista terminalis.

Teaching point

A prominent crista terminalis is common and can be identified by its characteristic location, smooth borders, and vertical orientation. It should not be mistaken for a right atrial mass.

REFERENCES

1. F. Saremi, S. Krishnan. Cardiac conduction system: anatomic landmarks relevant to interventional electrophysiologic techniques demonstrated with 64-detector CT. *Radiographics* 2007; **27**: 1539–65; discussion 1566–7.
2. L. S. Broderick, G. N. Brooks, J. E. Kuhlman. Anatomic pitfalls of the heart and pericardium. *Radiographics* 2005; **25**: 441–53.
3. J. R. Pharr, V. M. Figueredo. Lipomatus hypertrophy of the atrial septum and prominent crista terminalis appearing as a right atrial mass. *Eur J Echocardiogr* 2002; **3**: 159–61.
4. S. A. Mirowitz, F. R. Gutierrez. Fibromuscular elements of the right atrium: pseudomass at MR imaging. *Radiology* 1992; **182**: 231–3.

Pearls and Pitfalls in Cardiovascular Imaging, ed. Stefan L. Zimmerman and Elliot K. Fishman. Published by Cambridge University Press. © Cambridge University Press 2015.

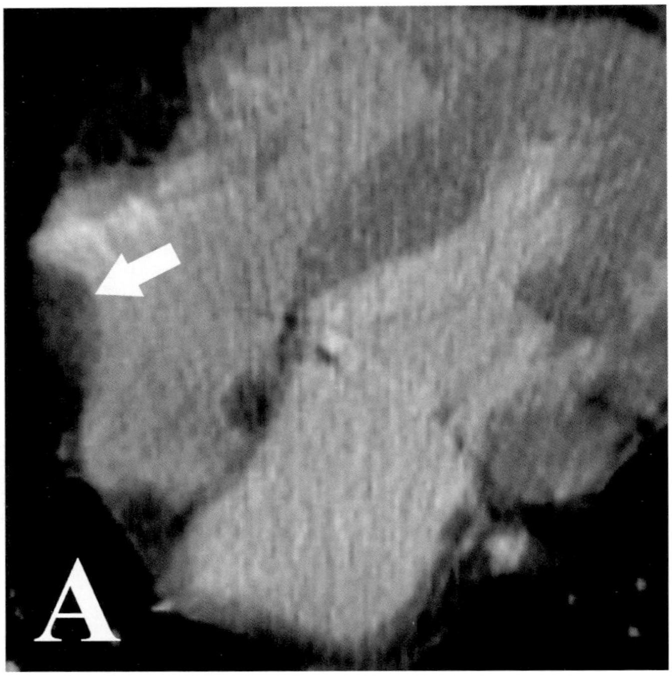

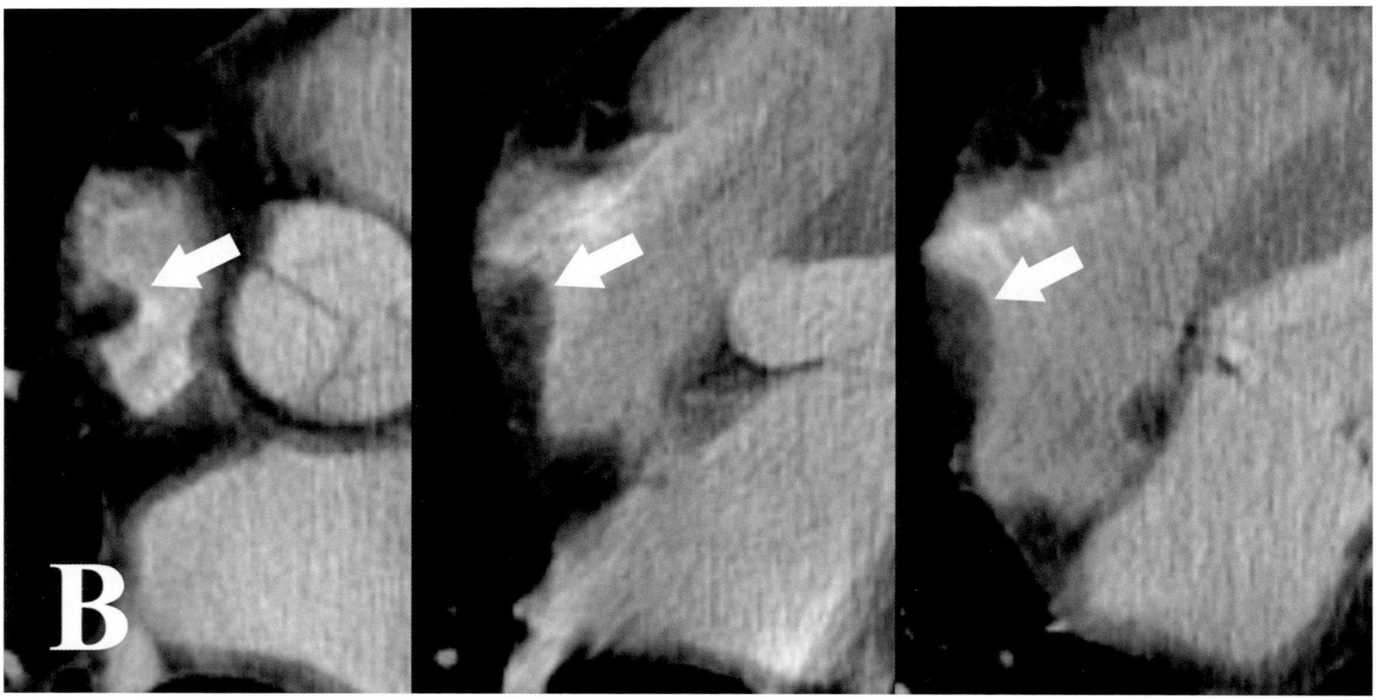

Figure 1.1 **A.** Axial contrast-enhanced CT image from a study performed in a 64-year-old male with lung cancer shows a prominent crista terminalis (arrow) that is low in attenuation due to fat content and located on the posterior wall of the right atrium. **B.** Multiple contiguous axial images in the same patient demonstrating the vertical course of the crista terminalis from superior to inferior along the posterior wall of the right atrium. **C.** Coronal oblique reformatted image shows the crista terminalis as a vertical, low-attenuation structure that courses superiorly to inferiorly (asterisks), just lateral to the connection of the superior vena cava (arrow) and inferior vena cava (arrowhead) to the right atrium. Note the partially visualized upper lung mass which is compressing the superior vena cava in this patient with known lung cancer.

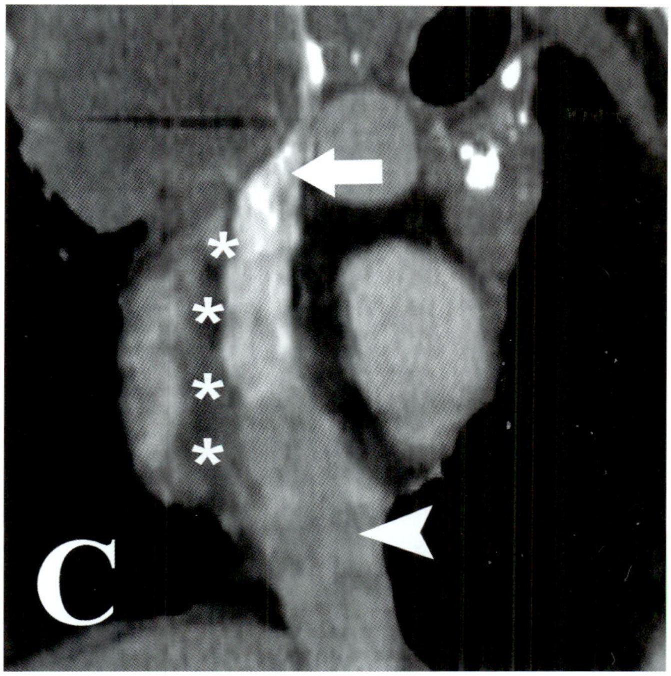

Figure 1.1 *(cont.)*

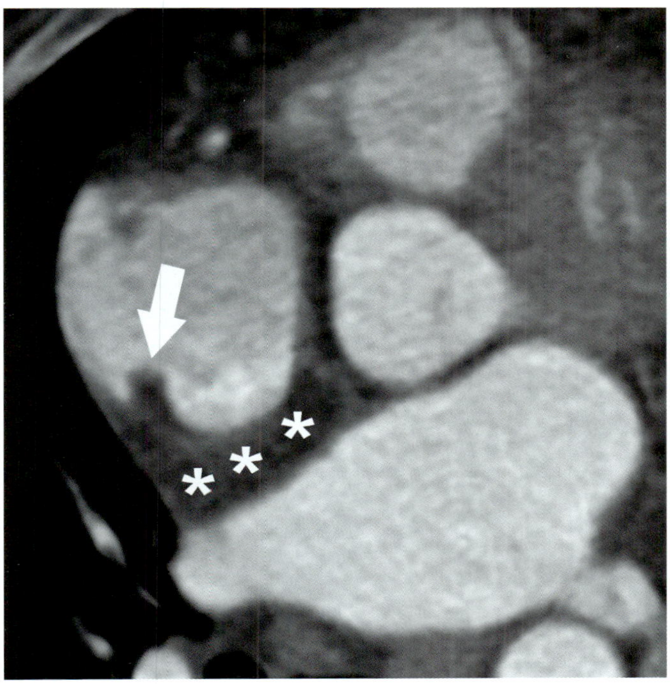

Figure 1.2 Axial image from contrast-enhanced CT in a 56-year-old woman with cardiac CT performed to evaluate chest pain demonstrates a prominent crista terminalis with a somewhat polypoid appearance (arrow). There is associated lipomatous hypertrophy of the interatrial septum (asterisks), which can be often seen in patients with a prominent crista.

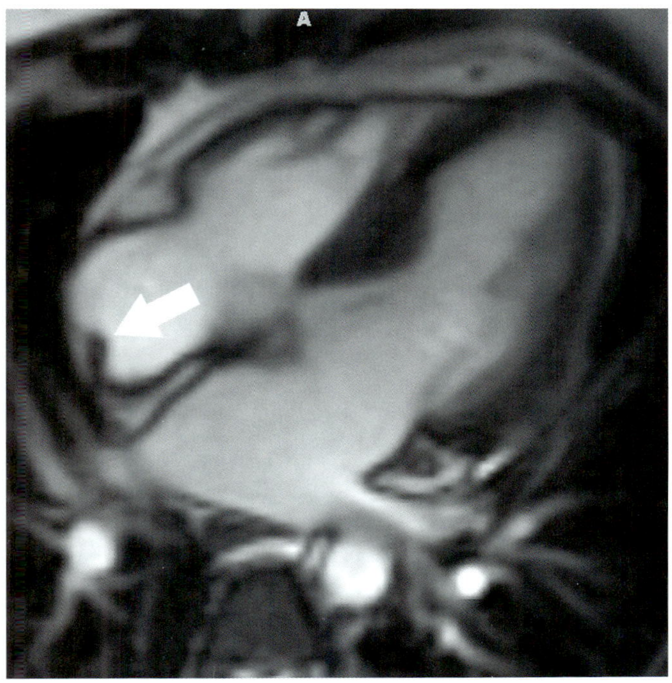

Figure 1.3 Horizontal long-axis bright blood steady-state free precession image from a cine cardiac MRI performed in a 35-year-old female with sarcoidosis shows a prominent crista terminalis (arrow), which has an internal high signal and a rim of low signal etching artifact due to the interface of fat with the right atrial wall. The fat of the crista is contiguous with fat within the interatrial septum, also surrounded by etching artifact.

CASE **2**

Cardiac pseudotumor due to lipomatous hypertrophy of the interatrial septum

Pejman Motarjem and Stefan L. Zimmerman

Imaging description

Lipomatous hypertrophy of the interatrial septum (LHIS) is a benign process of the heart characterized by fatty infiltration of the interatrial septum.[1] The diagnosis is made when fat in the interatrial septum measures greater than 20 mm in thickness and it is usually an incidental finding at cardiac imaging.[2]

At echocardiography, LHIS is recognized by echogenic thickening of the interatrial septum. On multiple detector computed tomography (MDCT) (with or without contrast) LHIS is a low-attenuation, < 0 Hounsfield units, bilobed mass with smooth margins that spares the fossa ovalis. It is this sparing of the fossa ovalis which gives this entity its characteristic bilobed or dumbbell-shaped morphology (Figure 2.1). Often, there is cranial extension to the level of the cavoatrial junction and fat may surround the distal superior vena cava (Figure 2.2).

On MRI the morphology of LHIS is similar to MDCT. The LHIS demonstrates hyperintensity on T1-weighted imaging with homogenous signal drop out on a fat-suppressed T1 sequence characteristic of macroscopic fat (Figure 2.2). On post-gadolinium sequences no enhancement is seen.[3]

FDG uptake within the atrial septum at positron emission tomography (PET) examinations may be seen, and is attributed to the variable presence of brown fat within LHIS (Figure 2.3).[4] It is important to note that the benign FDG uptake in LHIS must not be mistaken for a malignant process such adenopathy or metastatic tumor. Fusion PET-CT will help localize radiotracer uptake to the atrial septum and differentiate it from surrounding structures such as the right hilum, pleura or mediastinum. In difficult cases, it may be necessary to correlate PET-CT findings with either MRI or MDCT in order to prevent inappropriate staging of the patient.

Importance

The condition of LHIS is a benign incidental finding and typically does not cause any symptoms. Since it may demonstrate increased FDG uptake on PET/CT, it must not be confused with a malignant process, leading to misdiagnosis, inappropriate follow-up imaging or inappropriate biopsy.

Fat infiltration in the atrial septum increases with age, correlates with increased epicardial fat in obese patients and is contiguous with epicardial fat deposits.[5] The LHIS process has been associated with atrial arrhythmias, thought to be the result of disruption of atrial conduction pathways.[2] In rare cases, LHIS results in right atrial and superior vena cava partial obstructive symptoms requiring surgical resection.[6,7]

Typical clinical case scenario

Lipomatous hypertrophy of the interatrial septum is typically encountered incidentally on echocardiogram, MDCT, MRI, or PET/CT. It most often has a benign course with estimated prevalence of 1% at autopsies, 2–8% on echo[1] and 2.2% on MDCT.[2] Once encountered, no further follow-up imaging is recommended. As discussed above, in rare cases LHIS may lead to hemodynamic obstruction or may cause atrial arrhythmias, but in the overwhelming majority of the cases it is completely benign causing no symptoms.

Differential diagnosis

The main differential consideration of LHIS is cardiac lipoma (Figure 2.4). Unlike lipoma, LHIS lacks a true fibrous capsule. In addition, primary cardiac lipomas are exceedingly rare.

Liposarcoma is a malignant fatty lesion that is usually large and will present with aggressive features such as invasion into surrounding cardiac or mediastinal structures and mass effect.

Other benign tumors such as myxoma, fibroma and rhabdomyoma do not contain fat. Teratomas may have fat features on CT or MRI but they will usually have a mix of tissue types including soft tissue, bone or teeth. They also lack the typical bilobed morphology characteristic of LHIS.

Melanoma metastasis will demonstrate high signal on T1-weighted imaging similar to LHIS, but unlike LHIS it will not lose signal on the fat-suppressed sequence and will avidly enhance on post-contrast sequences.

Teaching point

Lipomatous hypertrophy of the interatrial septum is typically an incidental finding at cardiac imaging characterized by fat and a characteristic dumbbell or bilobed shape. In the overwhelming majority of the cases it is asymptomatic and requires no further follow-up. Although it may demonstrate FDG uptake due to presence of brown fat, it must not be mistaken for a malignant or neoplastic process.

REFERENCES

1. Meaney JF, Kazerooni EA, Jamadar DA, Korobkin M. CT appearance of lipomatous hypertrophy of the interatrial septum. *AJR* 1997; **168**:1081–1084.

2. Heyer CM, Kagel T, Lemburg SP, Bauer TT, Nicolas V. Lipomatous hypertrophy of the interatrial septum: a prospective study of incidence, imaging findings, and clinical symptoms. *Chest* 2003; **124**:2068–2073.

Pearls and Pitfalls in Cardiovascular Imaging, ed. Stefan L. Zimmerman and Elliot K. Fishman. Published by Cambridge University Press. © Cambridge University Press 2015.

3. Kozelj M, Angelski R, Dusan P. Lipomatous hypertrophy of the interatrial septum: diagnosis by echocardiography and magnetic resonance imaging. *Angiology* 1995; **46**:863–866.
4. Fan CM, Fischman AJ, Kwek BH, Abbara S, Aquino SL. Hypertrophy of the interatrial septum: increased uptake on FDG-PET. *AJR Am J Roentgenol* 2005; **184**:339–342.
5. Page DL. Lipomatous hypertrophy of the cardiac interatrial septum. *Human Pathol* 1970; **1**:151–163.
6. Tugcu A, Yildirimturk O, Rizaoglu E, Sagbas E, Akpinar B, Aytekin S. Lipomatous hypertrophy of the interatrial septum presenting as an obstructive right atrial mass in a patient with exertional dyspnea. *J Am Soc Echocardiogr* 2007; **20**:1319.
7. Breuer M, Wipperman J, Franke U, Wahlers T. Lipomatous hypertrophy of the interatrial septum and upper right atrial inflow obstruction. *Eur J Cardiothorac Surg* 2002; **22**:1023–1025.

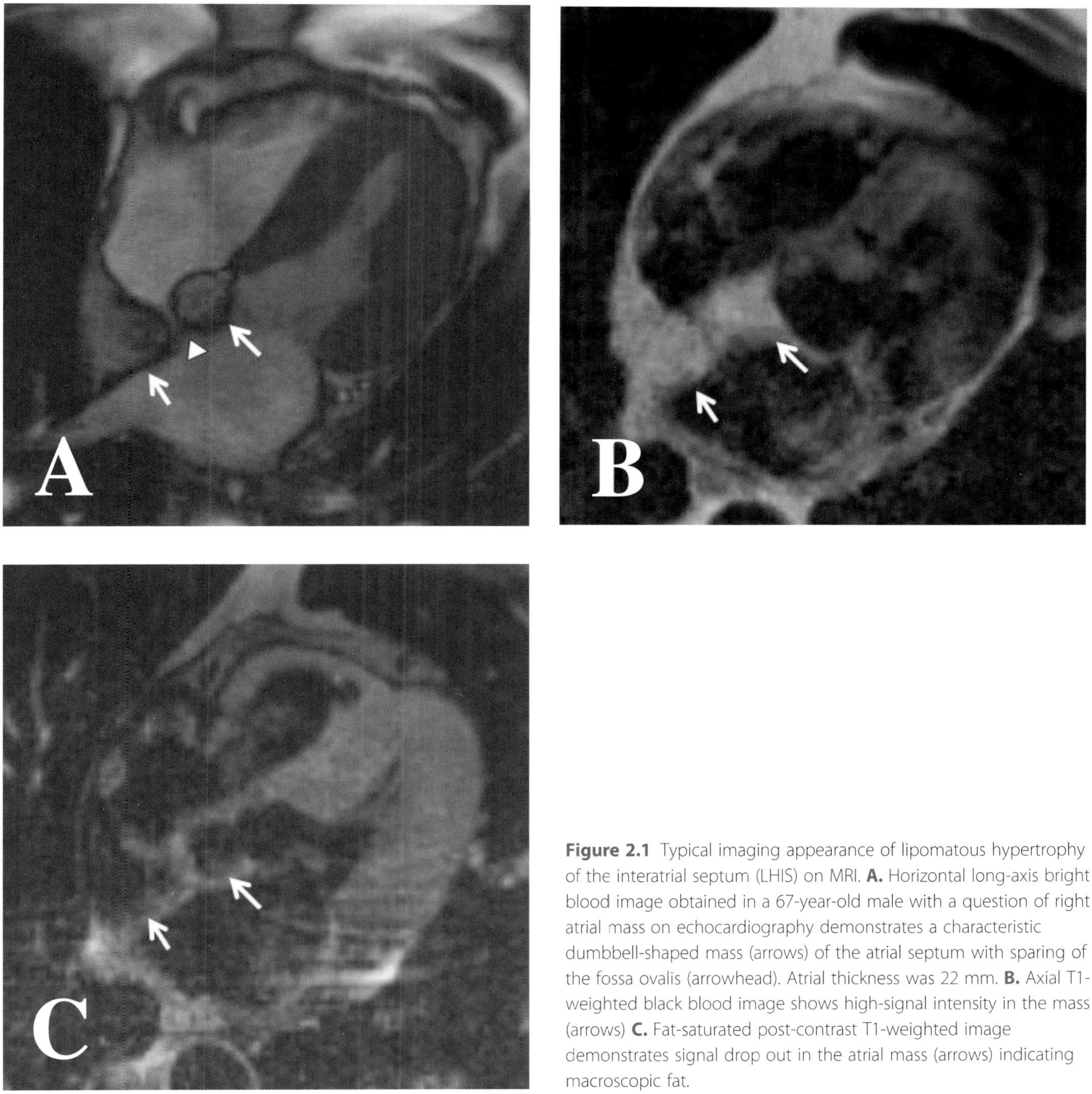

Figure 2.1 Typical imaging appearance of lipomatous hypertrophy of the interatrial septum (LHIS) on MRI. **A.** Horizontal long-axis bright blood image obtained in a 67-year-old male with a question of right atrial mass on echocardiography demonstrates a characteristic dumbbell-shaped mass (arrows) of the atrial septum with sparing of the fossa ovalis (arrowhead). Atrial thickness was 22 mm. **B.** Axial T1-weighted black blood image shows high-signal intensity in the mass (arrows) **C.** Fat-saturated post-contrast T1-weighted image demonstrates signal drop out in the atrial mass (arrows) indicating macroscopic fat.

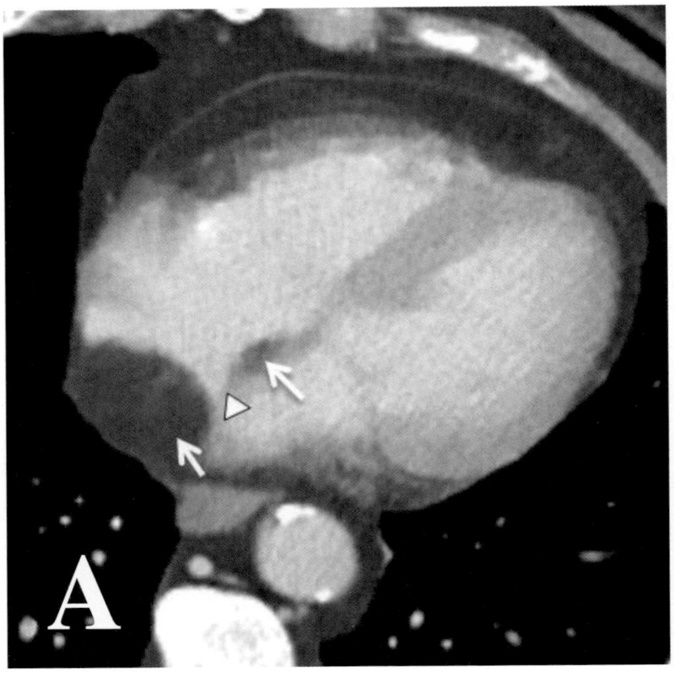

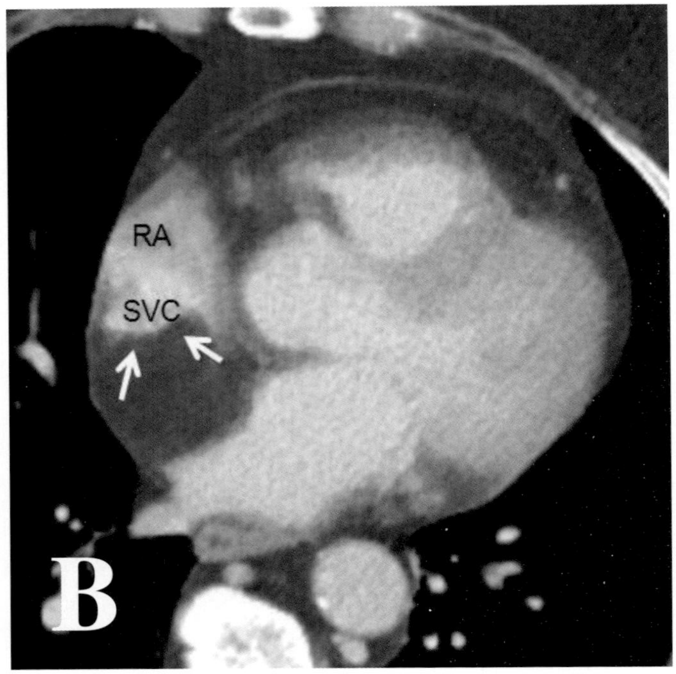

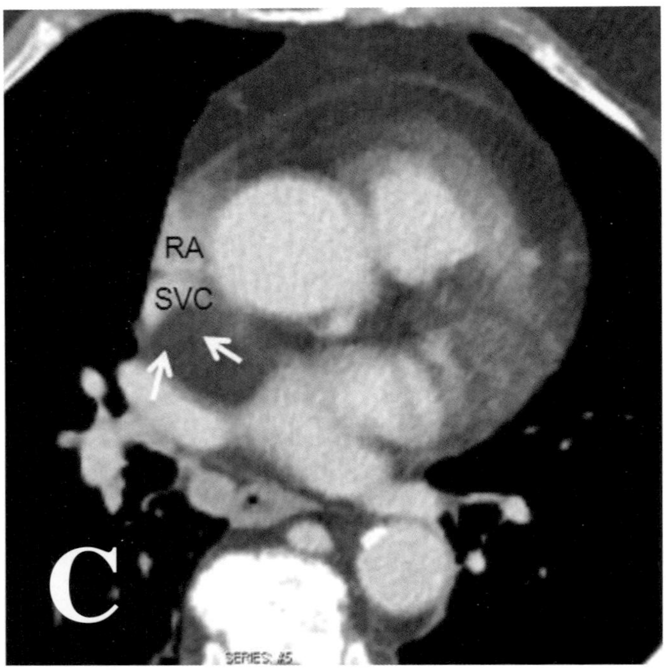

Figure 2.2 Incidental marked LHIS on CT. **A.** Axial contrast-enhanced CT image obtained in a 72-year-old female with Crohn's disease shows marked LHIS with typical dumbbell configuration (arrows) and sparing of the fossa ovalis (arrowhead). The degree of fat deposition in the portion adjacent to the posterior wall of the right atrium is much greater than the intracardiac portion, which is frequently seen. On more cranial axial images (**B, C**), fat abuts and narrows the junction of the superior vena cava (SVC) with the right atrium (RA) (arrows).

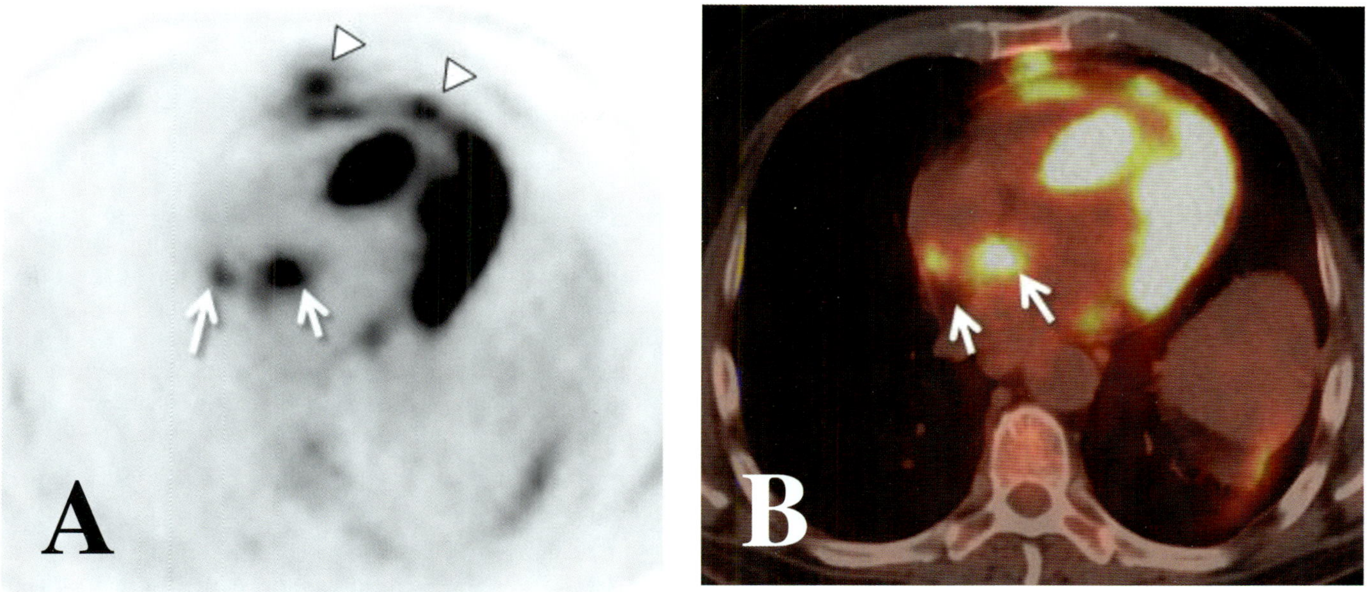

Figure 2.3 Atrial septal hypermetabolism due to brown fat. **A.** Axial image from FDG-PET examination performed in a 59-year-old male with lymphoma involving the pericardium demonstrates increased radiotracer uptake in the heart posteriorly (arrows) and along the pericardium anteriorly (arrowheads). **B.** On fused PET-CT images, the foci of increased uptake correlate with fat in the interatrial septum (arrows). These represent regions of hypermetabolic brown fat, not uncommonly seen in the interatrial septum, and should not be mistaken for malignancy.

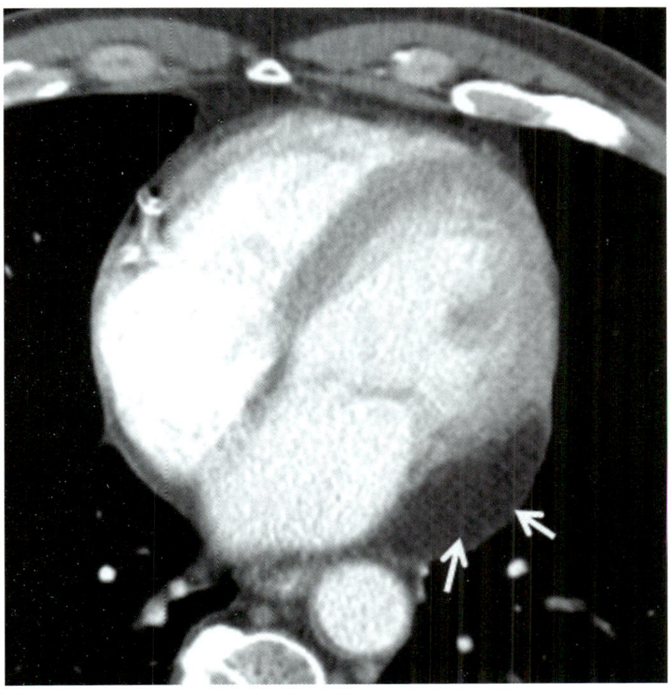

Figure 2.4 Cardiac lipoma. Axial contrast-enhanced CT image of the chest obtained in a 67-year-old male with abdominal pain demonstrates a well-encapsulated, ovoid-shaped fat density mass adjacent to the left atrioventricular groove compatible with cardiac lipoma (arrows).

CASE 3

Cardiac pseudotumor due to caseous mitral annular calcification

Stefan L. Zimmerman

Imaging description

At cardiac MRI (CMR), mitral annular calcification (MAC) is low in signal intensity on bright blood, T1- and T2-weighted images and can appear as a smooth, multilobulated mass or masses in the region of the atrioventricular groove (Figure 3.1). Caseous, also known as liquefactive, MAC is a rare variant that is typically a larger, rounded mass with central liquefactive necrosis, composed of calcium, inflammatory cells, and cholesterol.[1] Given that calcification is not well depicted by MRI, MAC can be mistaken for a cardiac tumor. Caseous MAC can occasionally be large – up to several centimeters in size – and may displace mitral valve leaflets, resulting in valvular dysfunction such as regurgitation or stenosis. On post-contrast images, there is occasionally a thin rim of enhancement due to fibrous tissue surrounding the calcification (Figure 3.2).[2,3] If CT is available, MAC is easy to identify on non-contrast images due to presence of high attenuation calcification (Figure 3.1).[3]

Importance

MAC at CMR can be mistaken for a cardiac tumor or other type of cardiac mass, leading to inappropriate additional testing as well as patient anxiety. Although benign, the presence of MAC is a marker of increased cardiovascular risk. MAC was associated with a 50% greater likelihood of cardiovascular events at follow-up in the Framingham Heart Study and predicted both increased all-cause and cardiovascular death.[4]

Typical clinical scenario

MAC is a common disorder. In the Multi-Ethnic Study of Atherosclerosis, MAC was detected by CT in 9% of a cohort of 6814 subjects from age 45–8.[5] Caseous MAC is more rare, affecting < 1% of subjects with MAC.[1] MAC is often discovered incidentally at echocardiography, and usually requires no further imaging. However, if the diagnosis is uncertain, patients may be referred to advanced imaging with MRI or CT.

Differential diagnosis

MAC should be differentiated from a true cardiac tumor. Location in the mitral annulus, low T1 and T2 signal intensity, and lack of enhancement are distinguishing characteristics. Myxomas are the most common primary cardiac tumor and can be located near valves; however, unlike MAC, will have increased T2 signal and heterogenous enhancement.[6] Cardiac fibroma can have a low signal on T1 and T2-weighted images due to fibrous content; however, it typically demonstrates either homogenous or heterogenous enhancement and is intramyocardial in location.[6]

Teaching point

Mitral annular calcification may be mass-like in appearance at CMR and can be mistaken for a cardiac tumor. The characteristic location, low signal, and lack of enhancement should suggest the correct diagnosis. For difficult cases, non-contrast CT demonstrating calcification can be used for confirmation.

REFERENCES

1. S. S. Srivatsa, M. D. Taylor, K. Hor, et al. Liquefaction necrosis of mitral annular calcification (LNMAC): review of pathology, prevalence, imaging and management: proposed diagnostic imaging criteria with detailed multi-modality and MRI image characterization. *Int J Cardiovasc Imaging* 2012; **28**: 1161–71.
2. L. Monti, E. Renifilo, M. Profili, L. Balzarini. Cardiovascular magnetic resonance features of caseous calcification of the mitral annulus. *J Cardiovasc Magn Reson* 2008; **10**: 25.
3. A. Gulati, C. Chan, A. Duncan, S. Raza, P. J. Kilner, J. Pepper. Multimodality cardiac imaging in the evaluation of mitral annular caseous calcification. *Circulation* 2011; **123**: e1–2.
4. C. S. Fox, R. S. Vasan, H. Parise, et al. Mitral annular calcification predicts cardiovascular morbidity and mortality: the Framingham Heart Study. *Circulation* 2003; **107**: 1492–6.
5. Y. S. Hamirani, K. Nasir, R. S. Blumenthal, et al. Relation of mitral annular calcium and coronary calcium (from the Multi-Ethnic Study of Atherosclerosis [MESA]). *Am J Cardiol* 2011; **107**: 1291–4.
6. K. Randhawa, A. Ganeshan, E. T. Hoey. Magnetic resonance imaging of cardiac tumors: Part 1, sequences, protocols, and benign tumors. *Curr Probl Diagn Radiol* 2011; **40**: 158–68.

Pearls and Pitfalls in Cardiovascular Imaging, ed. Stefan L. Zimmerman and Elliot K. Fishman. Published by Cambridge University Press. © Cambridge University Press 2015.

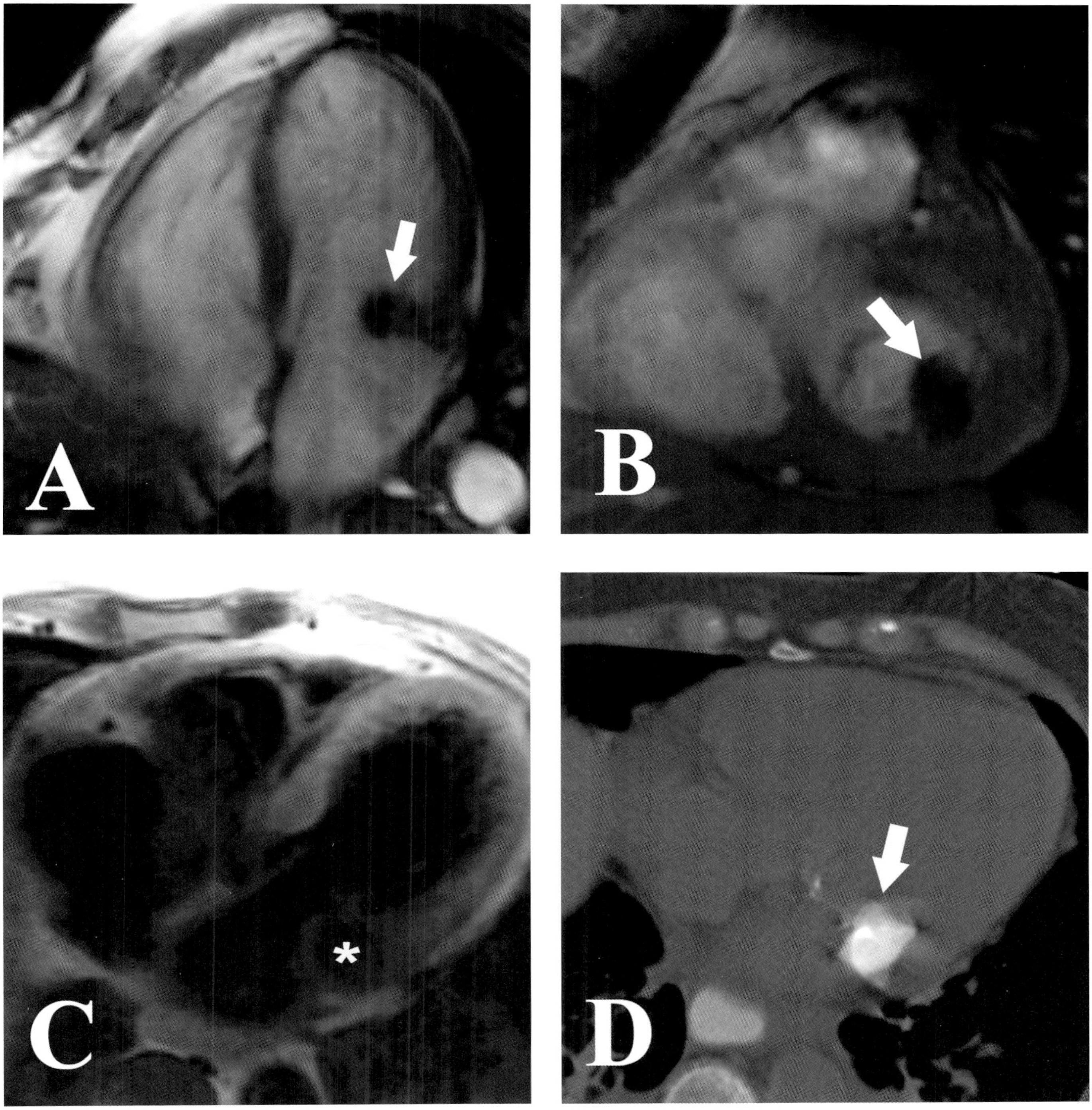

Figure 3.1 **A**. Four-chamber steady-state free precession bright blood image in an 81-year-old female referred to cardiac MRI for a mass found at echocardiography demonstrates a smooth, low signal mass in the region of the mitral annulus (arrow). **B**. Short-axis steady-state free precession bright blood image again demonstrates the low signal, round cardiac mass in the region of the mitral annulus (arrow). **C**. Axial T1-weighted dark blood image obtained demonstrates low signal within the mitral annular calcification (asterisk). **D**. Non-contrast CT examination performed in the same patient demonstrates calcification corresponding to the location of the mass on MRI, diagnostic of mitral annular calcification (arrow).

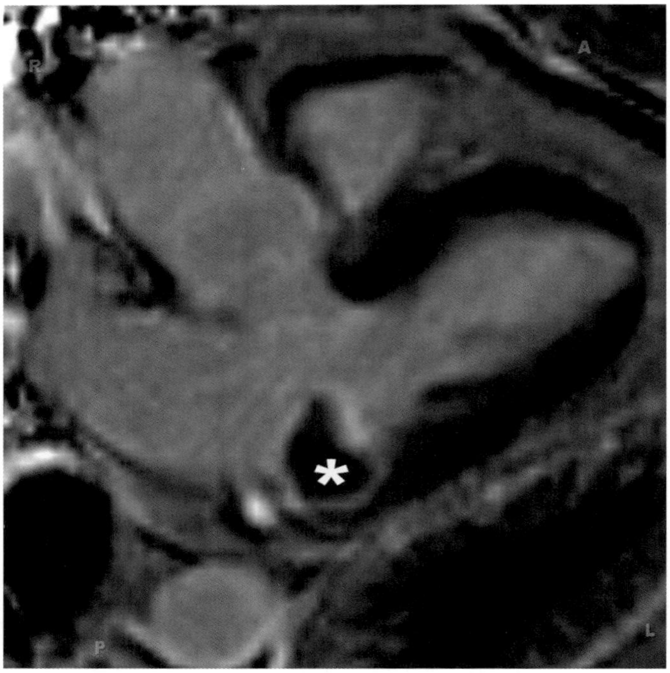

Figure 3.2 Three-chamber delayed enhancement image from an MRI performed in a 61-year-old male with mitral annular calcification demonstrates a low signal intensity mass (asterisk) in the mitral annulus with a characteristic thin rim of delayed enhancement related to fibrous tissue.

CASE

4 Cardiac pseudotumor due to focal hypertrophic cardiomyopathy

Celia P. Corona-Villalobos and Stefan L. Zimmerman

Imaging description

Focal left ventricular hypertrophy is a variant phenotype of hypertrophic cardiomyopathy (HCM) usually described as involvement of $\leq$ 2 cardiac segments.[1] Focal HCM can have a mass-like appearance, simulating tumors (Figures 4.1 and 4.2).[2] On cardiac MRI (CMR), mass-like HCM will generally be isointense to adjacent normal myocardium on dark blood spin echo T1- and T2-weighted images and bright blood steady-state free precession (SSFP) sequences. Occasionally, foci of an increased T2-weighted signal can be seen in hypertrophied segments on either dark blood or SSFP sequences, which will be mid-myocardial and patchy. On tagging images, displacement and deformation of tag lines will occur in both normal and hypertrophied myocardium due to myocyte contraction, although reduced contractility may be seen in thickened regions.[3] First-pass perfusion sequences will show homogeneous signal intensity and perfusion characteristics similar to adjacent myocardium.[2] Delayed enhancement has been reported in 45–80% of patients with HCM[1,2] and usually involves the thickest myocardium. The delayed enhancement pattern is typically patchy and mid-myocardial; however, it can be transmural in advanced cases.

Importance

Focal HCM can have a mass-like appearance and irregular delayed enhancement that may lead to incorrect diagnosis of a cardiac tumor such as metastasis, lymphoma, fibroma, or rhabdomyoma. This can lead to patient anxiety, inappropriate biopsies, or even surgery.

Typical clinical scenario

HCM is the most common primary genetic disease of the heart and has a prevalence of 1:500 in the general population.[2] In a large study of 333 individuals with HCM, 12% of patients had the focal pattern of hypertrophy.[1] Patients with a focal pattern of HCM may be initially detected by echocardiography, which can lead to further evaluation by cardiac MRI. Patients are often asymptomatic or may have symptomatic left ventricular outflow tract obstruction due to septal wall hypertrophy and/or systolic anterior motion of the anterior mitral valve leaflets.[2]

Differential diagnosis

The differential diagnosis includes metastatic and primary cardiac tumors. Given the occasional presence of patchy and irregular delayed enhancement, focal HCM can be mistaken for metastasis, which is far and away the most common type of cardiac tumor. However, metastases are typically aggressive in appearance and have signal characteristics on T1-weighted and T2-weighted imaging that are substantially different from normal myocardium. In addition, metastases will not show evidence of contraction on tagging images. Cardiac lymphoma is a rare cardiac mass that can result in wall thickening due to lymphocyte infiltration and may have signal intensity on precontrast T1- and T2-weighted images similar to normal myocardium; however, unlike focal HCM it has a very aggressive appearance, often involving several cardiac chambers, and is typically associated with pericardial effusion. In children, focal HCM can be mistaken for rhabdomyoma and fibroma, the two most common primary cardiac tumors in the pediatric age group. Rhabdomyomas are a homogeneous intramyocardial or intracavitary mass associated with tuberous sclerosis. They are mildly hyperintense on T2-weighted images, hypointense on SSFP and T1-weighted images and isointense to myocardium on delayed enhancement images.[4] Fibromas are solitary tumors well delineated by the surrounding myocardium. Fibromas often arise from the epicardium of the interventricular septum or lateral wall of the left ventricle. Generally they are hypointense compared to the normal myocardium in T1- and T2-weighted images and SSFP sequences due to fibrous content. Slow, gradual enhancement with low signal intensity on myocardial perfusion imaging and homogenous increased signal on delayed enhancement is typical for fibromas.[4] Finally, sarcomas can be considered in the differential diagnosis but are typically easily distinguished from focal HCM due to a highly aggressive appearance.[5]

Teaching point

Focal HCM can result in mass-like hypertrophy of the myocardium that should not be mistaken for a cardiac tumor. Signal intensity that is isointense to normal myocardium on precontrast pulse sequences and contractility on tagging images are characteristics that distinguish focal HCM from tumor.

REFERENCES

1. M. S. Maron, B. J. Maron, C. Harrigan, et al. Hypertrophic cardiomyopathy phenotype revisited after 50 years with cardiovascular magnetic resonance. *J Am Coll Cardiol* 2009; **54**: 220–8.

Pearls and Pitfalls in Cardiovascular Imaging, ed. Stefan L. Zimmerman and Elliot K. Fishman. Published by Cambridge University Press. © Cambridge University Press 2015.

2. M. W. Hansen, N. Merchant. MRI of hypertrophic cardiomyopathy: part I, MRI appearances. *AJR Am J Roentgenol* 2007; **189**: 1335–43.

3. P. D. Bergey, L. Axel. Focal hypertrophic cardiomyopathy simulating a mass: MR tagging for correct diagnosis. *AJR Am J Roentgenol* 2000; **174**: 242–4.

4. R. S. Beroukhim, A. Prakash, E. R. Buechel, et al. Characterization of cardiac tumors in children by cardiovascular magnetic resonance imaging: a multicenter experience. *J Am Coll Cardiol* 2011; **58**: 1044–54.

5. J. R. Dillman, G. C. Mueller, A. K. Attili, A. L. Dorfman, G. J. Ensing, D. Gordon. Case 153: atypical tumefactive hypertrophic cardiomyopathy. *Radiology* 2010; **254**: 310–13.

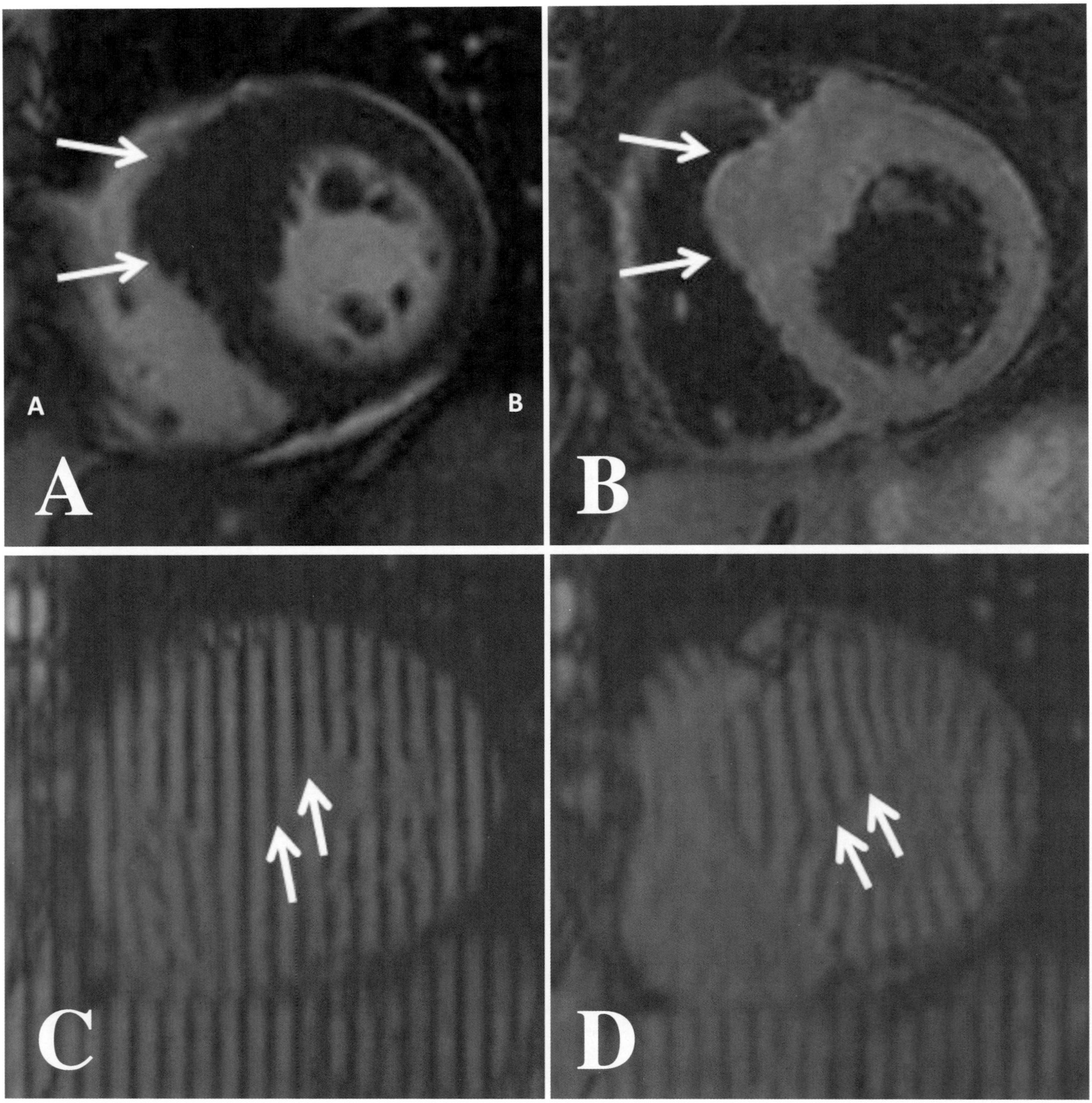

Figure 4.1 Focal HCM in a 56-year-old female with hypertrophic cardiomyopathy. Short-axis bright blood (**A**) and T2-weighted dark blood (**B**) images demonstrate mass-like wall thickening in the anteroseptum (arrows) with signal intensity identical to adjacent normal myocardium. Short-axis vertical tagging images acquired in diastole (**C**) and systole (**D**) show distortion of tag lines (arrows) within the thickened myocardium in systole, indicating active contraction, a feature that distinguishes hypertrophy from tumor. **E.** Short-axis delayed enhancement image showing patchy mid-myocardial delayed enhancement (arrows), a feature that can be seen in both focal hypertrophic cardiomyopathy and tumor. However, tumor enhancement would typically be more extensive and involving the entire mass-like region.

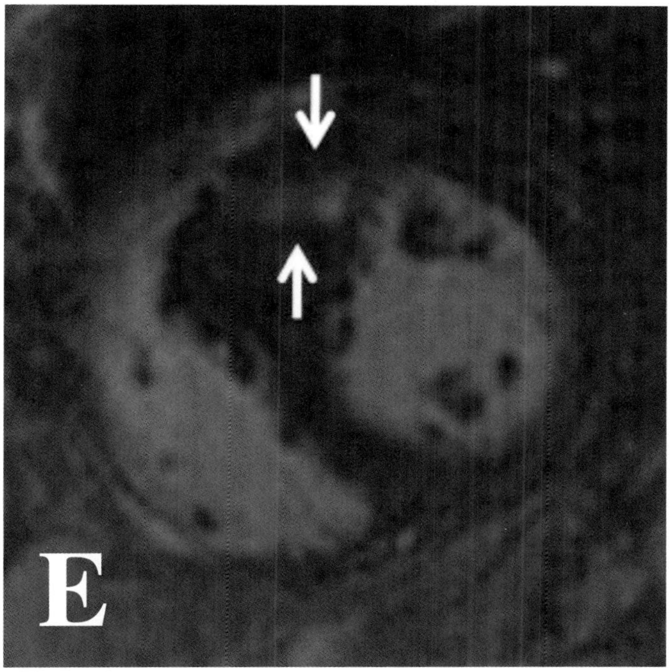

Figure 4.1 *(cont.)*

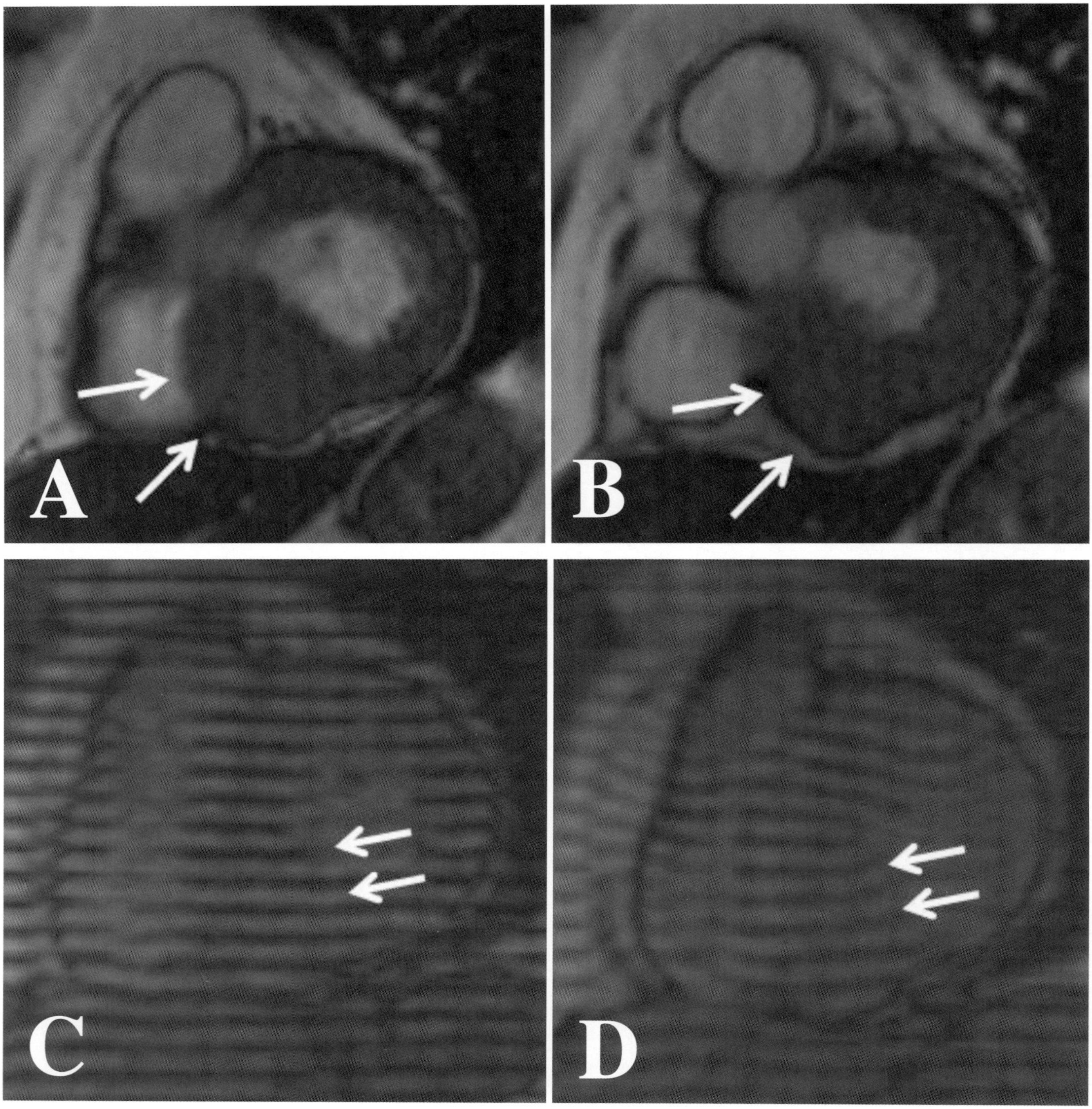

Figure 4.2 Focal HCM in a 46-year-old male. Short-axis bright blood images in end-diastole (**A**) and end-systole (**B**) show mass-like wall thickening in the basilar inferoseptum (arrows) that is identical in signal intensity to normal myocardium. Short-axis horizontal tagging images obtained in end-diastole (**C**) and end-sytole (**D**) in the same patient show distortion of tag lines in systole, indicating myocardial contraction, which distinguishes focal HCM from tumor. Short-axis T2-weighted dark blood (**E**), dynamic perfusion (**F**), and delayed enhancement (**G**) images show that the region of mass-like thickening (arrows) has identical T2 and perfusion characteristics to adjacent normal myocardium. On the delayed enhancement image, there is patchy focal increased signal in the center of the mass (short arrow) which is commonly found in HCM and is not pathognomonic for tumor.

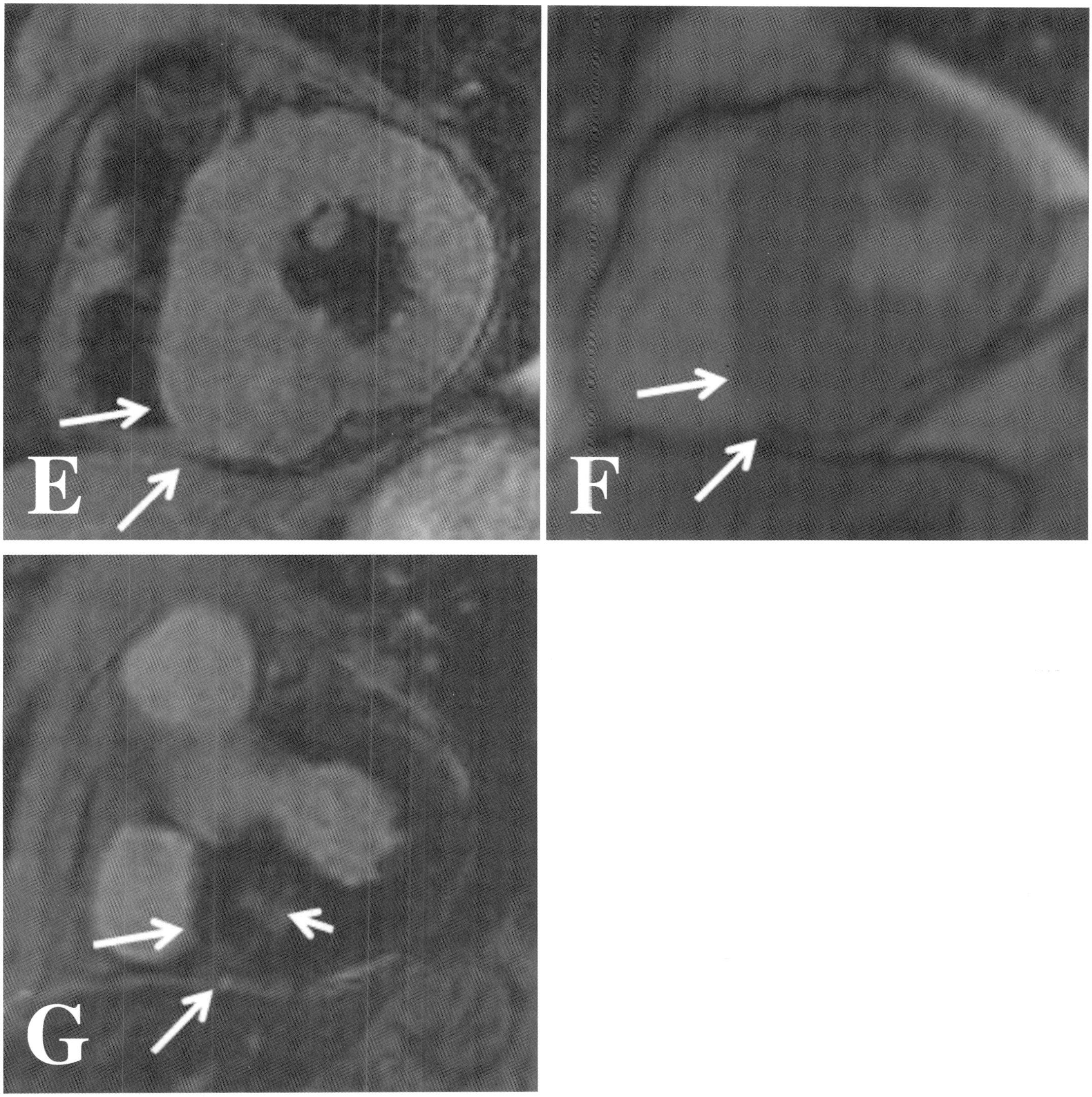

Figure 4.2 *(cont.)*

CASE

5 Psuedothrombus in the left ventricle due to microvascular obstruction

Stefan L. Zimmerman

Imaging description

A mass-like area of low signal intensity mimicking thrombus may be encountered in the setting of microvascular obstruction (MO) when cardiac MRI (CMR) is performed after acute myocardial infarction (MI). CMR is often used to assess viability after MI for prognosis and determining the need for possible revascularization. In the acute setting, large transmural MIs may demonstrate MO, which has been associated with poorer outcomes and adverse left venticular (LV) remodeling at follow-up imaging.[1] MO is subendocardial in location and low in signal intensity on late gadolinium enhancement (LGE) images, characteristically surrounded by a zone of increased myocardial signal intensity due to LGE (Figure 5.1).[2] MO represents a densely infarcted area of no-flow within the myocardium where gadolinium cannot reach due to severe microvascular damage. MO is recognized by its association with a wall motion abnormality, subendocardial decreased perfusion on dynamic post-contrast images, and a rim of delayed enhancement representing a zone of infarcted tissue with intact microvasculature that surrounds the infarct core with MO.[2]

Importance

MO is important to recognize given the fact that it is associated with poorer outcomes after MI.[1,3] MO must be correctly differentiated from thrombus, as this may require additional treatment such as anticoagulation therapy, which will expose the patient to additional bleeding risk in the inappropriate setting.

Typical clinical scenario

MO is encountered when viability MRI scans are performed in someone with recent MI. Differentiation of thrombus from MO is important as these patients with hypofunctioning myocardium in the setting of recent MI are at risk for thrombus due to blood stasis.

Differential diagnosis

Thrombus is the most important entity on the differential diagnosis of MO. The location of MO within the wall of the myocardium can help differentiate MO from thrombus. Myocardial location can be clarified by direct comparison of LGE and precontrast images (Figures 5.1, 5.2). Thrombus will be visible as a filling defect in the ventricular cavity adherent to the ventricular wall on precontrast images (Figure 5.3), whereas MO will not yet be visible on images without gadolinium. Both MO and thrombus do not enhance on post-contrast images, although the rim of myocardial LGE surrounding MO is characteristic. Calcification may also result in low signal intensity in a subendocardial location in association with LGE from MI;[4] however, it will be seen in association with chronic MI rather than in the acute setting.

> ### Teaching point
> MO is often seen in the setting of a large MI and portends a poor prognosis. It is important to distinguish from intracavitary thrombus through careful inspection of the location of the signal abnormality and its appearance on pre- and post-contrast images.

REFERENCES

1. K. C. Wu. CMR of microvascular obstruction and hemorrhage in myocardial infarction. *J Cardiovasc Magn Reson* 2012; **14**: 68.
2. V. Pineda, X. Merino, S. Gispert, P. Mahia, B. Garcia, R. Dominguez-Oronoz. No-reflow phenomenon in cardiac MRI: diagnosis and clinical implications. *AJR Am J Roentgenol* 2008; **191**: 73–9.
3. S. de Waha, S. Desch, I. Eitel, et al. Impact of early vs. late microvascular obstruction assessed by magnetic resonance imaging on long-term outcome after ST-elevation myocardial infarction: a comparison with traditional prognostic markers. *Eur Heart J* 2010; **31**: 2660–8.
4. F. Saremi, J. D. Grizzard, R. J. Kim. Optimizing cardiac MR imaging: practical remedies for artifacts. *Radiographics* 2008; **28**: 1161–87.

Pearls and Pitfalls in Cardiovascular Imaging, ed. Stefan L. Zimmerman and Elliot K. Fishman. Published by Cambridge University Press. © Cambridge University Press 2015.

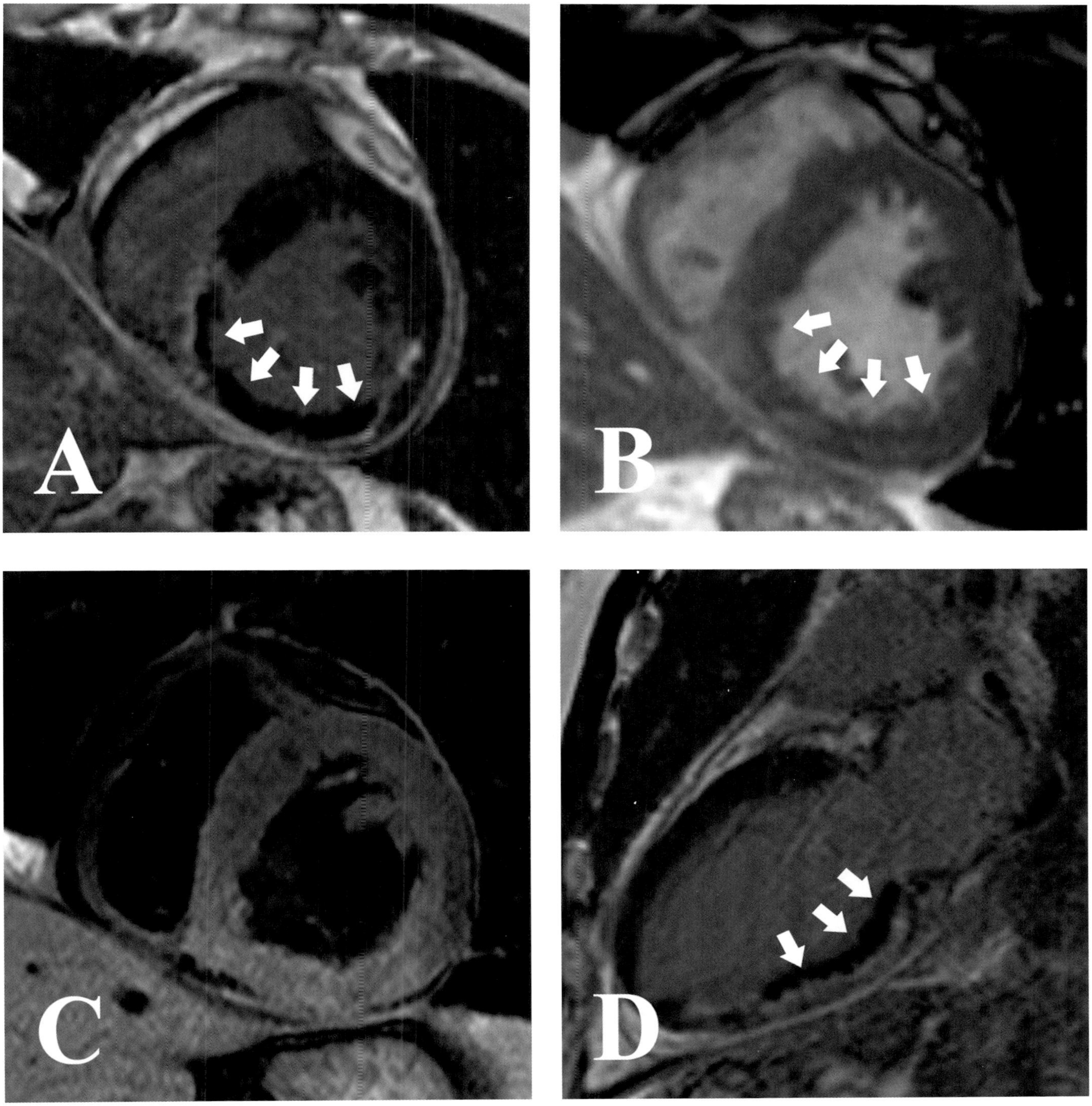

Figure 5.1 Short axis (**A**) and vertical long-axis (**D**) delayed enhancement images from a cardiac MRI performed to assess viability in a 61-year-old male with recent RCA territory myocardial infarction. There is extensive microvascular obstruction in the inferior wall (arrows), identified by the characteristic low signal intensity and surrounding rim of hyperenhancement. The low signal intensity microvascular obstruction has an appearance that could be mistaken for thrombus. Short-axis (**B**) and vertical long-axis (**E**) bright blood images and a short-axis T2-weighted dark blood (**C**) image obtained precontrast in the same patient demonstrates the affected wall with no intraluminal mass, excluding the possibility of thrombus, which should be apparent on both precontrast and post-contrast images.

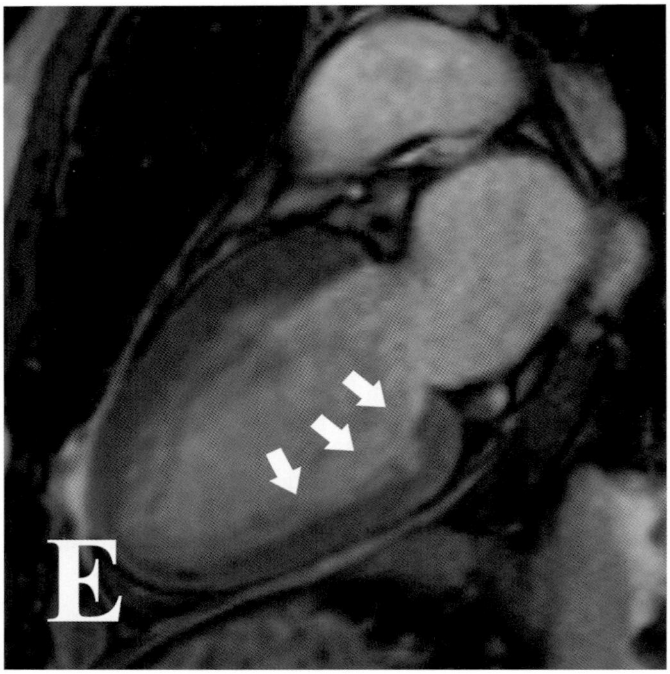

Figure 5.1 *(cont.)*

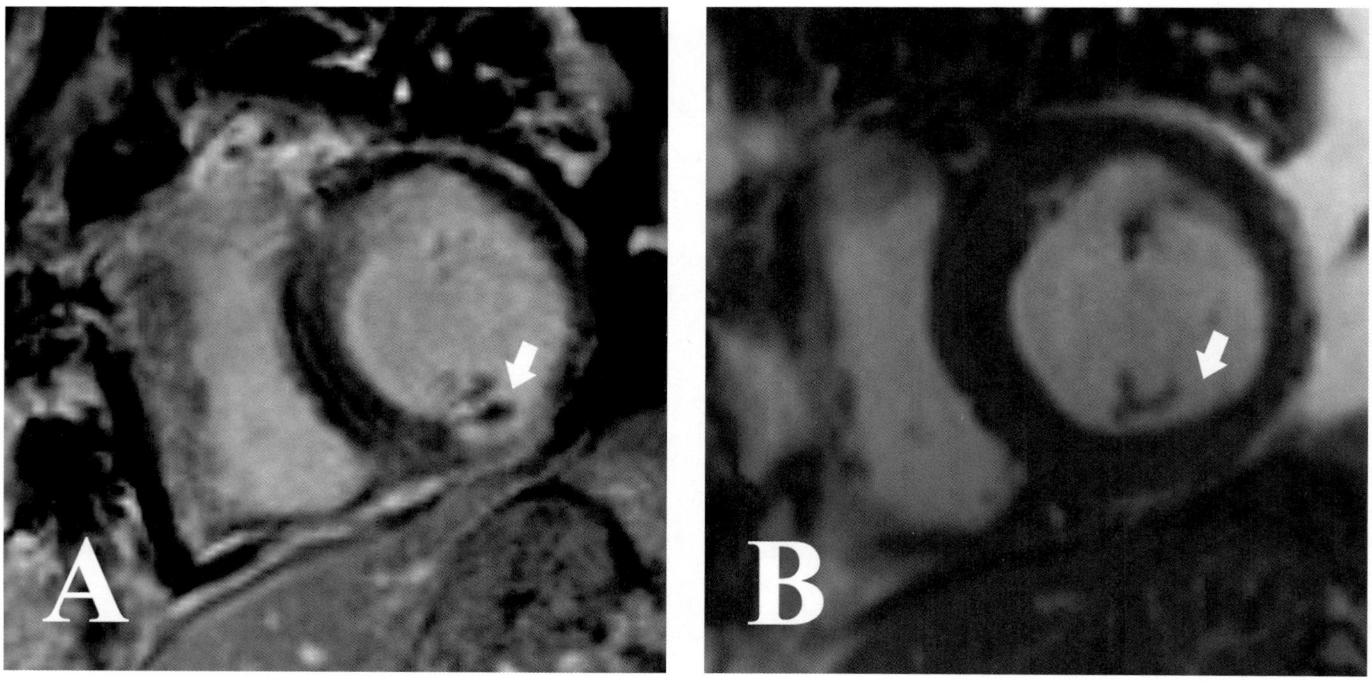

Figure 5.2 A. Short-axis delayed enhancement image from a cardiac MRI performed to assess viability in a 77-year-old male with recent RCA territory myocardial infarction. There is a small focus of microvascular obstruction in the inferior wall of the left ventricle (arrow). **B.** Comparison with the corresponding precontrast short-axis bright blood image confirms that this is not a thrombus, as no intraluminal mass is present in a similar location.

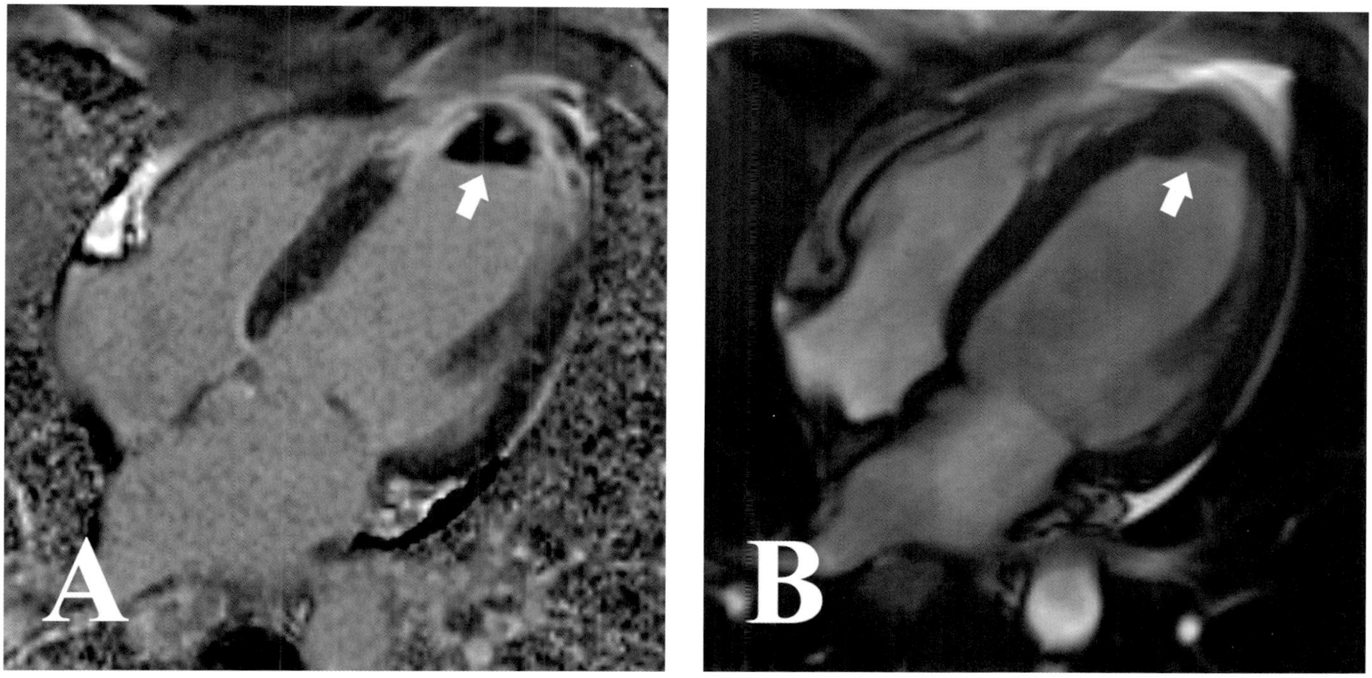

Figure 5.3 **A.** Horizontal long-axis delayed enhancement image from a 54-year-old male with history of left anterior descending coronary artery territory myocardial infarction demonstrates low signal intensity in the left ventricular apex (arrow) surrounded by hyperenhancing myocardial wall. **B.** Precontrast bright blood image confirms that this lesion is an apical thrombus (arrow), rather than microvascular obstruction, given that it is seen as a filling defect on both precontrast and delayed enhancement images.

CASE 6

Pseudothrombus in the left atrial appendage

Stefan L. Zimmerman

Imaging description

Left atrial appendage pseudothrombus is not uncommonly encountered in patients with left atrial enlargement and poor atrial function. In this entity, stasis of blood in the left atrium results in incomplete mixing, or underfilling, of non-opacified blood in the left atrial appendage with intravenous contrast. The result is a low-attenuation region in the tip of the appendage that can be mistaken for thrombus (Figure 6.1). At transesophageal echocardiography, the gold standard for evaluation of left atrial appendage thrombus, underfilling of the left atrial appendage on CT, usually corresponds to spontaneous echo contrast, a sign of blood stasis, with or without thrombus.[1]

Importance

Left atrial pseudothrombus is relatively common in patients with atrial fibrillation who undergo cardiac CT for pre-ablation mapping. In a large study of 402 atrial fibrillation patients with 64-slice contrast-enhanced CT, underfilling of the left atrial appendage was seen in 40 (10%), with nine of these patients having true thrombus detected by transesophageal echocardiography. The remaining patients had spontaneous echo contrast. Left atrial underfilling is also important to recognize in patients with a history of stroke, who may have emboli originating from the left atrium. If underfilling is recognized at the time of imaging, acquisition of additional delayed images can improve differentiation of thrombus from blood stasis (Figure 6.1).[2-4] Distinction of true left atrial thrombus from pseudothrombus is critical as ablation procedures should not be performed in the presence of thrombus, due to the risk of clot dislodgement and distal embolization during the procedure. Incorrect diagnosis of thrombus can result in unnecessary delay of ablation therapy and risks of anticoagulation medications.

Typical clinical scenario

Left atrial pseudothrombus can be seen in any patient, but is most commonly encountered in patients with dilated, poorly functioning atria. These patients have poor mixing of blood in the left atrial appendage due to stasis. Unfortunately, these same characteristics also put the patients at high risk for true left atrial thrombus, increasing the challenge of diagnosis.

Differential diagnosis

Left atrial pseudothrombus must be distinguished from true left atrial appendage thrombus. If delayed images are available, these will clearly show the homogenous enhancement of the appendage after time has passed to allow complete mixing to occur. In the absence of delayed images, pseudothrombus may be recognized by the presence of a smooth, graded transition of attenuation between opacified and non-opacified blood (Figure 6.1), unlike the sharp borders of thrombus (Figure 6.2). Pseudothrombus will typically have straight borders due to layering affects, whereas thrombus will be multilobulated in appearance (Figure 6.2). In some cases, it may be impossible to exclude true left atrial thrombus and in such a situation the patient should be recommended for transesophageal echocardiography for confirmation.

Teaching point

Left atrial appendage pseudothrombus is an artifact caused by incomplete mixing of unopacified blood in the left atrial appendage with intravenous contrast. In some cases, it may be distinguished from true clot by characteristic imaging findings or its disappearance on delayed images. In difficult cases, further evaluation with transesophageal echocardiography may be necessary to exclude a true thrombus.

REFERENCES

1. M. W. Martinez, J. Kirsch, E. E. Williamson, et al. Utility of nongated multidetector computed tomography for detection of left atrial thrombus in patients undergoing catheter ablation of atrial fibrillation. *JACC Cardiovasc Imaging* 2009; **2**: 69–76.
2. S. T. Sawit, A. Garcia-Alvarez, B. Suri, et al. Usefulness of cardiac computed tomographic delayed contrast enhancement of the left atrial appendage before pulmonary vein ablation. *Am J Cardiol* 2012; **109**: 677–84.
3. J. Hur, Y. J. Kim, H. J. Lee, et al. Left atrial appendage thrombi in stroke patients: detection with two-phase cardiac CT angiography versus transesophageal echocardiography. *Radiology* 2009; **251**: 683–90.
4. S. C. Kim, E. J. Chun, S. I. Choi, et al. Differentiation between spontaneous echocardiographic contrast and left atrial appendage thrombus in patients with suspected embolic stroke using two-phase multidetector computed tomography. *Am J Cardiol* 2010; **106**: 1174–81.

Pearls and Pitfalls in Cardiovascular Imaging, ed. Stefan L. Zimmerman and Elliot K. Fishman. Published by Cambridge University Press. © Cambridge University Press 2015.

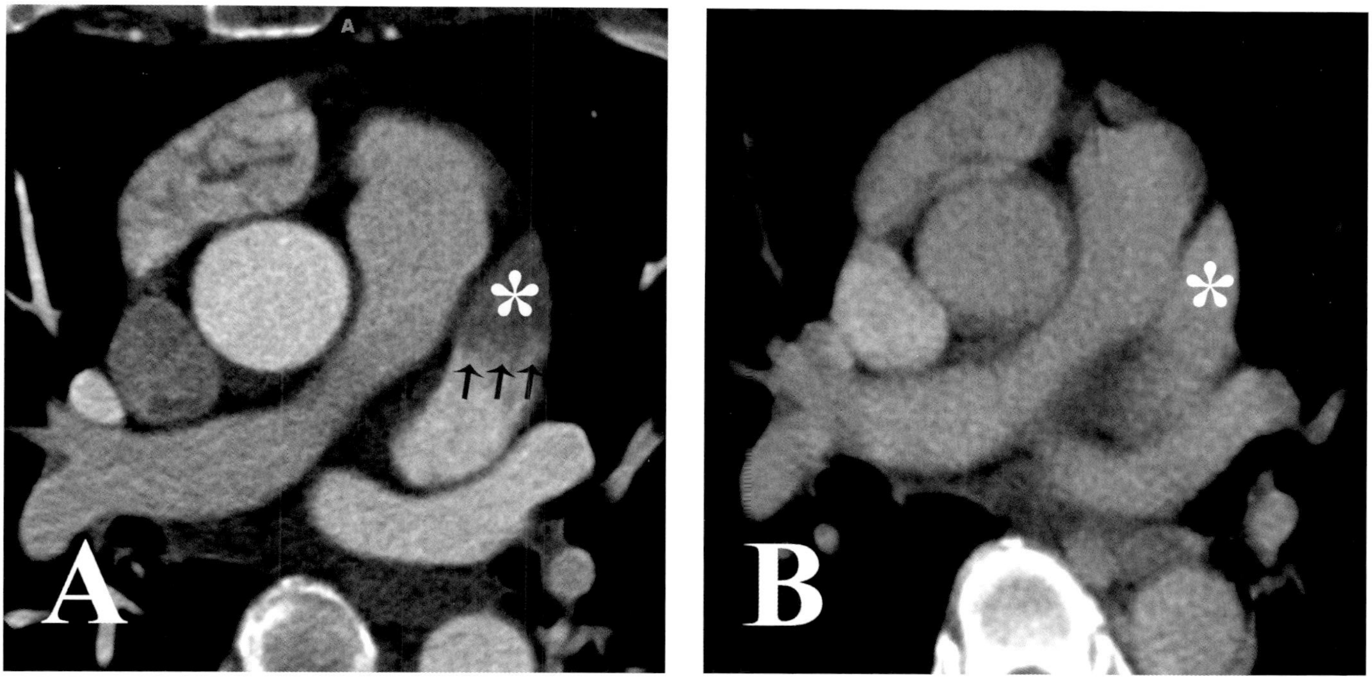

Figure 6.1 **A.** Axial contrast-enhanced image from a cardiac CT performed in a 74-year-old woman with a history of atrial fibrillation and chest tightness. There is low attenuation in the tip of the left atrial appendage (asterisk). This has the typical appearance of incomplete contrast opacification of the appendage with a horizontally oriented, gradual transition from enhanced left atrial lumen to non-enhanced appendage (black arrows). **B.** On a delayed scan performed as part of the same examination, there is complete enhancement of the entire atrial appendage, excluding the possibility of left atrial clot.

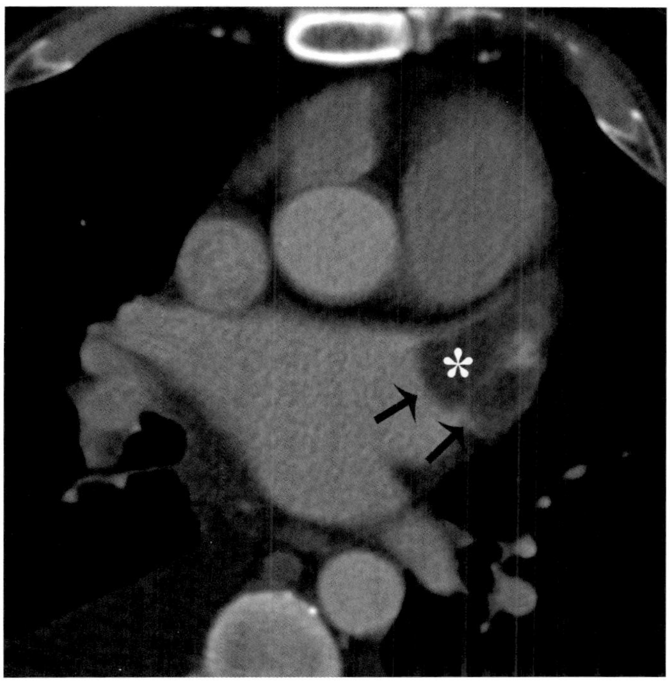

Figure 6.2 Axial contrast-enhanced CT image from a pulmonary embolism study performed in a 38-year-old male with atrial fibrillation and heart failure related to Graves' disease demonstrates a thrombus in the left atrial appendage (asterisk). There are sharp margins between the enhanced atrial lumen and the thrombus (black arrows), unlike the graded transition seen with underfilling of the appendage. In addition, the thrombus has lobulated margins, unlike the horizontal orientation seen with underfilling.

CASE 7

Pseudolymphadenopathy due to fluid in the pericardial recess

Satomi Kawamoto

Imaging description

Within the pericardial cavity, there are several recesses and sinuses where fluid can collect in close contiguity to the major vessels and lymph nodes, and can be misinterpreted as lymphadenopathy or mediastinal mass. The posterior portion of the superior aortic recess lies directly posterior to the ascending aorta, and is seen as a well-defined crescentic fluid collection on CT (Figure 7.1).[1] The superior aortic recess is usually caudal to the aortic arch, but sometimes extends cephalad and rightward into the right paratracheal region between the brachiocephalic vessels and the trachea (Figure 7.2), even in patients without pericardial effusion.[2] This is called the "high-riding" superior pericardial recess and may mimic hypodense paratracheal lymphadenopathy or a cystic mediastinal mass.[2] Fluid accumulation within the pericardial "sleeve" recess adjacent to the right inferior pulmonary vein can also mimic adenopathy (Figure 7.3).[3]

Importance

With recent technological advances that provide high temporal and spatial resolution there has been improved visualization of fine anatomic details of the pericardium, resulting in the routine visualization of the pericardial recesses.[1] A pericardial recess with prominent fluid may simulate hypodense lymphadenopathy or a cystic mass, especially in the setting of known primary malignancy.[1]

Typical clinical scenario

A pericardial recess is typically incidentally found on chest CT imaging. The pericardial cavity is a potential space between the parietal and visceral layers of the serous pericardium. It normally contains a small amount of serous fluid (15–25 ml).[1,4] The superior aortic recess is the upward extension of the transverse sinus of the pericardial cavity, and seen in 47% of patients without known pericardial disease.[5] The superior pericardial recess is the posterior division of the superior aortic recess, and is usually seen just caudal to the aortic arch.[2] However, it may extend more superiorly in the right paratracheal region, and may mimic a paratracheal lymph node or cystic mass.[2] A high-riding superior pericardial recess was diagnosed in 6 (2%) of 276 patients in a study by Choi et al.[2] A pericardial recess may change its size and shape due to redistribution of the fluid within a short interval. In a case report by Aribandi, "high-riding" superior pericardial recess seen on CT of the neck significantly decreased in size and changed its shape on subsequent chest CT performed 4 minutes later.[4]

During development, as the pulmonary veins penetrate the fibrous pericardium to enter the left atrium, a serosal sleeve of pericardium invests the veins.[3] Fluid can accumulate in this pericardial sleeve recess, and manifest as a well-circumscribed homogenous water attenuation structure located adjacent to the right inferior pulmonary vein.

Differential diagnosis

Differential diagnosis of fluid in the pericardial recess includes cystic/necrotic lymphadenopathy, and cystic mediastinal mass such as bronchogenic cyst and pericardial cyst. Unlike enlarged lymph nodes which tend to be round or oval, fluid in the pericardial recess tends to have a linear, crescent, or triangular shape.[4] Pericardial recesses demonstrate homogeneous fluid attenuation with no peripheral enhancement. The fat plane between the superior aortic recess and the aorta is usually absent.[4] Thin slice imaging with multiplanar reconstruction may also help to demonstrate communication between the "high-riding" portion and more inferior portion of the superior pericardial recess.[2]

Teaching point

Pericardial recess is occasionally prominent and may extend superiorly above the level of the aortic arch into the right paratracheal region, and may simulate lymphadenopathy or mass. Homogenous internal fluid attenuation, no enhancing rim, typical location and communication to the more inferior portion of the pericardial recess help to determine its diagnosis.

REFERENCES

1. Truong MT, Erasmus JJ, Gladish GW, et al. Anatomy of pericardial recesses on multidetector CT: implications for oncologic imaging. *AJR American Journal of Roentgenology* 2003;**181**:1109–1113.

Pearls and Pitfalls in Cardiovascular Imaging, ed. Stefan L. Zimmerman and Elliot K. Fishman. Published by Cambridge University Press. © Cambridge University Press 2015.

2. Choi YW, McAdams HP, Jeon SC, Seo HS, Hahm CK. The "high-riding" superior pericardial recess: CT findings. *AJR American Journal of Roentgenology* 2000;**175**:1025–1028.
3. Truong MT, Erasmus JJ, Sabloff BS, et al. Pericardial "sleeve" recess of right inferior pulmonary vein mimicking adenopathy: computed tomography findings. *Journal of Computer Assisted Tomography* 2004;**28**:361–365.
4. Aribandi M. High-riding superior pericardial recess: temporal change can help distinguish from mediastinal pathology. *Southern Medical Journal* 2007;**100**:407–408.
5. Groell R, Schaffler GJ, Rienmueller R. Pericardial sinuses and recesses: findings at electrocardiographically triggered electron-beam CT. *Radiology* 1999;**212**:69–73.

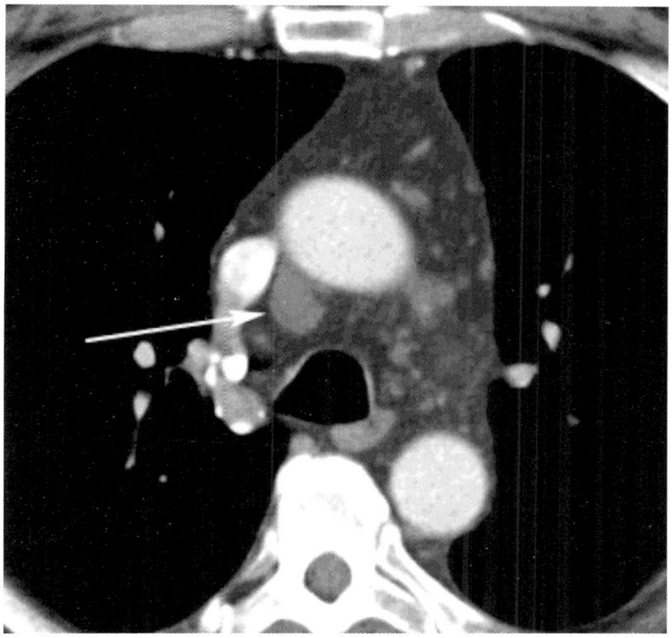

Figure 7.1 Axial contrast-enhanced CT in a 64-year-old man shows superior aortic recess (arrow) posterior to the ascending aorta.

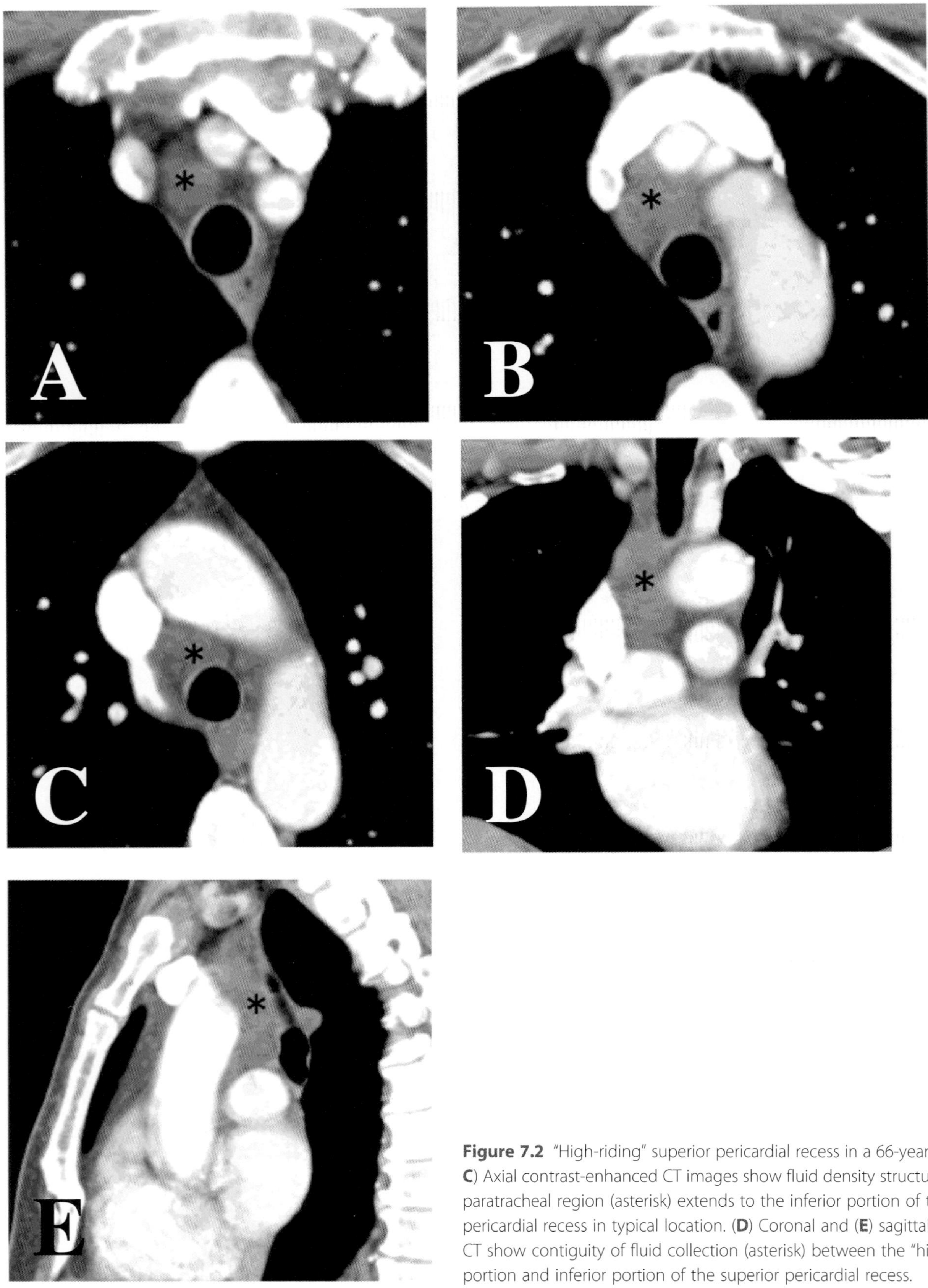

Figure 7.2 "High-riding" superior pericardial recess in a 66-year-old man. (**A–C**) Axial contrast-enhanced CT images show fluid density structure in the right paratracheal region (asterisk) extends to the inferior portion of the superior pericardial recess in typical location. (**D**) Coronal and (**E**) sagittal reformatted CT show contiguity of fluid collection (asterisk) between the "high-riding" portion and inferior portion of the superior pericardial recess.

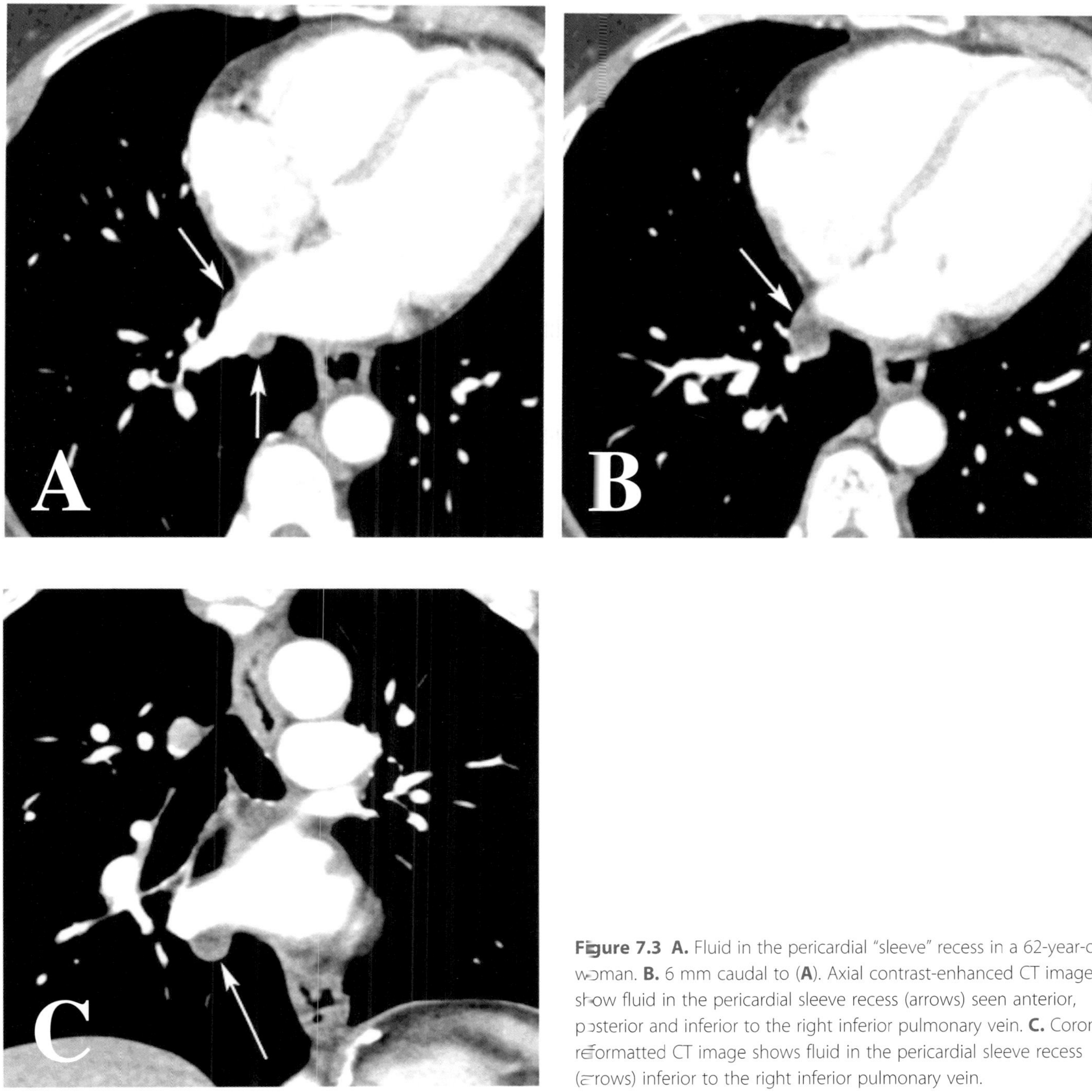

Figure 7.3 **A.** Fluid in the pericardial "sleeve" recess in a 62-year-old woman. **B.** 6 mm caudal to (**A**). Axial contrast-enhanced CT images show fluid in the pericardial sleeve recess (arrows) seen anterior, posterior and inferior to the right inferior pulmonary vein. **C.** Coronal reformatted CT image shows fluid in the pericardial sleeve recess (arrows) inferior to the right inferior pulmonary vein.

CASE **8**

Valvular masses

Stefan L. Zimmerman

Imaging description

Valvular masses can be challenging when encountered on cardiac CT or MRI. Echocardiography is the test of choice for evaluation of the valves; however, in some patients, CT or MRI may be requested due to lack of adequate imaging windows or need to evaluate for associated complications. Vegetations in the setting of infective endocarditis are more common than valvular tumors, are mobile during the cardiac cycle, low attenuation on CT (Figure 8.1), and low signal intensity on T1- and T2-weighted MRI. They are associated with valvular thickening or other sequelae of infectious endocarditis such as valvular regurgitation, perforation (Figure 8.1), fistulas between cardiac chambers, paravalvular abscesses, and pseudoaneurysms. Primary tumors of the valve are rare. Of these, the most commonly encountered valvular tumor is a papillary fibroelastoma which is commonly round with an irregular, frond-like surface. It will be low in attenuation on CT images (Figure 8.2), similar to the valve tissue, and will have intermediate T1 and high T2 signal intensity on MRI with homogenous delayed enhancement (Figure 8.3). Papillary fibroelastomas are usually mobile on a stalk, moving with the valve leaflets through the cardiac cycle. Involvement of the aortic and mitral valve is more common than the tricuspid and pulmonic valve.[1]

Importance

Although rare, valvular masses are important to recognize at cardiac imaging due to the fact that they pose a risk of distal embolization. In patients with infective endocarditis, neurologic complications develop in 20–40%.[2] Although benign, the treatment of choice for valvular tumors is surgical resection to avoid these complications. Antibiotic therapy may be used to treat vegetations; however, in complicated cases, such as those with fistulas or abscesses, surgical valve replacement may be necessary.

Typical clinical scenario

Valvular masses may be encountered incidentally or may be referred to advanced imaging after discovery at echocardiography. Coronary CT angiography may be used to preoperatively evaluate the coronary arteries in patients who are planned for valve replacement. Coronary CT angiography is highly accurate for detection of left-sided valve vegetations, with sensitivity and specificity of 96% and 97% when compared to pathologic findings after surgery.[3] The prevalence of infective endocarditis is estimated at 2–6 cases per 100,000 person-years.[2] The incidence is increased in intravenous drug abusers, diabetics, patients on hemodialysis and those with pre-existing valvular heart disease, the most common of which is mitral valve prolapse.[2] The aortic valve is involved in 50% of cases.[1] Papillary fibroelastomas are rare, most often found in older patients in their 60– 70s.[1] These are often discovered incidentally but may be found in symptomatic patients with embolic events.[1]

Differential diagnosis

The differential diagnosis for the valvular masses described also includes valvular or annular calcification, which can be low signal intensity and mass-like at MRI. Aortic valvular calcification is usually associated with aortic stenosis, resulting in high-velocity flow jets that should be evident on cine images. Calcification will be easily distinguished at CT by high attenuation appearance. Artifacts due to valve leaflet motion at coronary CT may occasionally result in an appearance that simulates a valvular mass, due to blurring of images in the setting of low temporal resolution. Valve leaflet thickening due to aging or rheumatic heart disease should also be considered; however, no discrete mass will be identified at imaging.

Teaching point

Although usually benign, valvular masses are important to recognize due to the risk of distal embolization. Vegetations and papillary fibroelastomas have characteristic clinical and imaging findings that help make the correct diagnosis.

REFERENCES

1. C. J. Bennett, J. J. Maleszewski, P. A. Araoz. CT and MR imaging of the aortic valve: radiologic-pathologic correlation. *Radiographics* 2012; **32**: 1399–420.
2. E. Mylonakis, S. B. Calderwood. Infective endocarditis in adults. *N Engl J Med* 2001; **345**: 1318–30.
3. G. M. Feuchtner, P. Stolzmann, W. Dichtl, et al. Multislice computed tomography in infective endocarditis: comparison with transesophageal echocardiography and intraoperative findings. *J Am Coll Cardiol* 2009; **53**: 436–44.

Pearls and Pitfalls in Cardiovascular Imaging, ed. Stefan L. Zimmerman and Elliot K. Fishman. Published by Cambridge University Press. © Cambridge University Press 2015.

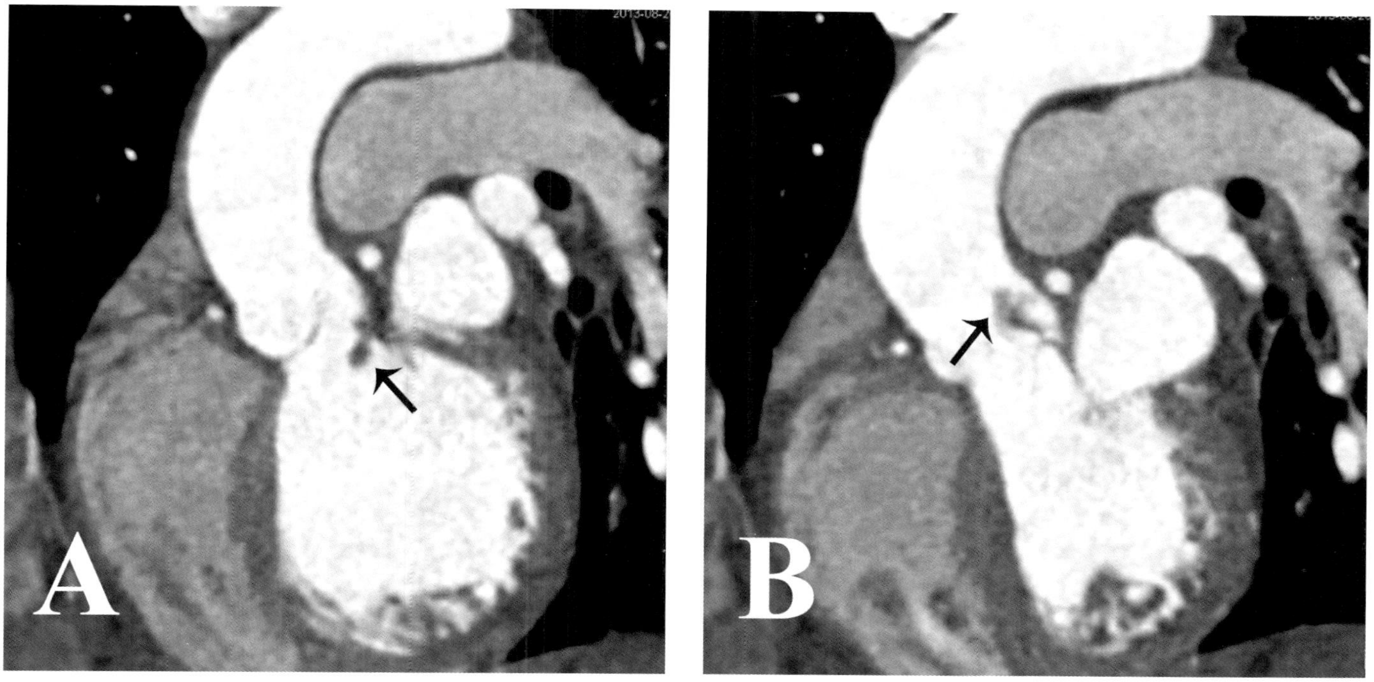

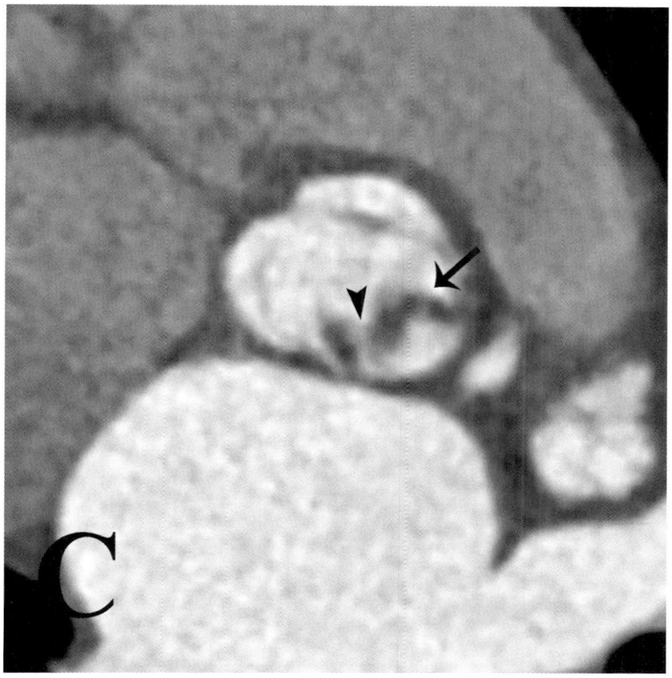

Figure 8.1 **A.** Coronal oblique end-diastolic image from a cardiac CT obtained in a 52-year-old male with a history of intravenous drug abuse and bacteremia demonstrates a large vegetation that extends inferiorly from the left coronary cusp into the left ventricular outflow tract (arrow). Vegetations are low in attenuation in CT and usually have a lobulated contour, usually attached to the valve leaflets as in this case. **B.** Coronal oblique image obtained in end-systole demonstrates prolapse of the vegetation into the proximal ascending aorta (arrow) as it is pulled upwards by the movement of the aortic valve leaflets. **C.** Short-axis image obtained through the aortic valve plane shows thickening of the left aortic valve cusp (arrow). There is a focal perforation of the valve leaflet (arrowhead), which was confirmed by echocardiography. Vegetations can be associated with complications such as valve perforation, perivalvular abscess, or formation of fistulas between cardiac chambers.

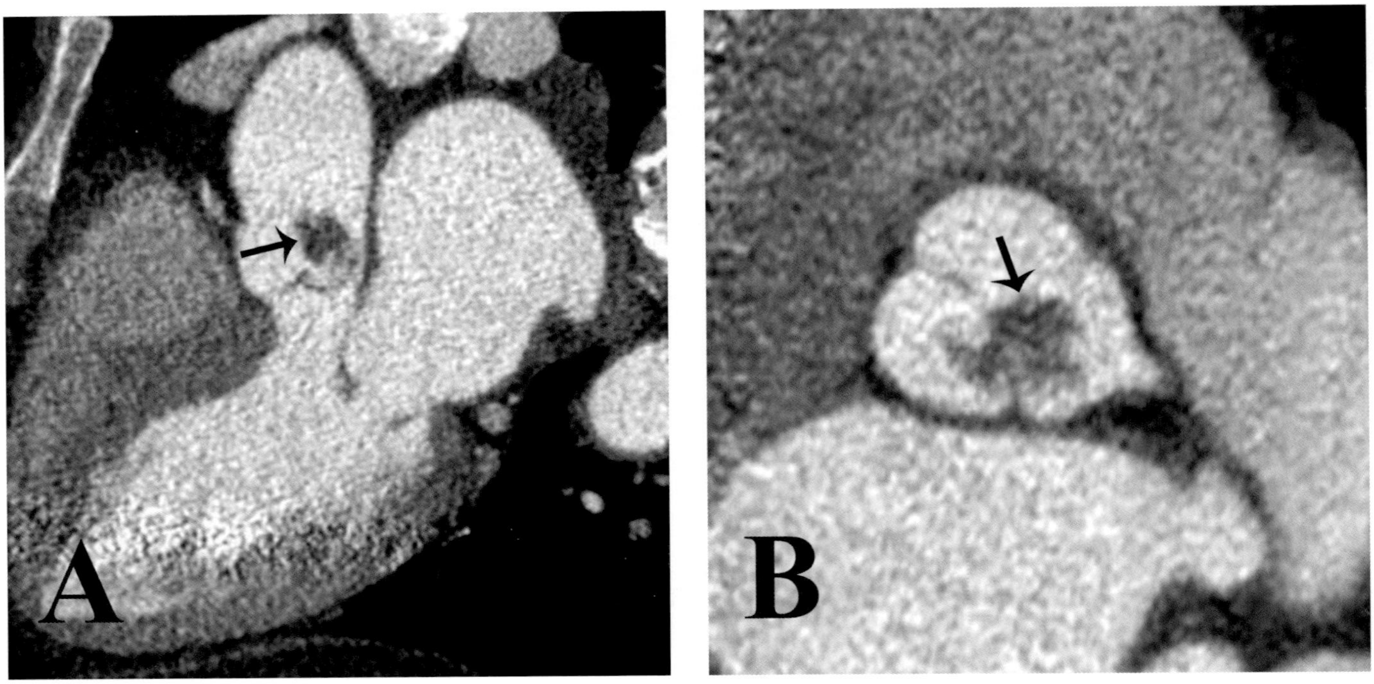

Figure 8.2 **A.** Three-chamber multiplanar reformatted image from a cardiac CT performed for preoperative evaluation of the coronary arteries in a patient with papillary fibroelastoma demonstrates a low-attenuation mass arising from the aortic valve with irregular, frond-like margins (arrow), typical for this entity. On dynamic cine images, not shown, the mass moved with the valve leaflet through the cardiac cycle, arising from a thin stalk. **B.** The short-axis image again demonstrates the frond-like margins of the mass and the association with the aortic valve (arrow). Papillary fibroelastomas are most commonly found in the left side of the heart, arising from the aortic or mitral valves.

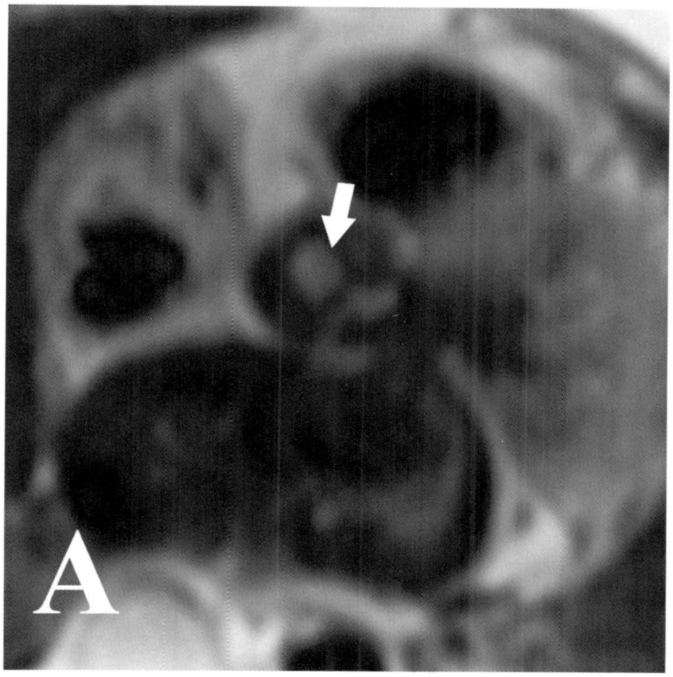

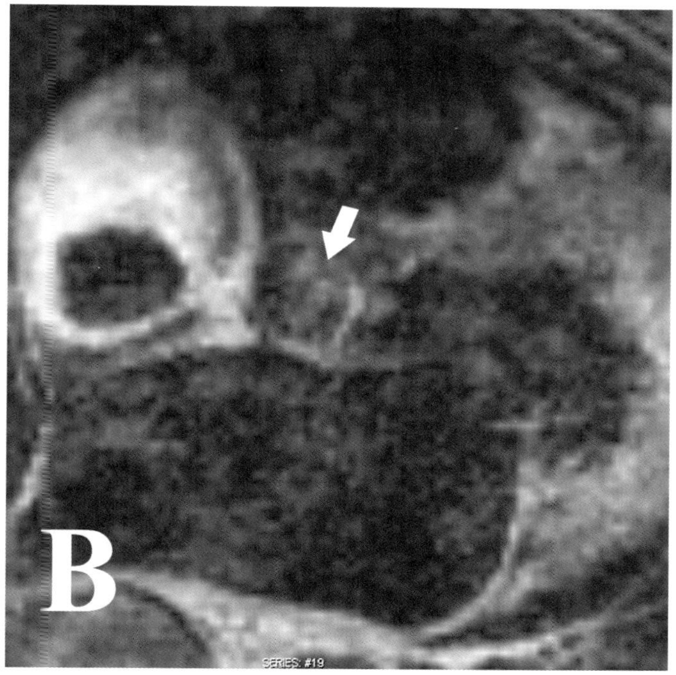

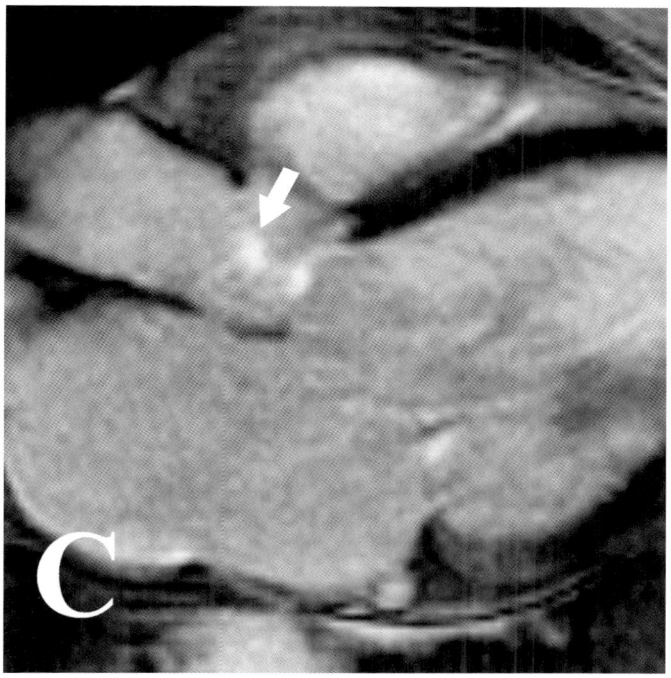

Figure 8.3 **A.** Axial dark blood T1-weighted MRI image (TR 2000 msec, TE 20 msec) obtained in an 83-year-old female for evaluation of a valvular mass demonstrates a round mass adjacent to the aortic valve with signal intensity isointense to myocardium (arrow). **B.** On T2-weighted triple-inversion recovery dark blood images the mass (arrow) is hyperintense, although images are somewhat blurred by motion. **C.** On a late gadolinium enhancement image obtained in the three-chamber plane the mass (arrow) demonstrates diffuse homogenous enhancement. These imaging features are typical for a papillary fibroelastoma.

CASE 9

Cardiac angiosarcoma

Stefan L. Zimmerman

Imaging description

Cardiac angiosarcoma is an aggressive, infiltrative mass that is most often found in the wall of the right atrium. On CT, they are typically low-attenuation, broad-based lobulated masses with heterogenous enhancement post-contrast (Figure 9.1).[1] On MRI, cardiac angiosarcoma is heterogenous due to presence of intralesional hemorrhage and necrosis; however, it is predominantly T2 hyperintense and T1 isointense to myocardium (Figure 9.2).[2] Flow voids within the mass may be seen due to extensive vascularity. Occasionally, tumors may be avidly enhancing with post-contrast tumor attenuation at CT and MRI nearly identical to the blood pool (Figure 9.1). Tumor infiltration into adjacent structures such as the pericardium, superior or inferior vena cava, or interatrial septum is common (Figure 9.3). Hemorrhagic pericardial effusions are typically seen and can be large.

Importance

Cardiac angiosarcomas may be difficult to diagnose at enhanced chest CT due to their hypervascularity (Figure 9.1). They can appear very similar in attenuation to the blood pool and may be overlooked if close attention is not paid to the heart. Early, small tumors may be also difficult to appreciate on non-gated CT examinations due to motion. The presence of a de novo hemorrhagic pericardial effusion should prompt close inspection of all cardiac chambers for this entity. Accurate diagnosis is critical for proper patient management.

Typical clinical scenario

Cardiac angiosarcomas are rare, although they are the most common primary cardiac malignancy. They represent 10% of all primary cardiac tumors.[2] Patients will most often present with chest pain, tamponade, or right heart failure.[1] The majority of patients will have metastastic disease at presentation. Prognosis is uniformly poor; patients do not usually survive beyond 12 months.[2]

Differential diagnosis

Cardiac metatastases are much more common than primary cardiac angiosarcoma and should always be considered. These will commonly be multiple and will be associated with additional sites of metastastic disease throughout the body. Lung, melanoma, and breast cancer are common tumors to metastasize to the heart.[3] Cardiac lymphoma can be infiltrative and aggressive; however, will typically be less intensely enhancing than cardiac angiosarcoma. Angiosarcoma can be distinguished from benign primary cardiac masses such as myxoma by aggressive imaging features such as invasion of adjacent structures and associated hemorrhagic effusion.

Teaching point

Cardiac angiosarcomas are rare, aggressive tumors that in some cases may be difficult to diagnose on non-gated imaging due to hypervascularity, resulting in attenuation identical to blood pool. Careful inspection of the cardiac chambers for masses should be performed in any patient presenting with a new hemorrhagic pericardial effusion.

REFERENCES

1. P. A. Araoz, H. E. Eklund, T. J. Welch, J. F. Breen. CT and MR imaging of primary cardiac malignancies. *Radiographics* 1999; **19**: 1421–34.
2. K. Randhawa, A. Ganeshan, E. T. Hoey. Magnetic resonance imaging of cardiac tumors: part 2, malignant tumors and tumor-like conditions. *Curr Probl Diagn Radiol* 2011; **40**: 169–79.
3. R. Bussani, F. De-Giorgio, A. Abbate, F. Silvestri. Cardiac metastases. *J Clin Pathol* 2007; **60**: 27–34.

Pearls and Pitfalls in Cardiovascular Imaging, ed. Stefan L. Zimmerman and Elliot K. Fishman. Published by Cambridge University Press. © Cambridge University Press 2015.

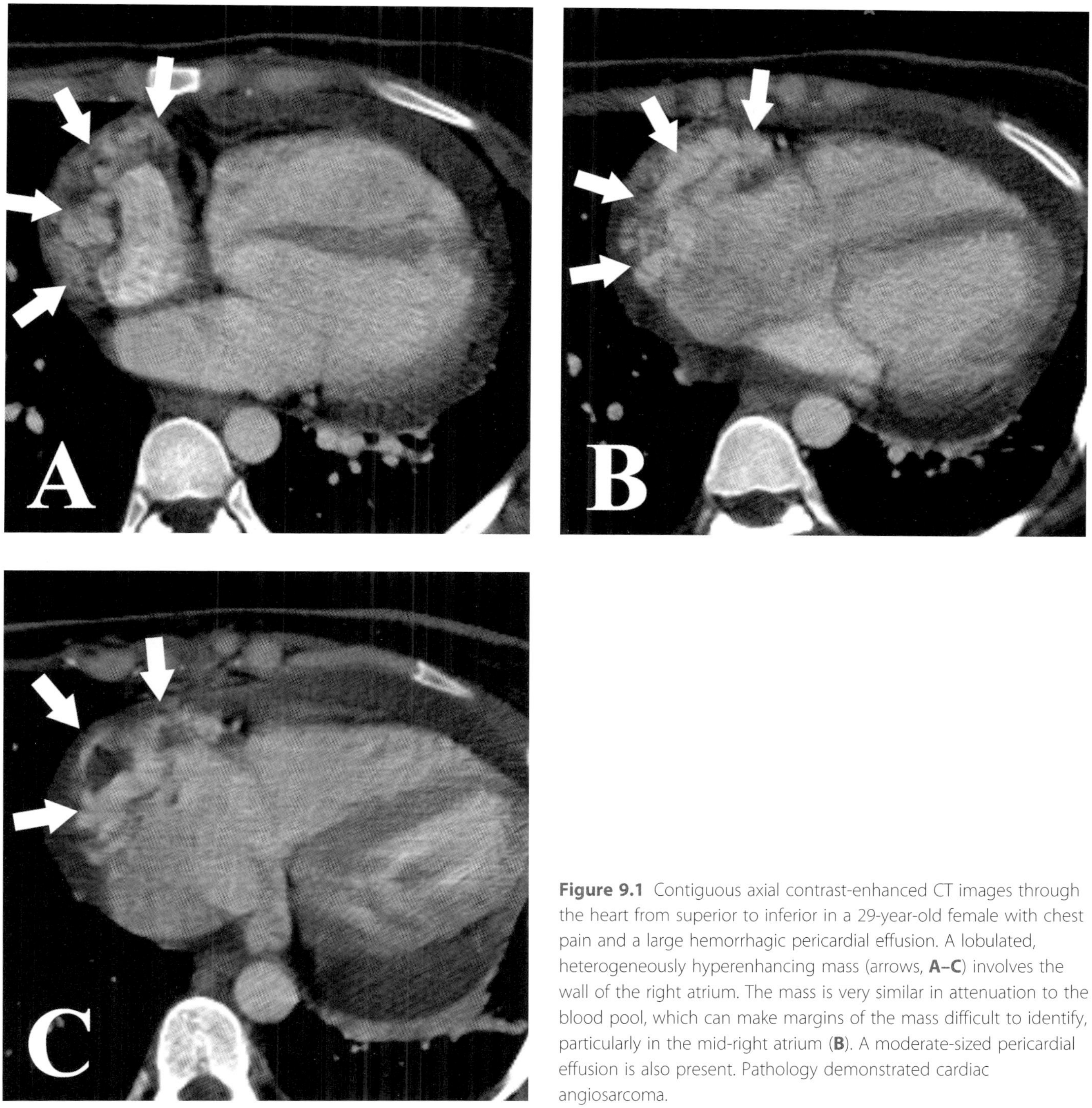

Figure 9.1 Contiguous axial contrast-enhanced CT images through the heart from superior to inferior in a 29-year-old female with chest pain and a large hemorrhagic pericardial effusion. A lobulated, heterogeneously hyperenhancing mass (arrows, **A–C**) involves the wall of the right atrium. The mass is very similar in attenuation to the blood pool, which can make margins of the mass difficult to identify, particularly in the mid-right atrium (**B**). A moderate-sized pericardial effusion is also present. Pathology demonstrated cardiac angiosarcoma.

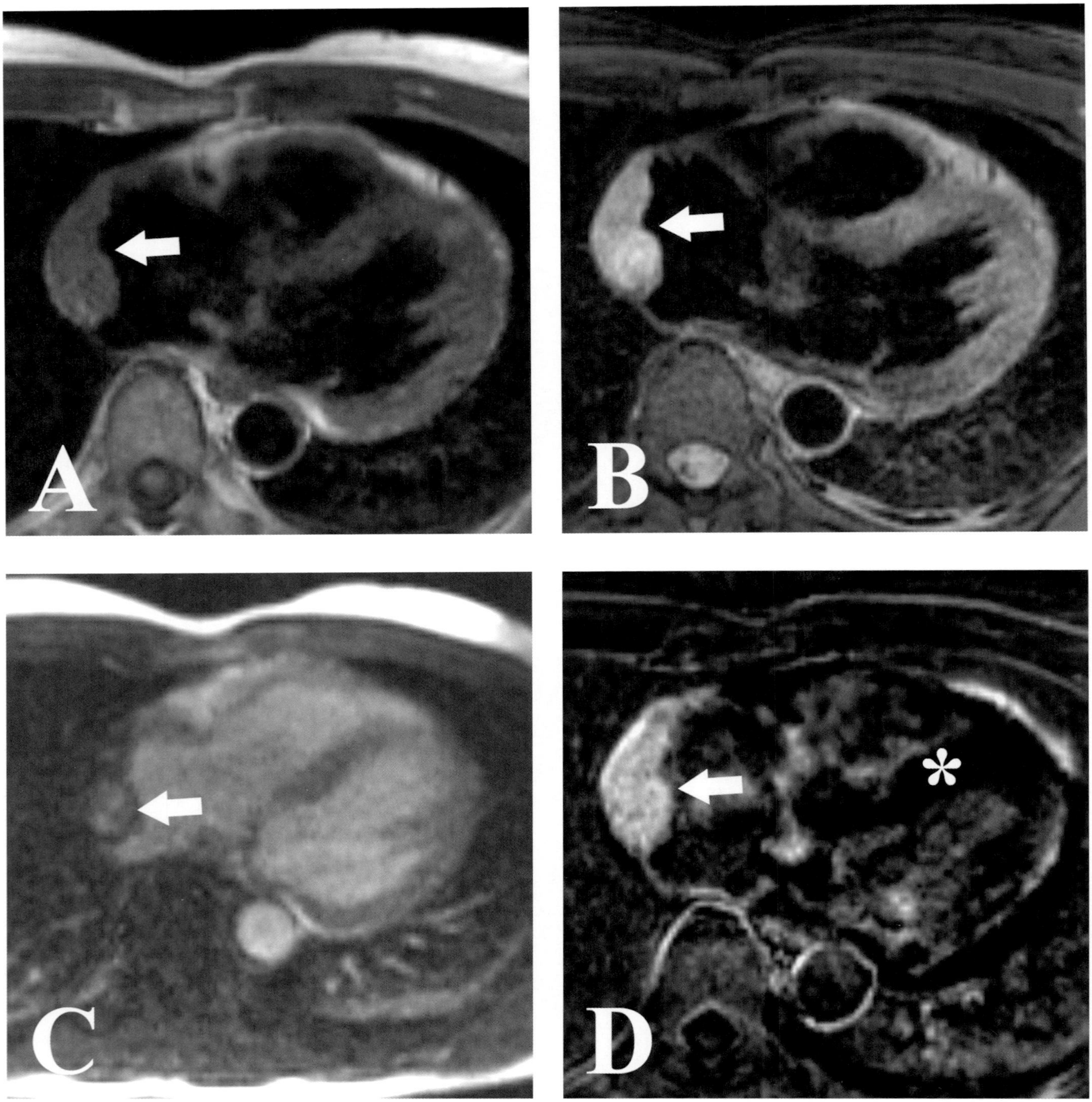

Figure 9.2 Contrast-enhanced MRI performed in a 52-year-old male who presented with tamponade and hemorrhagic pericardial effusion at pericardiocentesis. **A.** A lobulated mass is present in the right atrial wall that is isointense to normal myocardium on T1-weighted axial images (arrow). **B.** The mass is hyperintense on fat-saturated T2-weighted images (arrow). **C.** On axial dynamic perfusion imaging obtained post-contrast, there is early, heterogenous enhancement on the mass (arrow). **D.** On a T1-weighted post-contrast subtraction image, enhancement becomes more homogeneous (arrow) and is markedly hyperintense to ventricular myocardium (asterisk). Pathology was consistent with angiosarcoma.

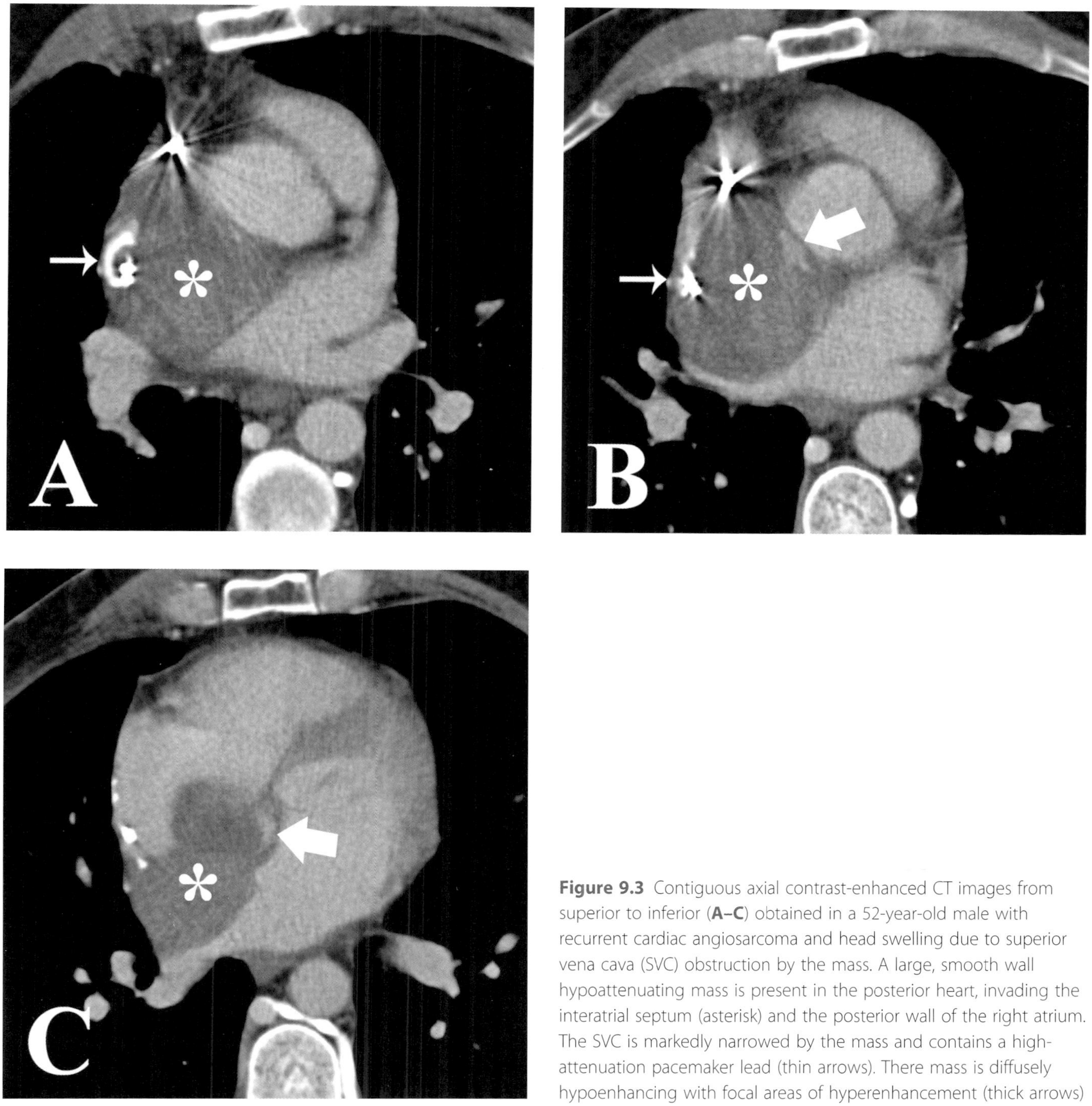

Figure 9.3 Contiguous axial contrast-enhanced CT images from superior to inferior (**A–C**) obtained in a 52-year-old male with recurrent cardiac angiosarcoma and head swelling due to superior vena cava (SVC) obstruction by the mass. A large, smooth wall hypoattenuating mass is present in the posterior heart, invading the interatrial septum (asterisk) and the posterior wall of the right atrium. The SVC is markedly narrowed by the mass and contains a high-attenuation pacemaker lead (thin arrows). There mass is diffusely hypoenhancing with focal areas of hyperenhancement (thick arrows)

CASE 10

Ventricular non-compaction

Nathan Johnson and Stefan L. Zimmerman

Imaging description

Non-compaction of the ventricular myocardium is a rare congenital cardiac disease characterized by excessive myocardial trabeculations and deep intertrabecular recesses. Non-compaction is thought to be the result of the arrest of normal cardiac development *in utero* during the 5th to 8th week of life, a time when loose myocardial fibers in the ventricles become organized and "compacted."[1] Non-compaction has been most often described in the left ventricle, but biventricular and isolated right ventricular involvement has also been reported.[1] The most common locations for non-compaction are the left ventricular apex, lateral wall, and inferior wall (Figure 10.1). Diagnostic criteria have been proposed for echocardiography that rely upon a comparison of the thickness of trabeculated and compacted myocardium,[2,3] or the number of prominent trabeculations.[4] By MRI, non-compaction has been defined as a ratio of trabeculated to compacted myocardium of greater than 2.3 in end-diastole.[5] However, recent studies in both normal subjects[6] and patients with heart failure[7] have suggested that current MRI criteria may be overly sensitive, resulting in overdiagnosis. Patients with non-compaction cardiomyopathy will often have myocardial dysfunction manifested by reduced ventricular ejection fraction and cavity dilation, sometimes complicated by intracavitary thrombus (Figure 10.2), which may aid in diagnosis. On dark blood images, high signal may be seen in between the prominent trabeculations due to slow blood flow. Delayed myocardial enhancement involving the prominent trabeculations may be present and has been associated with reduced ejection fraction and more advanced disease.[8]

Importance

Accurate diagnoses of LV non-compaction is challenging due to lack of clear diagnostic test for the disease and substantial overlap of current criteria with healthy subjects and those with heart failure from different causes.[6,7] True non-compaction cardiomyopathy is a serious disease with a poor prognosis.[9] Identification of these patients is important as they have a high rate of symptomatic heart failure, thromboembolic events, ventricular arrhythmias, and sudden death.[9] Some will eventually require heart transplant or placement of an implantable cardioverter defibrillator (ICD). A multifactorial approach to diagnosis that combines morphologic data with cardiac function, symptoms, and excludes other causes of heart failure has been suggested for improved diagnostic accuracy.[6]

Typical clinical scenario

Non-compaction can be seen in both children and adults. In the pediatric population, it may be associated with complex congenital heart disease.[1] Familial and sporadic cases of non-compaction have been reported, and gene mutations in proteins encoding for sarcomeric structural proteins have been implicated.[10] Initially thought of as an extremely rare disease, non-compaction is being increasingly recognized due to elevated awareness and perhaps overdiagnosis, and the true prevalence is unknown.[7] Patients may present with heart failure, embolic events, or arrhythmias. Asymptomatic cases may also be discovered by family member screening or imaging performed for other reasons.

Differential diagnosis

The differential diagnosis for non-compaction includes normal anatomic variation, dilated cardiomyopathy from another cause, and hypertrophic cardiomyopathy. Prominent trabeculations are commonly seen in healthy patients,[6] with 43% of healthy adults demonstrating at least one myocardial segment that meets proposed MRI criteria of a trabeculated to non-compacted ratio of $>$ 2.3. Therefore, the diagnosis of non-compaction should be made with caution in asymptomatic individuals with limited morphologic findings. Ischemic or non-ischemic cardiomyopathies of a variety of causes may have prominent trabeculations, which may be the result of LV cavity remodeling that occurs in the setting of chronically reduced low systolic function. Finally, hypertrophic cardiomyopathy, particularly with apical involvement, may be difficult to distinguish from non-compaction at echocardiography in cases with limited windows; however, these can be easily differentiated by cardiac MRI.

Teaching point

LV non-compaction should be considered in patients with cardiac dysfunction and prominent ventricular trabeculations on non-invasive imaging. Given the high prevalence of prominent trabeculations in healthy subjects, the diagnosis should be made with caution in asymptomatic individuals with limited morphologic findings. In the symptomatic patient, a multifactorial approach to diagnosis is recommended, combining clinical and imaging information, and excluding other causes of disease.

Pearls and Pitfalls in Cardiovascular Imaging, ed. Stefan L. Zimmerman and Elliot K. Fishman. Published by Cambridge University Press. © Cambridge University Press 2015.

REFERENCES

1. B. C. Weiford, V. D. Subbarao, K. M. Mulhern Noncompaction of the ventricular myocardium. *Circulation* 2004; **109**: 2965–71.

2. T. K. Chin, J. K. Perloff, R. G. Williams, K. Jue, R. Mohrmann. Isolated noncompaction of left ventricular myocardium. A study of eight cases. *Circulation* 1990; **82**: 507–13.

3. R. Jenni, J. Rojas, E. Oechslin. Isolated noncompaction of the myocardium. *N Engl J Med* 1999; **340**: 966–7.

4. C. Stollberger, J. Finsterer, G. Blazek. Left ventricular hypertrabeculation/ noncompaction and association with additional cardiac abnormalities and neuromuscular disorders. *Am J Cardiol* 2002; **90**: 899–902.

5. S. E. Petersen, J. B. Selvanayagam, F. Wiesmann, et al. Left ventricular non-compaction: insights from cardiovascular magnetic resonance imaging. *J Am Coll Cardiol* 2005; **46**: 101–5.

6. N. Kawel, M. Nacif, A. E. Arai, et al. Trabeculated (noncompacted) and compact myocardium in adults: the multi-ethnic study of atherosclerosis. *Circ Cardiovasc Imaging* 2012; **5**: 357–66.

7. S. K. Kohli, A. A. Pantazis, J. S. Shah, et al. Diagnosis of left-ventricular non-compaction in patients with left-ventricular systolic dysfunction: time for a reappraisal of diagnostic criteria? *Eur Heart J* 2008; **29**: 89–95.

8. J. D. Dodd, G. Holmvang, U. Hoffmann, et al. Quantification of left ventricular noncompaction and trabecular delayed hyperenhancement with cardiac MRI: correlation with clinical severity. *AJR Am J Roentgenol* 2007; **189**: 974–80.

9. E. N. Oechslin, C. H. Attenhofer Jost, J. R. Rojas, P. A. Kaufmann, R. Jenni. Long-term follow-up of 34 adults with isolated left ventricular noncompaction: a distinct cardiomyopathy with poor prognosis. *J Am Coll Cardiol* 2000; **36**: 493–500.

10. S. Klaassen, S. Probst, E. Oechslin, et al. Mutations in sarcomere protein genes in left ventricular noncompaction. *Circulation* 2008; **117**: 2893–901.

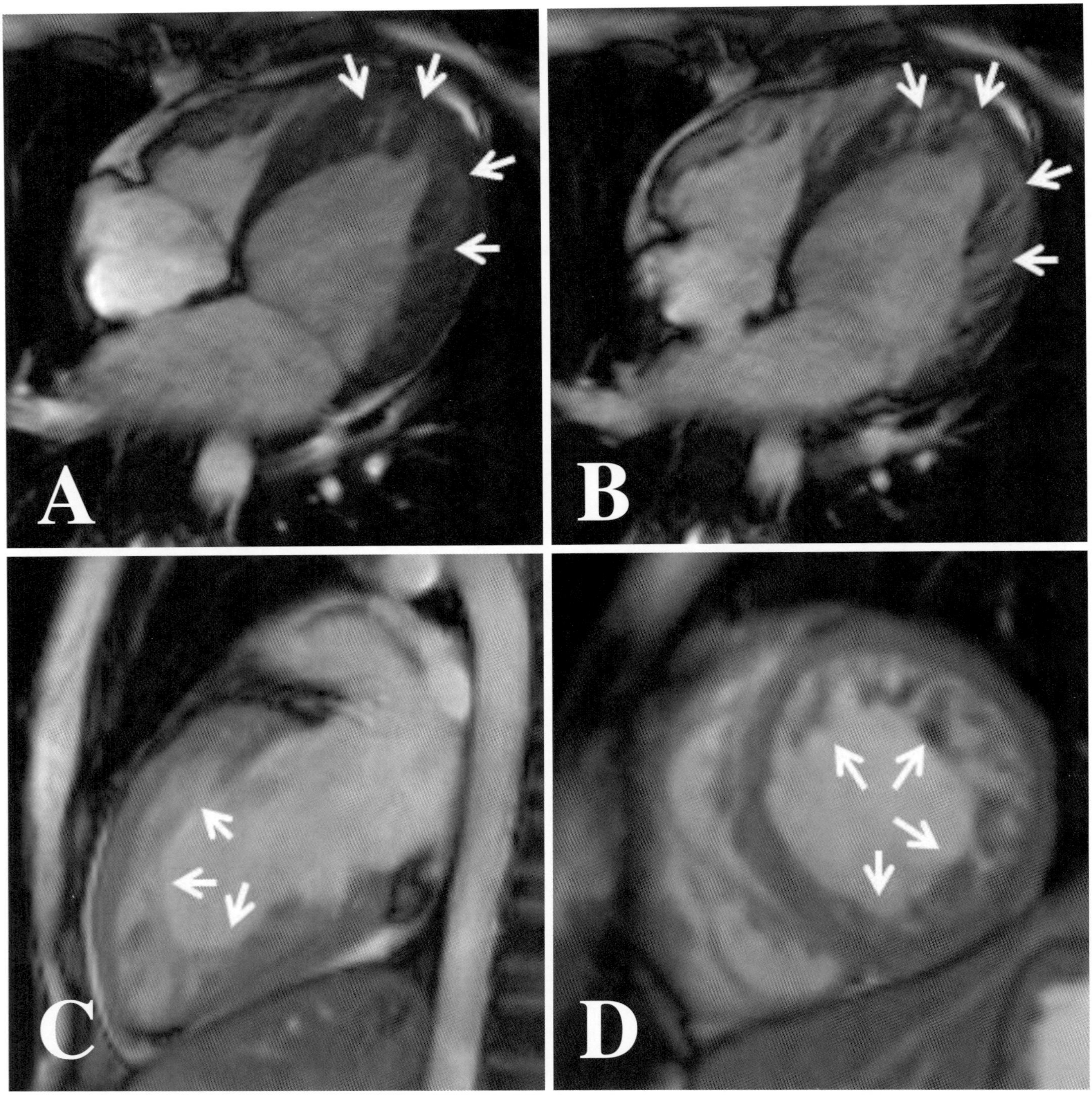

Figure 10.1 An 18-year-old male with non-compaction cardiomyopathy and Barth's syndrome. Bright blood cine MRI images in systole (**A**) and diastole (**B**) in the horizontal long-axis view and bright blood images obtained post-contrast in vertical long-axis (**C**) and short-axis (**D**) views. Prominent apical, anterior, inferior, and lateral wall trabeculations are seen (arrows), which are much more extensive than expected for a normal patient. Only the septum is spared. Ejection fraction was reduced, measuring 30%.

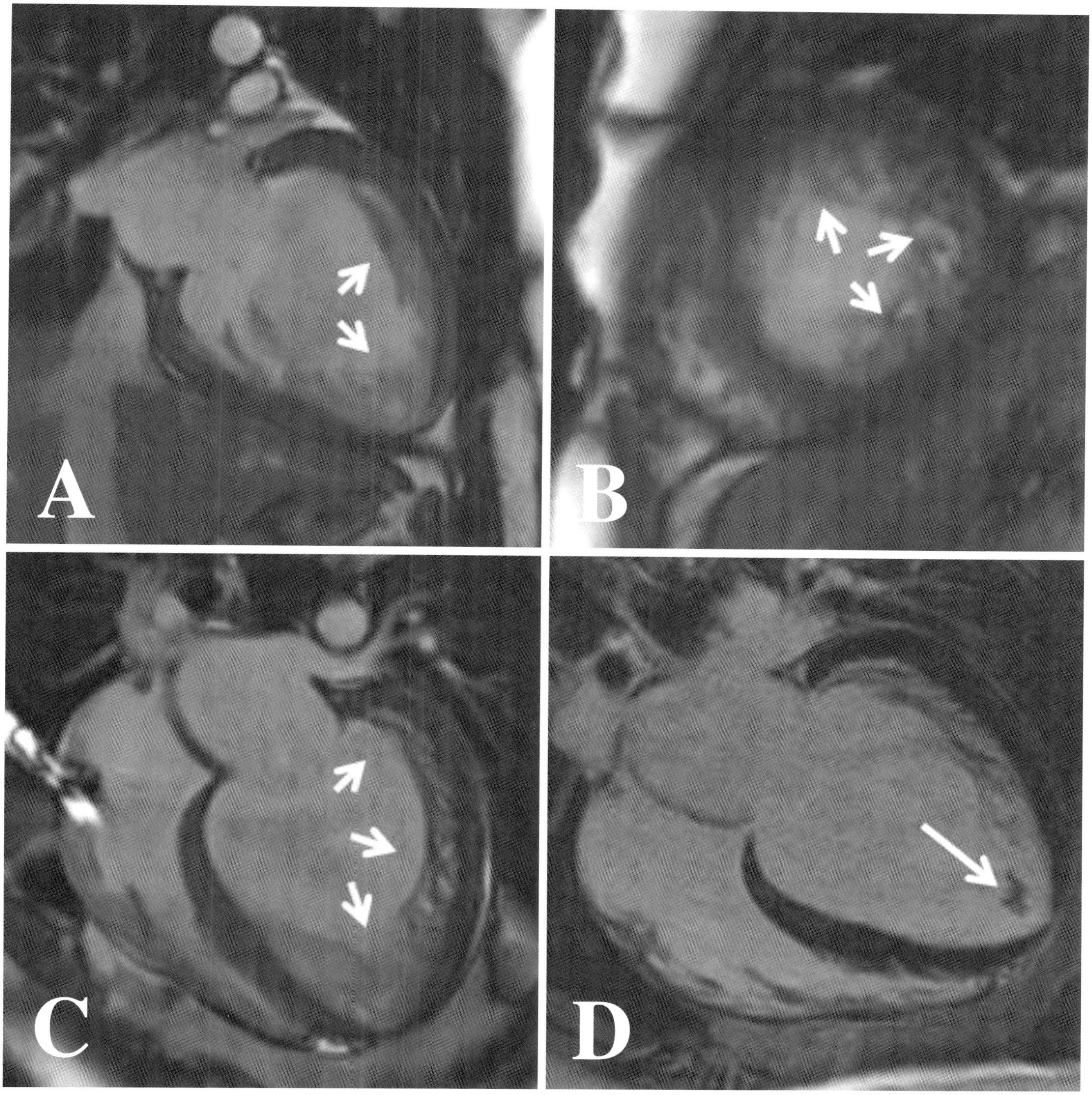

Figure 10.2 A 24-year-old male with heart failure and presumed non-compaction cardiomyopathy. Bright blood MRI images in the vertical long-axis (**A**), short-axis (**B**), and horizontal long-axis (**C**) views show extensive apical, anterior, inferior, and lateral wall trabeculations (arrows) in the setting of severe left ventricular dilation. Ejection fraction was 23%. On the post-contrast delayed enhancement images, there is a filling defect in the left ventricular blood pool (long arrow) (**D**), compatible with thrombus, which are not infrequently seen in patients with non-compaction and carry risk for stroke.

CASE **11**

Hypertrophic cardiomyopathy mimics

Stefan L. Zimmerman

Imaging description

Hypertrophic cardiomyopathy (HCM) is a diagnosis made when myocardial wall thickness exceeds 15 mm in the absence of any explanatory cardiac disease. Importantly, there are several uncommon reasons for cardiac hypertrophy that can mimic the appearance of HCM and should be considered whenever making the diagnosis. One such entity is cardiac amyloidosis. Cardiac amyloidosis is notable for concentric left and right ventricular hypertrophy in combination with diastolic dysfunction, features that overlap with HCM. Unlike the majority of HCM cases, however, hypertrophy in amyloid is diffuse and symmetric (Figure 11.1). Amyloid also has a characteristic pattern of late gadolinium enhancement (LGE), which is diffuse, concentric, and subendocardial, unlike the patch distribution of LGE seen in HCM (Figure 11.1).[1] In addition, amyloid causes alterations in the kinetics and distribution of gadolinium contrast, which results in poor differentiation between the myocardium and blood pool on LGE images due to absorption of gadolinium by amyloid proteins in both the blood and heart.[1] A second major diagnostic consideration when evaluating for HCM is a metabolic disorder such as Anderson-Fabry disease or, less commonly, Danon disease (Figure 11.2). These patients are typically young with left ventricular hypertrophy, similar to HCM, and midwall LGE, often confined to the basal inferolateral wall.[2]

Importance

Mimics of HCM are important to recognize given that their treatment and prognosis significantly differ from that of HCM. Referring clinicians should be made aware of the possibility of alternative diagnoses so that additional testing is ordered.

Typical clinical scenario

Mimics of HCM are less common than HCM itself. Amyloidosis is uncommon, affecting 10 per million person years in the United States.[3] The heart is involved in 90% of patients with systemic AL, or primary, amyloidosis, the most common of several types of amyloidosis.[3] More than half of patients will die from arrhythmia or heart failure.[3] Anderson-Fabry disease is the most common of the metabolic syndromes that result in myocardial hypertrophy. It is an x-linked disorder that is found in approximately 1:40,000 males; females are rarely affected.[4] In a large, multicenter study evaluating 1386 adult patients with unexplained left ventricular hypertrophy (males $>$ 35 years and females $>$ 40 years), Anderson-Fabry disease was identified in 0.5% of patients.[5] Other glycogen storage diseases such as Danon disease, Pompe disease, and *PRKAG2* cardiomyopathy can result in late-onset hypertrophy, but are even rarer.[4]

Differential diagnosis

In addition to amyloidosis and glycogen storage diseases, cardiac tumors can mimic focal hypertrophic cardiomyopathy. However, tumors will have an aggressive appearance and unlike HCM, will have T1 and T2 signal characteristics on cardiac MRI that significantly differ from adjacent normal myocardium. Athlete's heart can result in diffuse left ventricular hypertrophy that is sometimes mistaken for hypertrophic cardiomyopathy. Typically, these patients will not have wall thickness exceeding 15 mm; however, in difficult cases, a period of deconditioning may be required to document return to normal wall thickness.[6]

Teaching point

When evaluating a patient referred for the diagnosis of hypertrophic cardiomyopathy it is important to be aware of alternative diagnoses, such as amyloidosis and glycogen storage diseases, that can mimic the disease. Their recognition is critical given significant differences in prognosis and treatment.

REFERENCES

1. A. M. Maceira, J. Joshi, S. K. Prasad, et al. Cardiovascular magnetic resonance in cardiac amyloidosis. *Circulation* 2005; **111**: 186–93.
2. J. C. Moon, B. Sachdev, A. G. Elkington, et al. Gadolinium enhanced cardiovascular magnetic resonance in Anderson-Fabry disease. Evidence for a disease specific abnormality of the myocardial interstitium. *Eur Heart J* 2003; **24**: 2151–5.
3. J. B. Selvanayagam, P. N. Hawkins, B. Paul, S. G. Myerson, S. Neubauer. Evaluation and management of the cardiac amyloidosis. *J Am Coll Cardiol* 2007; **50**: 2101–10.
4. Z. Yousef, P. M. Elliott, F. Cecchi, et al. Left ventricular hypertrophy in Fabry disease: a practical approach to diagnosis. *Eur Heart J* 2013; **34**: 802–8.
5. P. Elliott, R. Baker, F. Pasquale, et al. Prevalence of Anderson-Fabry disease in patients with hypertrophic cardiomyopathy: the European Anderson-Fabry Disease survey. *Heart* 2011; **97**: 1957–60.
6. A. C. To, A. Dhillon, M. Y. Desai. Cardiac magnetic resonance in hypertrophic cardiomyopathy. *JACC Cardiovasc Imaging* 2011; **4**: 1123–37.

Pearls and Pitfalls in Cardiovascular Imaging, ed. Stefan L. Zimmerman and Elliot K. Fishman. Published by Cambridge University Press. © Cambridge University Press 2015.

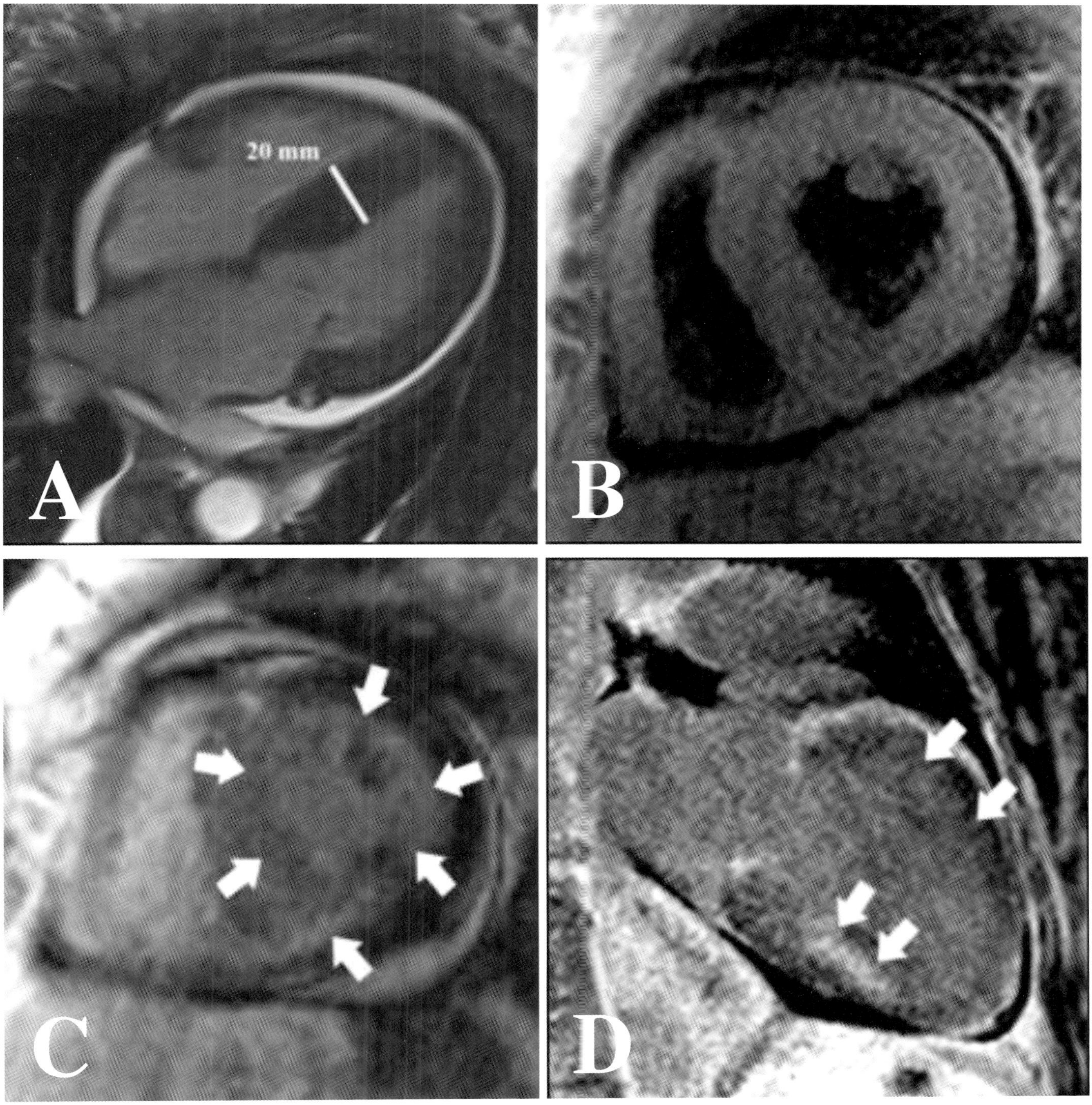

Figure 11.1 **A.** Four-chamber bright blood steady-state free precession image from a cardiac MRI obtained in a 69-year-old female with suspicion of cardiac amyloidosis, later confirmed by biopsy. There is diffuse left ventricular hypertrophy, with maximal septal wall thickness of 20 mm. Also note pleural and pericardial effusion, common in patients with amyloidosis and uncommon in hypertrophic cardiomyopathy (HCM). **B.** Short-axis dark blood image demonstrates diffuse thickening of the right and left ventricular walls, a pattern that would be uncommon in HCM but typical for amyloidosis. **C.** Short-axis late gadolinium enhancement image demonstrates diffuse subendocardial late gadolinium enhancement of the anterior, lateral, and inferior walls and near full-thickness late gadolinium enhancement in the septum (arrows). Notice the relatively poor contrast between blood pool and myocardium, typical for amyloidosis. **D.** Vertical long-axis late gadolinium enhancement image demonstrating subendocardial delayed enhancement, a pattern more typical for amyloidosis than HCM.

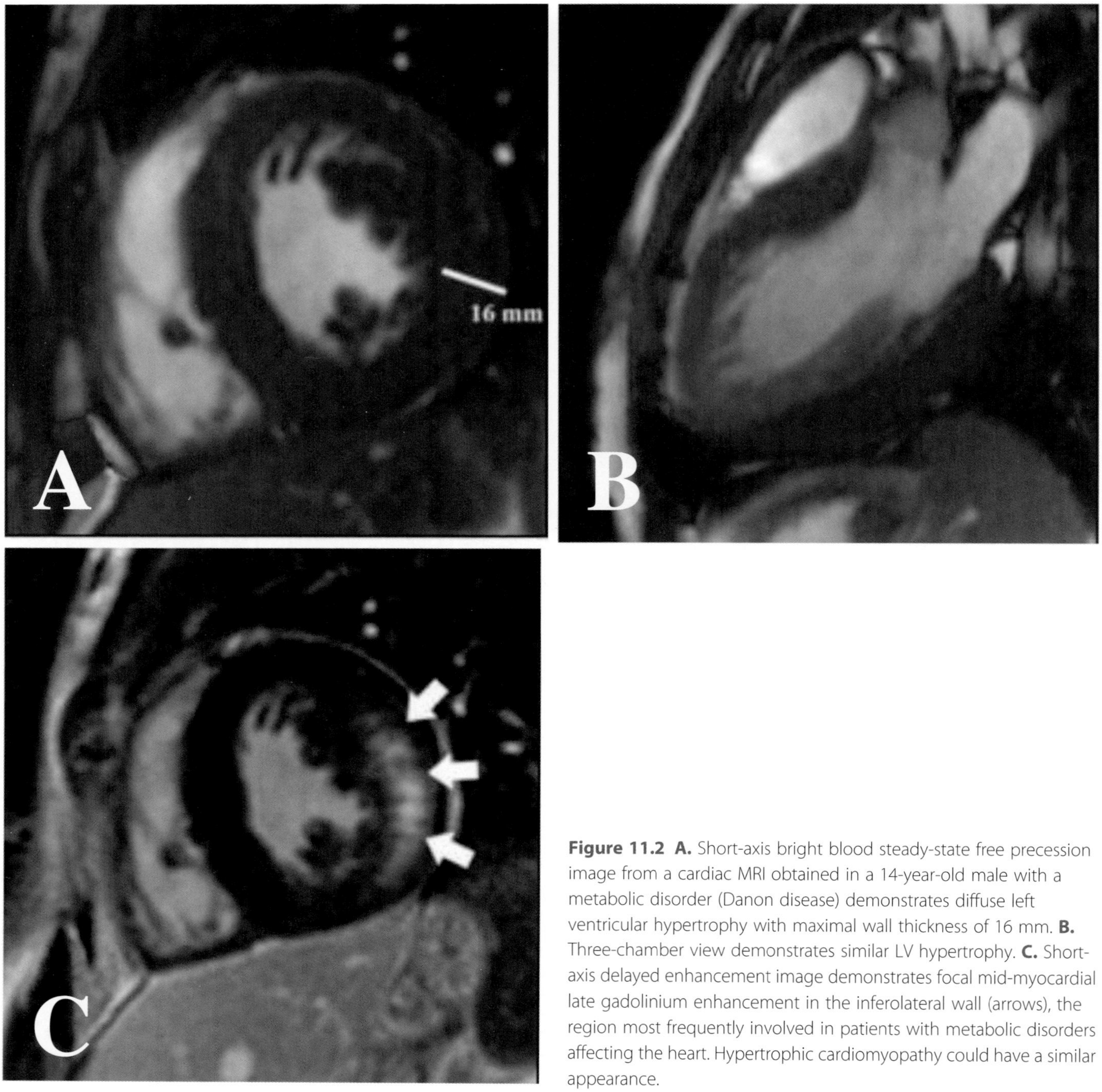

Figure 11.2 **A.** Short-axis bright blood steady-state free precession image from a cardiac MRI obtained in a 14-year-old male with a metabolic disorder (Danon disease) demonstrates diffuse left ventricular hypertrophy with maximal wall thickness of 16 mm. **B.** Three-chamber view demonstrates similar LV hypertrophy. **C.** Short-axis delayed enhancement image demonstrates focal mid-myocardial late gadolinium enhancement in the inferolateral wall (arrows), the region most frequently involved in patients with metabolic disorders affecting the heart. Hypertrophic cardiomyopathy could have a similar appearance.

CASE

12 Stress cardiomyopathy

Stefan L. Zimmerman

Imaging findings

Stress cardiomyopathy, also known as Takotsubo cardiomyopathy or apical ballooning syndrome, is a condition characterized by chest pain simulating acute coronary syndrome. There are severe ventricular wall motion abnormalities with a notable absence of obstructive coronary artery disease. Stress cardiomyopathy is a transient phenomenon, thought to be related to an acute increase in sympathetic activity due to severe physical or emotional stress, and the vast majority of patients will have complete normalization of cardiac abnormalities at follow-up.[1] Ventricular "ballooning" is the hallmark of the disease, characterized by akinesis or dyskinesis of ventricular walls during systole that is not confined to a single vascular territory (Figure 12.1). The ballooning occurs in the apex in more than 80% of patients.[2] Mid-ventricular, biventricular, and basilar ballooning patterns can also be seen, although much less frequently.[1,2] On cardiac MRI, transmural myocardial edema involving dyskinetic myocardial segments is present in the majority of patients. However, late gadolinium enhancement (LGE) is mostly absent. The prevalence of LGE reported in the literature ranges from 9–44% of patients,[2] and this variability is thought to be related to interstudy differences in the threshold used to define late gadolinium enhancement. In the largest study to date evaluating 239 patients, when a standard threshold of 5 SD above remote myocardium was used to define LGE not a single patient had detectable LGE.[1] When present, LGE may be patchy or transmural and will not conform to a vascular territory.[1,3] When evaluated by cardiac CT, multiphase retrospectively-gated images will demonstrate the typical ventricular ballooning pattern and coronary arteries will be free from significant plaque (Figure 12.2).[4]

Importance

The diagnosis of stress cardiomyopathy is challenging given its close resemblance to acute coronary syndrome, particularly since patients with stress cardiomyopathy may have EKG changes and elevated cardiac enzymes in addition to ventricular dysfunction. However, treatment and prognosis are very different between the two entities. Patients with stress cardiomyopathy will generally have complete recovery of symptoms in several weeks and only require supportive care, whereas those with acute coronary syndrome may require revascularization with surgery or percutaneous intervention.

Typical clinical scenario

Stress cardiomyopathy accounts for 2% of patients presenting with ST-elevation myocardial infarctions.[5] The majority of patients are women in the sixth to eighth decade, accounting for 88.8% of patients in a meta-analysis of 286 cases.[5] A history of recent physical or emotional stress is identified in two-thirds of patients.[5]

Differential diagnosis

The primary diagnosis to consider is acute myocardial infarction, which can have identical presenting signs and symptoms. Left anterior descending coronary artery infarction, in particular, can have apical dyskinesia that is very similar to stress cardiomyopathy. The key differentiating factor is the presence of obstructive coronary artery disease identified by either cardiac catheterization or cardiac CT. If cardiac MRI is performed, edema and LGE confined to a vascular territory will be seen in cases of acute myocardial infarction, whereas in stress cardiomyopathy LGE will be absent in the majority and most will have edema in a non-vascular distribution.

Teaching point

Stress cardiomyopathy is a challenging diagnosis with a presentation similar to acute coronary syndrome. It should be considered in patients with chest pain and ventricular wall motion abnormalities in the absence of significant coronary artery disease. Cardiac MRI may be helpful in difficult cases, where the presence of edema in a non-vascular distribution and the absence of late gadolinium enhancement are characteristic.

REFERENCES

1. I. Eitel, F. von Knobelsdorff-Brenkenhoff, P. Bernhardt, et al. Clinical characteristics and cardiovascular magnetic resonance findings in stress (Takotsubo) cardiomyopathy. *JAMA* 2011; **306**: 277–86.

2. A. Athanasiadis, B. Schneider, U. Sechtem. Role of cardiovascular magnetic resonance in Takotsubo cardiomyopathy. *Heart Fail Clin* 2013; **9**: 167–76, viii.

3. S. Nakamori, K. Matsuoka, K. Onishi, et al. Prevalence and signal characteristics of late gadolinium enhancement on contrast-enhanced magnetic resonance imaging in patients with Takotsubo cardiomyopathy. *Circ J* 2012; **76**: 914–21.

Pearls and Pitfalls in Cardiovascular Imaging, ed. Stefan L. Zimmerman and Elliot K. Fishman. Published by Cambridge University Press. © Cambridge University Press 2015.

4. J. W. Nance, U. J. Schoepf, L. Ramos-Duran. Takotsubo cardiomyopathy: findings on cardiac CT and coronary catheterisation. *Heart* 2010; **96**: 406–7.

5. M. Gianni, F. Dentali, A. M. Grandi, G. Sumner, R. Hiralal, E. Lonn. Apical ballooning syndrome or Takotsubo cardiomyopathy: a systematic review. *Eur Heart J* 2006; **27**: 1523–9.

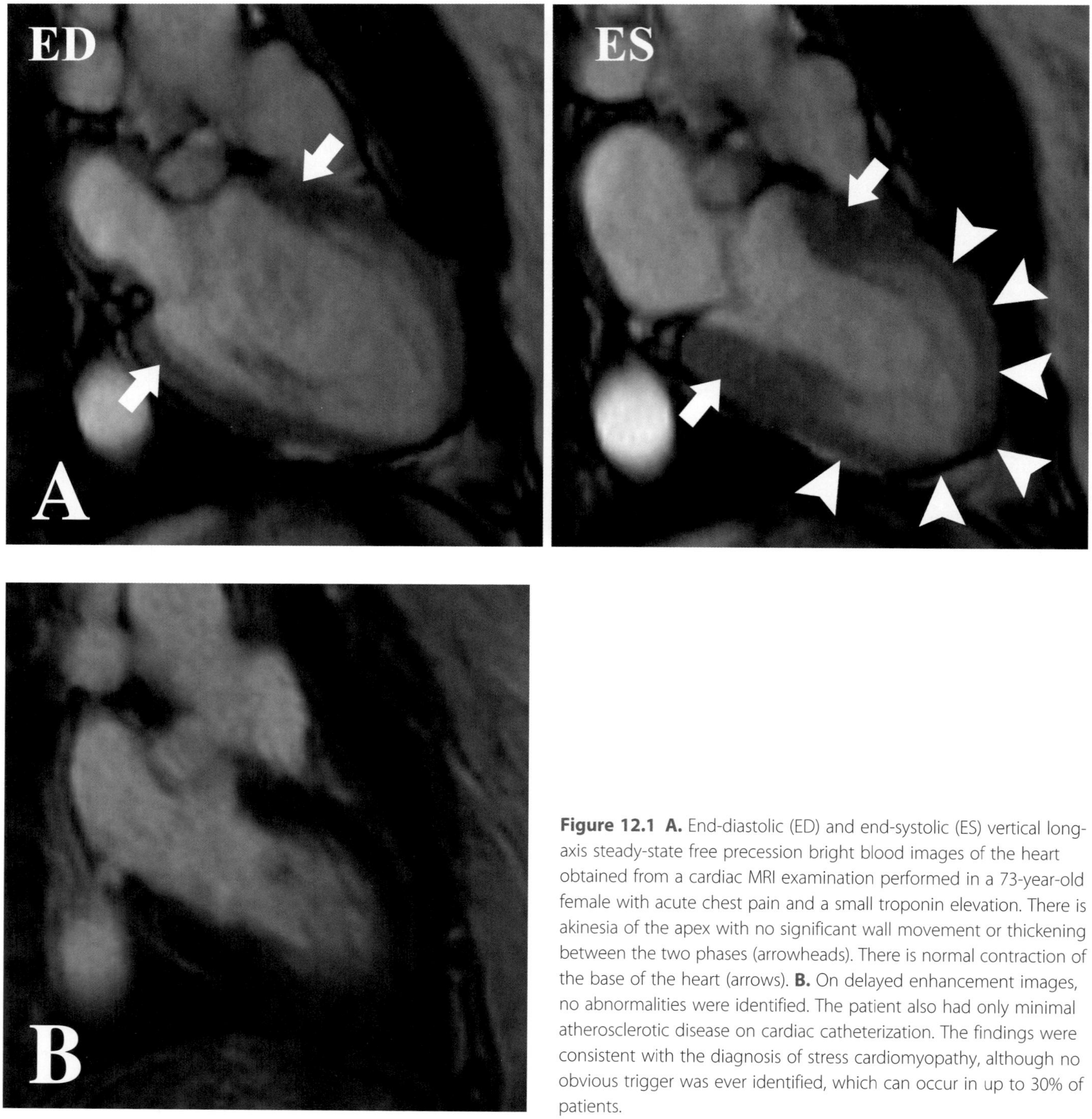

Figure 12.1 A. End-diastolic (ED) and end-systolic (ES) vertical long-axis steady-state free precession bright blood images of the heart obtained from a cardiac MRI examination performed in a 73-year-old female with acute chest pain and a small troponin elevation. There is akinesia of the apex with no significant wall movement or thickening between the two phases (arrowheads). There is normal contraction of the base of the heart (arrows). **B.** On delayed enhancement images, no abnormalities were identified. The patient also had only minimal atherosclerotic disease on cardiac catheterization. The findings were consistent with the diagnosis of stress cardiomyopathy, although no obvious trigger was ever identified, which can occur in up to 30% of patients.

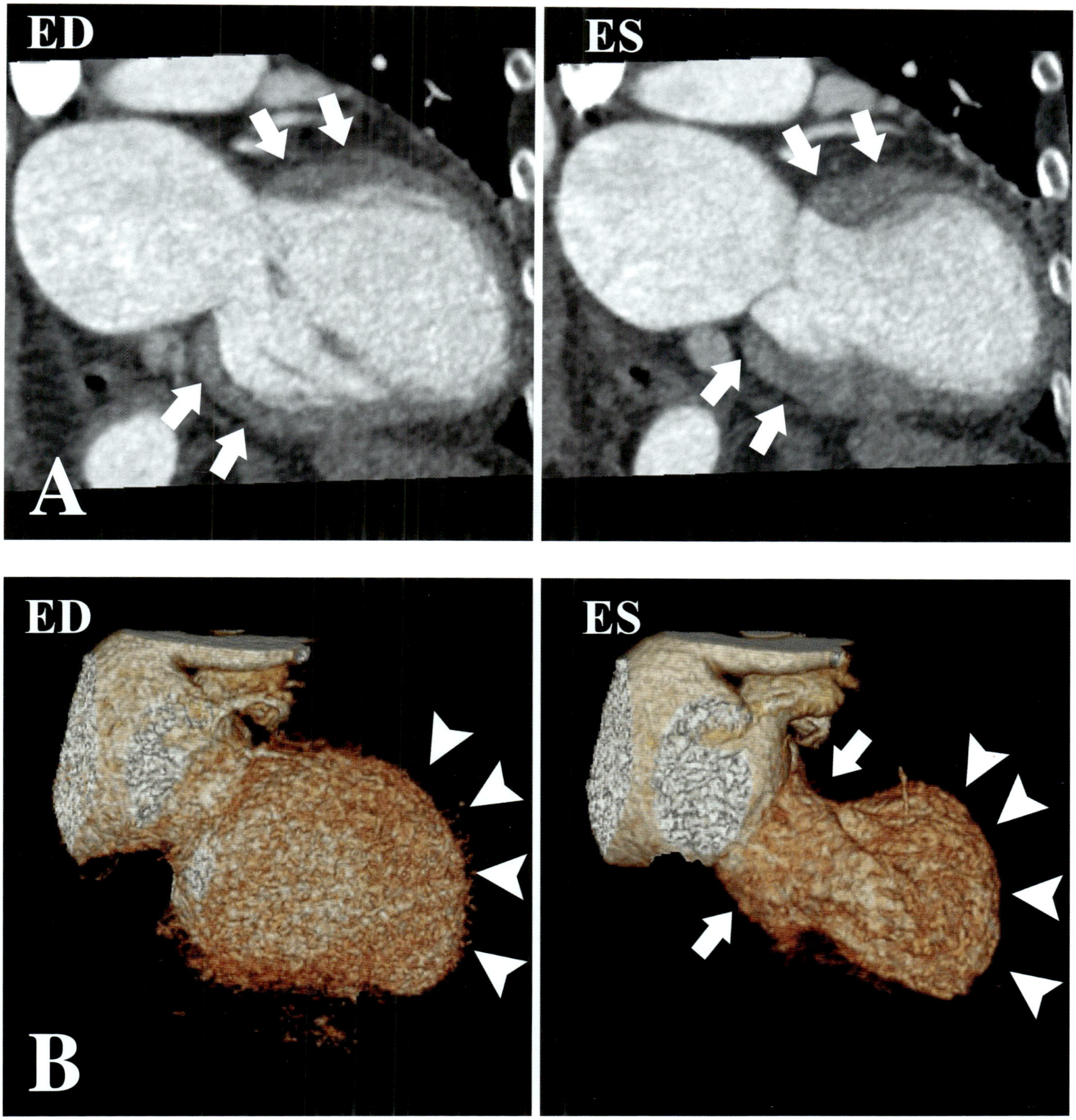

Figure 12.2 Multiple images obtained from a cardiac CT examination in a 56-year-old female with acute chest pain that began shortly after her son suffered a gunshot wound. Multiplanar reformatted images (**A**) and volume rendered images (**B**) in the vertical long-axis plane obtained in end-diastole (ED) and end-systole (ES) show contraction of the base of the heart (arrows), while the anterior and inferior walls from mid-cavity to apex are akinetic (arrowheads). **C.** Coronary arteries were entirely free of atherosclerotic disease, as demonstrated on curved planar reformatted images of the right coronary (RCA), left anterior descending (LAD), and circumflex (CX) coronary arteries. The patient was diagnosed with stress cardiomyopathy.

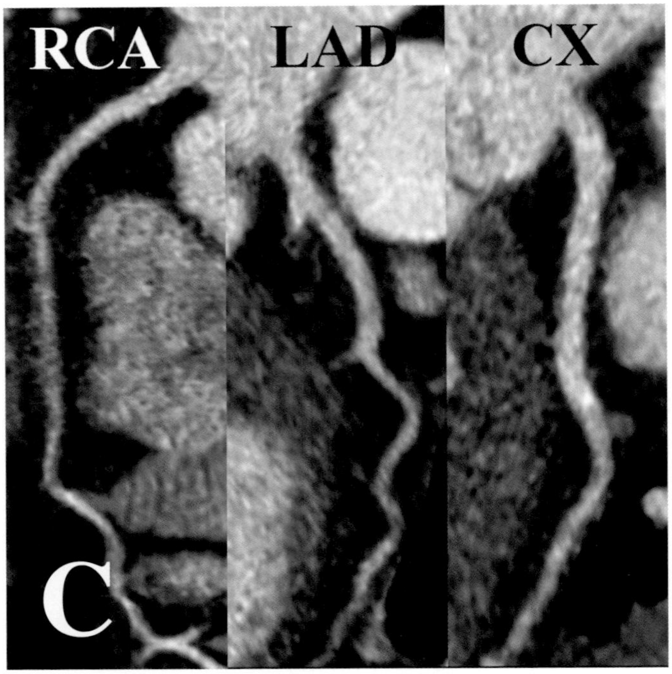

Figure 12.2 *(cont.)*

CASE 13

Epipericardial fat necrosis

Atif Zaheer

Imaging description

On CT, epipericardial fat necrosis appears as an encapsulated area of fat with surrounding inflammatory changes in the cardiophrenic region. The encapsulated fat has a high attenuation, thickened rim with adjacent fat stranding and possible thickening of the adjacent pericardium (Figure 13.1).[1] The surrounding capsule demonstrates enhancement after the administration of IV contrast. Multiplanar reconstructions help exclude any communication with abdominal fat due to diaphragmatic defects (Figure 13.2). The name epipericardial fat necrosis is currently preferred over pericardial fat necrosis, a term used in the past to describe this entity, given that the involved fat is located in the cardiophrenic space outside of the pericardium. Conservative treatment with anti-inflammatory medications and analgesics demonstrate resolution of these findings on imaging.[2]

Importance

Epipericardial fat necrosis is an uncommon benign condition presenting with acute pleuritic chest pain.[3] Possible etiologies include acute fat torsion or hemorrhagic necrosis from increased thoracic pressure after Valsalva maneuver resulting in increased capillary pressure.[4] Pathologic features are similar to fat necrosis in other locations such as the omentum, breast, and epiploic appendagitis.[3] Although uncommon, this entity can be easily diagnosed on CT or MRI due to its characteristic imaging findings. A correct diagnosis by the radiologist can avoid patients the risk of unnecessary invasive testing to exclude coronary artery disease such as catheter angiography.

Typical clinical scenario

Epipericardial fat necrosis may be identified on chest CT performed for the evaluation of acute onset pleuritic chest pain. Imaging follow-up after conservative management demonstrates complete resolution of the CT findings and is sufficient to confirm the diagnosis.[5]

Differential diagnosis

Diaphragmatic hernias through a diaphragmatic defect can be excluded using multiplanar reconstructions on CT. Lipoma usually does not have surrounding fat stranding. Malignant lesions such as liposarcoma, teratomas, and thymolipomas have a more aggressive appearance with presence of soft tissue components.[6] Infectious conditions such as mediastinal abscess are accompanied by a fluid collection.

Teaching point

In the setting of acute pleuritic chest pain, an encapsulated area of pericardial fat with surrounding inflammatory changes is highly suggestive of epipericardial fat necrosis. This is a benign self-limited disorder and resolution of imaging findings on follow-up confirms the diagnosis.

REFERENCES

1. V. Pineda, J. Caceres, J. Andreu, J. Vilar, M. L. Domingo. Epipericardial fat necrosis: radiologic diagnosis and follow-up. *AJR Am J Roentgenol* 2005; **185**: 1234–6.
2. D. Hernandez, J. Galimany, J. C. Pernas, J. Llauger. Case 170: Pericardial fat necrosis. *Radiology* 2011; **259**: 919–22.
3. R. C. Jackson, O. T. Clagett, J. R. McDonald. Pericardial fat necrosis; report of three cases. *J Thorac Surg* 1957; **33**: 723–9.
4. M. W. Webster, Jr., H. T. Bahnson. Pericardial fat necrosis. Case report and review. *J Thorac Cardiovasc Surg* 1974; **67**: 430–3.
5. V. Pineda, J. Andreu, J. Caceres, X. Merino, D. Varona, R. Dominguez-Oronoz. Lesions of the cardiophrenic space: findings at cross-sectional imaging. *Radiographics* 2007; **27**: 19–32.
6. N. Tomiyama, O. Honda, M. Tsubamoto, et al. Anterior mediastinal tumors: diagnostic accuracy of CT and MRI. *Eur J Radiol* 2009; **69**: 280–8.

Pearls and Pitfalls in Cardiovascular Imaging, ed. Stefan L. Zimmerman and Elliot K. Fishman. Published by Cambridge University Press. © Cambridge University Press 2015.

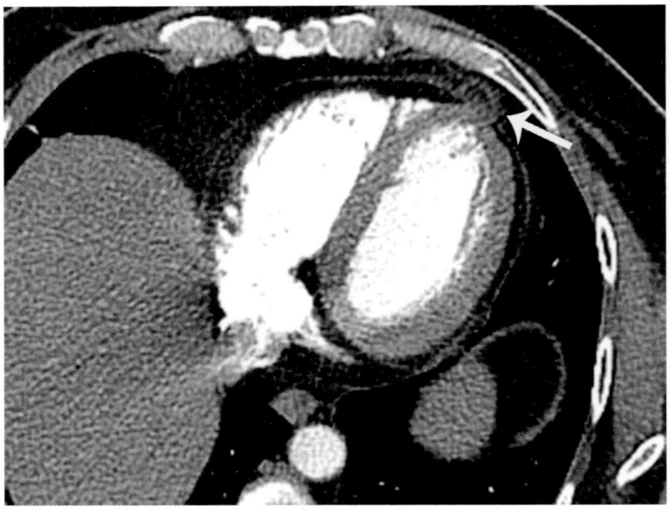

Figure 13.1 43-year-old man with severe sharp, left-sided chest pain radiating to the back. Physical examination revealed point tenderness in the left chest with pain increased on left arm abduction. Axial contrast-enhanced CT image demonstrates an encapsulated area of fat attenuation (arrow) abutting the pericardium fat.

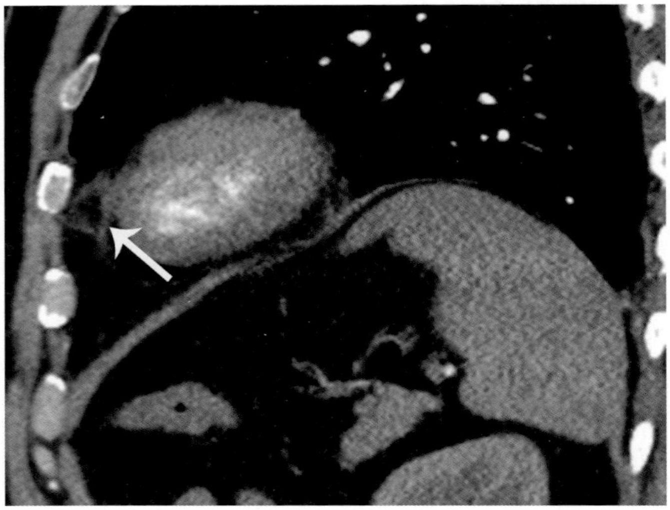

Figure 13.2 Sagittal reformatted CT image shows an encapsulated area of fatty attenuation in the anterior mediastinum with surrounding fat stranding (arrow). There is no evidence of omental fat herniation through a diaphragmatic defect. A diagnosis of epipericardial fat necrosis was made and the patient showed resolution of these findings on subsequent examination after conservative management.

CASE 14

True and false left ventricular aneurysms

Stefan L. Zimmerman

Imaging description

Ventricular aneurysms are defined as focal regions of abnormal diastolic contour with systolic bulging.[1] True left ventricular aneurysms are composed of all layers of the myocardial wall and are due to prior myocardial infarction and scarring (Figure 14.1). They most frequently occur in the LV anterior wall and apex in the LAD vascular territory.[2] True aneurysms can be recognized by thin walls, wide neck, and dyskinetic motion on dynamic functional imaging. On late gadolinium enhancement cardiac MRI images, true aneurysms will have transmural enhancement due to post-infarct fibrosis (Figure 14.1). On CT, chronic aneurysms may calcify (Figure 14.2). Thrombus formation within true aneurysms is common and is important to recognize (Figures 14.1, 14.2). False aneurysms, or pseudoaneurysms, do not contain all layers of the myocardium and are equivalent to a contained rupture of the myocardial wall, usually due to prior infarction. False aneurysms have a narrow neck (Figure 14.3) and are dyskinetic on functional imaging. False aneurysms most often occur in the inferior wall in the right coronary artery vascular territory or in the lateral wall in circumflex territory.

Importance

True aneurysms have a high risk of thrombus formation due to blood stasis, which can lead to stroke or other systemic embolization. False aneurysms are important to recognize due to their instability and high risk of rupture, which occurs in 30–45% of cases.[2] These aneurysms require prompt surgical treatment.

Typical clinical scenario

Left ventricular aneurysms usually occur in patients with prior myocardial infarction, and may be incidentally discovered at cross-sectional imaging performed for unrelated indications. False aneurysms can also be seen in the setting of prior surgery or trauma.[3]

Differential diagnosis

Takotsubo, or stress cardiomyopathy, presents with symptoms identical to myocardial infarction and will show apical dyskinesia on functional imaging. However, Takotsubo cardiomyopathy is a transient abnormality and patients have no significant coronary artery disease. Ventricular diverticula can mimic aneurysms due to outward bulging in diastole; however, unlike aneurysms they contract during systole.

Teaching point

True and false left ventricular aneurysms are important to recognize and accurately characterize due to important differences in treatment and prognosis. The presence of a narrow neck suggests a false aneurysm, which has a high risk of rupture and requires prompt treatment.

REFERENCES

1. E. T. Hoey, I. Nagra, A. Ganeshan. Cardiac aneurysms and diverticula: magnetic resonance and computed tomography appearances. *Curr Probl Diagn Radiol* 2011; **40**: 72–84.
2. J. S. Shambrook, R. Chowdhury, I. W. Brown, C. R. Peebles, S. P. Harden. Cross-sectional imaging appearances of cardiac aneurysms. *Clin Radiol* 2010; **65**: 349–57.
3. C. S. Restrepo, M. J. Lane, H. Murillo. Cardiac aneurysms, pseudoaneurysms, and diverticula. *Semin Roentgenol* 2012; **47**: 262–76.

Pearls and Pitfalls in Cardiovascular Imaging, ed. Stefan L. Zimmerman and Elliot K. Fishman. Published by Cambridge University Press. © Cambridge University Press 2015.

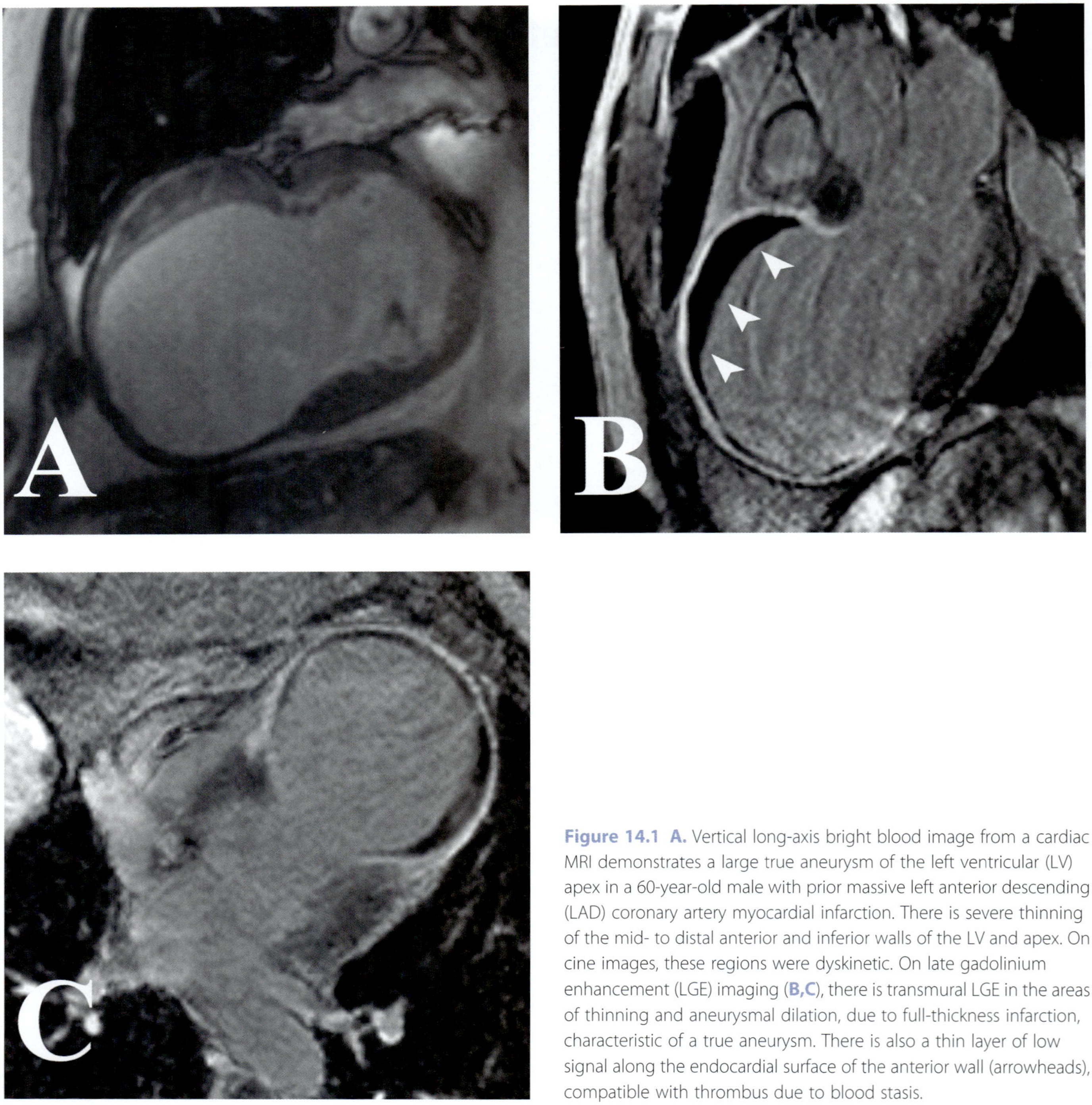

Figure 14.1 A. Vertical long-axis bright blood image from a cardiac MRI demonstrates a large true aneurysm of the left ventricular (LV) apex in a 60-year-old male with prior massive left anterior descending (LAD) coronary artery myocardial infarction. There is severe thinning of the mid- to distal anterior and inferior walls of the LV and apex. On cine images, these regions were dyskinetic. On late gadolinium enhancement (LGE) imaging (**B,C**), there is transmural LGE in the areas of thinning and aneurysmal dilation, due to full-thickness infarction, characteristic of a true aneurysm. There is also a thin layer of low signal along the endocardial surface of the anterior wall (arrowheads), compatible with thrombus due to blood stasis.

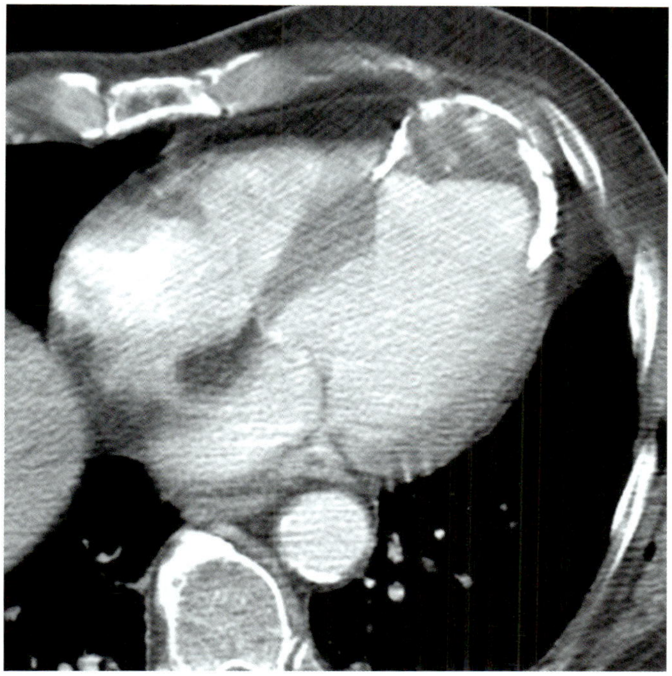

Figure 14.2 Axial CT image from an enhanced chest CT performed in a 75-year-old male with stroke demonstrates a large, calcified true aneurysm of the LV apex which is filled with low-attenuation thrombus. Calcification and thrombus formation are common in chronic LV aneurysms.

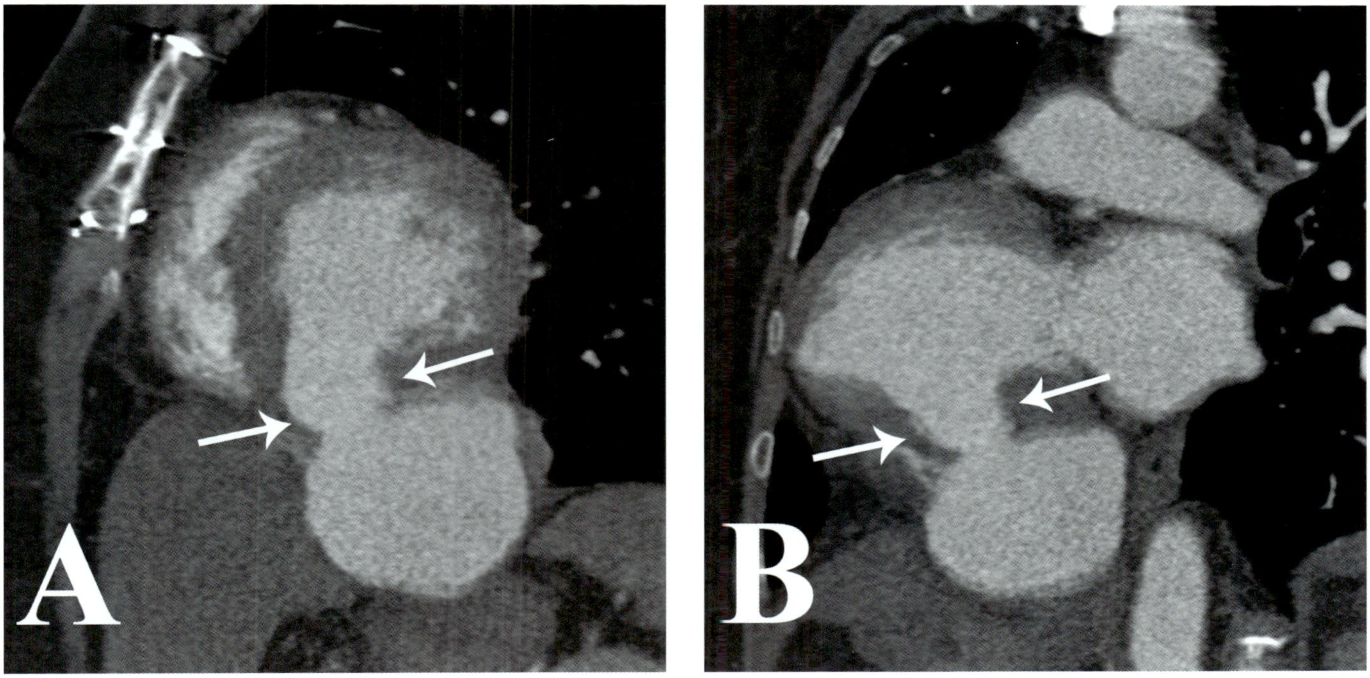

Figure 14.3 Short-axis (A) and vertical long-axis (B) multiplanar reformatted CT images from a CT angiogram performed in a 71-year-old female with prior inferior myocardial infarction demonstrate a large false aneurysm. There is a narrow-necked (arrows) communication with the inferior wall, which is the most common location for these aneurysms. False aneurysms are essentially contained ruptures of the ventricle and have a high mortality rate if untreated. This patient underwent attempted transcatheter repair with an occluder device.

CASE 15

Ventricular diverticula, clefts, and crypts

Stefan L. Zimmerman

Imaging description

Ventricular diverticula and clefts are rare congenital outpouchings of the ventricular cavity. No generally accepted formal definition of these entities exists, which has resulted in inconsistency in the nomenclature used in the literature. Recently, some authors have attempted to more precisely define these lesions, making a distinction between ventricular diverticula, clefts, and congenital aneurysms;[1,2] whereas prior reports have used the term diverticulum more broadly to include any type of congenital outpouching of the ventricular cavity.[3] Per the definitions suggested by Erol et al., diverticula are narrow-necked saccular outpouchings that extend beyond the confines of the myocardium, contain all three myocardial layers, and contract with the ventricle (Figures 15.1,15.2). Clefts are narrow fissure-like outpouchings of the ventricular cavity that do not extend beyond the margins of the myocardium and are obliterated during systolic contraction (Figure 15.3).[1,2] These are most often located in the left ventricular side of the septum or inferior wall. [3,4] Clefts are a confusing entity as several terms have been used to describe lesions of a similar description and imaging appearance within the literature, including diverticula, [3,4] clefts,[1,2] and crypts.[5] Finally, congenital aneurysms are defined as wide-mouthed, thin-walled outpouchings beyond the myocardial contour that show dyskinetic motion with ventricular contraction and contain fibrous tissue.[1] On cardiac MRI, clefts and diverticula will show contraction during systole on cine images and late gadolinium enhancement (LGE) is absent. Descriptions of cardiac MRI findings of congenital aneurysms are lacking, but presumably these lesions would show dyskinesia on cine images and LGE due to fibrous content.

Importance

Ventricular diverticula and clefts are important to distinguish from acquired ventricular aneurysms, particularly false aneurysms which carry a risk of rupture and require prompt attention. Outcomes were favorable in one series that followed children with left ventricular diverticula, unlike those with congenital aneurysms.[6] Ventricular clefts are considered to have no adverse prognostic significance.[1]

Typical clinical scenario

Ventricular diverticula are very rare and most often associated with congenital heart disease.[6] Lesions fitting the description of LV clefts are more common, found in approximately 2–3% of patients undergoing cardiac CT.[3,4] Clefts or crypts have been associated with hypertrophic cardiomyopathy and in one study were found with increased prevalence among genotype-positive, phenotype-negative carriers of hypertrophic cardiomyopathy-causing gene mutations, suggesting they may represent an early biomarker of the disease (Figure 15.4).[5]

Differential diagnosis

Ventricular diverticula should be distinguished from acquired left ventricular aneurysms. Contraction on cine images and a lack of LGE are important features characterstic of diverticula. Large diverticula may contain trabeculations. Acquired LV aneurysms are generally due to prior myocardial infarction and should be associated with wall motion abnormalties, myocardial thinning, and LGE in a vascular distribution and a history of coronary artery disease. Outpouchings or pseudoaneurysms of the LV apex that appear similar to diverticula can also occur in the setting of prior cardiac surgery utilizing LV apical venting (Figure 15.5).[7] Because these lesions represent scarring related to the procedure, when identified on MRI, they will be dyskinetic with transmural LGE on CMR.

Teaching point

Ventricular diverticula and clefts are contractile outpouchings of the ventricular cavity that are important to distinguish from acquired ventricular aneurysms, given differences in treatment and prognosis.

REFERENCES

1. C. Erol, M. Koplay, A. Olcay, et al. Congenital left ventricular wall abnormalities in adults detected by gated cardiac multidetector computed tomography: clefts, aneurysms, diverticula and terminology problems. *Eur J Radiol* 2012; **81**: 3276–81.
2. M. Wein, A. Wolf-Puetz, R. Niehues, T. Klein, P. J. Kilner, R. M. Klein. Multiple left ventricular inferoseptal clefts. Multimodality imaging appearance and differential diagnosis. *Herz* 2011; **36**: 438–43.
3. M. B. Srichai, E. M. Hecht, D. C. Kim, J. E. Jacobs. Ventricular diverticula on cardiac CT: more common than previously thought. *AJR Am J Roentgenol* 2007; **189**: 204–8.
4. T. Nakazono, J. Jeudy, C. S. White. Left and right ventricular diverticula: incidence and imaging findings on 256-slice multidetector computed tomography. *J Thorac Imaging* 2012; **27**: 179–83.
5. M. S. Maron, E. J. Rowin, D. Lin, et al. Prevalence and clinical profile of myocardial crypts in hypertrophic cardiomyopathy. *Circ Cardiovasc Imaging* 2012; **5**: 441–7.

Pearls and Pitfalls in Cardiovascular Imaging, ed. Stefan L. Zimmerman and Elliot K. Fishman. Published by Cambridge University Press. © Cambridge University Press 2015.

6. E. Marijon, P. Ou, L. Fermont, et al. Diagnosis and outcome in congenital ventricular diverticulum and aneurysm. *J Thorac Cardiovasc Surg* 2006; **131**: 433–7.

7. C. L. Kao, J. P. Chang. Left ventricular pseudoaneurysm secondary to left ventricular apical venting. *Tex Heart Inst J* 2003; **30**: 162–3.

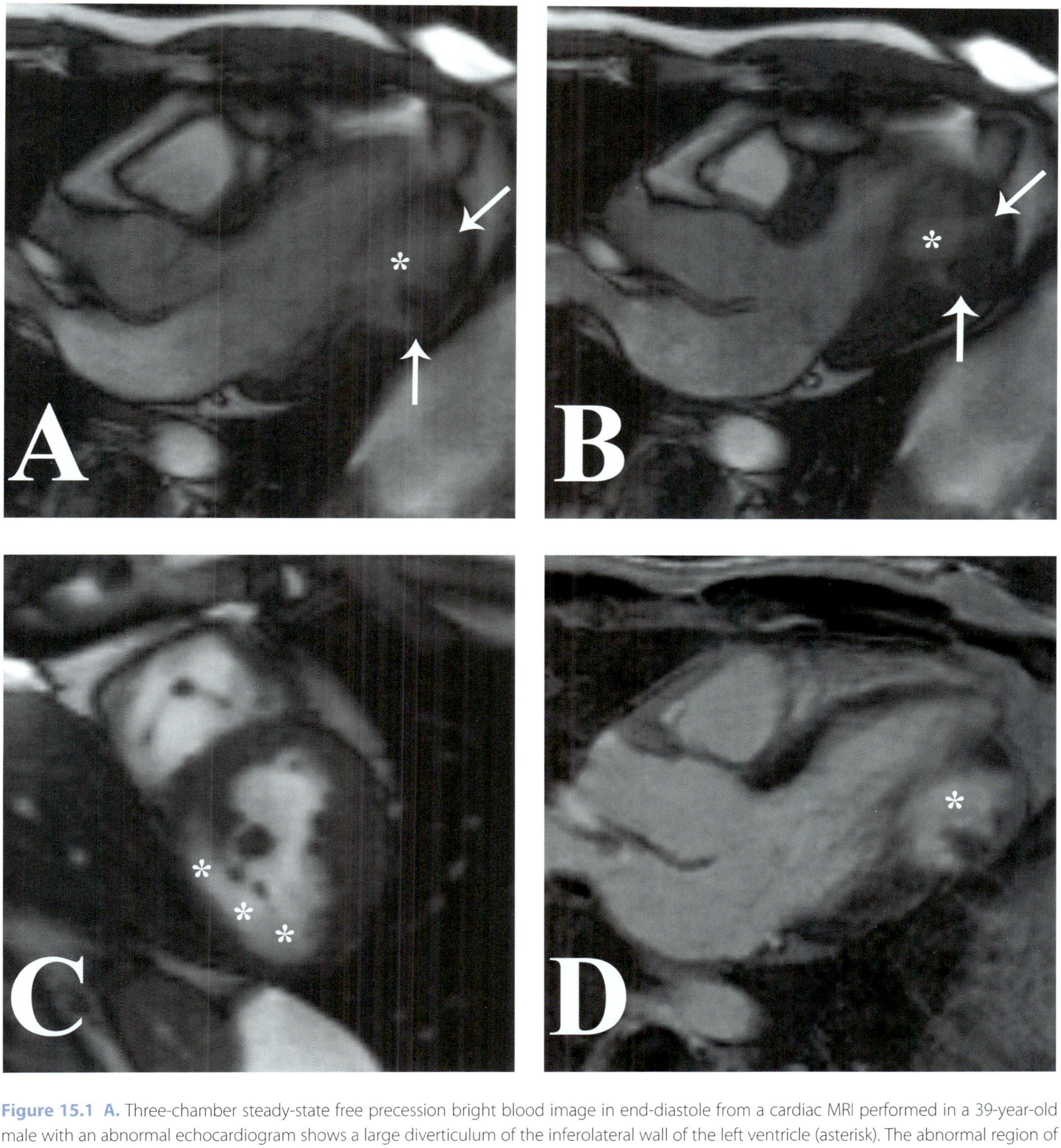

Figure 15.1 A. Three-chamber steady-state free precession bright blood image in end-diastole from a cardiac MRI performed in a 39-year-old male with an abnormal echocardiogram shows a large diverticulum of the inferolateral wall of the left ventricle (asterisk). The abnormal region of myocardium projects beyond the expected outer border of the myocardium. Within the diverticulum are deep trabecular recesses (arrows) which become smaller on end-systolic images (**B**), indicating contractile function within the diverticulum. The presence of contraction distinguishes this finding from a congenital aneurysm. **C.** Short-axis bright blood image demonstrates the diverticulum arising from the inferior and inferolateral region of the left ventricle. D. On post-contrast late gadolinium enhancement images, there is no enhancement to suggest fibrosis, further supporting the diagnosis of diverticulum rather than LV aneurysm.

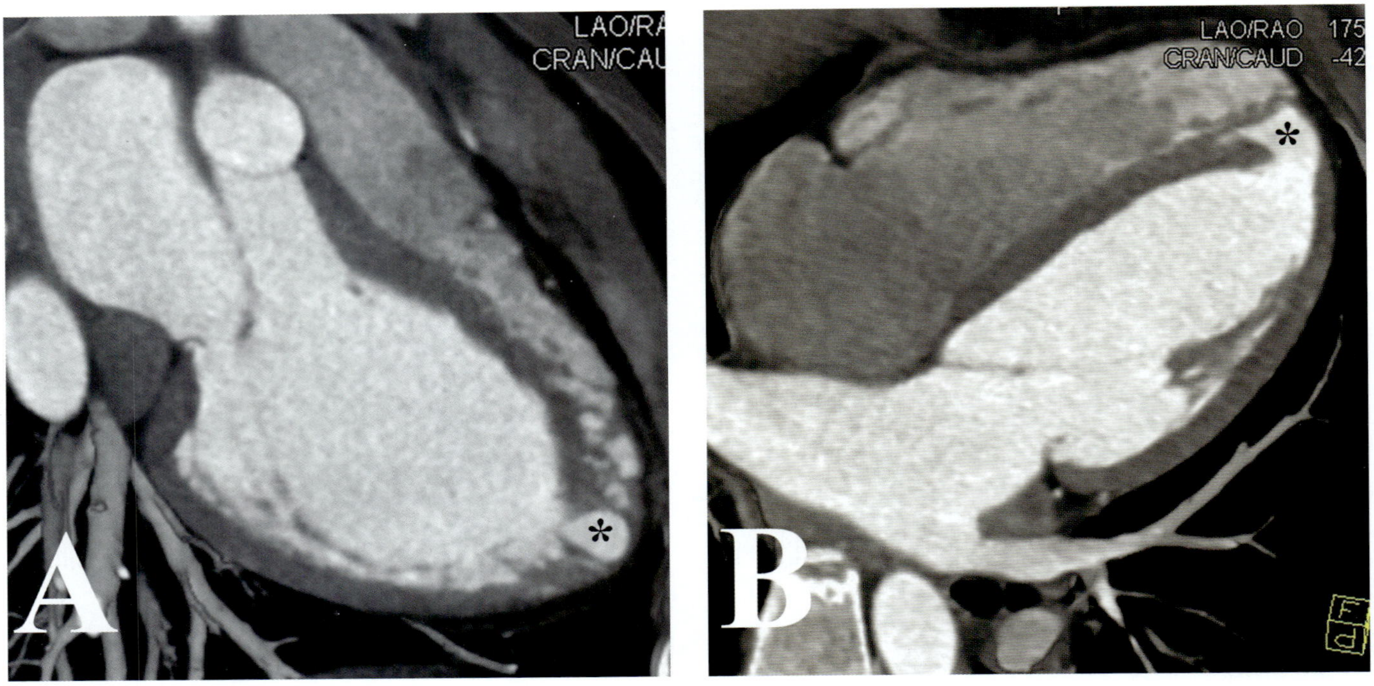

Figure 15.2 Incidental left ventricular apical diverticulum (asterisk) on a cardiac CT performed in a 20-year-old male with bicuspid aortic valve. The abnormality clearly projects beyond the expected contour of the left ventricle on the three-chamber view (**A**). On the four-chamber view (**B**), the abnormality is associated with thinning of the apical septum; however, the remainder of the myocardium is normal in appearance.

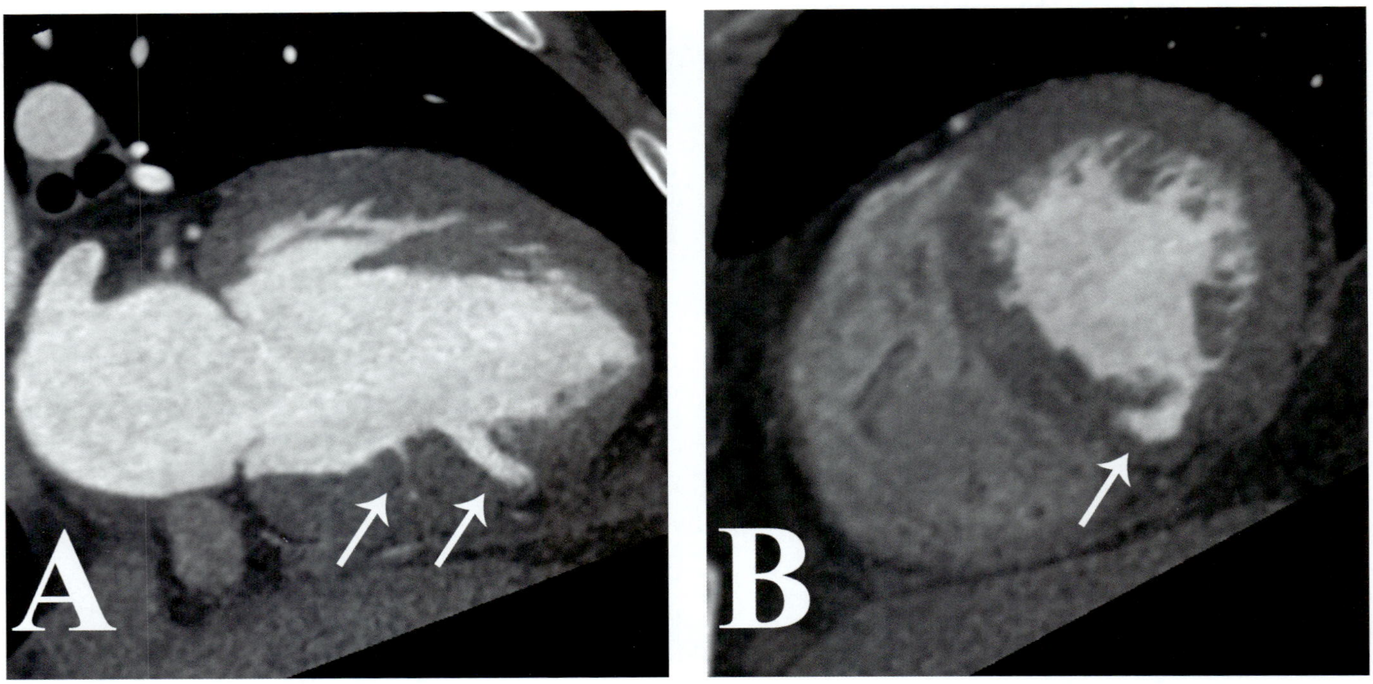

Figure 15.3 A. Vertical long-axis view of myocardial cleft or crypts (arrows) on a cardiac CT performed in a 53-year-old male with chest pain. Note the deep, thin channels that extend into the myocardium but do not extend beyond the normal expected outer contour of the left ventricle. **B.** Findings are confirmed on the short-axis view, which shows the cleft or crypt located within the inferoseptum (arrow) and communicating with the ventricular cavity.

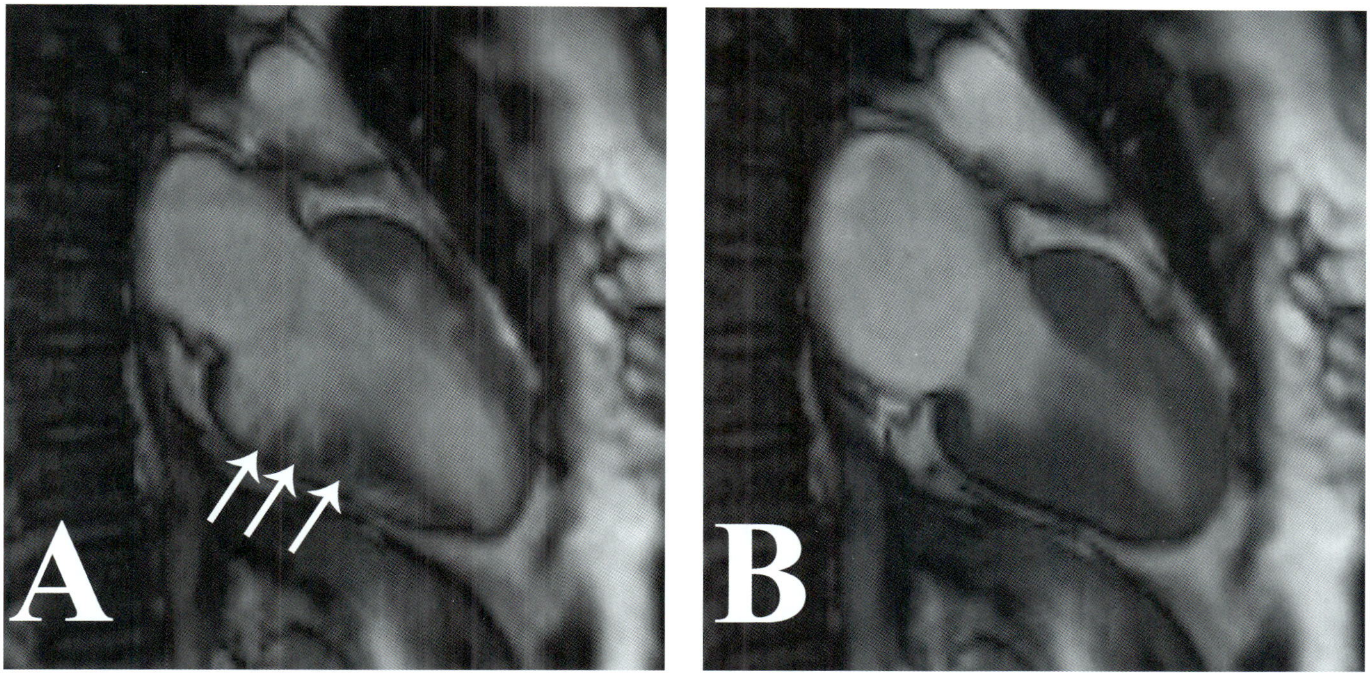

Figure 15.4 Myocardial crypts in a 23-year-old female with hypertrophic cardiomyopathy. A. Sagittal bright blood steady-state free precession cardiac MRI image shows multiple deep fissures in the basilar inferior wall (arrows) that extend outward from the LV cavity, perpendicular to the LV wall. B. At end-systole, the crypts are oblitered. Some groups have found an increased incidence of myocardial crypts in patients with hypertrophic cardiomyopathy and phenotype-negative HCM-gene carriers.

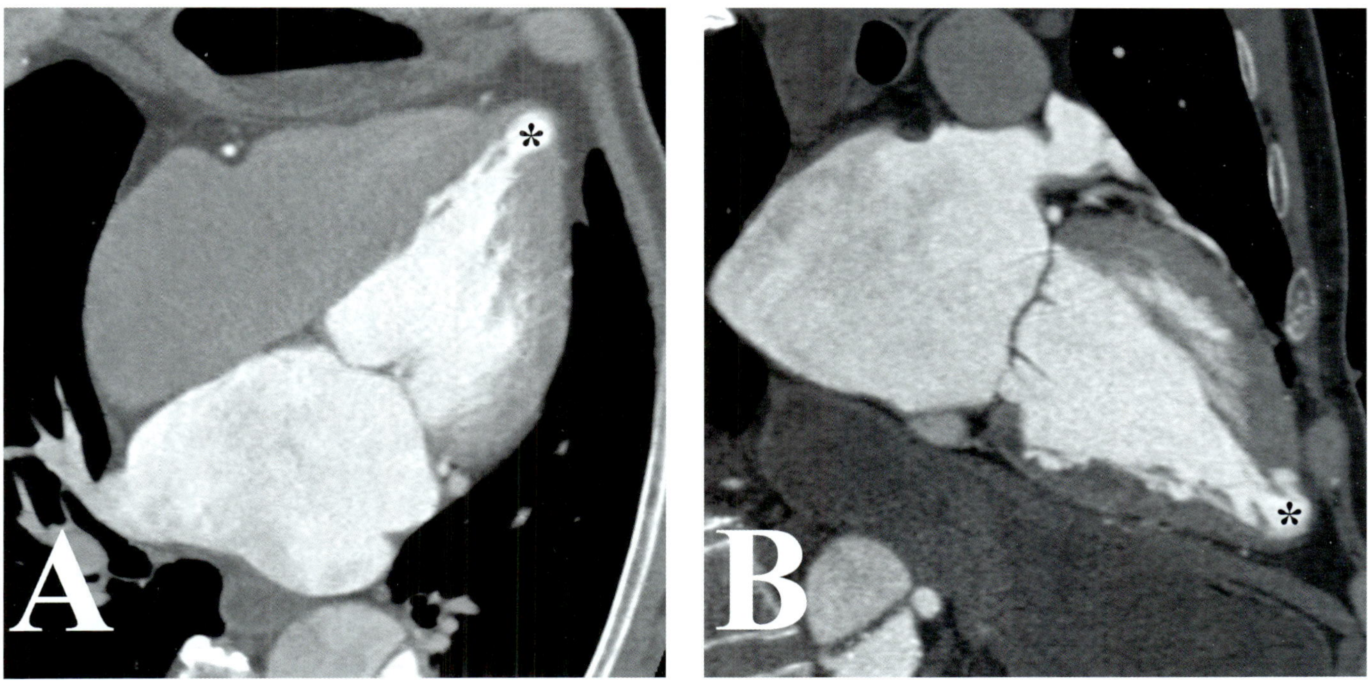

Figure 15.5 Small post-operative pseudoaneurysm of the LV apex (asterisk) in a 71-year-old male with prior type A dissection repair demonstrated by four-chamber (A) and vertical long-axis (B) images from a cardiac CT. These small pseudoaneurysms are due to scarring at the site of an LV apical vent and are generally of no clinical consequence. Rarely, they can be large and will be repaired due to risk of rupture.

CASE 16

Left atrial diverticula

Stefan L. Zimmerman

Imaging description

Left atrial diverticula are outpouchings of the left atrial wall that communicate with the left atrial lumen. They are usually less than 1 cm in size (Figure 16.1),[1,2] although rarely large diverticula may be encountered (Figure 16.2).[3] Left atrial diverticula are usually lobulated in contour and may contain internal trabeculations (Figure 16.3). Some authors have made a distinction between left atrial diverticula, which are internally smooth, and accessory left atrial appendages, which have internal trabculations similar to the left atrial appendage.[4] However, the distinction can sometimes be difficult given the small size of these structures. The most common location for left atrial diverticula is the right anterior–superior wall of the left atrium.[1,2,4]

Importance

Left atrial diverticula can be important in patients who undergo atrial ablation procedures. Left atrial diverticula may be a source for ectopic arrhythmogenic foci,[5] and can also be a cause for post-procedural thrombus formation.[6] There is also a potential risk for perforation if diverticula occur adjacent to ablation lines or if catheters are inadvertently lodged within the diverticulum,[7] given the relative thinness of the diverticular wall compared to the normal left atrial wall.[2]

Typical clinical scenario

Left atrial diverticula are common, identified in 36% of atrial fibrillation patients undergoing pre-ablation cardiac CT.[2] No differences have been found in the prevalence of diverticula among patients with atrial fibrillation and healthy controls.[1,2]

Differential diagnosis

Left atrial diverticula should be distinguished from false aneurysms of the left atrial wall which could occur in the setting of prior trauma or surgery.

Teaching point

Left atrial diverticula are small outpouchings from the left atrial wall which are generally of no clinical importance. However, in patients who undergo ablation procedures they may be a source for arrhythmia or may carry a risk of perforation or thrombus formation.

REFERENCES

1. O. Lazoura, T. Reddy, M. Shriharan, et al. Prevalence of left atrial anatomical abnormalities in patients with recurrent atrial fibrillation compared with patients in sinus rhythm using multi-slice CT. *J Cardiovasc Comput Tomogr* 2012; **6**: 268–73.
2. L. Q. Peng, J. Q. Yu, Z. G. Yang, et al. Left atrial diverticula in patients referred for radiofrequency ablation of atrial fibrillation: assessment of prevalence and morphologic characteristics by dual-source computed tomography. *Circ Arrhythm Electrophysiol* 2012; **5**: 345–50.
3. C. Gao, R. Wang, G. Wang, Y. Wang. Giant left atrial diverticulum. *J Card Surg* 2011; **26**: 70.
4. S. Abbara, J. A. Mundo-Sagardia, U. Hoffmann, R. C. Cury. Cardiac CT assessment of left atrial accessory appendages and diverticula. *AJR Am J Roentgenol* 2009; **193**: 807–12.
5. R. P. Killeen, S. A. O'Connor, D. Keane, J. D. Dodd. Ectopic focus in an accessory left atrial appendage: radiofrequency ablation of refractory atrial fibrillation. *Circulation* 2009; **120**: e60–2.
6. T. Nagai, A. Fujii, K. Nishimura, et al. Large thrombus originating from left atrial diverticulum: a new concern for catheter ablation of atrial fibrillation. *Circulation* 2011; **124**: 1086–8.
7. L. Olivotti, A. Nicolino, G. Succio, M. Ghidara, G. Serafini, S. Moshiri. Left atrial diverticulum : "Thin ice" for interventionalists. *Herz* 2013; **38**: 943–4.

Pearls and Pitfalls in Cardiovascular Imaging, ed. Stefan L. Zimmerman and Elliot K. Fishman. Published by Cambridge University Press. © Cambridge University Press 2015.

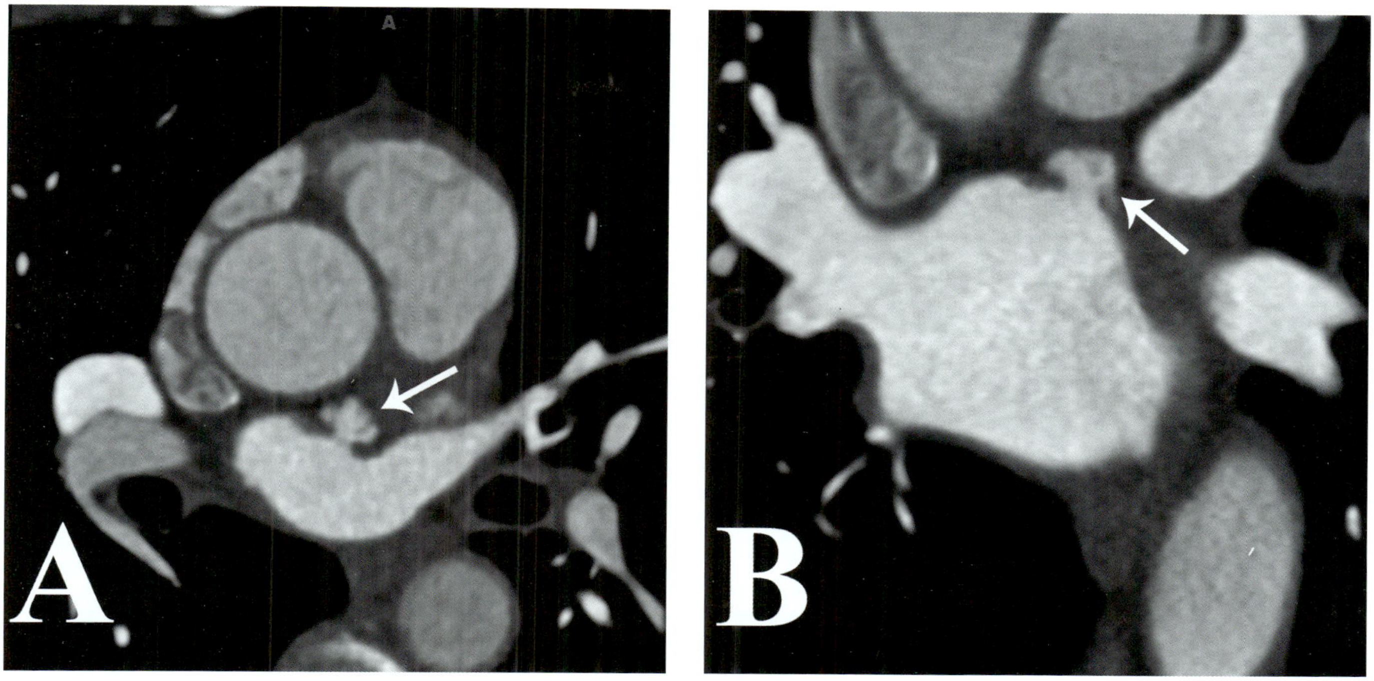

Figure 16.1 **A.** Axial image from a cardiac CT performed in a 49-year-old male with chest pain demonstrates the typical appearance of a small left atrial diverticulum (arrow) arising from the superior left atrium. There is a lobulated outer contour with internal trabeculations. Some authors would describe this finding as an accessory left atrial appendage, due to the presence of trabeculations. **B.** Oblique coronal multiplanar reformatted image redemonstrates the findings (arrow). As in this case, the majority of atrial diverticula are small, typically less than 1 cm in size, and located in the anterior–superior aspect of the left atrium.

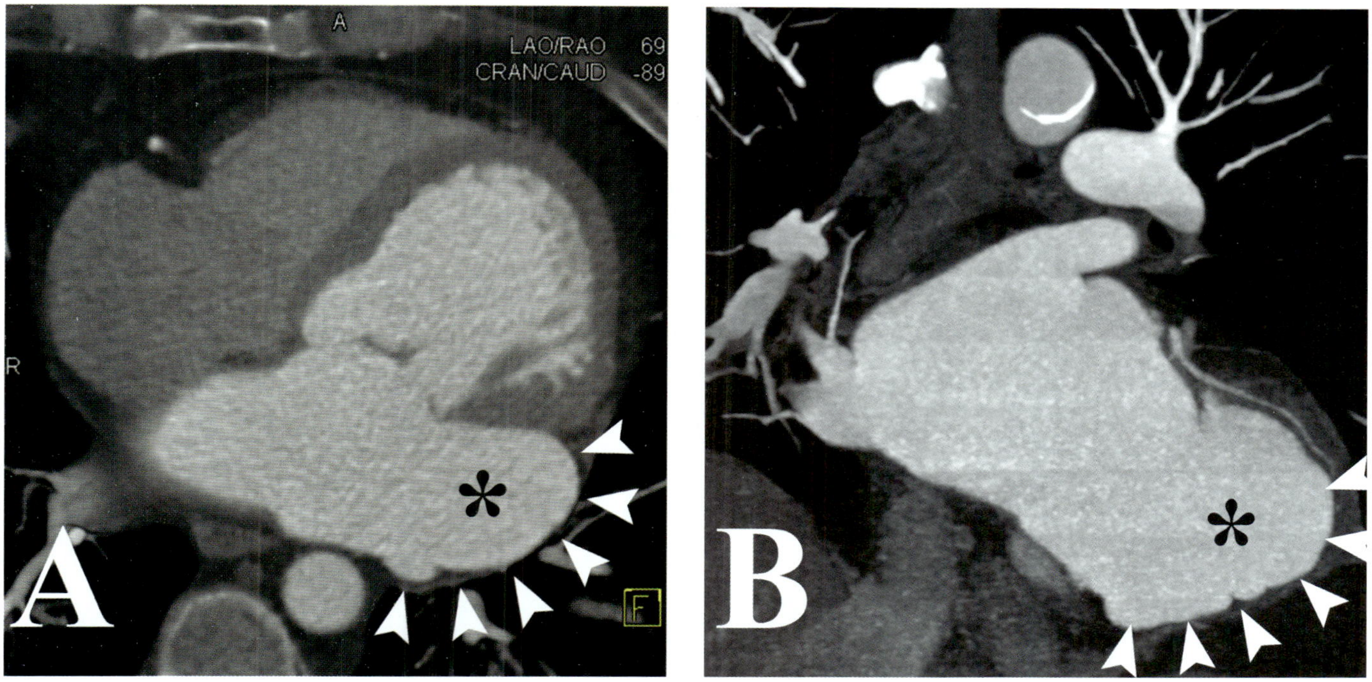

Figure 16.2 Large atrial diverticulum demonstrated on an axial volume-rendered image (**A**) and coronal maximum intensity projection image (**B**) obtained from a cardiac CT performed in a 56-year-old male with arrhythmia and abnormal echocardiogram. The diverticulum (asterisk) has a wide-mouthed communication with the lumen of the left atrium and smooth, well-defined borders (arrowheads). Diverticula this large are rarely encountered.

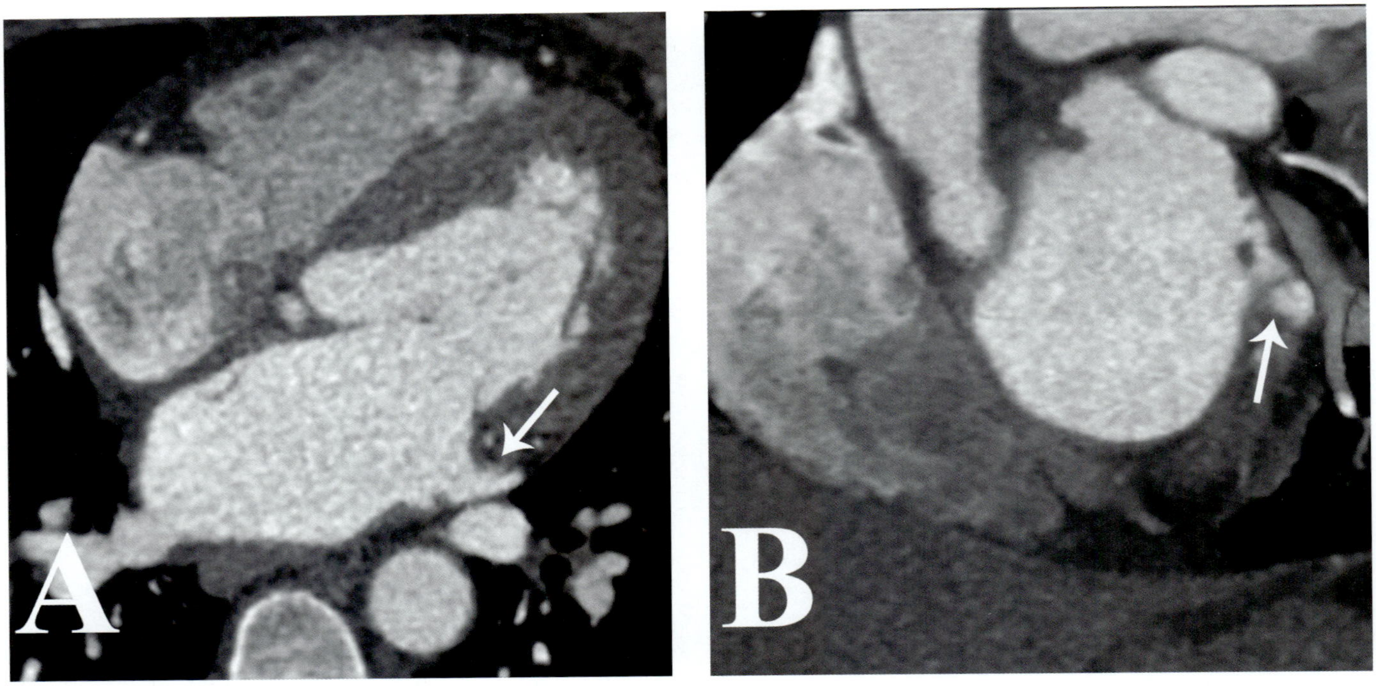

Figure 16.3 Typical appearance of a left atrial diverticulum arising from the lateral wall (arrow) demonstrated by axial (**A**) and coronal volume rendered (**B**) images from a cardiac CT performed in a patient with chest pain. The diverticulum is small and contains a few internal trabeculations.

CASE **17**

Aneurysm of the membranous ventricular septum

Stefan L. Zimmerman

Imaging description

Aneurysm of the membranous ventricular septum appears as a thin-walled, round or lobulated outpouching of the basilar ventricular septum just inferior to the aortic valve annulus (Figure 17.1). It bulges into the right ventricle because of higher left ventricular pressure; however, it may change in size dynamically during the cardiac cycle. Signal characteristics on imaging match the left ventricular blood pool (Figure 17.2), unless complicated by thrombus. Membranous septal aneurysms (MSA) are wide-necked and typically measure 10–15 mm in size; however, much larger aneurysms have been reported.[1]

Importance

Membranous ventricular septal aneurysms may be incorrectly diagnosed as sinus of Valsalva aneurysms or cardiac masses, potentially leading to inappropriate surgery and patient anxiety.[2,3] Membranous septal aneurysms generally have a benign course; however, thrombus formation, right ventricular outflow tract (RVOT) obstruction, rupture, and infection have been reported.[4]

Typical clinical scenario

Membranous septal aneurysms are typically incidentally diagnosed at echocardiography, cardiac CT, or cardiac MRI. They are rare congenital malformations and when found in children, are often associated with other types of congenital heart disease with an estimated prevalence of 0.3% in children with congenital heart disease.[2] When diagnosed in children, membranous septal aneurysms are associated with a ventricular septal defect (VSD) and left-to-right shunt in approximately 20% of cases and some experts believe they may play a role in spontaneous closure of these shunts.[4] Given this association, identification of a membranous septal aneurysm should prompt evaluation for membranous defect and left-to-right shunt. There is an increased incidence of atrioventricular block in patients with membranous septal aneurysms.[2]

Differential diagnosis

The primary differential diagnosis is a sinus of Valsalva aneurysm. These originate above the level of the aortic valve annulus; however, similar to MSA they can protrude into the right ventricular outflow tract.[5] Periaortic pseudoaneurysm due to endocarditis may also have a similar appearance; however, patients will have an abnormal aortic valve and will be quite ill. In patients with prior VSD repair, the patch material located at the membranous septum can bulge into the RVOT with an identical appearance to MSA, except the surgical material is usually calcified.

Teaching point

Membranous septal aneurysm should be considered when a thin-walled bulging of the basilar septum is present on left ventricular outflow tract (LVOT) views and should not be mistaken for sinus of Valsalva aneurysm or a cardiac mass.

REFERENCES

1. Sugioka K., Watanabe H., Gersony D.R., et al. Giant aneurysm of the membranous ventricular septum extending outside the heart: diagnosis by transthoracic color flow Doppler echocardiography. *J Am Soc Echocardiogr* 2002; **15**:188–191.
2. Choi M., Jung J.I., Lee B.Y., Kim. H.R. Ventricular septal aneurysms in adults: findings of cardiac CT images and correlation with clinical features. *Acta Radiologica* 2011; **52**:619–623.
3. Dodd J.D., Aquino S.L., Holmvang G., et al. Cardiac septal aneurysm mimicking pseudomass: appearance on ECG-gated cardiac MRI and MDCT. *Am J Roentgenol* 2007; **188**:550–553.
4. Loukas M., Tubbs R.S., Louis Jr. R.G., Curry B. Pseudoaneurysm of the membranous septum, case report and review of the literature. *Surg Radiol Anat* 2006; **28**:564–568.
5. Shambrook J.S., Chowdhury R., Brown I.W., Peebles C.R., Harden S.P. Cross-sectional imaging appearances of cardiac aneurysms. *Clin Radiol* 2010; **65**:349–357.

Pearls and Pitfalls in Cardiovascular Imaging, ed. Stefan L. Zimmerman and Elliot K. Fishman. Published by Cambridge University Press. © Cambridge University Press 2015.

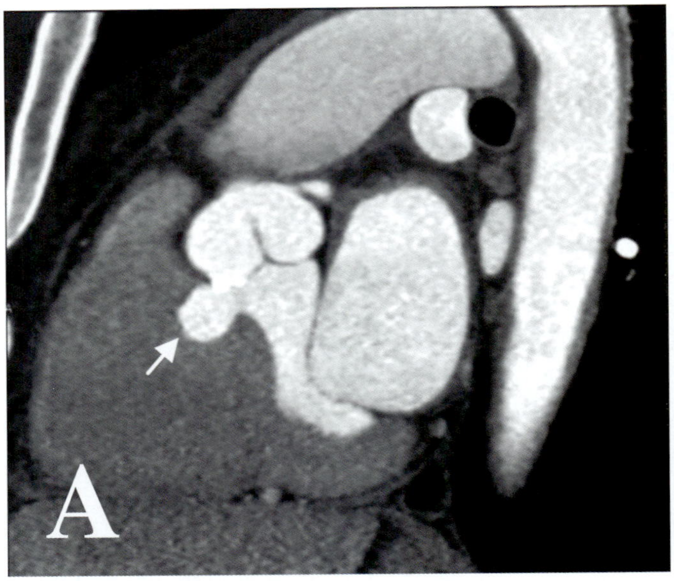

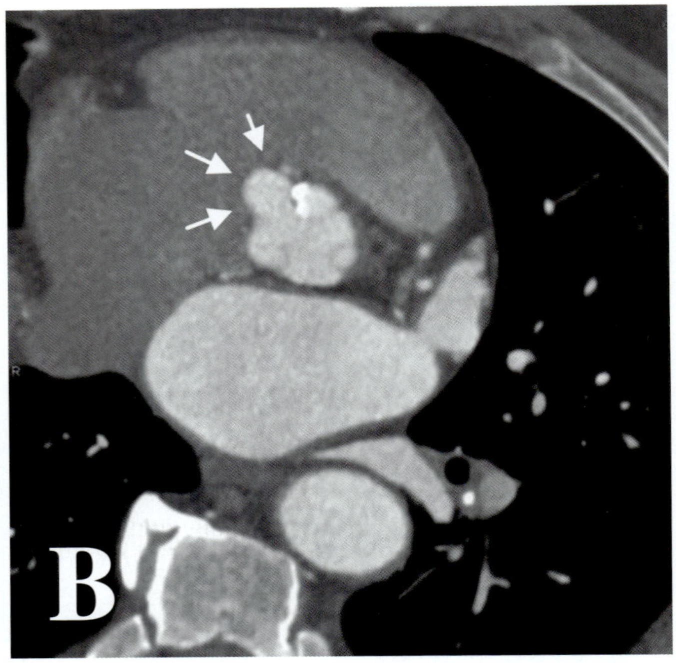

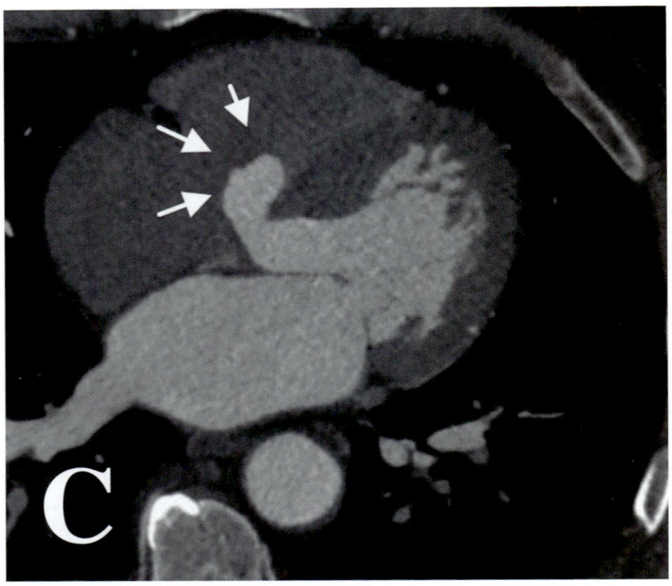

Figure 17.1 **A.** Asymptompatic 64-year-old male participant in a research study with family history of coronary artery disease. Image demonstrates a typical round, smooth-walled aneurysm of the membranous ventricular septum located below the aortic annulus and separate from the sinuses of Valsalva (arrow). The attenuation of the aneurysm matches the blood pool of the left ventricle. **B.** Short-axis image in the plane of the aortic valve just below the aortic valve annulus demonstrates the bulging aneurysm between the insertion of the non-coronary and right coronary cusps to the aortic annulus (arrows). **C.** Axial image in the same patient demonstrates a slightly lobulated contour with homogenous enhancement of the aneurysm with attenuation identical to blood pool (arrows).

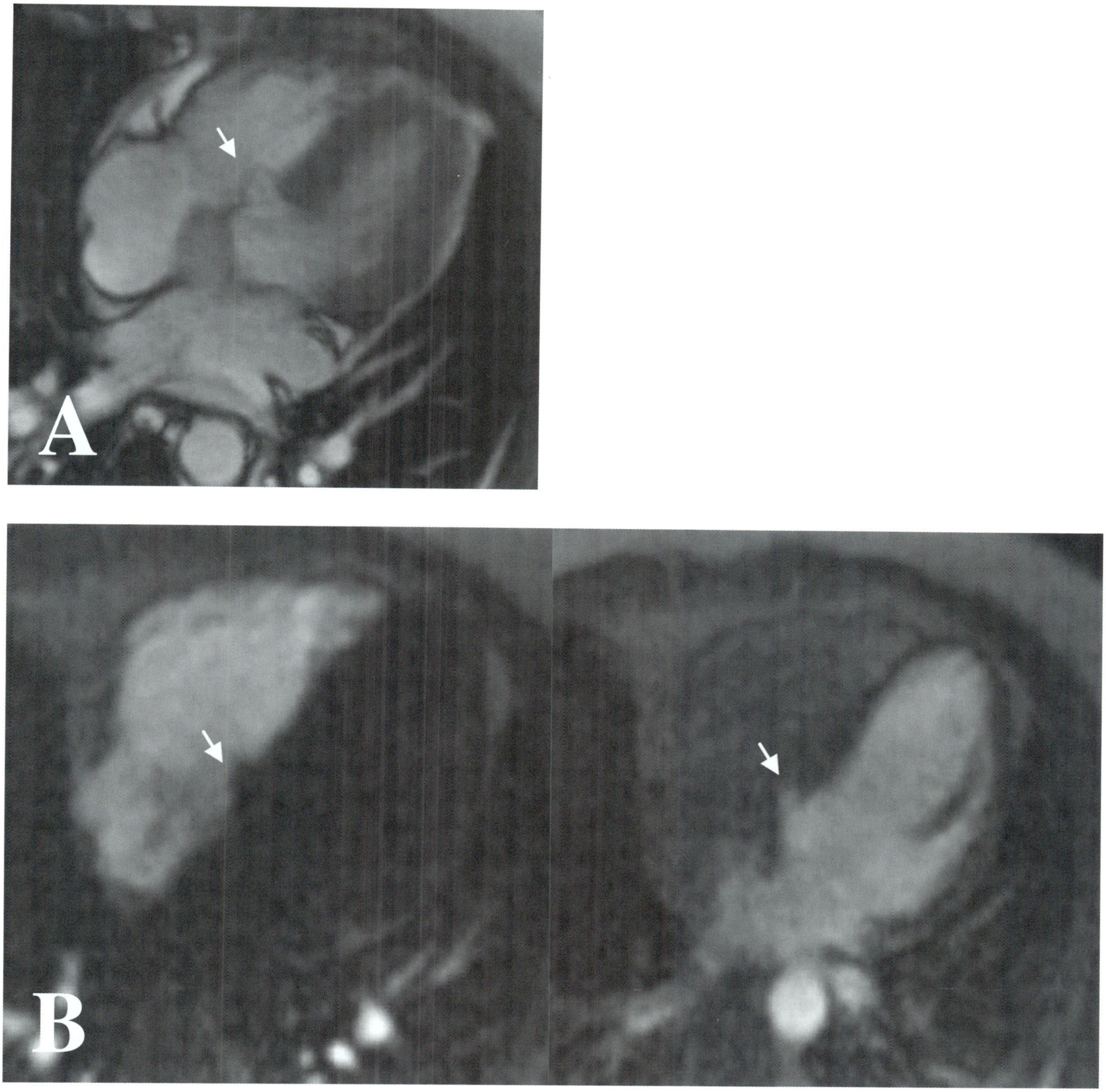

Figure 17.2 **A.** Bright blood cine axial image from a cardiac MRI in a 54-year-old male demonstrates a small membranous septal aneurysm in the LVOT region, just below the aortic valve annulus. The aortic valve leaflets are partially visualized (arrow). **B.** Four-chamber images from dynamic contrast-enhanced perfusion MRI obtained in the same patient demonstrate the basilar septal aneurysm enhancing with the signal intensity identical to left ventricular blood pool during the first pass of contrast through the right and left ventricles (arrows).

CASE 18

Aneurysm of the interatrial septum

Stefan L. Zimmerman

Imaging description

Atrial septal aneurysms (ASA) appear as a thin-walled, round or lobulated outpouching located at the fossa ovalis. They are formed by redundant tissue of the fossa ovalis that protrudes ≥ 10–15 mm beyond the plane of the interatrial septum with a base ≥ 15 mm in width (Figure 18.1).[1–4] ASAs bulge into either the left or right atrium depending upon the prevailing atrial pressure gradient and often have a "to-and-fro" motion throughout the cardiac cycle (Figure 18.2).[2] Signal characteristics on imaging match the adjacent left or right atrial blood pool (Figure 18.3). For instance, if the aneurysm is protruding into the left atrium, signal characteristics will match the right atrial blood pool, and vice versa. Diagnosis is straightforward with echocardiography and cardiac MRI, given the ability to visualize the characteristic motion of the ASA during the cardiac cycle (Figure 18.4). Diagnosis can be challenging on enhanced CT examinations of the chest that use a saline chaser following the contrast bolus. The right atrium is low attenuation in these cases due to the saline flush. ASAs directed into the left atrium will appear as hypoattenuating masses in the enhanced left atrial blood pool (Figure 18.5).[1] Conversely, septal aneurysms directed into the right atrium could be mistaken for a right atrial mass on acquisitions timed for the pulmonary arteries. Injection protocols that utilize dilute contrast in the second phase of the injection for opacification of right-sided heart structures are helpful to avoid this pitfall.[1,2] In addition, if available, multiphase ECG-gated images are helpful to visualize the characteristic motion of septal aneurysms.[2]

Importance

ASAs may be incorrectly mistaken for cardiac tumors, particularly atrial myxomas, during enhanced CT of the chest.[1] Misdiagnosis or uncertainty in diagnosis can lead to unnecessary follow-up examinations, patient anxiety, or worse, inappropriate surgery. ASAs generally have a benign course; however, patients with ASA have an increased prevalence of patent foramen ovale, present in 50–70% cases (Figure 18.1), and cerebral ischemic events (stroke or transient ischemic attack).[3,5] Surgical or percutaneous closure should be considered in patients with evidence of emoblization and left-to-right shunting.[3]

Typical clinical scenario

ASAs are typically incidentally diagnosed at echocardiography, CT, or cardiac MRI. ASA prevalence is estimated at 2% in the general population and 8% among patients with cerebral ischemic events (stroke or transient ischemic attack).[5] There is also an increased association of atrial arrhythmias, mitral valve prolapse, atrial septal defect, and sinus venosus defect.[2,3]

Differential diagnosis

The primary differential diagnosis is an atrial tumor such as myxoma. These will also originate from the fossa ovalis; however, they have subtle differences at imaging. Myxomas will have round or lobulated margins, are heterogenous due to presence of mixed tissue elements, and may be attached to the septum via a stalk.[6] On cine imaging, atrial myxomas may prolapse through the atrioventricular valve, whereas atrial septal aneurysms will display characteristic "to-and-fro" motion. Atrial myxomas will show heterogenous enhancement at post-contrast imaging, whereas ASAs will have signal characteristics identical to the blood pool.[6]

Teaching point

Atrial septal aneurysm should be considered when encountering a round, well-circumscribed atrial mass located at the fossa ovalis and should not be mistaken for a cardiac myxoma.

REFERENCES

1. Dodd J.D., Aquino S.L., Holmvang G., et al. Cardiac septal aneurysm mimicking pseudomass: appearance on ECG-gated cardiac MRI and MDCT. *AJR Am J Roentgenol* 2007; **188**:550–3.
2. Rojas C.A., Jaimes C.E., El-Sherief A.H., et al. Cardiac CT of non-shunt pathology of the interatrial septum. *J Cariovasc Comput Tomogr* 2011; **5**:93–100.
3. Shambrook J.S., Chowdhury R., Brown I.W., Peebles C.R., Harden S.P. Cross-sectional imaging appearances of cardiac aneurysms. *Clin Radiol* 2010; **65**:349–57.
4. Zeina A.R., Orlov I., Sharif D., Barmeir E. Detection of atrial septal aneurysm by ECG-gated MDCT. *AJR* 2006; **187**:W229–30.
5. Agmon Y., Khandheria B.K., Meissner I., et al. Frequency of atrial septal aneurysms in patients with cerebral ischemic events. *Circulation* 1999; **99**:1942–4.
6. Grebenc M.L., Rosado-de-Christenson M.L., Green C.E., Burke A.P., Galvin J.R. Cardiac myxoma: imaging features in 83 patients. *Radiographics* 2002; **22**:673–89.

Pearls and Pitfalls in Cardiovascular Imaging, ed. Stefan L. Zimmerman and Elliot K. Fishman. Published by Cambridge University Press. © Cambridge University Press 2015.

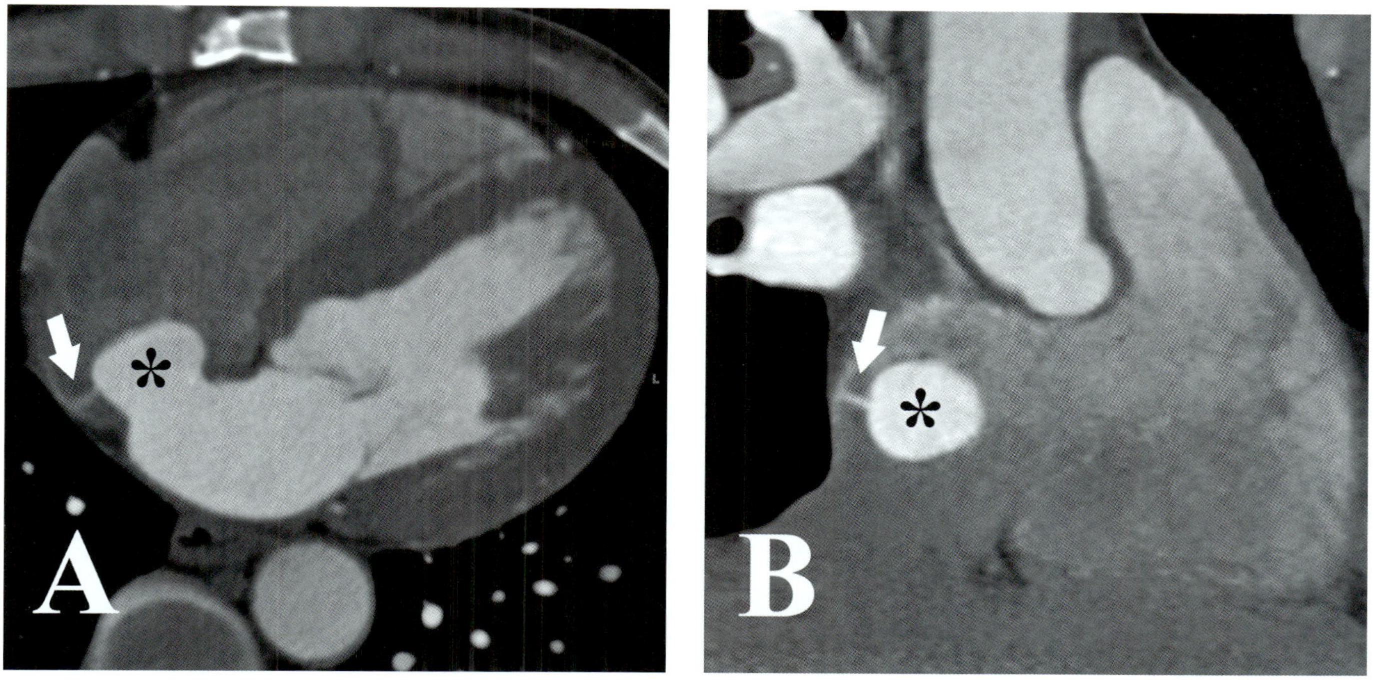

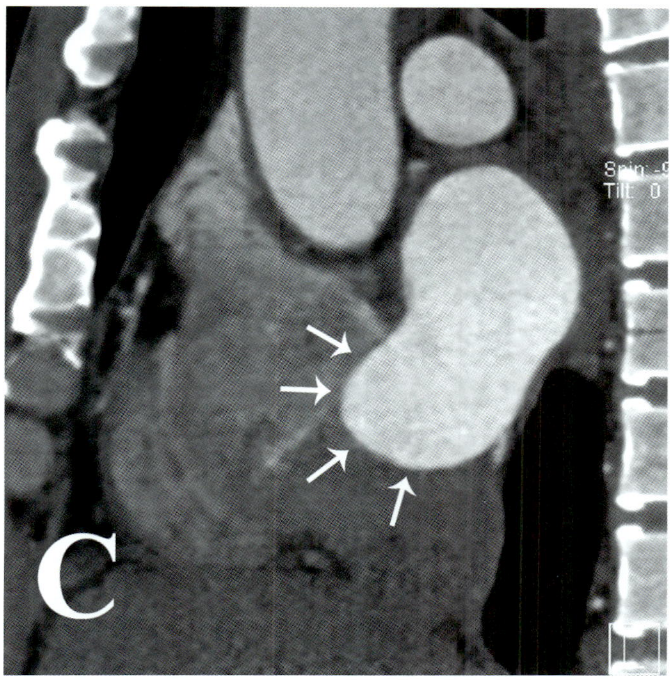

Figure 18.1 **A.** Axial image from contrast-enhanced cardiac CT demonstrates a large atrial septal aneurysm (asterisk), which is located in the center of the atrial septum at the fossa ovalis. The aneurysm is round with smooth margins and attenuation matching the left atrial blood pool. A posteriorly directed jet of contrast (arrow) travels through a small patent foramen ovale, which has an increased incidence in patients with atrial septal aneurysms. **B.** Oblique coronal image parallel to the plane of the interatrial septum shows the atrial septal aneurysm (asterisk) at the center of the interatrial septum with a posteriorly directed jet of contrast flow through a patent foramen ovale (arrow). **C.** Oblique sagittal image in the same patient demonstrates a slightly lobulated contour with homogenous enhancement of the aneurysm with attenuation identical to blood pool (arrows).

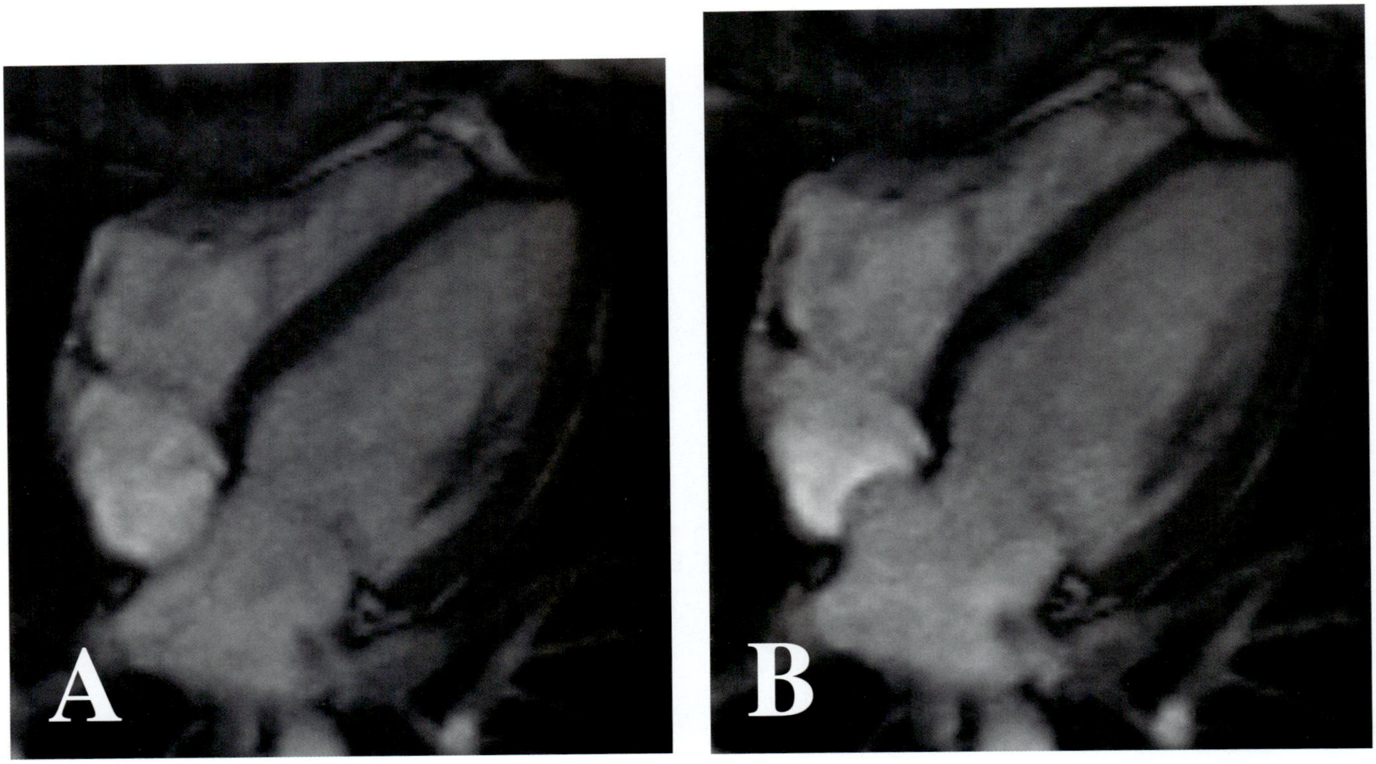

Figure 18.2 Four-chamber cine axial images obtained at two different points of the cardiac cycle demonstrate to-and-fro motion of a small atrial septal aneurysm. On early diastolic images, the aneurysm bulges into the right atrium (**A**) and then on late diastolic images the septum flattens and minimally bulges into the left atrium (**B**).

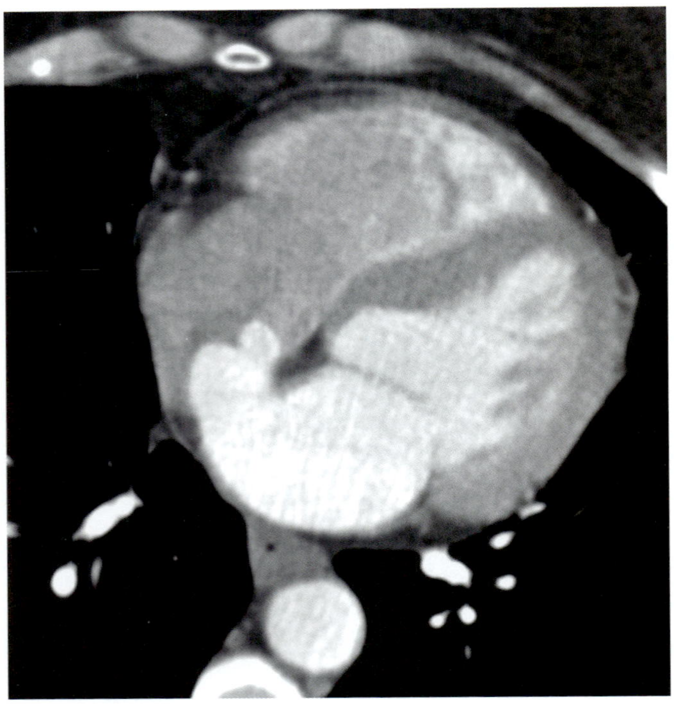

Figure 18.3. Axial image from a contrast-enhanced cardiac CT examination demonstrates a large, bilobed atrial septal aneurysm protruding into the right atrium.

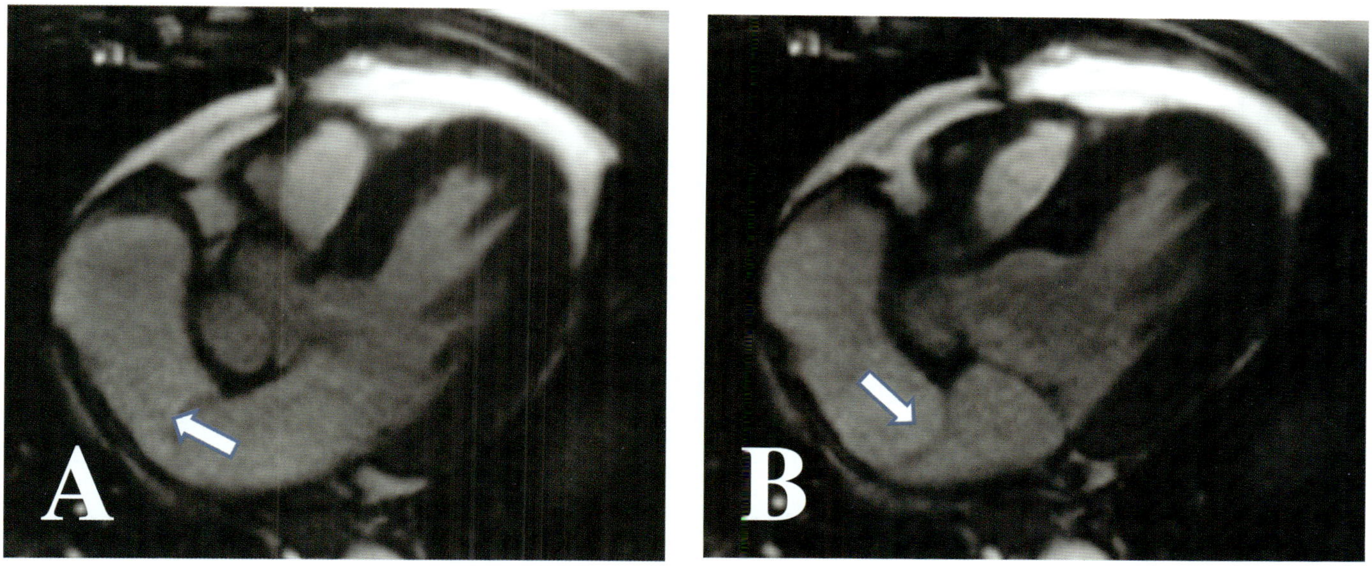

Figure 18.4 A. and B. Images from an axial cine bright blood sequence obtained in a patient being evaluated for cardiac sarcoidosis demonstrates "to-and-fro" motion of an atrial septal aneurysm (arrows).

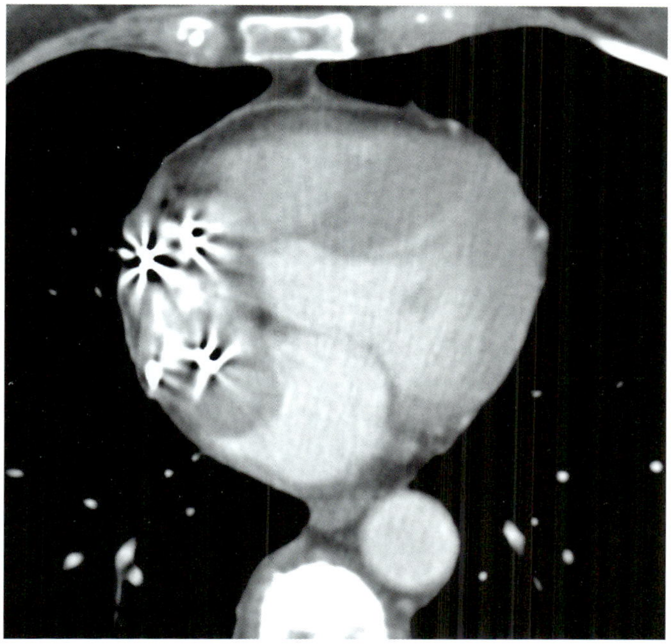

Figure 18.5 Axial image from contrast-enhanced CT of the chest demonstrates an atrial septal aneurysm bulging into the left atrium, which could potentially be mistaken for a left atrial mass originating from the atrial septum.

CASE 19

Sinus of Valsalva aneurysm

Vivek Halappa and Atif Zaheer

Imaging description

The sinuses of Valsalva are focal expansions forming the walls of the aortic root. Sinus of Vasalva aneurysm (SVA) is a rare congenital anomaly with involvement of the right sinus in 65–85% of instances, and less commonly originating from non-coronary (10–30%) and left sinuses (< 5%).[1] Most SVA are congenital due to deficiency of the normal elastic tissue and abnormal development of the bulbus cordis.[1] Acquired SVA can be seen with infective endocarditis, trauma, tuberculosis, and Behçet disease. Up to 21% of reported cases of SVA are clinically asymptomatic,[2] and may be incidentally found at necropsy or during a diagnostic test for evaluation of unrelated non-cardiac or cardiac abnormalities. SVA are found in association with ventricular septal defects in 30–60% of patients.[3] SVA can be identified on all modalities used for imaging the heart and aorta including catheter angiography, echocardiography, multidetector computed tomography (MDCT) and cardiac magnetic resonance (CMR). Currently transthoracic followed by transesophageal echocardiography is recommended for the initial assessment of both ruptured or non-ruptured SVA,[4] as they offer advantage in color flow and spectral Doppler to demonstrate the presence and direction of turbulent jets at the point of rupture. MDCT and CMR generate high-resolution multiplanar images to facilitate three-dimensional visualization and provide imaging of the coronary arteries, which is useful when surgical correction is being considered. On cardiac MRI, sinus of Valsalva aneurysms manifest as thin-walled outpouchings that are contiguous with the aortic root on sequential slices. Rupture can be identified by a turbulent flow jet from the sinus into the adjacent cardiac chamber on cine bright blood images.[3] Large SVA can project into the right atrium and mimic an atrial mass, particularly if thrombosed (Figures 19.1 and 19.2). Partial or complete thrombosis is often seen with SVA due to blood stasis.

Importance

SVA may mimic a right-sided cardiac mass, particularly if thrombosed, which could lead to incorrect diagnosis and may alter surgical planning. Both ruptured and non-ruptured Valsalva sinus aneurysms are associated with potentially fatal complications. Ruptured aneurysms can result in shunting and cardiac failure. Complications in non-ruptured aneurysms are the result of mass effect on adjacent coronary arteries, resulting in ischemia, or obstruction of the right ventricular outflow tract.[3]

Typical clinical scenario

SVA are often encountered incidentally on cross-sectional imaging such as CT or CMR or on echocardiography performed for other indications. Patients with symptomatic SVA often present with shortness of breath and murmur related to the left-to-right shunt from the aortic root to the right heart. Small SVA need no immediate treatment and can be followed.

Differential diagnosis

A non-thrombosed SVA can mimic an aneurysm of the membranous ventricular septum; however, these can be distinguished by location above (SVA) or below (membranous septal aneurysm) the aortic annulus on reformatted images (Figures 19.3 and 19.4). Differential diagnosis for a thrombosed SVA includes intracardiac tumors, such as myxoma or metastatic disease. Thrombosed SVA can be differentiated from a cardiac mass anatomically as thrombosed aneurysm will appear contiguous with the aortic root on multiplanar reformatted cross-sectional images (Figures 19.1 and 19.2). Blood within the SVA will have attenuation and signal identical to the adjacent blood pool on both CT and cardiac MRI, unless thrombosed. Thrombus will be low attenuation on post-contrast CT and may show high signal on T1-weighted MR imaging. Lack of enhancement seen within a thrombus compared to heterogeneous enhancement seen in myxomas and metastatic disease can be a distinguishing feature.[5]

Teaching point

SVA incidentally seen on CT or MRI should not be mistaken for an intracardiac mass, and may be correctly identified by careful evaluation of its relationship with the aortic root on high-resolution multiplanar images.

REFERENCES

1. W. S. Ring. Congenital Heart Surgery Nomenclature and Database Project: aortic aneurysm, sinus of Valsalva aneurysm, and aortic dissection. *Ann Thorac Surg* 2000; **69**: S147–63.

2. S. Moustafa, F. Mookadam, L. Cooper, et al. Sinus of Valsalva aneurysms – 47 years of a single-center experience and systematic overview of published reports. *Am J Cardiol* 2007; **99**: 1159–64.

3. A. O. Bricker, B. Avutu, T. L. Mohammed, et al. Valsalva sinus aneurysms: findings at CT and MR imaging. *Radiographics* 2010; **30**: 99–110.

Pearls and Pitfalls in Cardiovascular Imaging, ed. Stefan L. Zimmerman and Elliot K. Fishman. Published by Cambridge University Press. © Cambridge University Press 2015.

4. D. N. Feldman, M. J. Roman. Aneurysms of the sinuses of Valsalva. *Cardiology* 2006; **106**: 73–81.

5. P. J. Sparrow, J. B. Kurian, T. R. Jones, M. U. Sivananthan. MR imaging of cardiac tumors. *Radiographics* 2005; **25**: 1255–76.

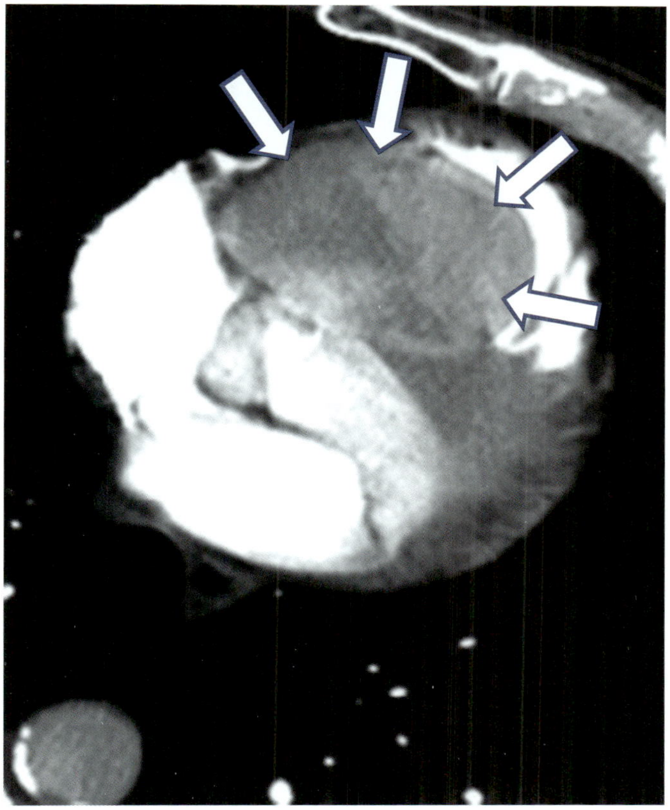

Figure 19.1 A 67-year-old man with thrombosed sinus of Valsalva aneurysm. Axial contrast-enhanced CT performed for evaluation of shortness of breath demonstrates a mass-like low-attenuation lesion in the right ventricular outflow tract (arrows).

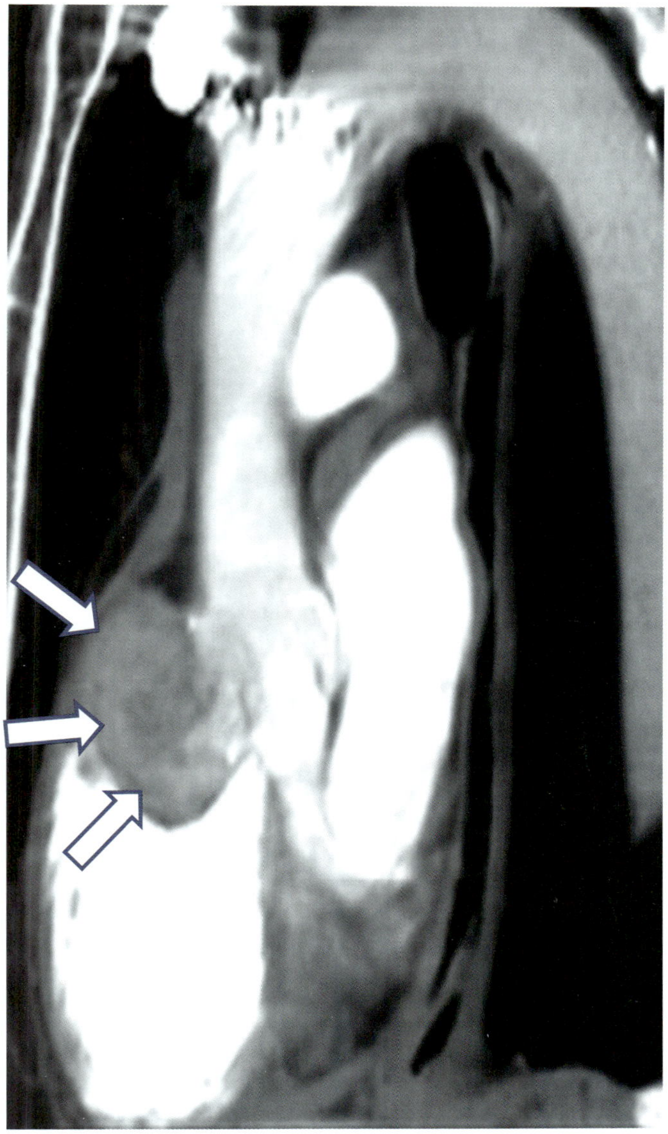

Figure 19.2 A 67-year-old man with thrombosed sinus of Valsalva aneurysm. Sagittal reconstruction CT image demonstrates an expanded right coronary sinus filled with thrombus (arrows). On the reformatted images the mass is clearly in continuity with the aortic root and located above the aortic valve annulus.

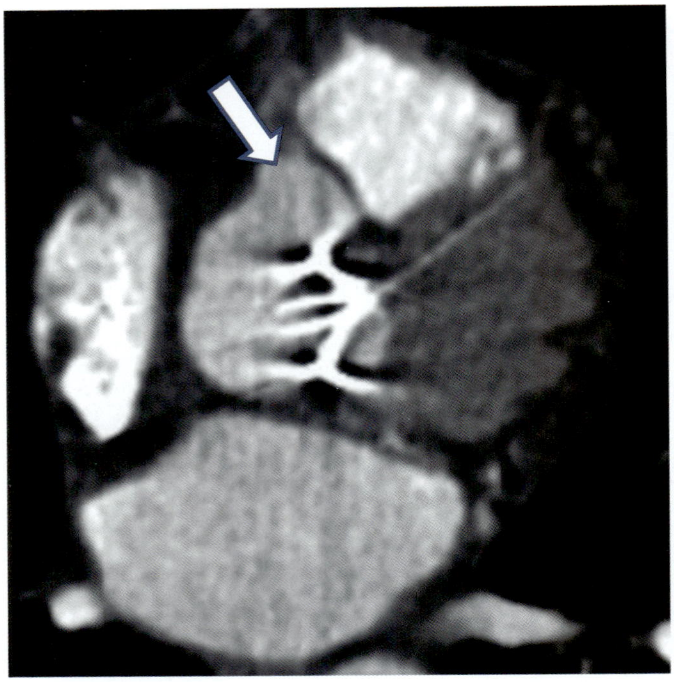

Figure 19.3 Axial image from a contrast-enhanced CT obtained in a 55-year-old male with prior mechanical aortic valve replacement for bacterial endocarditis shows a small sinus of Valsalva aneurysm (arrow). On axial images, the relationship with the aortic valve annulus and aortic root can be difficult to assess.

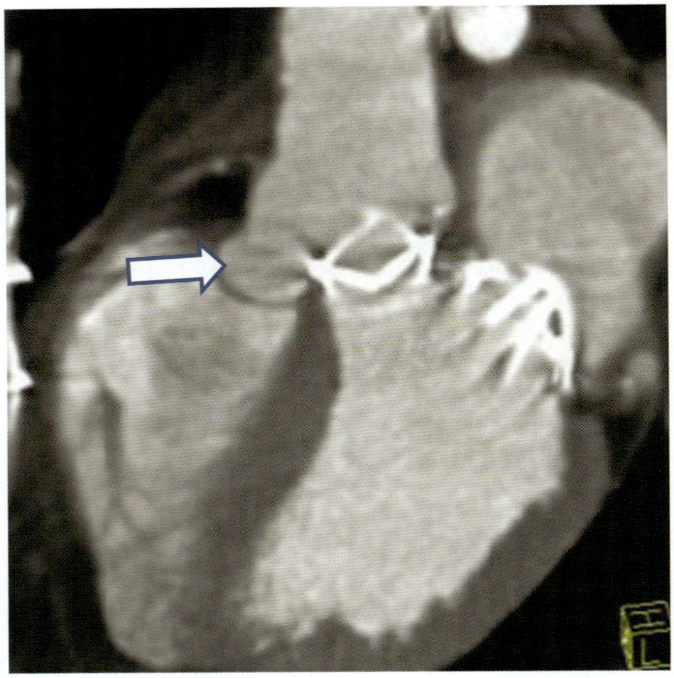

Figure 19.4 Reformatted oblique sagittal image from a contrast-enhanced CT obtained in a 55-year-old male with prior mechanical aortic valve replacement for bacterial endocarditis shows a small sinus of Valsalva aneurysm. There is no evidence of thrombosis and the relationship of the aneurysm above the aortic valve annulus and contiguous with the aortic root is clearly seen (arrow).

CASE **20**

Patent foramen ovale and left atrial septal pouch

Stefan L. Zimmerman

Imaging description

A patent foramen ovale (PFO) occurs when the two components of the atrial septum, the septum primum and septum secundum, fail to fuse after birth. The result is a persistent valve-like potential pathway between the left and right atria. In fetal life, this pathway allows blood from the inferior vena cava to cross into the left atrium, bypassing the lungs. In adults, there is potential for blood to cross from right to left if there is reversal of the normal interatrial pressure gradient, which can occur during straining or a Valsalva maneuver. On imaging, a patent foramen ovale can occasionally be identified by cardiac CT, which demonstrates a slit-like, vertically oriented channel in the atrial septum between the left and right atria.[1] A jet of contrast will often be seen exiting the channel into the right atrium inferiorly (Figure 20.1). Occasionally, a jet of unopacified blood will result in a blush of negative contrast in the left atrium if there is right-to-left flow across the PFO during the exam. Similar findings may be seen on dynamic contrast-enhanced MRI. The atrial septal pouch is a related anatomic structure created by partial fusion of the septum primum and septum secundum.[2] This can be recognized at cardiac CT by a small channel in the left atrial side of the atrial septum that fills with contrast but does not communicate with the right side (Figure 20.2).

Importance

Some studies have found an increased incidence of PFO in patients with cryptogenic stroke, suggesting a causative role in thromboembolism.[3] However, results from other studies have been contradictory and currently the role of PFO in management of patients with stroke is uncertain.[3] A potential for blood stasis and thrombus within atrial septal pouches (ASP) has been suggested,[2] and case reports have found thrombus within ASP in patients with embolic stroke.[4,5] However, a larger case-control study of 187 patients with first-ever stroke and 157 controls found no increased incidence of atrial septal pouch in patients with stroke.[5] Further studies will be necessary to define the association between ASP and stroke risk.

Typical clinical scenario

Patent foramen ovale is common, occurring in approximately 30% of the general population.[1] They are frequently incidentally identified at cardiac CT performed for other reasons. The atrial septal pouch is also quite common, reported to occur in approximately 60% of autopsy specimens.[1]

Differential diagnosis

Secundum atrial septal defects (ASD) should also be considered when making the diagnosis of PFO. Unlike PFO, which is a transient communication between the atria, a secundum ASD is always open with constant communication between the two chambers. In these cases, there is more prominent left-to-right flow and patients will often have some degree of right cardiac chamber dilation due to volume overload. Left atrial band can also be considered in the differential diagnosis of an atrial septal pouch, both of which result in thin linear filling defects in the left atrial chamber. They can be distinguished by location – the atrial septal pouch will attach to the fossa ovalis, abutting the atrial septum – whereas atrial bands originate from the fossa ovalis and connect to other walls of the left atrium.[1]

Teaching point

Patent foramen ovale and atrial septal pouches are normal anatomic variants frequently identified incidentally at cardiac CT. Whether or not these entities confer increased risk of cerebral emboli is uncertain and further studies will be necessary to clearly define the association with cryptogenic stroke.

REFERENCES

1. O. Balli, K. Aytemir, M. Karcaaltincaba. Multidetector CT of left atrium. *Eur J Radiol* 2012; **81**: e37–46.
2. S. C. Krishnan, M. Salazar. Septal pouch in the left atrium: a new anatomical entity with potential for embolic complications. *JACC Cardiovasc Interv* 2010; **3**: 98–104.
3. B. Irwin, S. Ray. Patent foramen ovale – assessment and treatment. *Cardiovasc Ther* 2012; **30**: e128–35.
4. S. Buchholz, D. Robaei, N. H. Jacobs, M. O'Rourke, M. P. Feneley. Thromboembolic stroke with concurrent left atrial appendage and left atrial septal pouch thrombus. *Int J Cardiol* 2012; **162**: e16–17.
5. A. Tugcu, K. Okajima, Z. Jin, et al. Septal pouch in the left atrium and risk of ischemic stroke. *JACC Cardiovasc Imaging* 2010; **3**: 1276–83.

Pearls and Pitfalls in Cardiovascular Imaging, ed. Stefan L. Zimmerman and Elliot K. Fishman. Published by Cambridge University Press. © Cambridge University Press 2015.

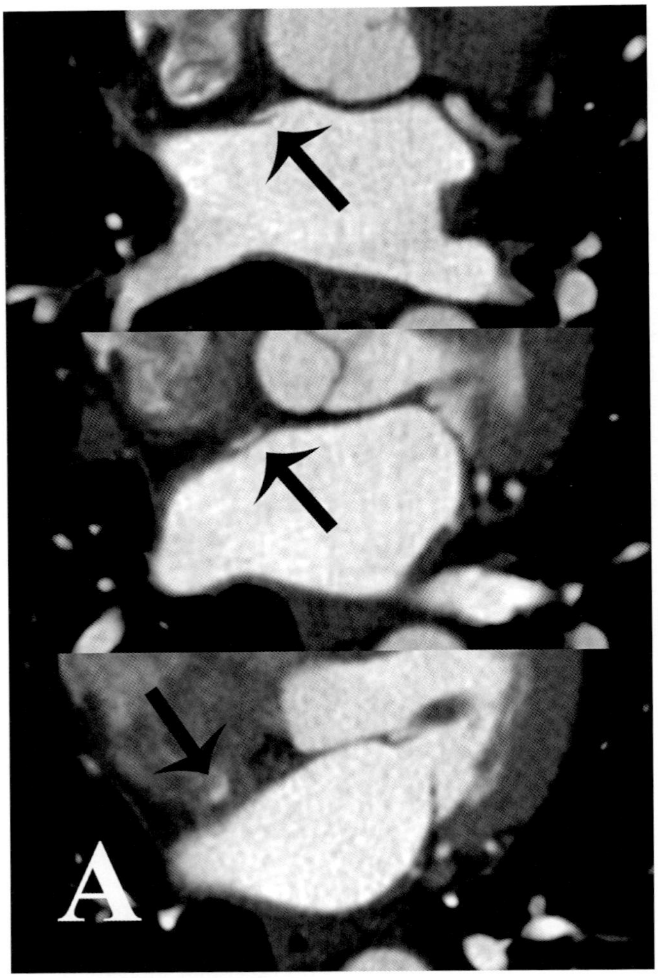

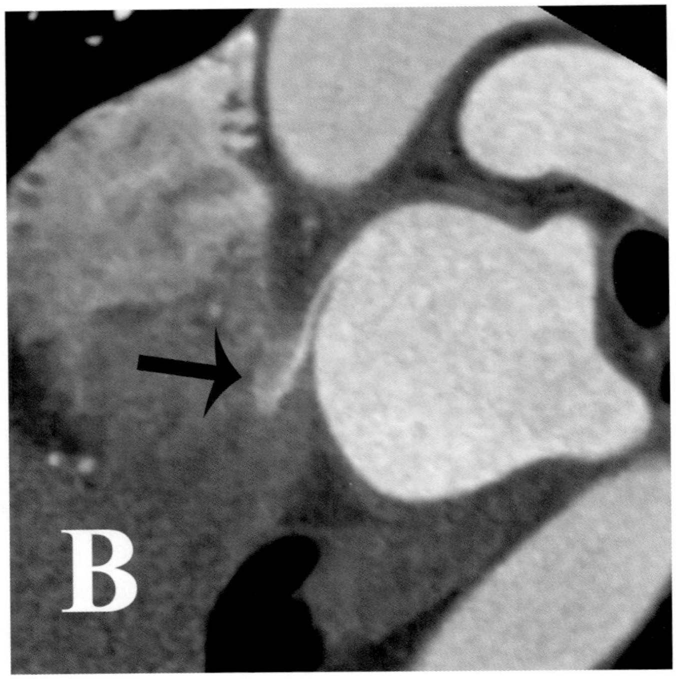

Figure 20.1 A. Contiguous cranial (top) to caudal (bottom) axial CT images from an ECG-gated CT angiogram of the chest performed in a 50-year-old male with an aneurysm of the ascending aorta demonstrates a small patent foramen ovale (PFO, black arrow). There is a thin channel of contrast that connects the left atrium superiorly to the right atrium inferiorly. **B.** Oblique coronal multiplanar reformatted image from the same study confirms the presence of a PFO, demonstrating a blush of contrast in the right atrium (black arrow).

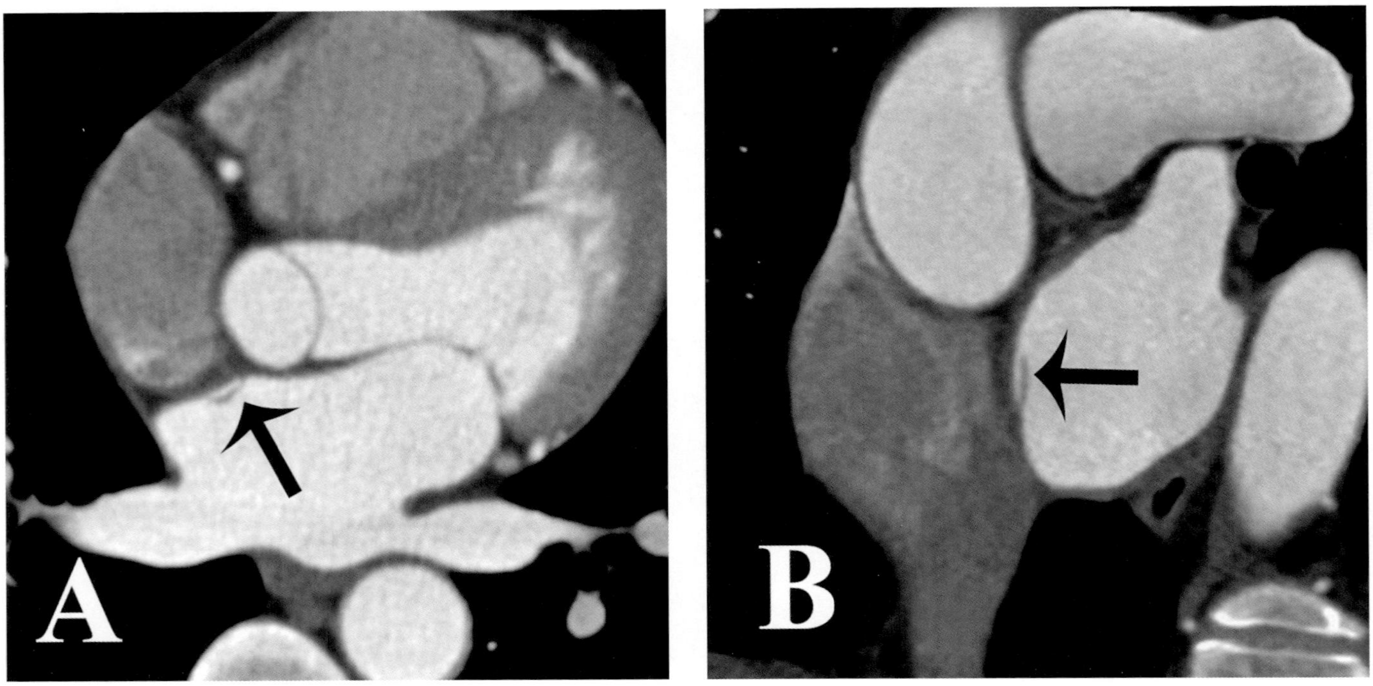

Figure 20.2 A. Incidental identification of an atrial septal pouch in a 52-year-old male with cardiac CT performed for atypical chest pain. On the axial image, there is a small, curvilinear filling defect in the left atrium attached to the left atrial side of the atrial septum (black arrow). **B.** On an oblique coronal image, unlike PFO, there is no communication with the right atrial chamber, suggesting this represents an atrial septal pouch due to incomplete fusion of the foramen ovale.

CASE **21**

Partial cor triatriatum

Stefan L. Zimmerman

Imaging description

Cor triatriatum, also known as cor triatriatum sinister, is a congenital abnormality of the left atrium in which a fibromuscular membrane separates the atrium into anterior and posterior chambers (Figure 21.1). The membrane appears as a low-attenuation structure on cardiac CT extending from the atrial septum medially to the ridge of tissue between left pulmonary vein ostia and the left atrial appendage laterally. Cor triatriatum is the result of incomplete fusion of a common pulmonary vein chamber posteriorly with the anterior mitral valve and left atrial appendage during fetal life.[1] The result is a fibromuscular membrane within the left atrium which usually contains one or multiple openings that allow communication between anterior and posterior chambers. Depending on the size of the opening(s) of the membrane, there may be obstruction of pulmonary venous outflow, resulting in symptoms similar to mitral stenosis. Cor triatriatum with larger defects may present with symptoms late in adulthood or can be entirely asymptomatic (Figures 21.1, 21.2).[2,3]

Importance

Cor triatriatum is an uncommon abnormality, which in adults is frequently misdiagnosed at initial presentation as mitral valve disease or pulmonary hypertension.[3] If identified, it is important to draw attention to the abnormality and recommend further non-invasive evaluation with echocardiography to assess for any functionally significant obstruction that might require surgical treatment.

Typical clinical scenario

Cor triatriatum is a rare abnormality, accounting for less than 1% of all congenital cardiac malformations.[1] The majority of patients with cor triatriatum present in infancy; however, a minority of patients will present in adulthood.[3]

Differential diagnosis

Cor triatriatum should be differentiated from a complete total anomalous pulmonary venous return, in which pulmonary veins connect to a common venous chamber that drains separately into the heart. Chronic left atrial clot can sometimes have angular or web-like appearances that may simulate cor triatriatum; however, it will often be associated with a mass-like thrombus or calcifications.

Teaching point

Cor triatriatum is a rare abnormality characterized by a fibromuscular membrane in the left atrium that separates the pulmonary venous outflow from the mitral valve. If recognized, further evaluation with echocardiography is recommended to evaluate for the presence of pulmonary venous obstruction, which can result in symptoms similar to mitral stenosis and pulmonary hypertension.

REFERENCES

1. N. Alphonso, M. A. Norgaard, A. Newcomb, Y. d'Udekem, C. P. Brizard, A. Cochrane. Cor triatriatum: presentation, diagnosis and long-term surgical results. *Ann Thorac Surg* 2005; **80**: 1666–71.
2. S. Basavarajaiah, D. Oxborough, M. Wilson, S. Sharma. Incidental finding of cor triatriatum in an asymptomatic elite athlete. *J Am Soc Echocardiogr* 2007; **20**: 771: e9–12.
3. Q. Chen, S. Guhathakurta, G. Vadalapali, Z. Nalladaru, R. N. Easthope, A. K. Sharma. Cor triatriatum in adults: three new cases and a brief review. *Tex Heart Inst J* 1999; **26**: 206–10.

Pearls and Pitfalls in Cardiovascular Imaging, ed. Stefan L. Zimmerman and Elliot K. Fishman. Published by Cambridge University Press. © Cambridge University Press 2015.

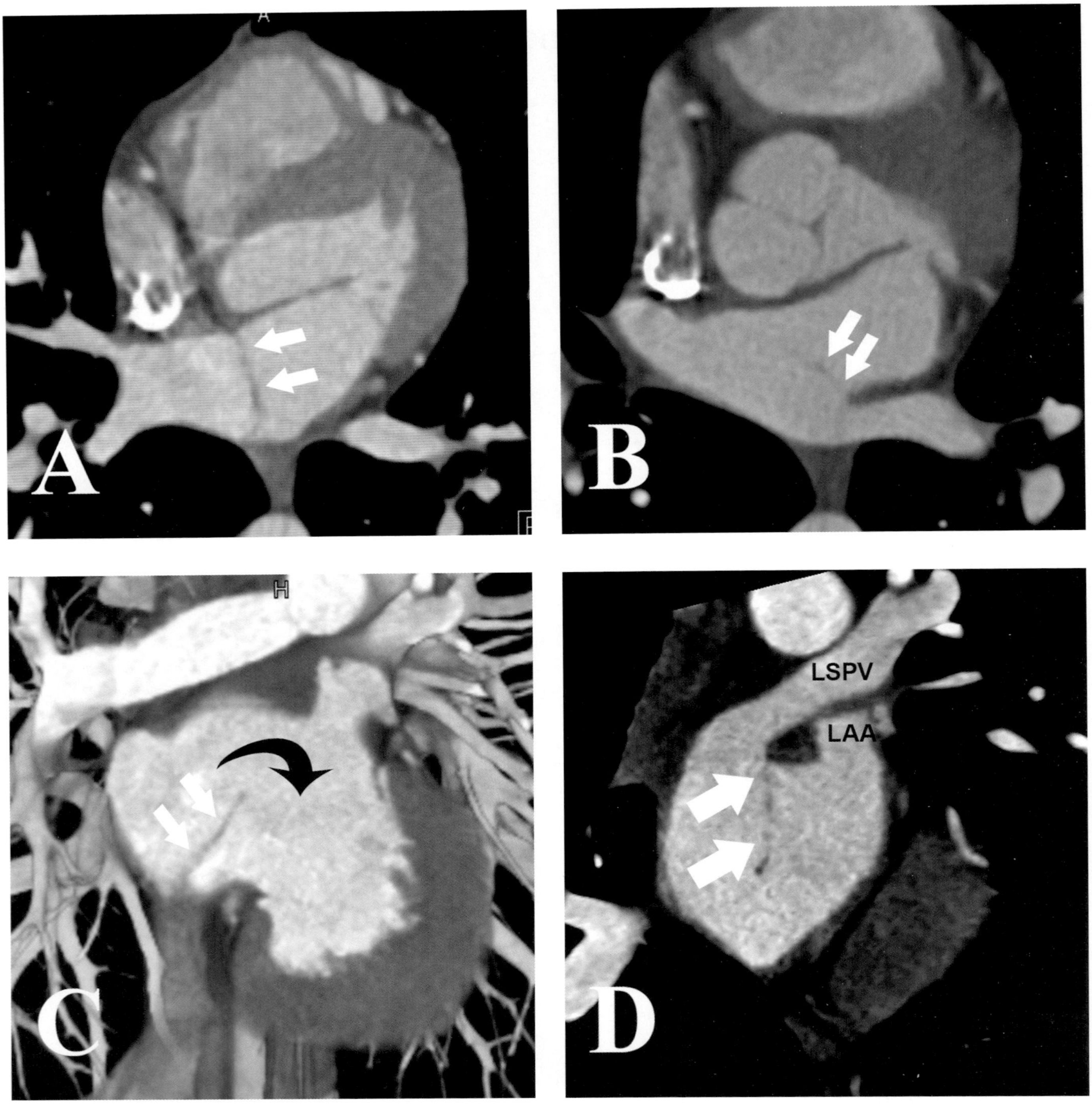

Figure 21.1 A. Axial image from cardiac CT performed in a 15-year-old male with non-obstructive cor triatriatum incidentally diagnosed during work-up for rheumatic fever. There is a thin low-attenuation membrane in the left atrium (white arrows) which attaches to the interatrial septum medially. **B.** Laterally, the membrane attaches to the left atrial wall just anterior to the left superior pulmonary vein. **C.** On a coronal volume-rendered image, a wide orifice between the posterior and anterior chambers (curved black arrow) can be seen, explaining the lack of clinical symptoms of obstruction. **D.** On an oblique sagittal multiplanar reformatted image, the superolateral attachment site of the membrane to the ridge between the left superior pulmonary vein (LSPV) and the left atrial appendage (LAA) is clearly identified.

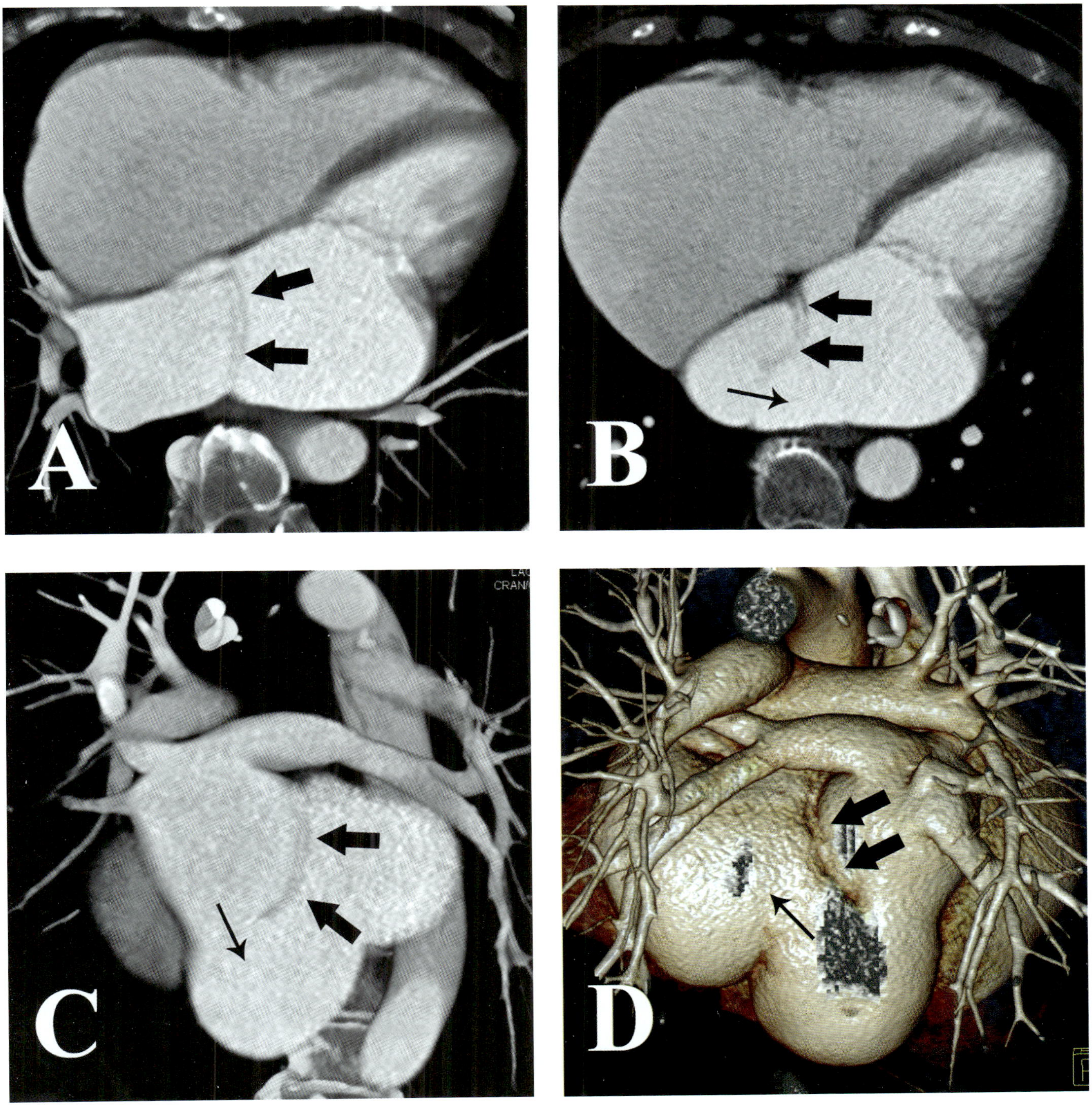

Figure 21.2 A. Axial volume-rendered image from a contrast-enhanced CT of the chest performed in a 67-year-old female with recurrent liposarcoma and long-standing history of atrial fibrillation and pulmonary hypertension demonstrates a clinically unsuspected cor triatriatum. A low-attenuation membrane separates the left atrium into anterior and posterior chambers (black arrow). **B.** On an axial image obtained more inferior than image A, there is a connection between anterior and posterior chambers (thin black arrow). **C.** This connection is also demonstrated on a coronal volume-rendered image, showing the posterior chamber superiorly receiving the pulmonary veins, and the membrane (thick black arrow), with communication via a small orifice (thin black arrow). **D.** Volume-rendered image obtained in a posterior view again demonstrates marked dilation of the left atrium as well as the left atrial membrane (thick black arrows) and orifice between the two atrial chambers (thin black arrow).

CASE 22

Congenital absence of the pericardium

Tessa S. Cook

Imaging description

Congenital absence of the pericardium is most easily diagnosed on axial CT or MR images. The heart appears rotated into the left hemithorax (Figure 22.1). Lung can be seen interposed between the aorta and the pulmonary artery, where normally there is fat covered by a layer of pericardium (Figure 22.2). In some cases, pericardium will be clearly visible along the right heart but not along the left heart (Figure 22.3). If the pericardial defect is small, focal herniation of a portion of the heart or great vessels may occur, increasing the risk for strangulation.

Importance

Distinguishing between complete and partial absence of the pericardium can be difficult when the normal, thin pericardium is generally difficult to visualize. Identifying absence of the pericardium is particularly important when the defect is partial, as this can result in herniation and strangulation of a portion of the heart or adjacent great vessels, which necessitates surgical correction.

Typical clinical scenario

Congenital absence of the pericardium occurs in approximately 0.002–0.004% of individuals.[1] Partial absence of the left pericardium only (the most common form) results from atrophy of the left common cardinal vein, which interferes with development of the pericardium on that side.[2]

It is most commonly incidentally detected during thoracic imaging ordered for unrelated reasons. Additionally, most cases are asymptomatic, although positional dyspnea and non-exertional chest pain have been reported, as has right bundle branch block.[3] In 30% of patients, it is associated with congenital heart disease, such as tetralogy of Fallot, atrial septal defect, bicuspid aortic valve or patent ductus arteriosus.[4]

Differential diagnosis

The differential diagnosis falls within two major categories: causes of levoposition of the heart or focal outpouchings from the heart. Volume loss in the left hemithorax due to atelectasis, prior lobectomy or left-sided bronchial atresia can also lead to levoposition of the heart in the setting of an intact pericardium. Enlargement of the right heart due to valvular disease or other causes can displace the heart into the left hemithorax. Focal outpouchings from the heart such as atrial or ventricular diverticula or left ventricular pseudoaneurysms can mimic the focal herniation of a cardiac chamber through a pericardial defect.[5]

Teaching point

Congenital absence of the pericardium, whether complete or partial, may be incidentally discovered during cross-sectional imaging and is commonly asymptomatic. The diagnosis should be considered when the heart appears to be displaced into the left hemithorax in the absence of pathology affecting the left lung.

REFERENCES

1. P. Psychidis-Papakyritsis, A. de Roos, L. J. Kroft. Functional MRI of congenital absence of the pericardium. *AJR Am J Roentgenol* 2007; **189**: W312–4.
2. S. Chassaing, C. Bensouda, O. Bar, C. Barbey, D. Blanchard. A case of partial congenital absence of pericardium revealed by MRI. *Circ Cardiovasc Imaging* 2010; **3**: 632–4.
3. M. Scheuermann-Freestone, E. Orchard, J. Francis, et al. Images in cardiovascular medicine. Partial congenital absence of the pericardium. *Circulation* 2007; **116**: e126–9.
4. A. E. Abbas, C. P. Appleton, P. T. Liu, J. P. Sweeney. Congenital absence of the pericardium: case presentation and review of literature. *Int J Cardiol* 2005; **98**: 21–5.
5. F. Verde, P. T. Johnson, S. Jha, E. K. Fishman, S. L. Zimmerman. Congenital absence of the pericardium and its mimics. *J Cardiovasc Comput Tomogr* 2013; **7**: 11–17.

Pearls and Pitfalls in Cardiovascular Imaging, ed. Stefan L. Zimmerman and Elliot K. Fishman. Published by Cambridge University Press. © Cambridge University Press 2015.

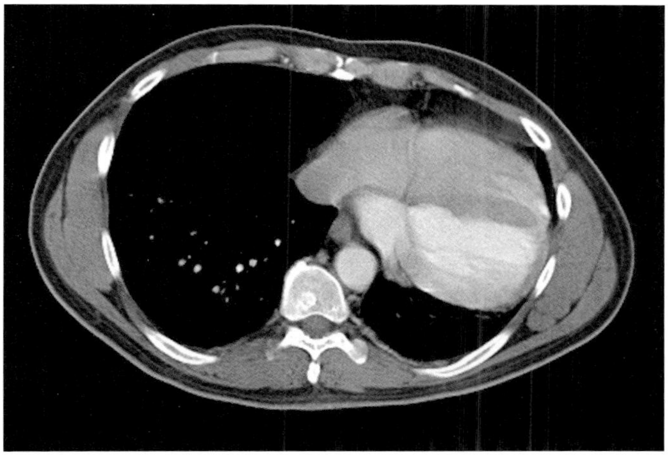

Figure 22.1. Asymptomatic 62-year-old male found to have rotation of the heart into the left hemithorax on enhanced chest CT, raising suspicion for absence of the pericardium. No focal herniation of the heart was seen through a pericardial defect in this case.

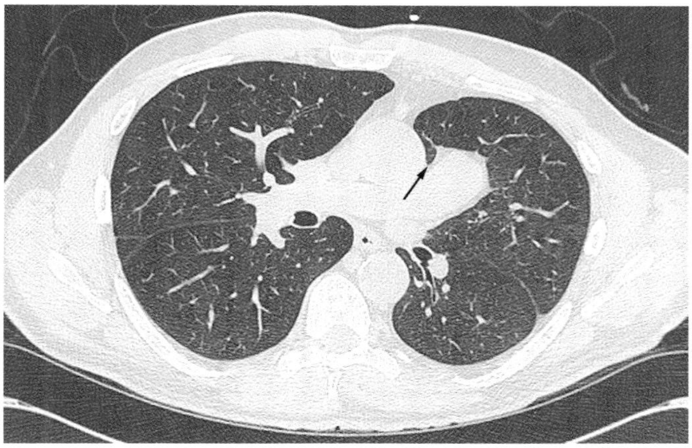

Figure 22.2. Axial non-contrast CT from the same patient demonstrates lung interposed between the ascending aorta and the main pulmonary artery (arrow), in a location that normally contains fat covered by pericardium.

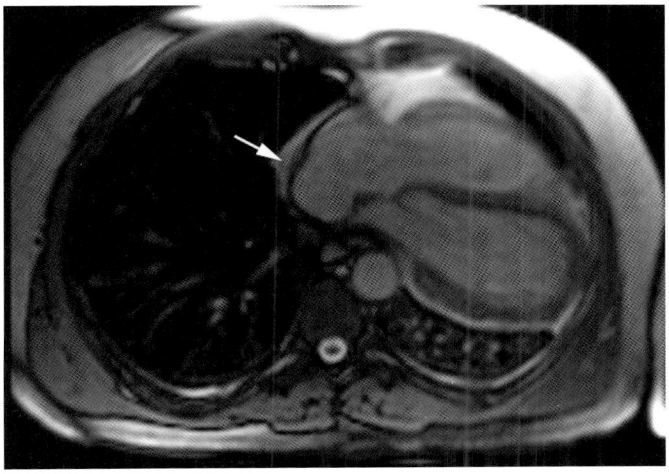

Figure 22.3. Axial bright blood MR image from a 57-year-old male with known congenital absence of the pericardium demonstrates a small rim of hypointense pericardium (arrow) adjacent to the right atrium but no pericardium adjacent to either ventricle.

CASE **23**

Partial anomalous pulmonary venous return

Tessa S. Cook

Imaging description

Partial anomalous pulmonary venous return (PAPVR) is characterized by the inappropriate drainage of one or more pulmonary veins into the systemic venous circulation. Anomalous drainage of the left superior pulmonary vein to the left brachiocephalic vein or the right superior pulmonary vein to the superior vena cava (Figures 23.1 and 23.2) are the most common incidentally encountered forms of PAPVR in adults undergoing chest CT exams.[1] Right upper lobe PAPVR is associated with a sinus venosus type atrial septal defect in 42% of patients (Figure 23.2).[1] Scimitar syndrome is a specialized form of PAPVR that predominantly involves the right-sided pulmonary veins (Figure 23.3). In this scenario, the right inferior pulmonary vein drains below the diaphragm to join the IVC just distal to the hepatic vein confluence (Figure 23.1). Scimitar syndrome is often associated with right-sided thoracic anomalies, such as a hypoplastic right lung (Figure 23.2). PAPVR is a left-to-right shunt, and depending on the volume of shunting, right-sided cardiac chamber enlargement and pulmonary artery enlargement may be present (Figure 23.1).

Importance

PAPVR occurs in many forms, which together have a prevalence of less than 1%.[2] Although rare, PAPVR can be detected incidentally in asymptomatic patients, which may prompt further evaluation to assess need for repair. In addition, in patients being evaluated for an occult shunt due to right-sided chamber enlargement, PAPVR is an important subtype of shunt that may be missed by echocardiography. Cross-sectional imaging becomes important for characterization of the anatomy, particularly in patients who are symptomatic and are undergoing preoperative evaluation. Surgical therapy is generally considered if the Qp:Qs is at least 1.5:1, because of the risk of pulmonary hypertension and right ventricular failure.[3]

Typical clinical scenario

The timing of diagnosis of PAPVR is closely related to the degree of symptoms and number of associated anomalies. Patients who are incidentally found to have PAPVR as adults are rarely symptomatic and have few associated anomalies, while those who are diagnosed earlier in life typically have more severe symptoms and a higher number of associated congenital malformations.[1] Symptoms associated with PAPVR are non-specific, and include chest pain, shortness of breath, tachycardia, palpitations, and electrophysiologic abnormalities.

Differential diagnosis

PAPVR is on the differential diagnosis for left-to-right shunts, including atrial or ventricular septal defects, as well as a patent ductus arteriosus.

Teaching point

PAPVR is one cause of left-to-right shunt that can remain undetected until adulthood and should be considered in patients with enlarged right-sided cardiac chambers and pulmonary hypertension of unclear etiology. The chronic shunt physiology can increase the risk of pulmonary hypertension and right ventricular failure.

REFERENCES

1. M. L. Ho, S. Bhalla, A. Bierhals, F. Gutierrez. MDCT of partial anomalous pulmonary venous return (PAPVR) in adults. *J Thorac Imaging* 2009; **24**: 89–95.
2. J. R. Dillman, S. G. Yarram, R. J. Hernandez. Imaging of pulmonary venous developmental anomalies. *AJR Am J Roentgenol* 2009; **192**: 1272–85.
3. E. H. Sears, J. M. Aliotta, J. R. Klinger. Partial anomalous pulmonary venous return presenting with adult-onset pulmonary hypertension. *Pulm Circ* 2012; **2**: 250–5.

Pearls and Pitfalls in Cardiovascular Imaging, ed. Stefan L. Zimmerman and Elliot K. Fishman. Published by Cambridge University Press. © Cambridge University Press 2015.

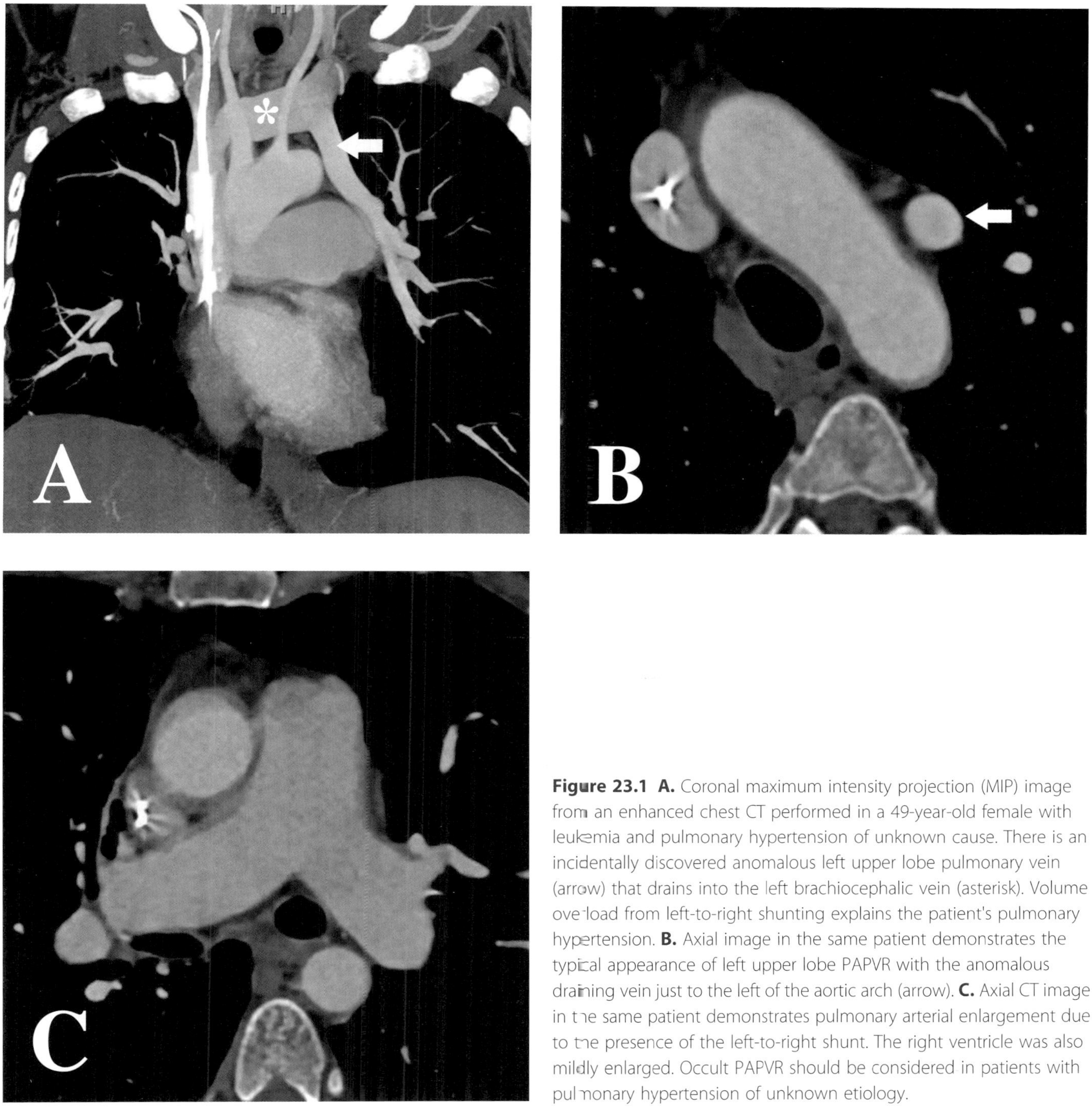

Figure 23.1 **A.** Coronal maximum intensity projection (MIP) image from an enhanced chest CT performed in a 49-year-old female with leukemia and pulmonary hypertension of unknown cause. There is an incidentally discovered anomalous left upper lobe pulmonary vein (arrow) that drains into the left brachiocephalic vein (asterisk). Volume overload from left-to-right shunting explains the patient's pulmonary hypertension. **B.** Axial image in the same patient demonstrates the typical appearance of left upper lobe PAPVR with the anomalous draining vein just to the left of the aortic arch (arrow). **C.** Axial CT image in the same patient demonstrates pulmonary arterial enlargement due to the presence of the left-to-right shunt. The right ventricle was also mildly enlarged. Occult PAPVR should be considered in patients with pulmonary hypertension of unknown etiology.

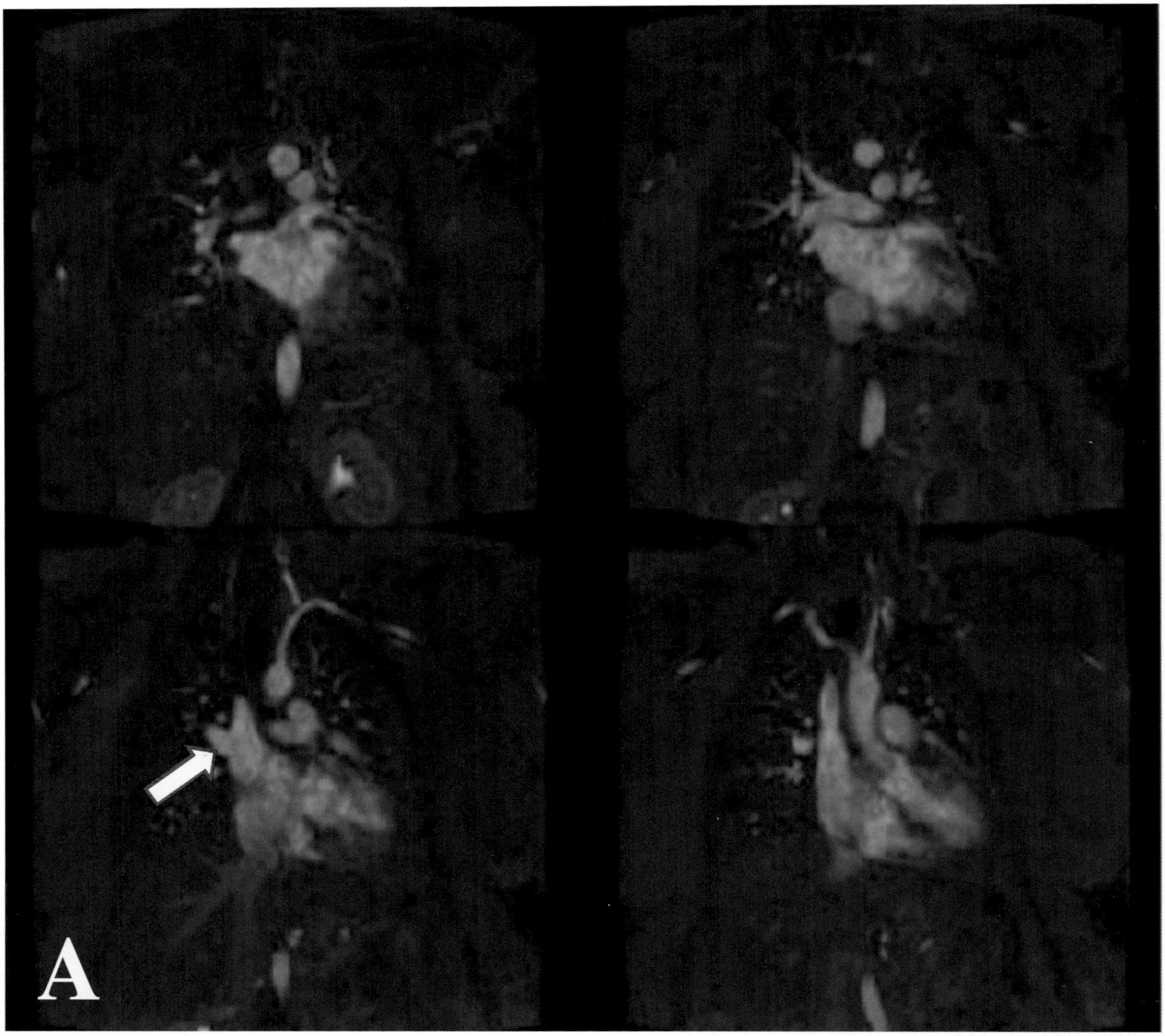

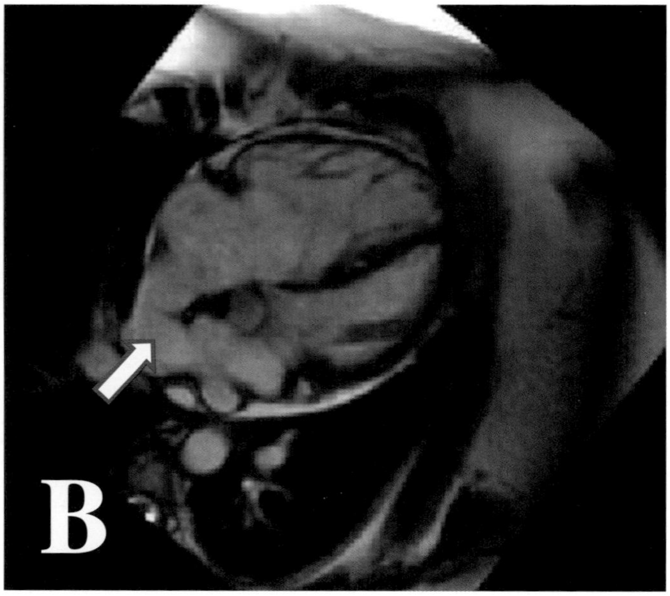

Figure 23.2 A. Coronal images from an MR angiogram performed in a 66-year-old female with cardiomegaly and a newly diagnosed left-to-right shunt. The right upper lobe pulmonary vein drains into the IVC (arrow), while the remaining pulmonary veins drain into the left atrium. **B.** On a bright blood steady-state free precession image obtained in the four-chamber view, a sinus venosus atrial septal defect (arrow) is also detected in the same 66-year-old female patient, consistent with the left-to-right shunt. The sinus venosus ASD is commonly associated with right upper lobe PAPVR due to the "unroofing" of the pulmonary vein into the superior vena cava. The right ventricle is dilated with bowing of the interventricular septum due to volume overload.

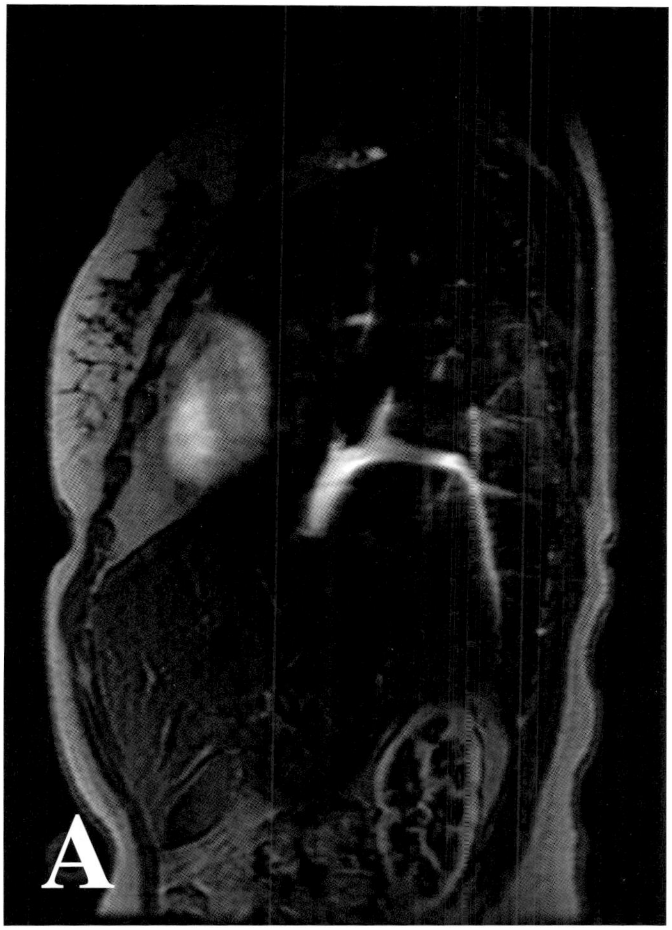

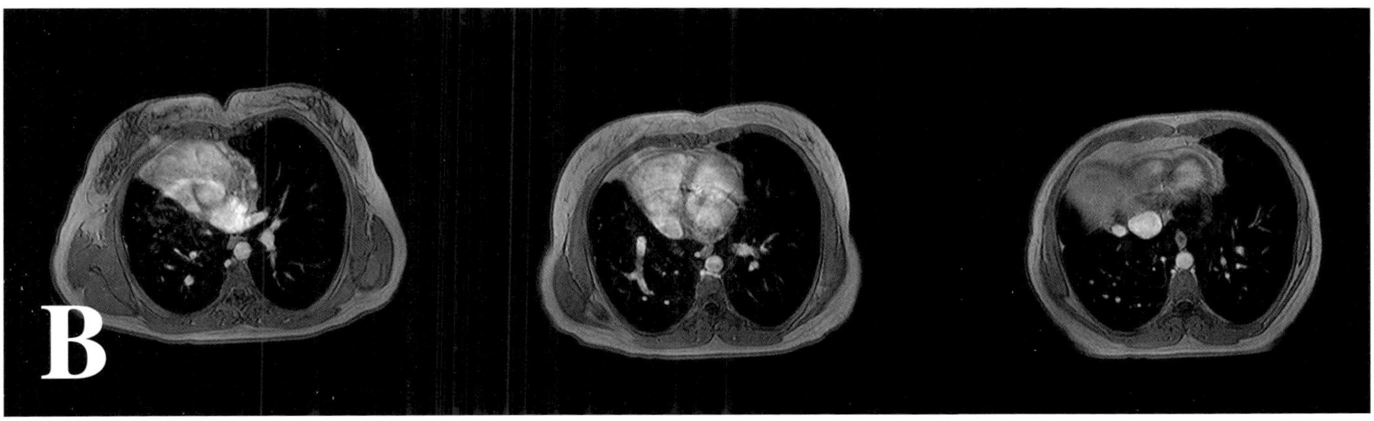

Figure 23.3 **A.** Sagittal MR angiogram in a 39-year-old female with known pulmonary vein anomaly demonstrating vessels from the right lower lobe draining toward an infradiaphragmatic vessel that is not seen on this image. **B.** Sequential axial images from an MR angiogram in the same patient demonstrate a hypoplastic right lung and paucity of pulmonary veins draining to the right hilum and a pulmonary vein approaching the IVC. These findings are consistent with scimitar syndrome, a form of PAPVR that specifically affects the right-sided pulmonary veins and is associated with hypoplasia of the right lung, right pulmonary artery, and other right-sided musculoskeletal anomalies.

CASE **24**

Unroofed coronary sinus

Mark Stellingworth and Stefan L. Zimmerman

Imaging description

Unroofed coronary sinus is a communication between the coronary sinus and left atrium. The result is a left-to-right shunt that allows flow of oxygenated blood from the left atrium into the coronary sinus. In the normal situation, the coronary sinus courses inferior to the undersurface of the left atrium in the left atrioventricular groove, emptying into the right atrium. In unroofed coronary sinus there is a variably sized communication between the two structures (Figure 24.1). In partial unroofing, a single or several small orifices are seen. In complete unroofing, there is total absence of the tissue separating the left atrium and coronary sinus. At cross-sectional imaging, defects are optimally visualized in a short-axis plane parallel to the atrioventricular groove (Figure 24.2).[1] Associated signs include enlargement of the right atrium and right ventricle due to shunting, which can be quantified using phase-contrast MRI.[1,2] In the case of small restrictive defects, turbulent flow jets may be visualized in the left atrium on cardiac MRI.

Importance

Unroofed coronary sinus is a rare cause for left-to-right shunt. It may be challenging to make the diagnosis on transthoracic echocardiography due to limited imaging windows,[3] resulting in referral of patients to cardiac CT or MRI to evaluate for occult shunt. Diagnosis is important due to potential for transient right-to-left shunting that can result in systemic emboli or brain abscess.[1]

Typical clinical scenario

Unroofed coronary sinus is a rare disorder that is the least common type of atrial septal defect, representing less than 1% of these anomalies.[3] There is a frequent association with left-sided superior vena cava, which is seen in approximately 63–75% of cases.[1,2] Many patients will have additional congenital cardiac defects.[2]

Differential diagnosis

Unroofed coronary sinus should be distinguished from other types of potentially difficult to diagnose left-to-right shunts, such as sinus venosus atrial septal defects and partial anomalous pulmonary venous return. Normal enlargement of the coronary sinus can occur in the setting of a left-sided superior vena cava, and does not imply the presence of a shunt if no defect is seen.

Teaching point

Unroofed coronary sinus is a rare cause of left-to-right shunt that should be considered in patients presenting for occult shunt evaluation.

REFERENCES

1. H. Kim, Y. H. Choe, S. W. Park, et al. Partially unroofed coronary sinus: MDCT and MRI findings. *AJR Am J Roentgenol* 2010; **195**: W331–6.
2. S. S. Shah, S. D. Teague, J. C. Lu, A. L. Dorfman, E. A. Kazerooni, P. P. Agarwal. Imaging of the coronary sinus: normal anatomy and congenital abnormalities. *Radiographics* 2012; **32**: 991–1008.
3. A. El-Eshmawi, G. H. Tang, A. Pawale, A. C. Anyanwu, D. H. Adams. Unroofed coronary sinus in an adult. *J Card Surg* 2013; **28**: 19–22.

Pearls and Pitfalls in Cardiovascular Imaging, ed. Stefan L. Zimmerman and Elliot K. Fishman. Published by Cambridge University Press. © Cambridge University Press 2015.

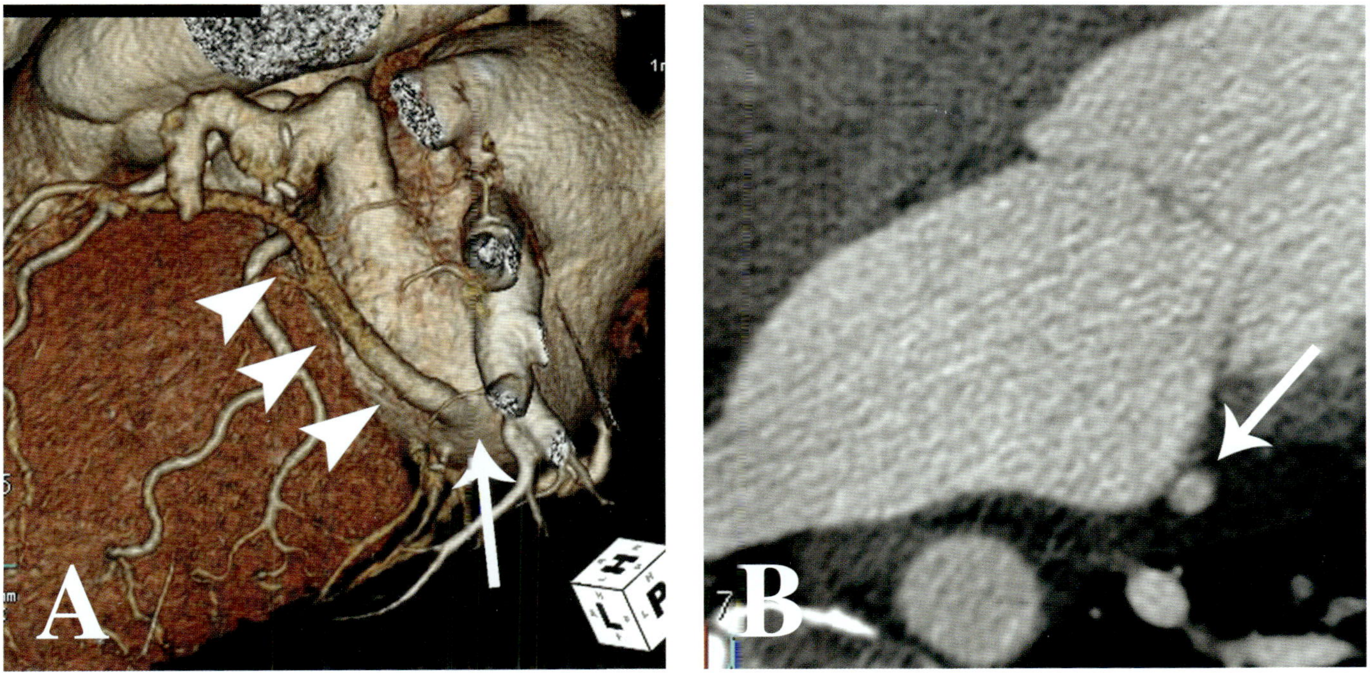

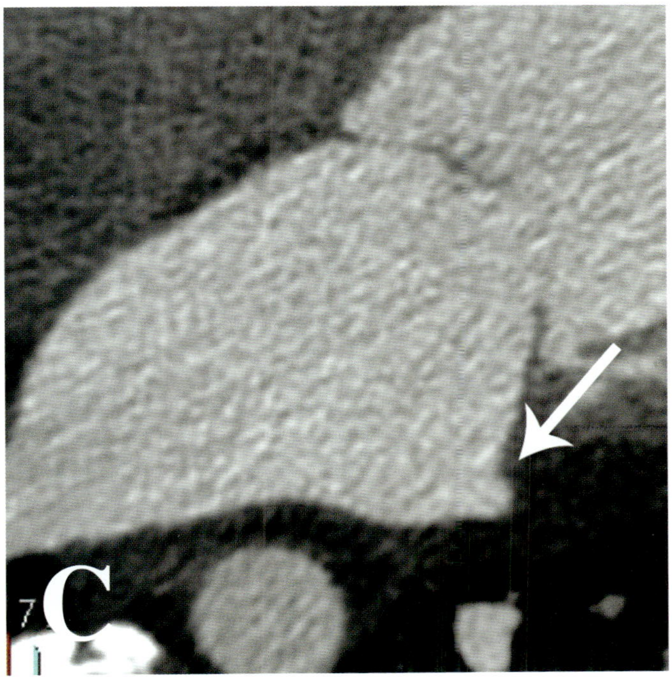

Figure 24.1 A. Sagittal volume rendered image from a cardiac CT performed in a 46-year-old female being evaluated for suspected right-to-left shunt. There is an unroofed coronary sinus (arrowheads) which drains directly into the left atrium (long arrow). This finding is confirmed on contiguous axial source images (**B,C**) which show the coronary sinus (long arrow) draining into the left atrium.

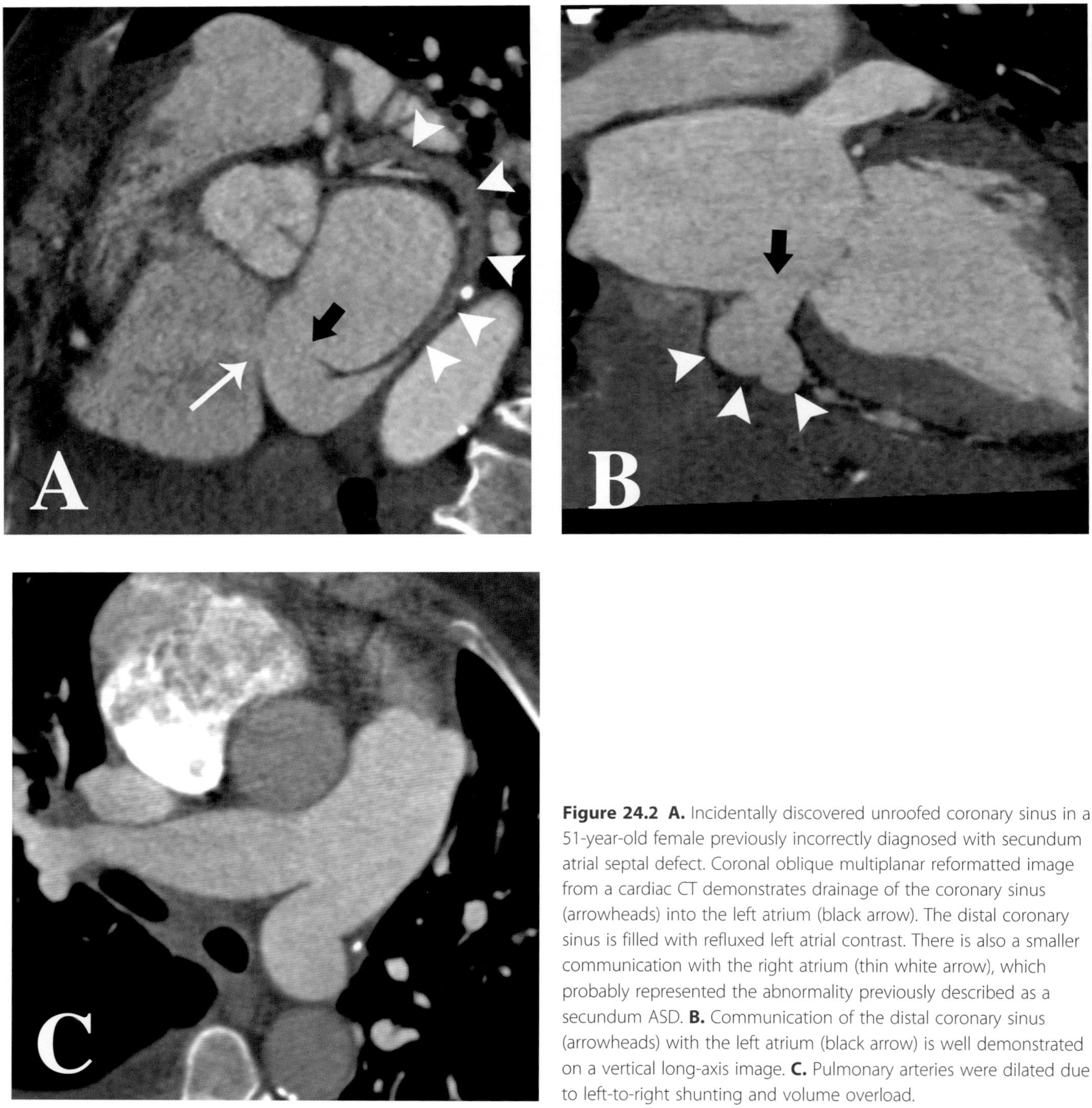

Figure 24.2 **A.** Incidentally discovered unroofed coronary sinus in a 51-year-old female previously incorrectly diagnosed with secundum atrial septal defect. Coronal oblique multiplanar reformatted image from a cardiac CT demonstrates drainage of the coronary sinus (arrowheads) into the left atrium (black arrow). The distal coronary sinus is filled with refluxed left atrial contrast. There is also a smaller communication with the right atrium (thin white arrow), which probably represented the abnormality previously described as a secundum ASD. **B.** Communication of the distal coronary sinus (arrowheads) with the left atrium (black arrow) is well demonstrated on a vertical long-axis image. **C.** Pulmonary arteries were dilated due to left-to-right shunting and volume overload.

CASE 25

Patent ductus arteriosus

Tessa S. Cook

Imaging description

A tubular connection between the proximal descending aorta and the main pulmonary artery which opacifies after intravenous contrast administration (Figure 25.1) most likely represents a patent ductus arteriosus (PDA). The luminal diameter of the PDA is typically larger at the aortic end than at the pulmonic end (Figure 25.2). Cine imaging can be used to confirm that there is flow through the vessel from the aorta to the pulmonary artery, rather than just a pseudoaneurysm of the aorta that abuts the main pulmonary artery. Sagittal oblique MR images through the aorta demonstrate the PDA and confirm its patency by capturing the flow jet (dark signal) caused by flow into the main pulmonary artery (Figure 25.3).

Importance

The significance of a patent ductus arteriosus detected on imaging depends on its effect on the patient. Evaluation of the functional significance of a PDA is ideally performed with a cardiac MRI that can quantify not only cardiac ejection fraction but also shunt fraction and direction. An incidentally discovered PDA may not need further imaging evaluation in an asymptomatic individual.

Typical clinical scenario

The ductus arteriosus (DA) is an embryological connection between the proximal descending aorta and the main pulmonary artery (MPA). It exists to shunt deoxygenated blood away from the pulmonic circulation (which is high resistance *in utero*) back into the aorta so that it can travel to the placenta for oxygenation. The incidence of patent ductus arteriosus is low in term infants (57 per 100,000 live births) but can be very high in preterm infants (1 in 3 live births).[1]

Normally the DA closes within 24–48 hours of birth, although it can be kept open pharmacologically with the administration of prostaglandins, particularly in the case of congenital heart disease where a left-to-right shunt is necessary to survive until surgery (Figure 25.4).[2] When it closes normally, the DA becomes the ligamentum arteriosum, a fibrous connection between the two great vessels without any lumen. In preterm infants, the DA can remain open and may require pharmacologic closure with the administration of NSAIDs such as indomethacin or ibuprofen, or surgical closure with a device or coils.

Individuals with a PDA may present with a murmur or worsening heart failure, as a result of the left-to-right shunt. Many, however, are asymptomatic and the presence of a PDA is discovered only when thoracic imaging is ordered for other reasons.[3]

Differential diagnosis

The differential diagnosis of an apparent anatomic connection between the aorta and main pulmonary artery includes a PDA or pseudoaneurysm of the aorta or pulmonary artery in that location. The differential diagnosis of heart failure or suspected left-to-right shunt is much broader, and includes atrial or ventricular septal defects, patent foramen ovale, and anomalous pulmonary venous return.

Teaching point

The patent ductus arteriosus is more common in preterm infants than term infants. It may be completely asymptomatic or cause symptoms ranging from a systolic murmur to severe heart failure and pulmonary volume overload. Identification of a PDA on imaging should be correlated to symptoms suggestive of a left-to-right shunt.

REFERENCES

1. S. E. Hamrick, G. Hansmann. Patent ductus arteriosus of the preterm infant. *Pediatrics* 2010; **125**: 1020–30.
2. D. J. Schneider, J. W. Moore. Patent ductus arteriosus. *Circulation* 2006; **114**: 1873–82.
3. O. Goitein, C. R. Fuhrman, J. M. Lacomis. Incidental finding on MDCT of patent ductus arteriosus: use of CT and MRI to assess clinical importance. *AJR Am J Roentgenol* 2005; **184**: 1924–31.

Pearls and Pitfalls in Cardiovascular Imaging, ed. Stefan L. Zimmerman and Elliot K. Fishman. Published by Cambridge University Press. © Cambridge University Press 2015.

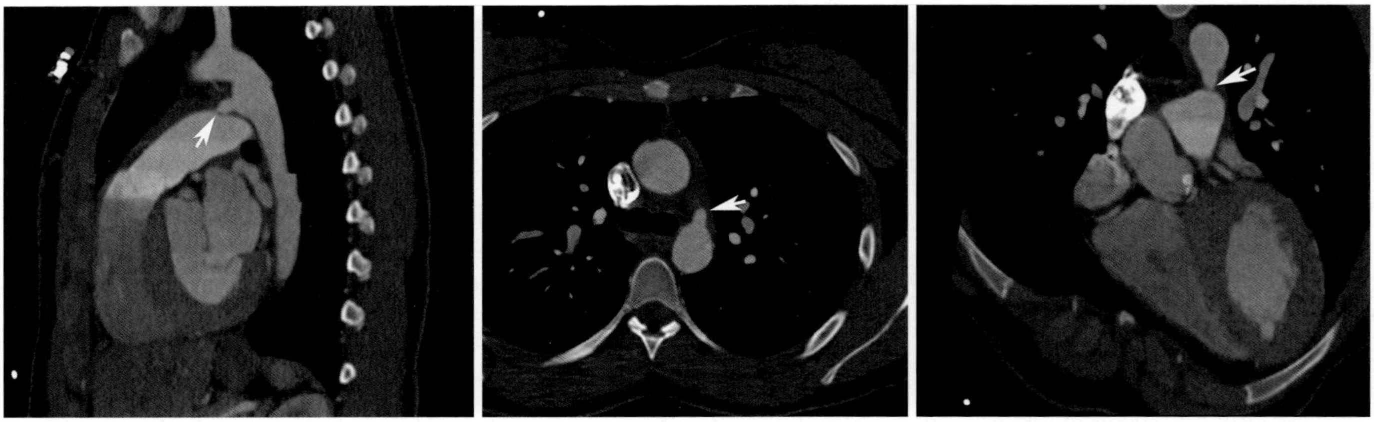

Figure 25.1 Orthogonal planes through the gated CTA from a 22-year-old female patient imaged for evaluation of a bicuspid aortic valve showing a focal outpouching (arrows) arising from the left inferior aspect of the proximal descending aorta and extending toward the main pulmonary artery.

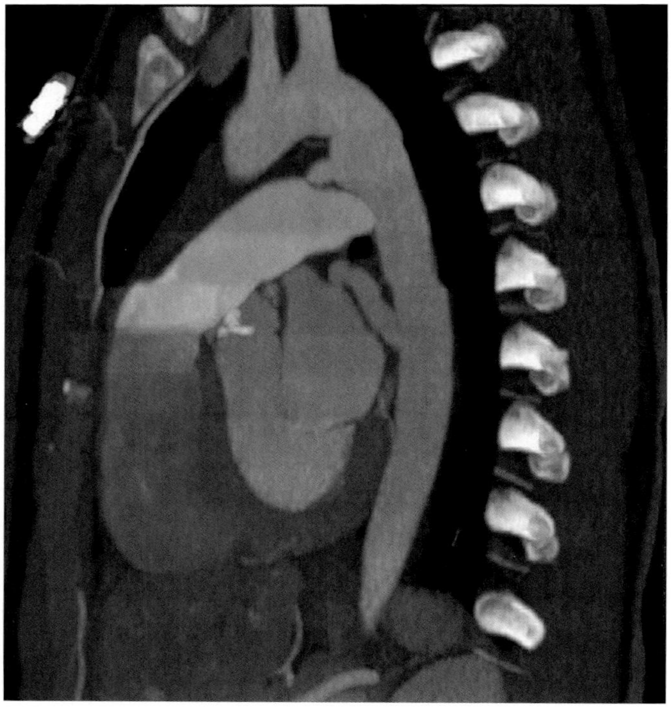

Figure 25.2 Sagittal oblique maximum intensity projection from the same patient as in Figure 25.1, demonstrating the connection between the descending aorta and the main pulmonary artery, in keeping with a PDA. Note that the conduit is wider at the aortic end compared to the pulmonic end, where it appears extremely narrow.

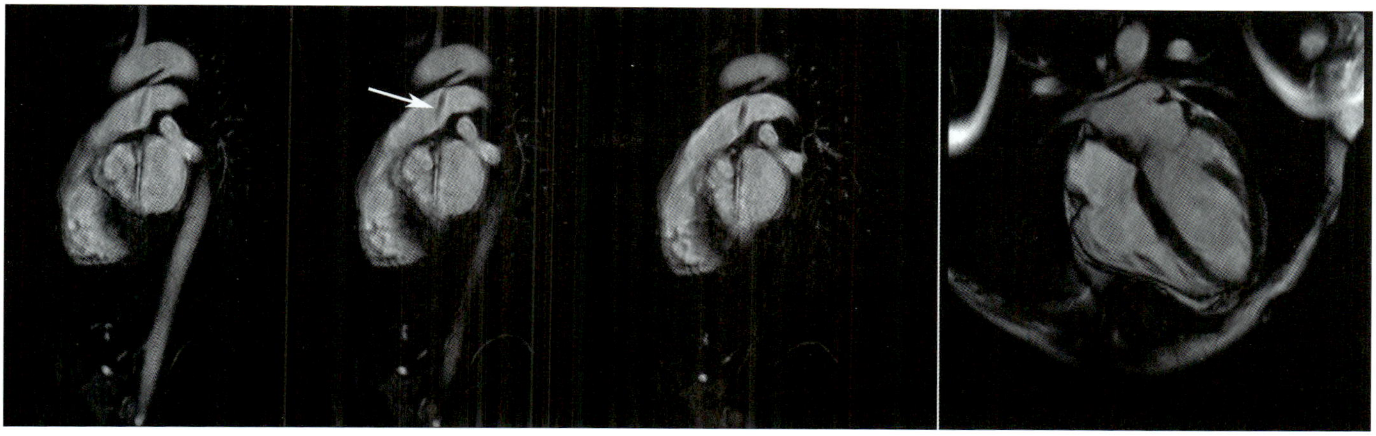

Figure 25.3 Sagittal oblique MR images (left) from a 47-year-old female with a possible PDA seen on echocardiography demonstrate a PDA connecting the descending aorta to the main pulmonary artery. The patency of the conduit is confirmed by the flow jet within the pulmonary artery (arrow). Four-chamber bright blood image (right) demonstrates normal left and right ventricular sizes, without significant dilation of the right heart. Cine imaging can be helpful to confirm patency and assess the functional impact of a PDA.

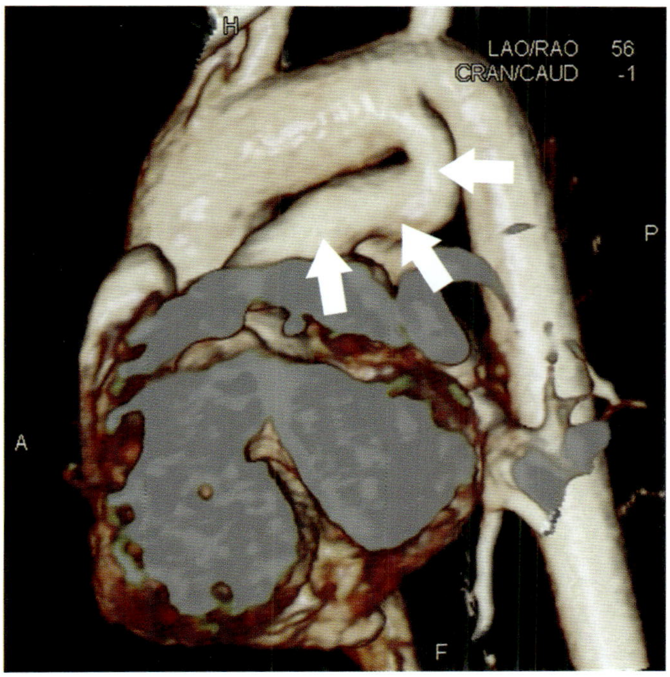

Figure 25.4 Sagittal oblique volume rendered image from a CT angiogram obtained in a 4-day-old premature infant with tetralogy of Fallot and main pulmonary artery hypoplasia demonstrates a large patent ductus arteriosus (white arrows) connecting the aorta to the main pulmonary artery (not pictured). In this patient, ductal patency was maintained pharmacologically to preserve lung perfusion.

CASE 26 Bicuspid aortic valve with raphe mimicking tricuspid valve

Stefan L. Zimmerman

Imaging description

Bicuspid aortic valves are congenital malformations of the aortic valve that result in two functional aortic valve leaflets. In the majority of cases, the right and left aortic cusps are fused with a central raphe, or ridge, that is variable in size.[1] On static images of the aortic valve acquired in diastole with either cardiac CT or MRI, a bicuspid valve with prominent raphe will have an appearance that mimics a tricuspid valve (Figure 26.1). However, dynamic images obtained during systole will reliably demonstrate the restricted motion of the fused valve and typical fish-mouth appearance of the aortic valve orifice using either modality.[2,3] Bicuspid valves are also typically morphologically abnormal with leaflet thickening and calcification commonly identified, that can suggest further investigation (Figure 26.2). Fusion occurs between the left and right cusps in the majority of patients.[4]

Importance

Recognition of a bicuspid valve is important given the increased risk of aortic stenosis, regurgitation, aneurysm, and dissection.[1] Patients with bicuspid valve are closely followed with serial echocardiography to assess valve and ventricular function.[1]

Typical clinical scenario

Bicuspid aortic valve is the most common congenital cardiovascular abnormality, affecting 1–2% of the population.[4] Bicuspid valve morphology is highly variable; however, fusion of the right and left cusps with a midline raphe is the most common pattern, found in 59% of cases in one large series.[5] Patients with bicuspid valve may be referred to cardiac CT or MRI for assessment of coronary arteries, ventricular function, or aortic size. Bicuspid valves may also be an incidental finding on cardiac imaging exams performed for other indications.

Differential diagnosis

Tricuspid aortic valve with acquired cusp fusion due to senile degeneration can be difficult to distinguish from congenitally bicuspid aortic valve with raphe given similar morphologies. Central calcification of the midline raphe, unequal cusp size, and the presence of an ascending aortic aneurysm are more commonly associated with bicuspid valves and can suggest the diagnosis.[6]

Teaching point

Bicuspid aortic valves with a prominent central raphe can be mistaken for tricuspid valves on static images acquired in diastole. Clinical suspicion for a bicuspid valve or identification of valve thickening and calcification should prompt further investigation with functional cardiac imaging. Bicuspid valves will then be easily recognized by the characteristic fish-mouthed opening in systole.

REFERENCES

1. S. C. Siu, C. K. Silversides. Bicuspid aortic valve disease. *J Am Coll Cardiol* 2010; **55**: 2789–800.
2. H. Alkadhi, S. Leschka, P. T. Trindade, et al. Cardiac CT for the differentiation of bicuspid and tricuspid aortic valves: comparison with echocardiography and surgery. *AJR Am J Roentgenol* 2010; **195**: 900–8.
3. T. G. Gleeson, I. Mwangi, S. J. Horgan, A. Cradock, P. Fitzpatrick, J. G. Murray. Steady-state free-precession (SSFP) cine MRI in distinguishing normal and bicuspid aortic valves. *J Magn Reson Imaging* 2008; **28**: 873–8.
4. C. J. Bennett, J. J. Maleszewski, P. A. Araoz. CT and MR imaging of the aortic valve: radiologic–pathologic correlation. *Radiographics* 2012; **32**: 1399–420.
5. B. M. Schaefer, M. B. Lewin, K. K. Stout, et al. The bicuspid aortic valve: an integrated phenotypic classification of leaflet morphology and aortic root shape. *Heart* 2008; **94**: 1634–8.
6. I. Joo, E. A. Park, K. H. Kim, W. Lee, J. W. Chung, J. H. Park. MDCT differentiation between bicuspid and tricuspid aortic valves in patients with aortic valvular disease: correlation with surgical findings. *Int J Cardiovasc Imaging* 2012; **28**: 171–82.

Pearls and Pitfalls in Cardiovascular Imaging, ed. Stefan L. Zimmerman and Elliot K. Fishman. Published by Cambridge University Press. © Cambridge University Press 2015.

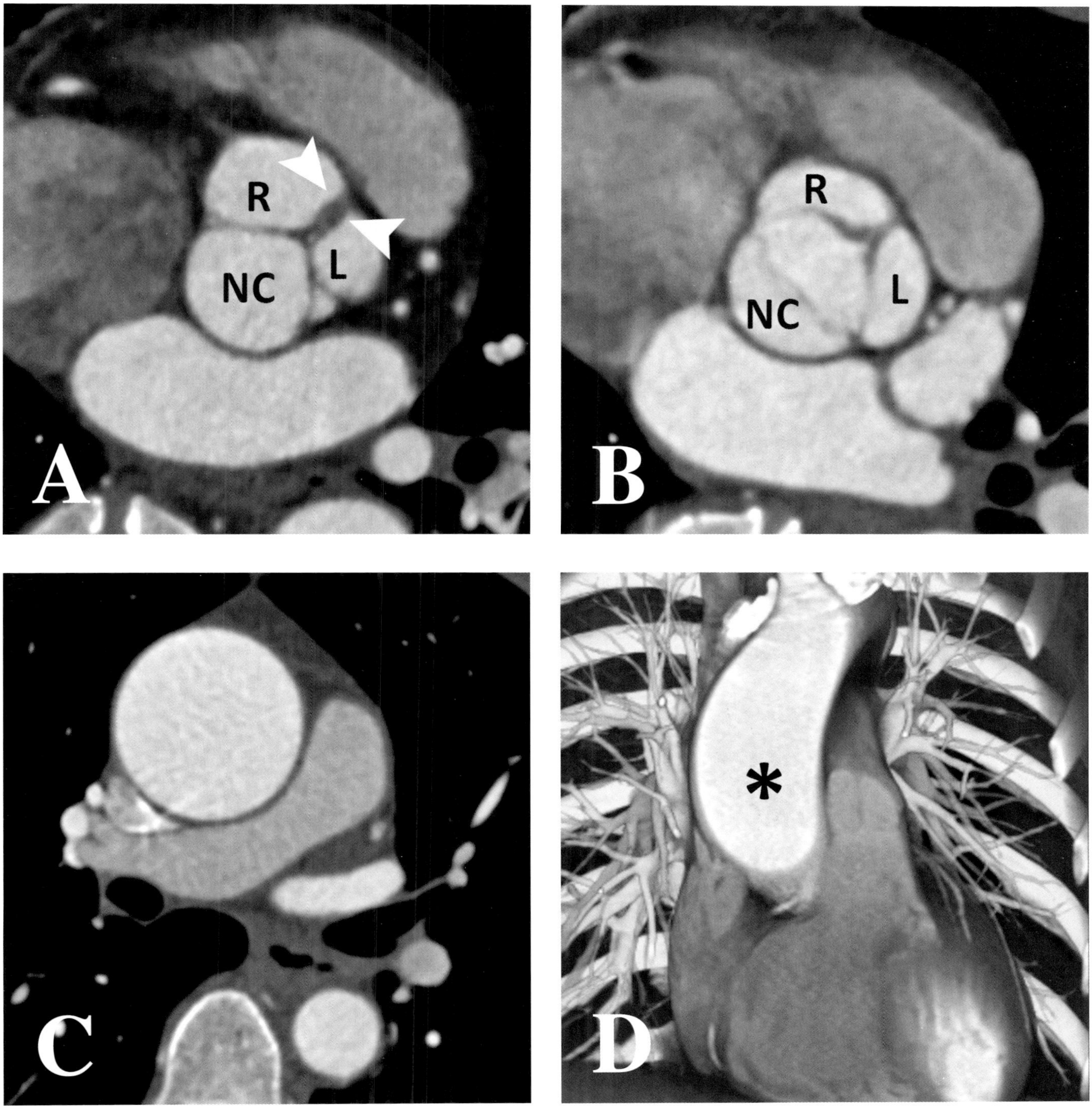

Figure 26.1 **A.** Short-axis end-diastolic image of the aortic valve from a cardiac CT obtained in a 50-year-old female with ascending aortic aneurysm demonstrates three distinct valve cusps (R = right, L= left, and NC = non-coronary). The cusps are unequal in size and there is thickening between the right and the left cusps (arrowheads), findings which should suggest the possibility of bicuspid valve with raphe. **B.** On systolic images from the same study, there is a fish-mouthed opening of the aortic valve, diagnostic of bicuspid aortic valve. The thickening between right and left cusps is due to a prominent raphe at the point of cusp fusion. This can be mistaken for a tricuspid valve on static diastolic images. Axial (**C**) and volume rendered coronal (**D**) images demonstrate the aneurysm of the ascending aorta (asterisk) which is typical in patients with bicuspid valves.

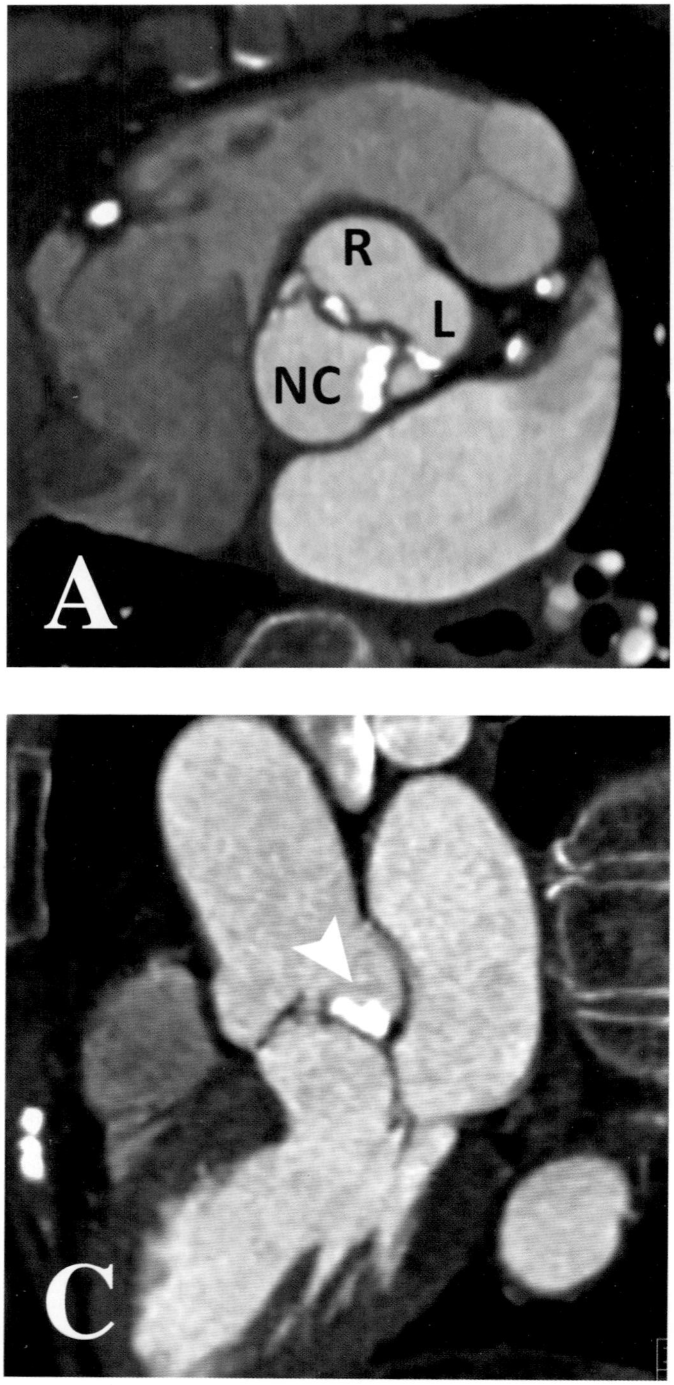

Figure 26.2 **A.** Short-axis end-diastolic image of the aortic valve from a cardiac CT obtained in an 80-year-old female with severe aortic stenosis demonstrates a bicuspid aortic valve with complete fusion of right and left cusps and no midline raphe. The valve leaflets are thickened and calcified, common findings associated with bicuspid valves. **B.** On systolic images, there is restricted opening of the valve, compatible with a history of aortic stenosis. **C.** Left venticular outflow tract view shows severe aortic valvular calcification (arrowhead).

CASE 27

Pseudocoarctation due to aortic tortuosity

Vivek Halappa and Atif Zaheer

Imaging description

Pseudocoarctation is characterized by pseudostenoses of the descending thoracic aorta just distal to the origin of the left subclavian artery at the level of the ligamentum arteriosum.[1] Both contrast-enhanced CT and magnetic resonance angiography are useful diagnostic imaging tests with distinct diagnostic advantages for non-invasive assessment of the abnormality. Multiplanar reformatted images are particularly helpful in differentiating this entity from true coarctation with demonstration of "kinking and buckling" and an elongated descending aorta with absence of collateral circulation (Figures 27.1 and 27.2).[2] MRI has the added advantage of providing measurement of the pressure gradient before and after the area of pseudocoarctation using phase-contrast imaging as well as estimates of collateral flow volume.[3] In cases of pseudocoarction, the pressure gradient should be negligible, whereas it will be elevated in coarctation with intervention considered at a threshold of 15–20 mmHg.[3]

Importance

Pseudocoarctation, a rare congenital anomaly, manifests as kinking of the aortic arch due to its redundancy. Recognition of this abnormality is important since it may be mistaken for true coarctation, aneurysm, or mediastinal neoplasm. Additionally, pseudocoarctation is associated with other abnormalities such as bicuspid aortic valve, patent ductus arteriosus, ventricular septal defect, and anomalies of the left subclavian artery (Figure 27.3).[4,5]

Typical clinical scenario

Pseudocoarctation is usually asymptomatic and may be an incidental finding on imaging. Findings of esophageal compression with dysphagia and weight loss may also be seen.[2] Patients may be monitored for aneursymal dilatation in the affected areas.[6]

Differential diagnosis

Differential diagnosis for pseudocoarctation includes true coarctation, aneurysm, and mediastinal neoplasm. Pseudocoarctation is differentiated from true coarctation of the aorta by the absence of significant hemodynamic obstruction and collateral vessels.

Teaching point

Accurate diagnosis of pseudocoarctation is important and follow-up is recommended for asymptomatic patients without associated anomalies and treatment is recommended for symptomatic patients and those with associated anomalies.

REFERENCES

1. C. Sebastia, S. Quiroga, R. Boye, M. Perez-Lafuente, E. Castella, A. Alvarez-Castells. Aortic stenosis: spectrum of diseases depicted at multisection CT. *Radiographics* 2003; **23** Spec No: S79–91.
2. R. M. Kessler, K. B. Miller, S. Pett, J. A. Wernly. Pseudocoarctation of the aorta presenting as a mediastinal mass with dysphagia. *Ann Thorac Surg* 1993; **55**: 1003–5.
3. J. J. Hom, K. Ordovas, G. P. Reddy. Velocity-encoded cine MR imaging in aortic coarctation: functional assessment of hemodynamic events. *Radiographics* 2008; **28**: 407–16.
4. I. Steinberg, M. A. Engle, G. R. Holswade, J. W. Hagstrom. Pseudocoarctation of the aorta associated with congenital heart disease: report of ten cases. *Am J Roentgenol Radium Ther Nucl Med* 1969; **106**: 1–20.
5. D. A. Bluemke. Pseudocoarctation of the aorta. *Cardiol J* 2007; **14**: 205–6.
6. K. Kimura, H. Ohtake, H. Kato, N. Yashiki, S. Tomita, G. Watanabe. Pseudocoarctation of the aorta complicated by thoracic aortic aneurysm. *Asian Cardiovasc Thorac Ann* 2011; **19**: 265–7.

Pearls and Pitfalls in Cardiovascular Imaging, ed. Stefan L. Zimmerman and Elliot K. Fishman. Published by Cambridge University Press. © Cambridge University Press 2015.

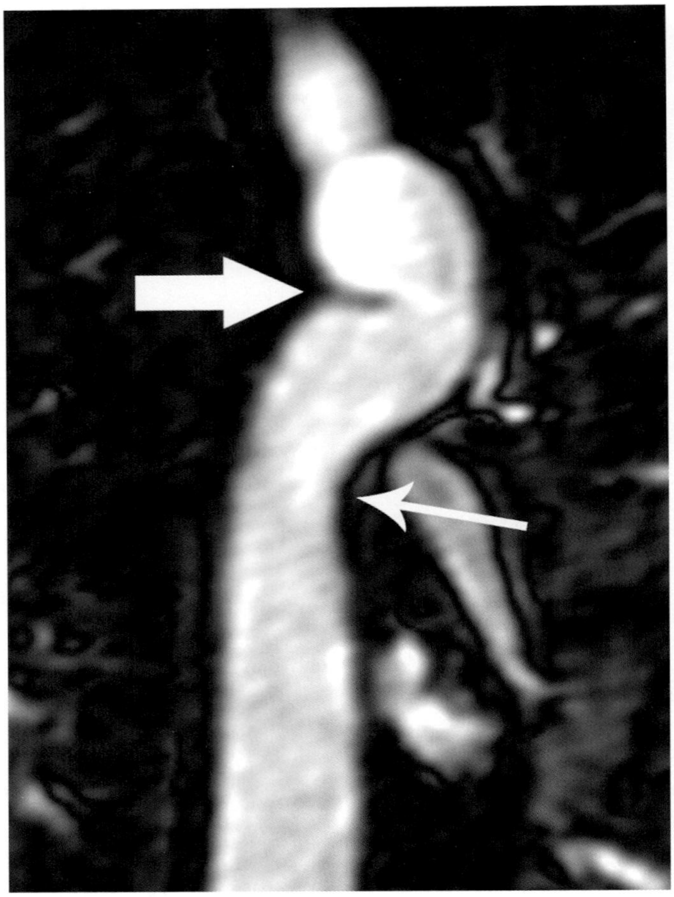

Figure 27.1 A 50-year-old man with pseudocoarctation of the aorta. Post-contrast coronal MRA image demonstrates a tortuous aorta with kinking of the arch (large arrow) and redundancy of the aorta immediately below the area of kinking.

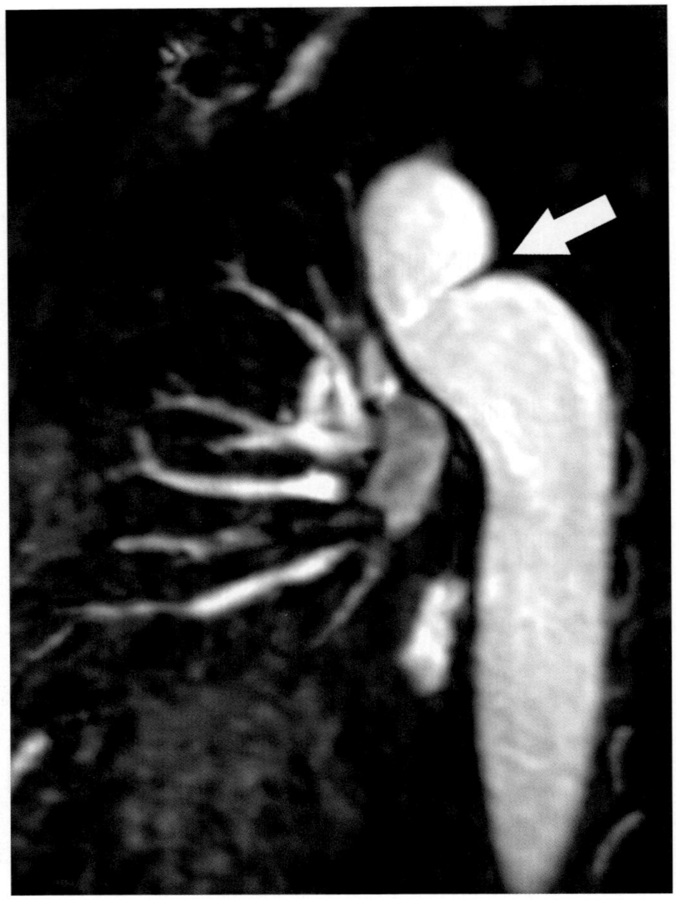

Figure 27.2 A 50-year-old man with pseudocoarctation of the aorta. Post-contrast sagittal MRA maximal intensity projection image demonstrates kinking of the arch (arrow). Note the absence of collateral circulation, a point of differentiation from true coarctation.

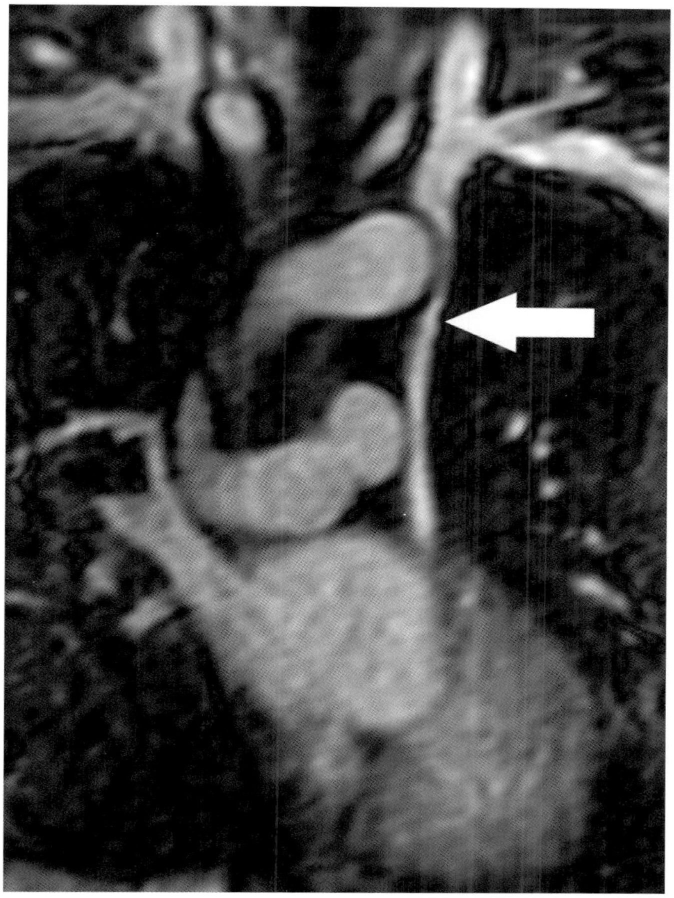

Figure 27.3 A 50-year-old man with pseudocoarctation of the aorta. Post-contrast coronal MRA image demonstrates a persistent left-sided SVC (arrow) draining into the coronary sinus.

CASE 28

Respiratory and cardiac gating artifacts in cardiac CT

Tessa S. Cook

Imaging description

Respiratory motion and heart rate variability are two of the primary causes for image artifacts on a gated thoracic computed tomographic angiography (CTA).[1] Respiratory motion artifacts affect both the heart and adjacent structures, such as the sternum anteriorly and the descending aorta posteriorly (Figures 28.1 and 28.2), and are best identified using sagittal multiplanar reformats (MPRs). On sagittal MPRs, respiratory motion will cause stair-step artifacts and discontinuity of the sternum, aorta, and cardiac chambers. Blurring of lung parenchyma will also be visible on axial images in lung windows. Coronary segments may appear blurred or absent altogether (Figure 28.3). Cardiac gating artifacts can be distinguished from respiratory motion as they only affect the heart (Figure 28.4); no sternal discontinuity will result on sagittal MPRs. The appearance of cardiac gating artifacts will vary depending on whether the study is being acquired with prospective triggering or retrospective gating. With prospective triggering, the stair-step or stepladder artifact may occur due to heart rate irregularity or arrhythmias resulting in capture of a different segment of the heart than is desired. With retrospective gating in combination with tube current modulation, gating artifacts may result in stair-step artifacts combined with a band of noisy data being reconstructed (Figure 28.5).

Importance

Obtaining a diagnostic coronary CTA depends on heart rate optimization and the patient's ability to breath-hold during the image acquisition. In the absence of one or both of these factors, the resulting artifacts may lead to suboptimal evaluation or even complete non-visualization of certain coronary segments. Effective protocoling of a coronary CTA should include assessment of the patient's heart rate and breathing, and implementation of necessary interventions, such as beta blockade, to decrease high heart rates or accommodate known arrhythmias. The ability to successfully acquire a diagnostic gated thoracic CTA examination can be affected by irregular heart rates or arrhythmias such as atrial fibrillation. Studies must be carefully protocoled in order to make sure that diagnostic-quality images can be obtained. Prospective triggering with ECG-gated acquisitions in end-systole (200–450 milliseconds after the R wave) may improve quality of exams in this challenging patient population.[2]

Typical clinical scenario

Respiratory and cardiac gating artifacts can affect the diagnostic quality of a gated CTA. These artifacts typically occur when the patient's heart rate is not well controlled, or the patient is unprepared for the potential transient discomfort associated with an intravenous contrast injection. Both respiratory motion and heart rate variability can occur in the same patient (Figure 28.6). In addition to protocoling the image acquisition portion of a gated CTA, it is important to determine a priori the patient's heart rate and consider beta blockade or other alternatives for heart rate control in order to minimize cardiac motion artifact and heart rate variability.[3] In a patient with atrial fibrillation, the feasibility of a gated study must also be gauged. Rehearsing breath-holding with the patient immediately before the study as well as identifying and addressing issues that may affect breath-holding (such as anxiety, claustrophobia, or respiratory conditions) can help to decrease the likelihood of respiratory motion artifacts.

Differential diagnosis

The differential diagnosis for indistinct or non-visualized segments of coronary arteries includes artifacts caused by different types of motion. Respiratory motion is most commonly due to a patient's inability to hold his or her breath for the duration of the trigger delay and the CT acquisition. In some cases, patients may be startled or experience significant discomfort associated with the contrast injection. As a result, patients may shift or try to readjust themselves on the scanner table, resulting in global patient motion. This can also sometimes lead to an unanticipated increase in heart rate, particularly if beta blockade has not been administered. Unexpected heart rate variability will cause motion of the coronary arteries during imaging and can occur as a result of anxiety, discomfort or arrhythmia.

Teaching point

Both respiratory and cardiac motion can result in indistinct or non-visualized portions of the heart, aorta, and coronary arteries. Sagittal multiplanar reformats are the best means for determining the cause of the motion.

Pearls and Pitfalls in Cardiovascular Imaging, ed. Stefan L. Zimmerman and Elliot K. Fishman. Published by Cambridge University Press. © Cambridge University Press 2015.

REFERENCES

1. H. S. Choi, B. W. Choi, K. O. Choe, et al. Pitfalls, artifacts, and remedies in multi-detector row CT coronary angiography. *Radiographics* 2004; **24**: 787–800.

2. M. B. Srichai, M. Barreto, R. P. Lim, R. Donnino, J. S. Babb, J. E. Jacobs. Prospective-triggered sequential dual-source end-systolic coronary CT angiography for patients with atrial fibrillation: a feasibility study. *J Cardiovasc Comput Tomogr* 2013; **7**: 102–9.

3. C. Hong, C. R. Becker, A. Huber, et al. ECG-gated reconstructed multi-detector row CT coronary angiography: effect of varying trigger delay on image quality. *Radiology* 2001; **220**: 712–17.

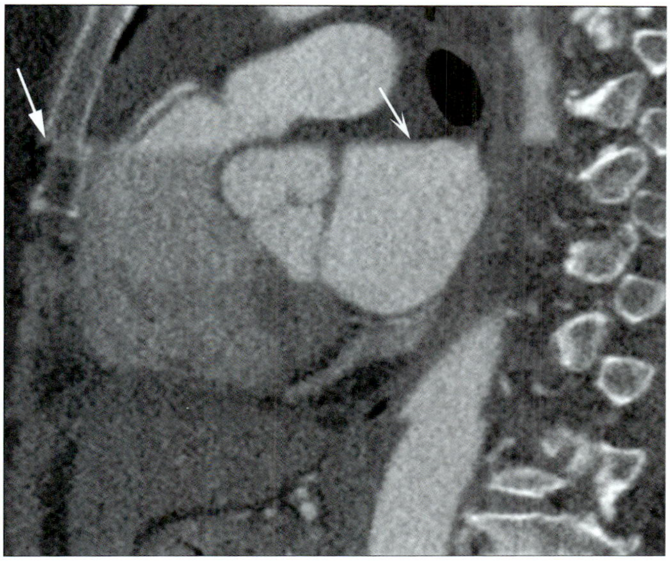

Figure 28.1 Respiratory motion in a 65-year-old male with chest pain causing discontinuity of the sternum and anterior chest wall (closed arrow) on this sagittal reformat of a coronary CTA. Note the discontinuity of the left atrium (open arrow), which is also captured on this slice.

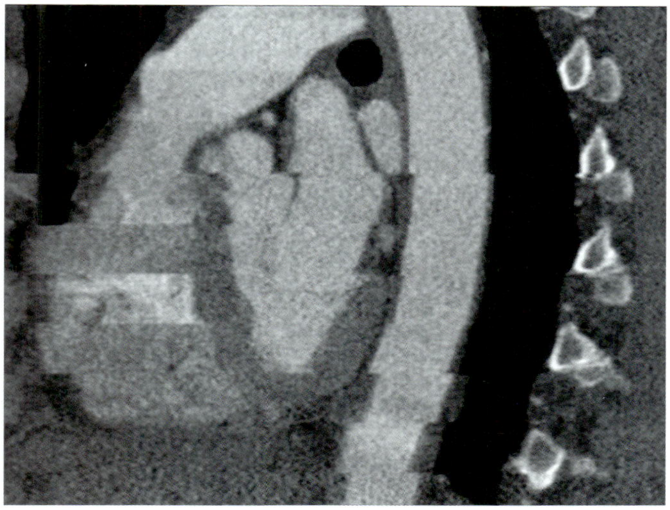

Figure 28.2 The extent of respiratory motion is much appreciated on this sagittal reformat from a 50-year-old male with chest pain, which demonstrates the stair-step artifact that occurs when the intrathoracic structures are displaced by respiratory motion during the coronary CTA.

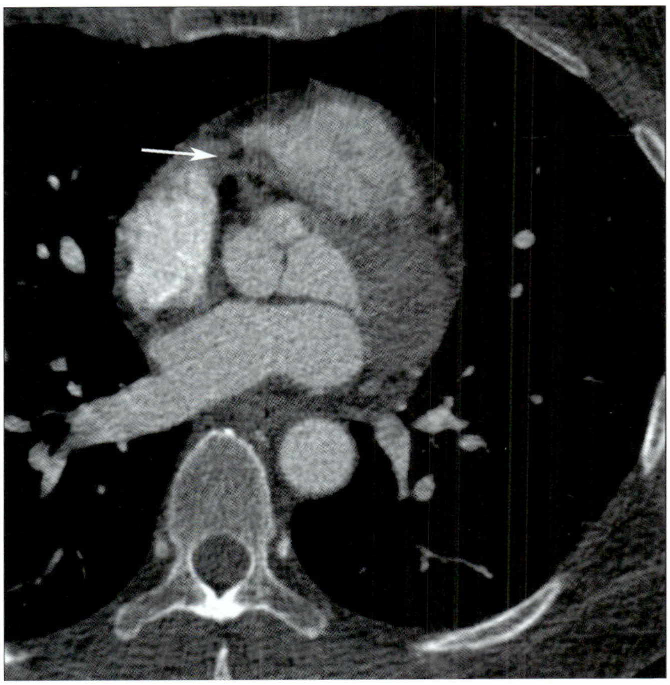

Figure 28.3 Axial coronary CT image from the same patient as Figure 28.2 demonstrating the effect of respiratory motion on the ability to distinguish the proximal segment of the right coronary artery (RCA). The RCA is blurred (arrow) and incorrectly appears to be branching just distal to the right coronary cusp.

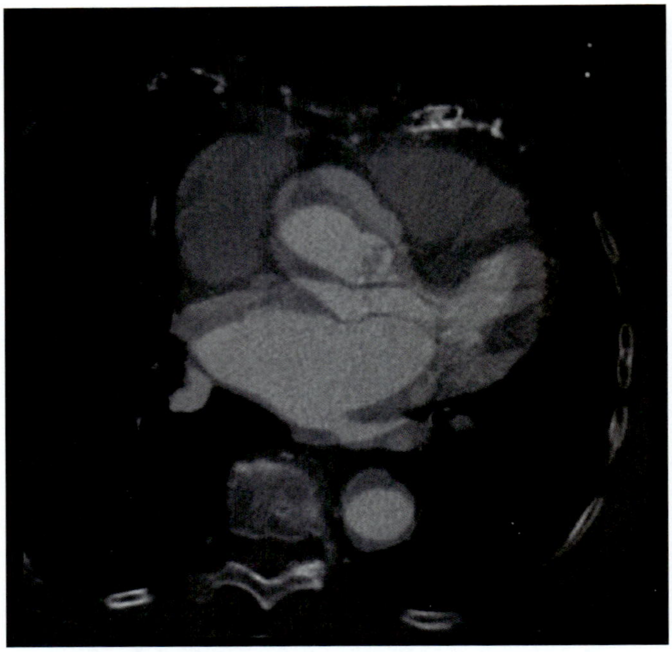

Figure 28.4 Axial image from a gated thoracic CT angiogram of a 62-year-old male with known dilation of the aortic root demonstrating cardiac gating artifact due to heart rate variability. The location of this artifact was particularly troublesome as it precluded accurate measurement of the aortic root.

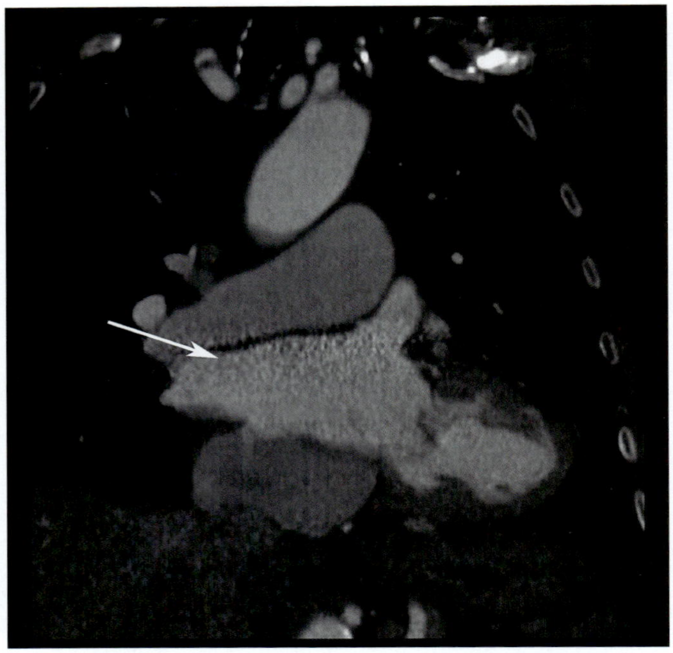

Figure 28.5 Coronal reformat from the same patient as in Figure 28.4, demonstrating a band of noisy data which was incorporated into the reconstructed data as a result of heart rate variability during a retrospectively gated study.

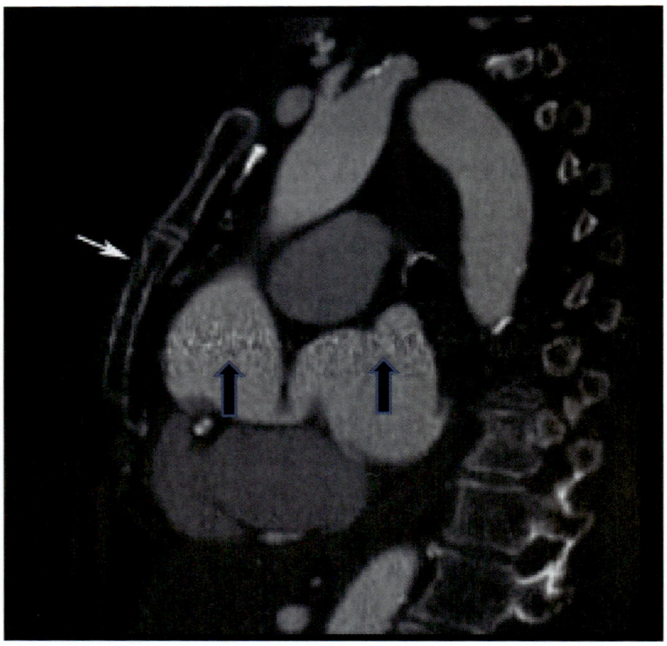

Figure 28.6 Sagittal reformat from the same patient as in Figure 28.4, demonstrating both cardiac gating artifact (black arrows) and respiratory motion (white arrow).

CASE

29 Overestimation of coronary artery stenosis due to calcified plaque

Stefan L. Zimmerman

Imaging description

Coronary artery calcification is routinely encountered at coronary CT angiography. In some cases, large amounts of calcium may obscure the lumen of the vessel, limiting the accuracy of evaluation. The true severity of coronary artery stenosis in the presence of large plaques is frequently overestimated by CT secondary to blooming artifact and beam hardening,[1] leading to false positive diagnoses. Use of a wide window and level at the workstation, sharp reconstruction kernels, and iterative reconstruction techniques are recommended to limit these artifacts as much as possible (Figures 29.1 and 29.2).[2,3]

Importance

Heavy coronary calcification limits the accuracy of coronary CT, sometimes leading to overcalling of severity of disease. This may lead to unnecessary testing such as cardiac catheterization or stress testing, and the risks and expenses associated with those procedures.

Typical clinical scenario

Coronary artery calcification is very common, particularly in older patients with risk factors for coronary artery disease. Several studies have shown an increase in false positive coronary CT angiography (CCTA) results in the setting of extensive coronary calcium. In a meta-analysis of 19 published studies, specificity of coronary CT compared to the gold standard of catheter angiography was reduced to 42% in patients with calcium scores $\geq$ 400, as compared to 90% for patients with scores $<$ 10 and 88.5% for those with scores $<$ 100.[4] In another study comparing calcified plaques evaluated by coronary CT and catheter angiography, concordance between the two modalities was reduced from 95% and 91% for small- (occupying less than 50% of vessel diameter on CT) and moderate-(occupying 50–90% vessel diameter) sized plaques to 67% for large plaques (occupying more than 90% of vessel diameter).[1] Despite the reduction in specificity, however, sensitivity of CCTA for detection of significant stenosis remains high ($>$ 95%) in patients with extensive calcium.[4,5]

Differential diagnosis

In the presence of extensive calcification, truly obstructive lesions ($>$ 50% luminal stenosis) may be difficult to differentiate from pseudostenosis. Sharp reconstructions or iterative reconstruction should be used to reduce blooming artifacts; however, in some cases catheter angiography or functional evaluation for coronary artery disease with stress testing may be required for further evaluation (Figure 29.3).

Teaching point

Coronary artery calcification, when extensive, can limit the accuracy of coronary CT for assessment of the severity of coronary artery stenosis. Use of sharp reconstruction kernels or iterative reconstruction may help; however, in some cases alternative tests, such as catheter angiography, may be necessary.

REFERENCES

1. S. Zhang, D. C. Levin, E. J. Halpern, D. Fischman, M. Savage, P. Walinsky. Accuracy of MDCT in assessing the degree of stenosis caused by calcified coronary artery plaques. *AJR Am J Roentgenol* 2008; **191**: 1676–83.
2. M. Renker, J. W. Nance, Jr., U. J. Schoepf, et al. Evaluation of heavily calcified vessels with coronary CT angiography: comparison of iterative and filtered back projection image reconstruction. *Radiology* 2011; **260**: 390–9.
3. J. W. Hoe, K. H. Toh. A practical guide to reading CT coronary angiograms – how to avoid mistakes when assessing for coronary stenoses. *Int J Cardiovasc Imaging* 2007; **23**: 617–33.
4. J. Abdulla, K. S. Pedersen, M. Budoff, K. F. Kofoed. Influence of coronary calcification on the diagnostic accuracy of 64-slice computed tomography coronary angiography: a systematic review and meta-analysis. *Int J Cardiovasc Imaging* 2012; **28**: 943–53.
5. M. A. den Dekker, K. de Smet, G. H. de Bock, R. A. Tio, M. Oudkerk, R. Vliegenthart. Diagnostic performance of coronary CT angiography for stenosis detection according to calcium score: systematic review and meta-analysis. *Eur Radiol* 2012; **22**: 2688–98.

Pearls and Pitfalls in Cardiovascular Imaging, ed. Stefan L. Zimmerman and Elliot K. Fishman. Published by Cambridge University Press. © Cambridge University Press 2015.

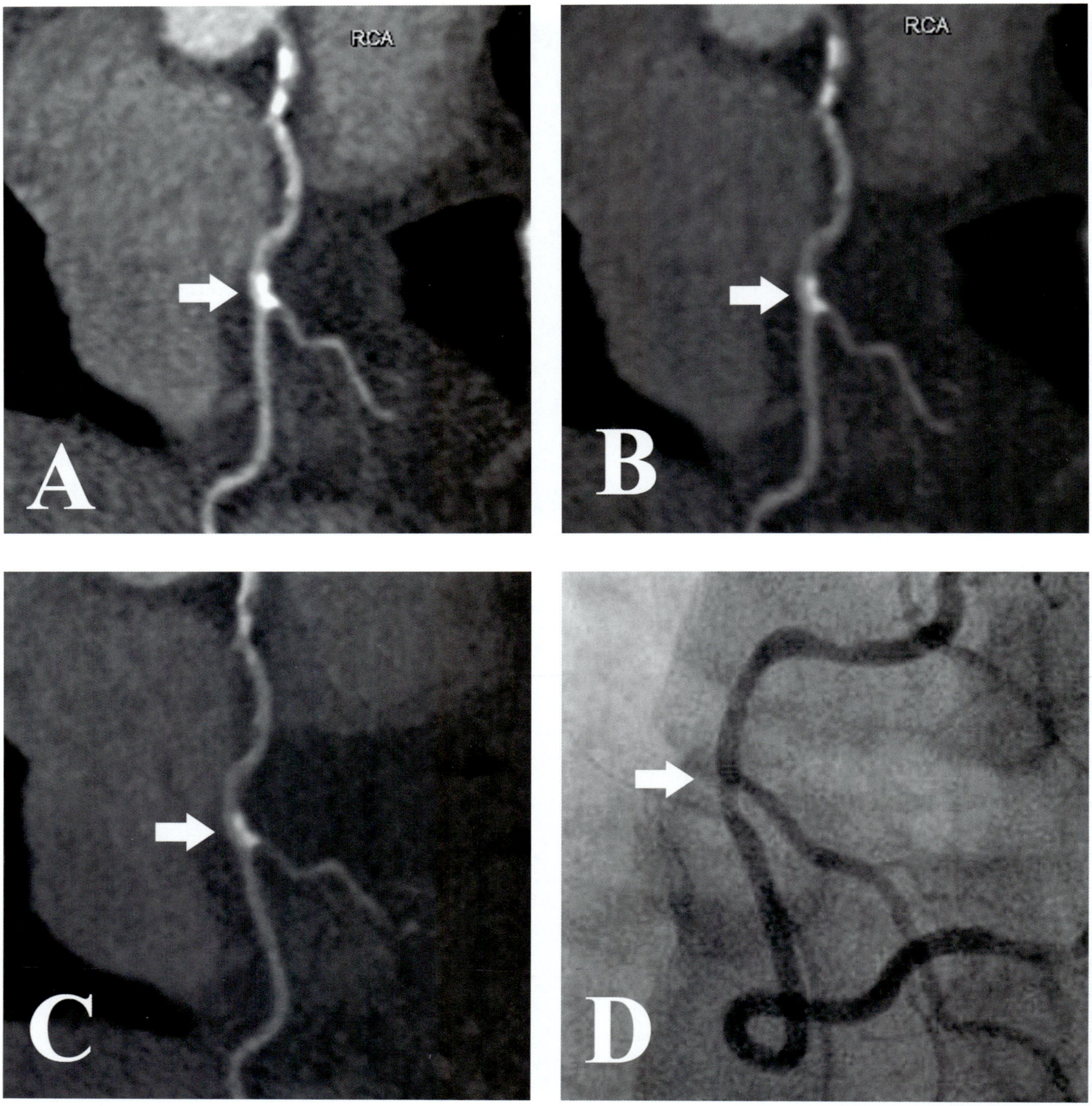

Figure 29.1 **A**. Curved planar reformatted (CPR) image of the right coronary artery (RCA) in a 63-year-old male being evaluated with coronary CT in the emergency department for symptoms of atypical chest pain. A large calcified plaque is present in the mid-RCA at the acute marginal origin. On standard imaging windows (window 900, level 180), degree of stenosis appears at least 50% in severity (arrow). **B.** A wider window and level (window 1500, level 450) results in decreased size of the calcified plaque relative to the vessel lumen, suggesting that the true degree of stenosis is less than 50% (arrow). **C.** Iterative reconstruction technique and a sharp reconstruction kernel demonstrate slight decrease in size of the calcified plaque relative to the vessel lumen, supporting the diagnosis of non-obstructive plaque (arrow). **D.** Screen capture from catheter angiography of the RCA in the same patient shows the same region of the mid-RCA with no visible stenosis to correspond to the abnormality seen on CT (arrow). Calcified plaques often appear more significant on CT than catheter angiography due to blooming artifacts.

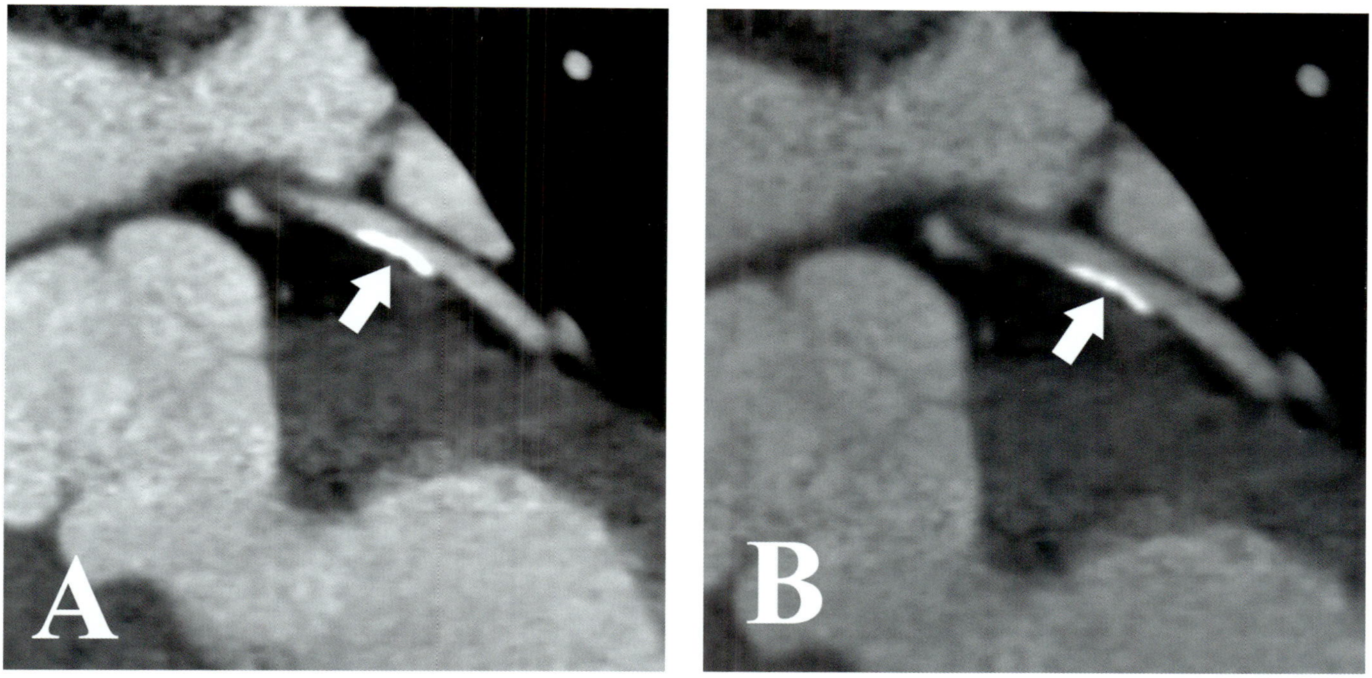

Figure 29.2 A. Sagittal multiplanar reformatted image (MPR) from a cardiac CT performed in a 43-year-old male for preoperative evaluation of the coronary arteries prior to bicuspid aortic valve replacement. On standard imaging windows from a filtered back projection reconstruction (window 650, level 220, kernel B26), the calcium occupies 30–40% of the lumen of the left anterior descending coronary artery (LAD, arrow). B. With iterative reconstruction, there is significant decrease in the size of the calcified plaque, which now appears mostly eccentric in location relative to the lumen, with no significant stenosis. Use of iterative reconstruction, sharp reconstruction kernels, and wide window/level settings will minimize the blooming artifact due to calcium and minimize overestimation of stenosis.

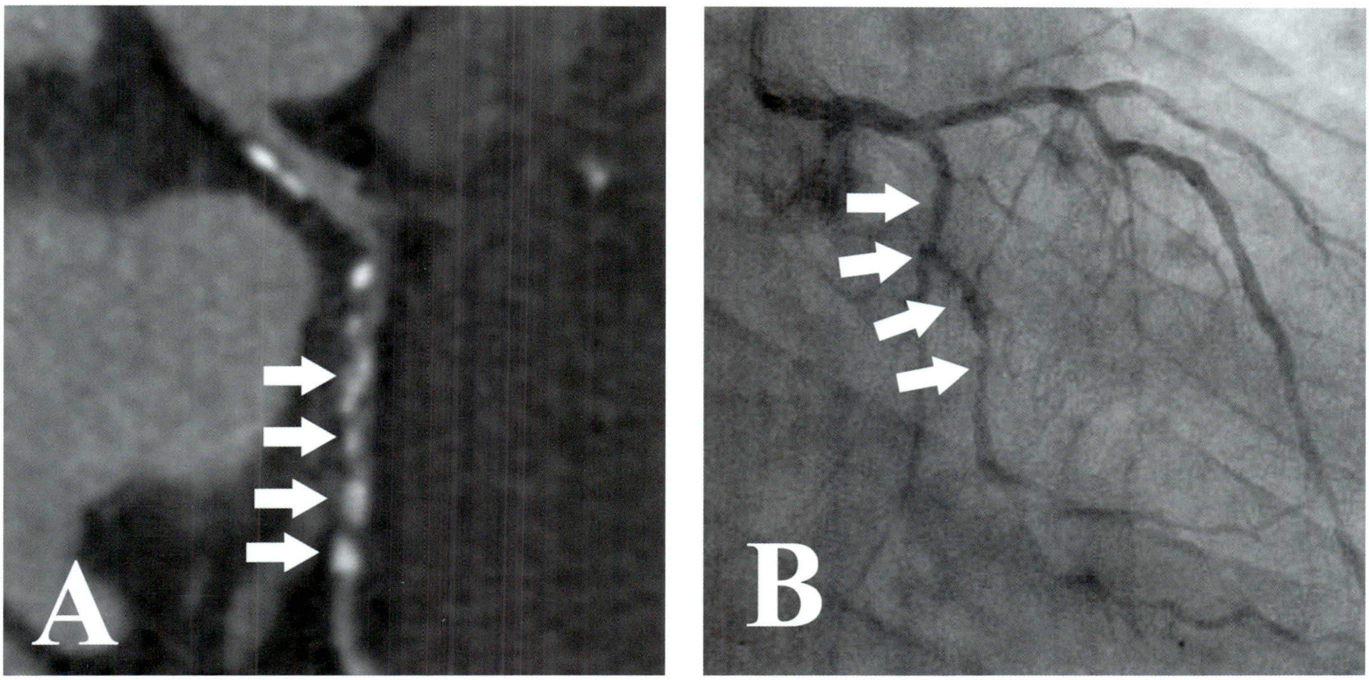

Figure 29.3 A. Curved planar reformatted image of the circumflex coronary artery through the proximal first obtuse marginal branch obtained from a cardiac CT performed in a 75-year-old male with atypical chest pain. There are multiple large calcified plaques (arrows) that obscure the lumen of the vessel, suggesting these may be obstructive lesions. B. Screen capture image from a cardiac catheterization performed in the same patient demonstrating injection of the left main coronary artery with contrast. Mild luminal irregularity is seen in the proximal circumflex coronary artery and first obtuse marginal; however, there is no significant stenosis to correspond to the calcified lesions seen at CT. Calcified lesions on CT often overestimate the degree of stenosis due to blooming effects, particularly problematic in smaller vessels where the lumen can be entirely obscured.

CASE 30

Right coronary artery pseudostenosis due to streak artifact

Stefan L Zimmerman

Imaging description

Streak, or beam hardening, related either to highly concentrated intravenous contrast or to metal from devices within the superior vena cava/right atrium, may result in artifacts that overlap the course of the right coronary artery (RCA) and limit accurate evalution at coronary CT.[1] These artifacts may be either high attenuation or low attenuation in appearance (Figures 30.1 and 30.2). They are often linear- or starburst-shaped in appearance. They are recognized by their origin from a region of highly concentrated, hyperattenuating contrast material or a metallic device in an adjacent right-sided cardiac structure.

Importance

Streak artifact can limit diagnostic quality of coronary CT examinations. In some cases, diagnostic visualization of the RCA may be impossible. In other cases, streak artifacts may simulate stenoses or calcification, leading to misdiagnosis and potentially inappropriate treatment or therapies.

Typical clinical scenario

Right coronary artery streak artifact can occur when highly concentrated intravenous contrast has not cleared the superior vena cava or right atrium at the time of the coronary CT acquisition. Dual-bolus or triple-bolus injection techniques use a saline flush that is designed to push the contrast out of the right cardiac structures and eliminate streak artifact. In the dual-bolus technique, contrast is followed by a saline flush that is intended to clear the right-sided cardiac structures of any contrast.[1] The disadvantage of this technique is that qualitative and quantitative assessment of the right ventricle is limited due to lack of contrast in the RV cavity. In the triple-bolus technique, also known as split-bolus, the initial injection of contrast is followed by a mix of contrast and saline, then finished with a pure saline flush.[2] The objective is to fill left-sided structures (left atrium and ventricle, coronaries, aorta) with high-attenuation contrast, fill right-sided structures with a moderate amount of dilute contrast to allow better visualization, and to clear the superior vena cava of high-attenuation contrast to avoid streak. Streak artifact related to metal from internal cardioverter defibrillator (ICD) or pacemaker leads cannot be avoided and may render some segments of the RCA uninterpretable.

Differential diagnosis

The differential diagnosis for streak artifact in the right coronary artery includes true coronary artery disease such as calcified and non-calcified plaque. Streak artifact can be differentiated by the linear appearance described above and the association with high-attenuation contrast. In this scenario, the abnormality will be absent on precontrast calcium-scoring images. If there is any question, repeat examination with dual- or triple-bolus technique can be considered. Motion artifacts may cause blurring of the right coronary artery that can cause low- and high-attenuation regions similar to streak artifacts and should also be considered.

Teaching point

Streak artifact due to highly concentrated intravenous contrast or metal in the superior vena cava or right atrium may cause the artifactual appearance of stenosis or calcification in the right coronary artery. Dual- or triple-bolus injection techniques should be considered to prevent the accumulation of contrast in right-sided cardiac structures.

REFERENCES

1. M. A. Auler, T. Heagy, L. Aganovic, R. Brothers, P. Costello, U. J. Schoepf. Saline chasing technique with dual-syringe injector systems for multi-detector row computed tomographic angiography: rationale, indications, and protocols. *Curr Probl Diagn Radiol* 2006; **35**: 1–11.
2. J. M. Kerl, J. G. Ravenel, S. A. Nguyen, et al. Right heart: split-bolus injection of diluted contrast medium for visualization at coronary CT angiography. *Radiology* 2008; **247**: 356–64.

Pearls and Pitfalls in Cardiovascular Imaging, ed. Stefan L. Zimmerman and Elliot K. Fishman. Published by Cambridge University Press. © Cambridge University Press 2015.

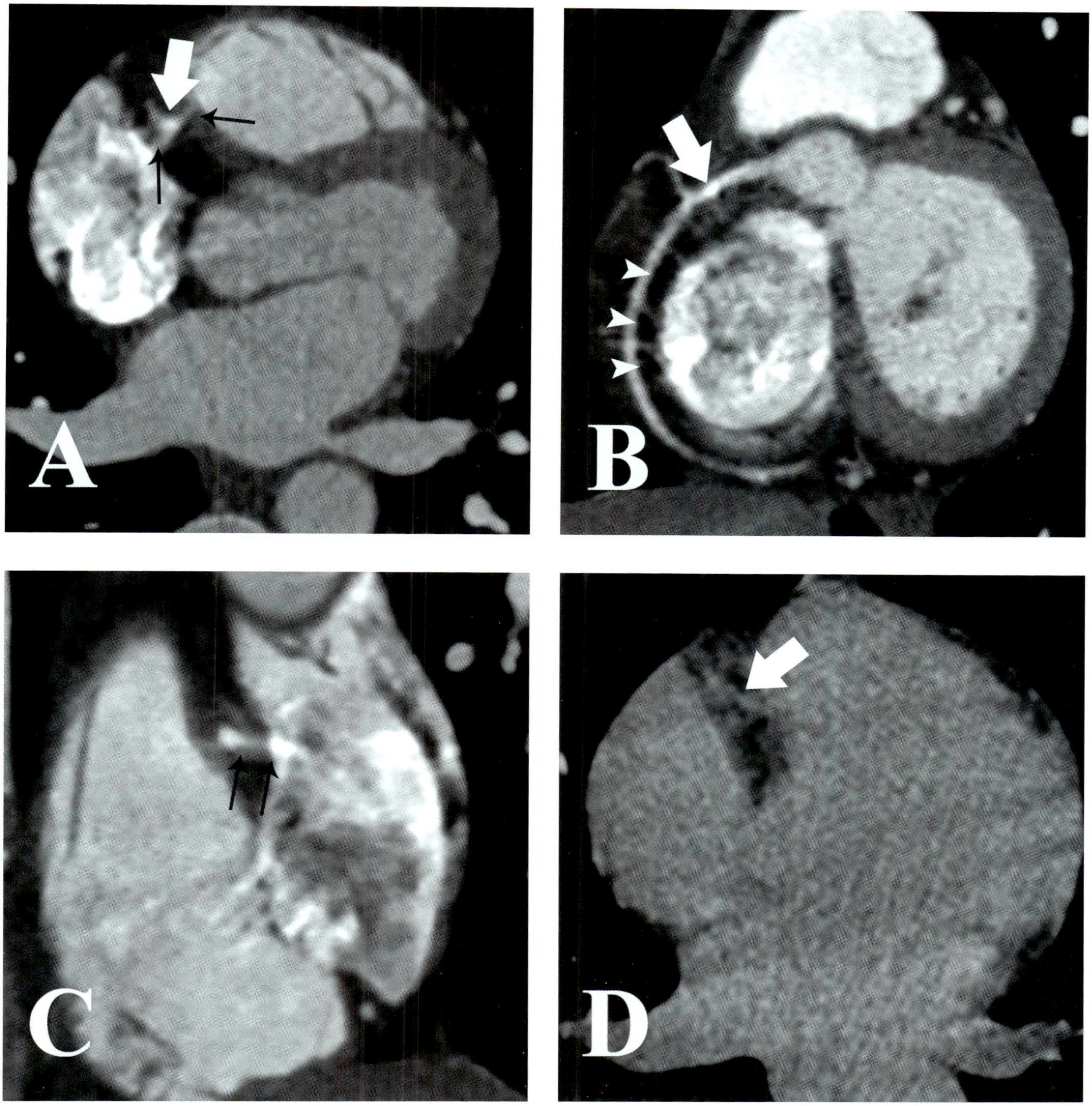

Figure 30.1 **A.** Axial image from cardiac CT performed in a 44-year-old female with chest pain as part of a triple-rule-out protocol. There is high attenuation in the proximal right coronary artery (RCA, white arrow), mimicking calcified plaque. Linear high attenuation also extends from the right atrium through the right coronary artery and adjacent fat (black arrows), suggesting this is a streak artifact related to concentrated intravenous contrast. **B.** Short-axis image of the RCA from the same patient demonstrates the pseudolesion in the proximal RCA (white arrow) and several low-attenuation regions adjacent to the right atrium, also related to streak artifact (arrowheads). **C.** Oblique sagittal image again demonstrates high-attenuation streak from the right atrium to the RCA (black arrows), creating the pseudolesion that mimics calcified plaque. **D.** Axial image from a calcium-scoring sequence performed in the same patient confirms the absence of calcification in the location of the RCA pseudolesion (white arrow).

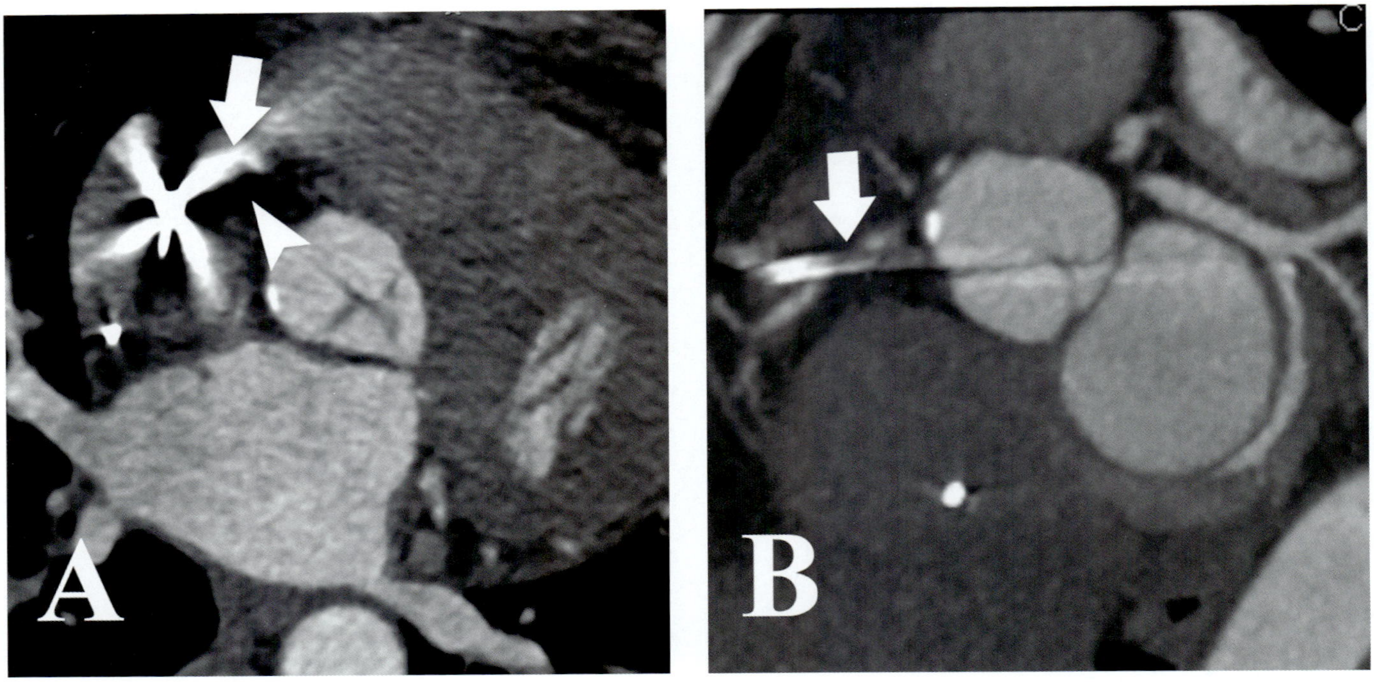

Figure 30.2 **A.** Axial image from a cardiac CT performed in a 77-year-old with chest pain and a dual-chamber pacemaker. There is extensive streak artifact from the pacemaker lead that results in alternating bright and dark regions radiating outward (arrow, arrowhead). **B.** Short-axis reformatted image from the same patient shows the artifact obscuring evaluation of the proximal RCA (arrow). In the presence of such an artifact, diagnostic evaluation of this segment of the RCA is not possible.

CASE 31

Pseudostenosis from stair-step reconstruction artifact

Stefan L. Zimmerman

Imaging description

Stair-step reconstruction artifacts occur with ECG-gated CT scanning techniques. Bands of data in the z-direction are acquired at sequential heart beats in the cardiac cycle as the patient moves through the scanner and are reconstructed into a single image.[1] If there is an irregular heart rhythm, the coronary arteries are not in the exact same location for the acquisition of each band of data, and then a phase misregistration, or stair-step artifact will be seen at the interface between these bands (Figure 31.1).[2] These artifacts have a horizontal orientation and can range from mild to severe, rendering images non-diagnostic in the worst cases. Mild cases of stair-step artifact can be quite misleading, and may result in artifactual appearance of significant stenoses (Figures 31.1 and 31.2).[1,2] However, on multiphase reconstructions acquired at different points in the cardiac cycle, these artifacts generally disappear or change in location (Figure 31.2). Routine confirmation of any significant coronary stenoses using these additional reconstructed phases is recommended to avoid misdiagnosis.[3] Additionally, the absence of visible atherosclerotic plaque in association with a stenosis should serve as a clue that the lesion may be an artifact.[3]

Importance

Stair-step artifacts are common and can be quite misleading. Inadvertent overestimation of coronary artery stenosis due to these artifacts may lead to unnecessary additional tests such as catheter angiography or stress testing and the risks and costs associated with these procedures.

Typical clinical scenario

Stair-step artifacts can be seen in nearly any coronary CT examination; however, they are particularly problematic in patients with irregular heart rates. Beta blockade may help reduce heart rate variability during coronary CT. ECG-editing may help improve quality of examinations if patients have ventricular ectopy. If the arrhythmia is limited to one or several ectopic beats, the image data related to these ectopic beats can be deleted from the image dataset and may be able to salvage the examination.[1] There is a limit, however, to how much of the data can be excluded without creating data gaps that result in incomplete coverage of the cardiac anatomy. Large-volume detector and high-pitch acquisition techniques do not suffer from stair-step artifacts given that the entire dataset is acquired during a single heart beat.

Differential diagnosis

Stair-step artifacts must be distinguished from true coronary artery stenoses. When several phases of the cardiac cycle are interrogated, a true stenosis should persist, while stair-step artifacts will disappear or change in location.

Teaching point

Stair-step reconstruction artifacts can be a source of false positive diagnosis of a significant stenosis at coronary CT. To avoid this problem, multiphase datasets should be used to confirm any significant lesions.

REFERENCES

1. J. R. Lesser, B. J. Flygenring, T. Knickelbine, T. Longe, R. S. Schwartz. Practical approaches to overcoming artifacts in coronary CT angiography. *J Cardiovasc Comput Tomogr* 2009; **3**: 4–15.
2. L. J. Kroft, A. de Roos, J. Geleijns. Artifacts in ECG-synchronized MDCT coronary angiography. *AJR Am J Roentgenol* 2007; **189**: 581–91.
3. J. W. Hoe, K. H. Toh. A practical guide to reading CT coronary angiograms – how to avoid mistakes when assessing for coronary stenoses. *Int J Cardiovasc Imaging* 2007; **23**: 617–33.

Pearls and Pitfalls in Cardiovascular Imaging, ed. Stefan L. Zimmerman and Elliot K. Fishman. Published by Cambridge University Press. © Cambridge University Press 2015.

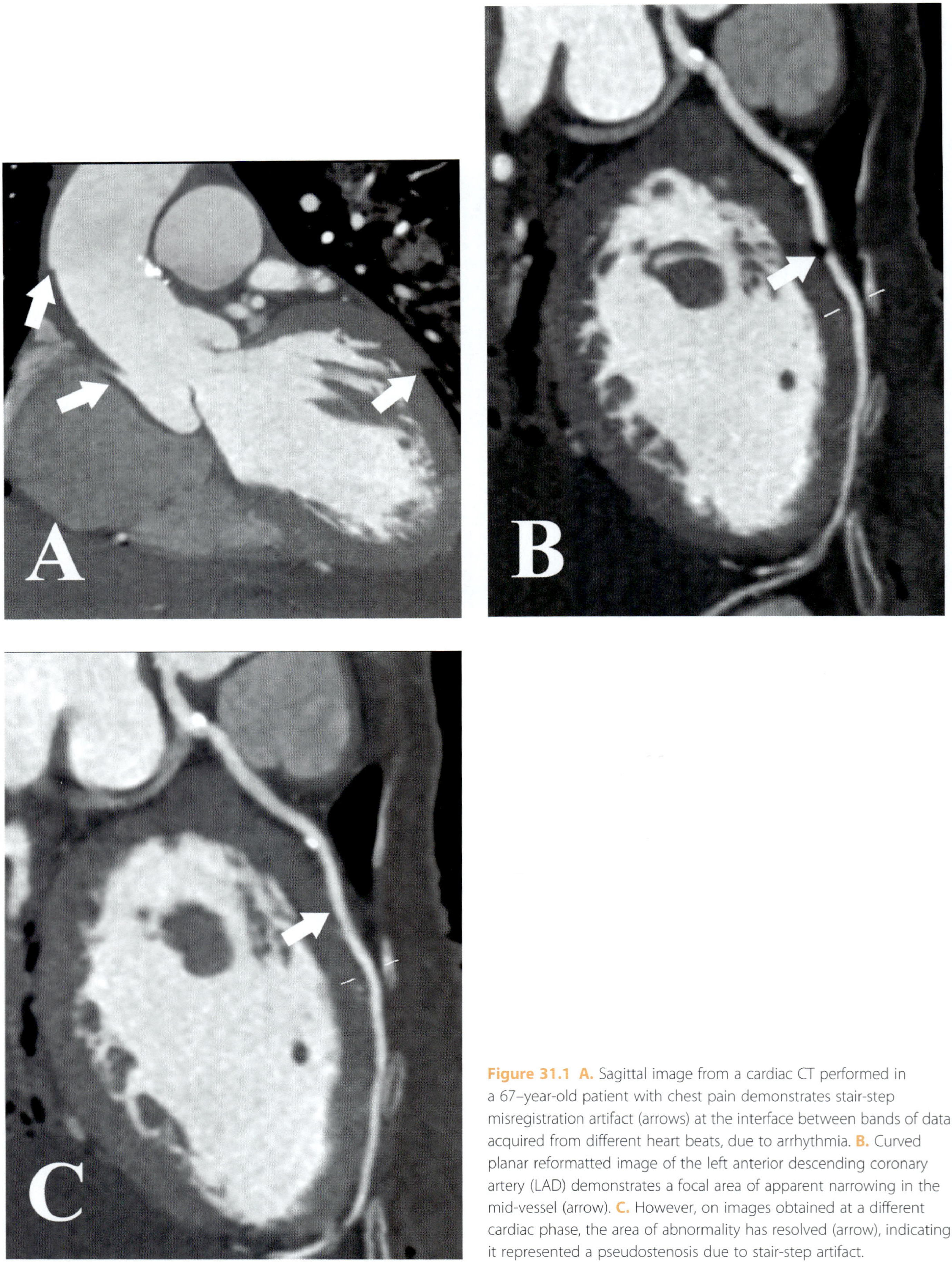

Figure 31.1 **A.** Sagittal image from a cardiac CT performed in a 67-year-old patient with chest pain demonstrates stair-step misregistration artifact (arrows) at the interface between bands of data acquired from different heart beats, due to arrhythmia. **B.** Curved planar reformatted image of the left anterior descending coronary artery (LAD) demonstrates a focal area of apparent narrowing in the mid-vessel (arrow). **C.** However, on images obtained at a different cardiac phase, the area of abnormality has resolved (arrow), indicating it represented a pseudostenosis due to stair-step artifact.

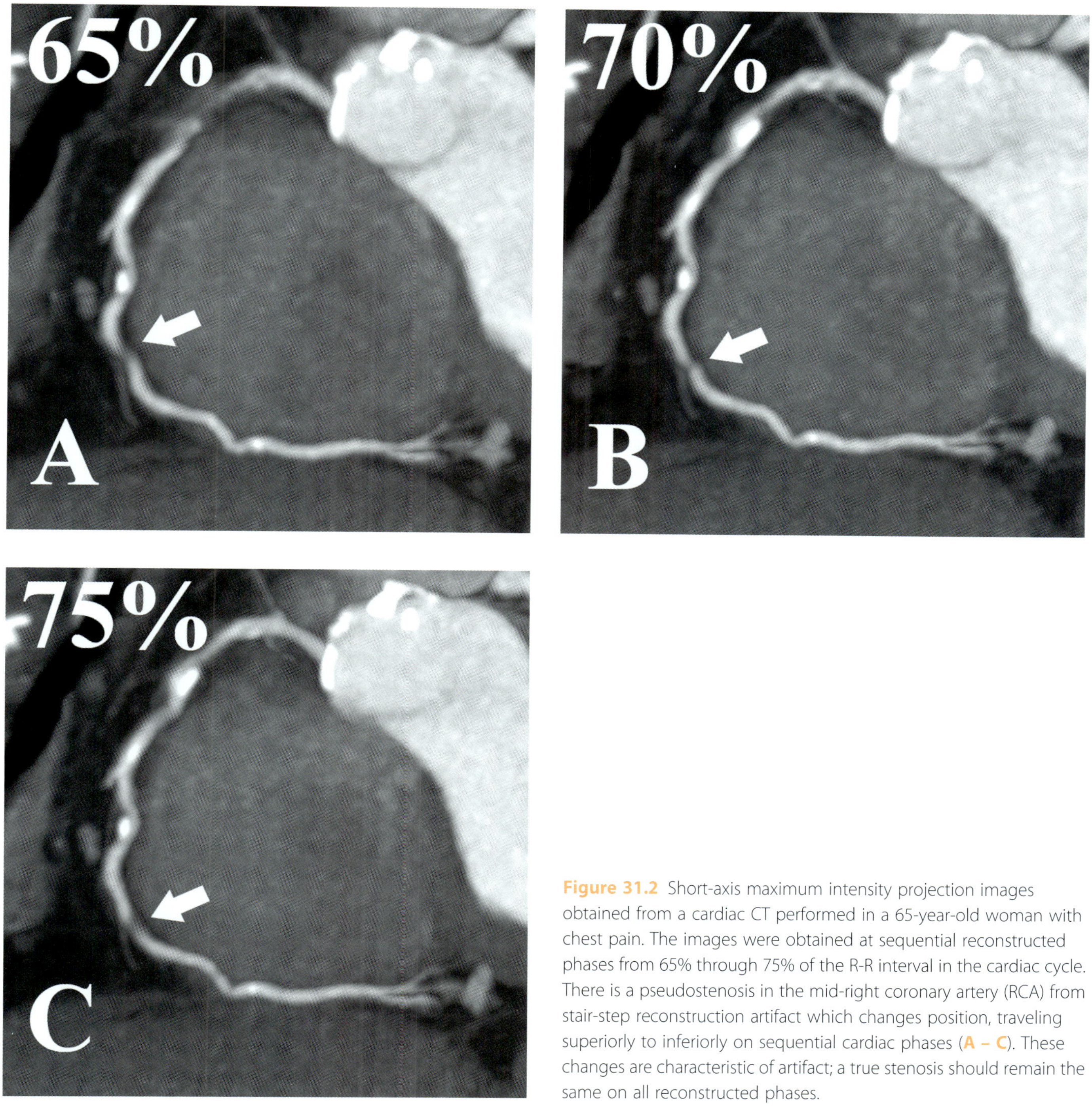

Figure 31.2 Short-axis maximum intensity projection images obtained from a cardiac CT performed in a 65-year-old woman with chest pain. The images were obtained at sequential reconstructed phases from 65% through 75% of the R-R interval in the cardiac cycle. There is a pseudostenosis in the mid-right coronary artery (RCA) from stair-step reconstruction artifact which changes position, traveling superiorly to inferiorly on sequential cardiac phases (**A – C**). These changes are characteristic of artifact; a true stenosis should remain the same on all reconstructed phases.

CASE 32

Pseudostenosis in the coronary arteries due to motion artifact

Stefan L. Zimmerman

Imaging description

Motion artifact in coronary CT angiography (CCTA) occurs when the temporal resolution of the acquisition is inadequate to resolve moving cardiac structures. A temporal resolution of < 50 msec is required to permit imaging of cardiac structures during any point in the cardiac cycle without blurring.[1] Current scanner technology has not yet achieved this benchmark, and therefore imaging is targeted to portions of the cardiac cycle that have the least motion, mid-diastole (60–70% of R-R interval) and end-systole (30–40% of R-R interval). Motion artifacts can affect any vessel, but are most pronounced in the RCA, the vessel with the highest displacement velocity and range during the cardiac cycle.[2] Motion artifacts may have one of several appearances. In some cases, low-attenuation blurring of the coronary artery lumen and wall may be seen, simulating segmental high-grade stenosis or occlusion (Figure 32.1). In other cases, arcs or rounded regions of high and low attenuation may be seen adjacent to the coronary arteries (Figure 32.1). Recognition of blurring of the walls of cardiac chambers, such as the left atrium or ventricle, can provide a clue that the images are degraded by motion and should be interpreted with caution (Figure 32.1). In the setting of elevated heart rates (> 70 beats per minute), reconstructed phases obtained in end-systole at approximately 30–40% of the R-R interval have the greatest chance of diagnostic images.[3] For motion-degraded CCTA examinations, multiple reconstructed phases can often be used to piece together a comprehensive assessment of the coronary arteries.[3] In this scenario, not all vessel segments will be best visualized on a single phase, but each segment is well visualized on at least one phase.

Importance

Motion blurring can simulate coronary artery stenosis. The motion leads to blurring of the coronary lumen and adjacent low-attenuation fat, resulting in an appearance mimicking high-grade stenosis. Reconstructed phases from different points in the cardiac cycle should be evaluated to confirm or disprove any significant coronary artery stenosis (Figure 32.2). Motion artifact is the major reason for non-diagnostic scans.[2] On 64-slice MDCT, the rate of non-diagnostic coronary artery segments is approximately 3–11%.[2] With next generation dual-source and wide-area detector scanner technology, the rate of non-diagnostic segments has further decreased, ranging from 0.8–3% in a recent meta-analysis of 22 studies using dual-source CT.[4] In the setting of either false positive or non-diagnostic scans, patients may require additional testing to evaluate for coronary artery disease and incur the risks and costs associated with those procedures.

Typical clinical scenario

Motion artifact is most often seen in patients with elevated heart rates, typically > 70 bpm. The use of beta blockers prior to the examination will reduce the risk of motion-degraded images by both decreasing heart rate and reducing heart rate variability during the scan.[2]

Differential diagnosis

Stenosis due to motion artifact should be distinguished from true obstructive lesions due to coronary artery plaque. Evaluation of multiphase datasets will often allow distinction of these two entities. Motion artifacts will often change positions from phase to phase, whereas a true stenosis should remain fixed on every phase.

Teaching point

Motion artifacts can simulate coronary artery stenosis or lead to non-diagnostic exams. Beta blockade to reduce heart rate prior to the examination and interrogation of multiphase datasets after the examination can reduce the likelihood of misdiagnosis.

REFERENCES

1. J. R. Lesser, B. J. Flygenring, T. Knickelbine, T. Longe, R. S. Schwartz. Practical approaches to overcoming artifacts in coronary CT angiography. *J Cardiovasc Comput Tomogr* 2009; **3**: 4–15.
2. L. J. Kroft, A. de Roos, J. Geleijns. Artifacts in ECG-synchronized MDCT coronary angiography. *AJR Am J Roentgenol* 2007; **189**: 581–91.
3. J. W. Hoe, K. H. Toh. A practical guide to reading CT coronary angiograms – how to avoid mistakes when assessing for coronary stenoses. *Int J Cardiovasc Imaging* 2007; **23**: 617–33.
4. A. Salavati, F. Radmanesh, K. Heidari, B. A. Dwamena, A. M. Kelly, P. Cronin. Dual-source computed tomography angiography for diagnosis and assessment of coronary artery disease: systematic review and meta-analysis. *J Cardiovasc Comput Tomogr* 2012; **6**: 78–90.

Pearls and Pitfalls in Cardiovascular Imaging, ed. Stefan L. Zimmerman and Elliot K. Fishman. Published by Cambridge University Press. © Cambridge University Press 2015.

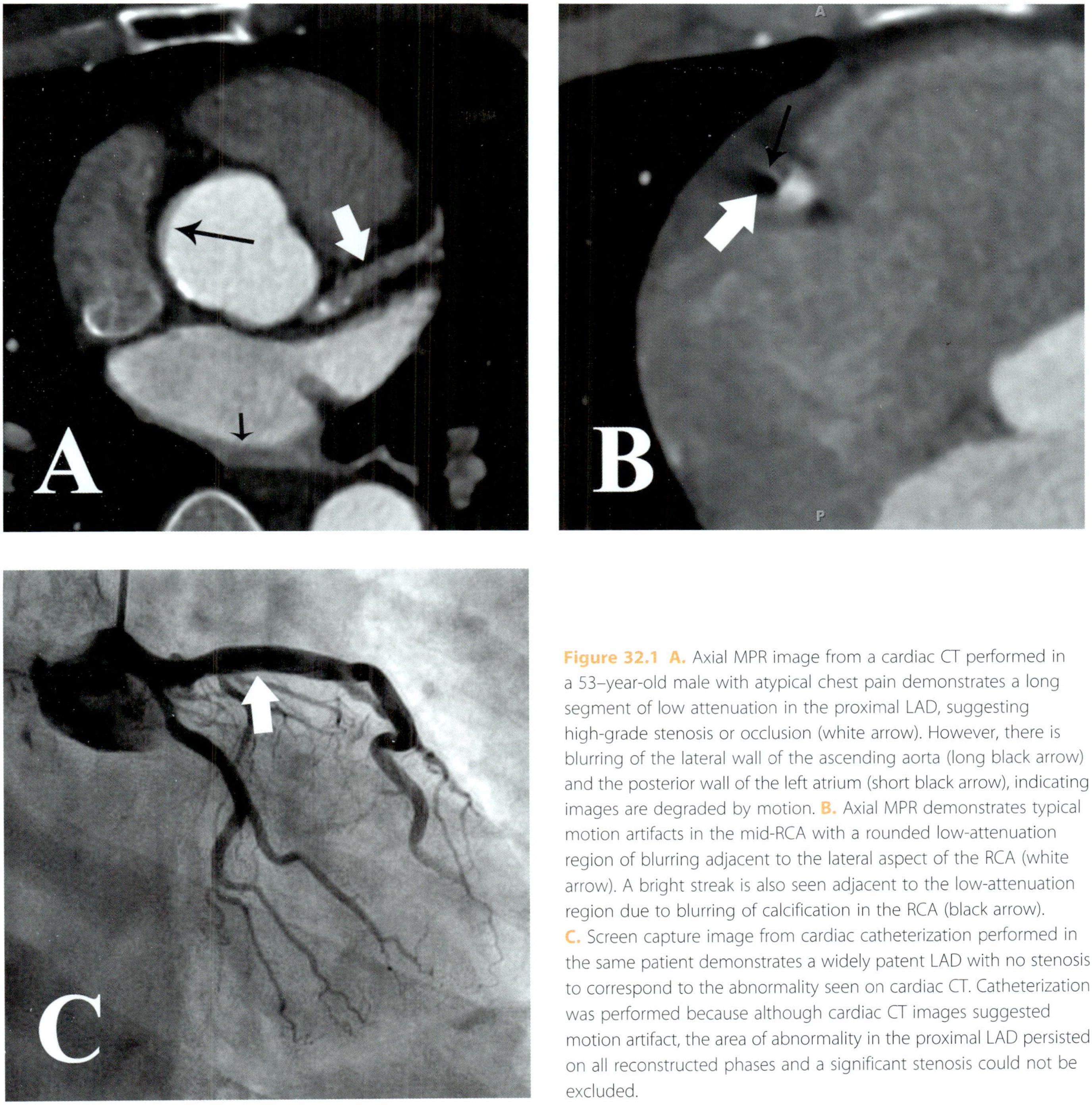

Figure 32.1 **A.** Axial MPR image from a cardiac CT performed in a 53-year-old male with atypical chest pain demonstrates a long segment of low attenuation in the proximal LAD, suggesting high-grade stenosis or occlusion (white arrow). However, there is blurring of the lateral wall of the ascending aorta (long black arrow) and the posterior wall of the left atrium (short black arrow), indicating images are degraded by motion. **B.** Axial MPR demonstrates typical motion artifacts in the mid-RCA with a rounded low-attenuation region of blurring adjacent to the lateral aspect of the RCA (white arrow). A bright streak is also seen adjacent to the low-attenuation region due to blurring of calcification in the RCA (black arrow). **C.** Screen capture image from cardiac catheterization performed in the same patient demonstrates a widely patent LAD with no stenosis to correspond to the abnormality seen on cardiac CT. Catheterization was performed because although cardiac CT images suggested motion artifact, the area of abnormality in the proximal LAD persisted on all reconstructed phases and a significant stenosis could not be excluded.

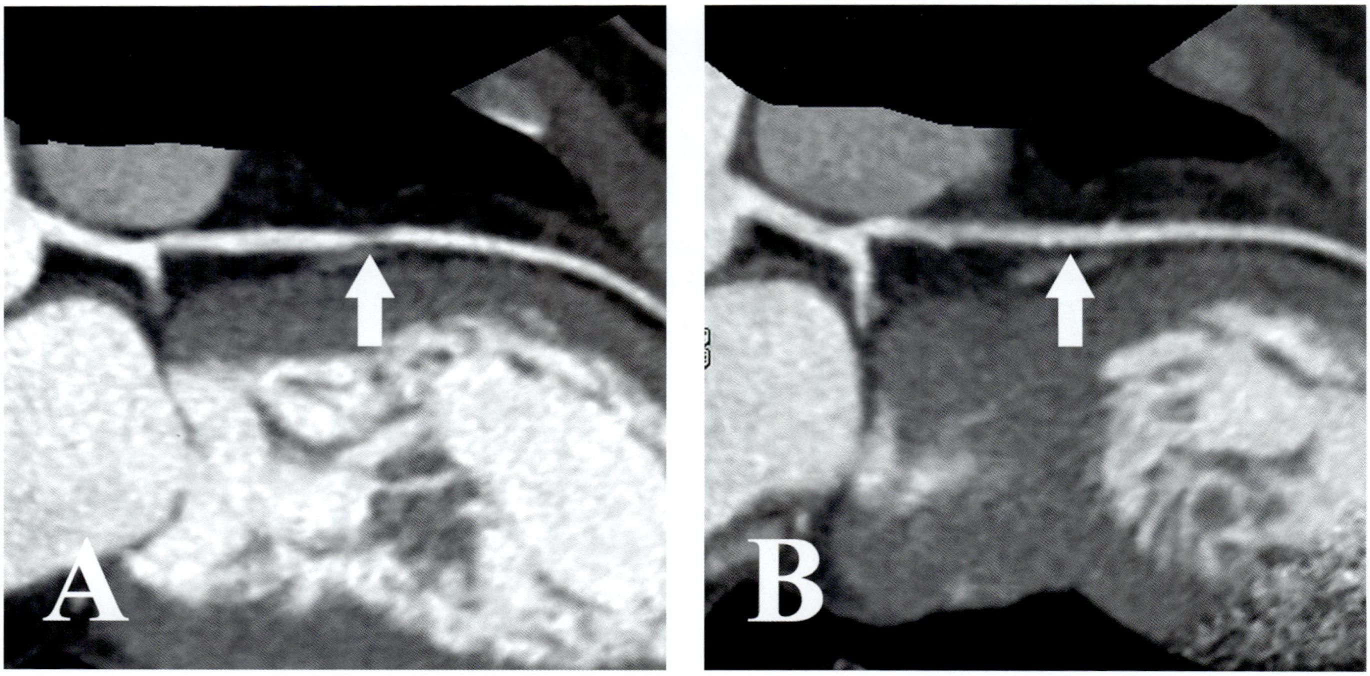

Figure 32.2 A. Curved planar reformatted image of the left anterior descending coronary artery (LAD) from a cardiac CT performed in a 37-year-old female with atypical chest pain demonstrates what appears to represent a high-grade stenosis in the proximal LAD (arrow). **B.** Curved planar reformatted image reconstructed in a different cardiac phase clearly shows that the lesion was an artifact due to motion and the LAD is patent and free of disease (arrow). Significant stensoses should always be confirmed on multiple reconstructed phases to exclude artifacts.

CASE 33

Pseudostenosis on curved planar reformatted images

Stefan L. Zimmerman

Imaging description

Curved planar reformatted (CPR) images are a form of post-processing whereby the lumen of a vessel of interest is tracked automatically by dedicated 3D software and a centerline is created through the vessel. Reformatted images created orthogonal to the centerline then allow the entire vessel to be visualized on one imaging plane. This technique is very useful for providing a comprehensive view of the entire vessel of interest on a single image. However, occasionally these automated techniques can result in artifactual lesions in the coronaries due to difficulties with vessel tracking.[1] This seems to occur most often when the vessel takes an acute turn and the software is unable to completely straighten the tortuous segment, resulting in truncation of portions of the vessels. The result is a discontinuity in the vessel at the location of incorrect vessel tracking that can mimic a stenosis (Figure 33.1).

Importance

Misdiagnosis of coronary artery stenosis due to inappropriate vessel tracking could result in additional diagnostic testing, such as invasive cardiac catheterization, and further risks and costs that are unnecessary.

Typical clinical scenario

CPR images are used routinely for evaluation of the coronary arteries by many centers. Vessel tracking errors are most frequent in tortuous vessels, which are more likely in older patients.

Differential diagnosis

Pseudostenosis from incorrect vessel tracking should be distinguished from true coronary artery stenoses caused by atherosclerotic disease. These entities can be differentiated by inspection of the unprocessed source images with manual multiplanar reformatting.

Teaching point

Incorrect vessel tracking on automated CPR images can result in a pseudostenosis of the coronary arteries. It is important to always confirm stenoses identified with automated post-processing techniques on the source images.

REFERENCES

1. L. J. Kroft, A. de Roos, J. Geleijns. Artifacts in ECG-synchronized MDCT coronary angiography. *AJR Am J Roentgenol* 2007; **189**: 581–91.

Pearls and Pitfalls in Cardiovascular Imaging, ed. Stefan L. Zimmerman and Elliot K. Fishman. Published by Cambridge University Press. © Cambridge University Press 2015.

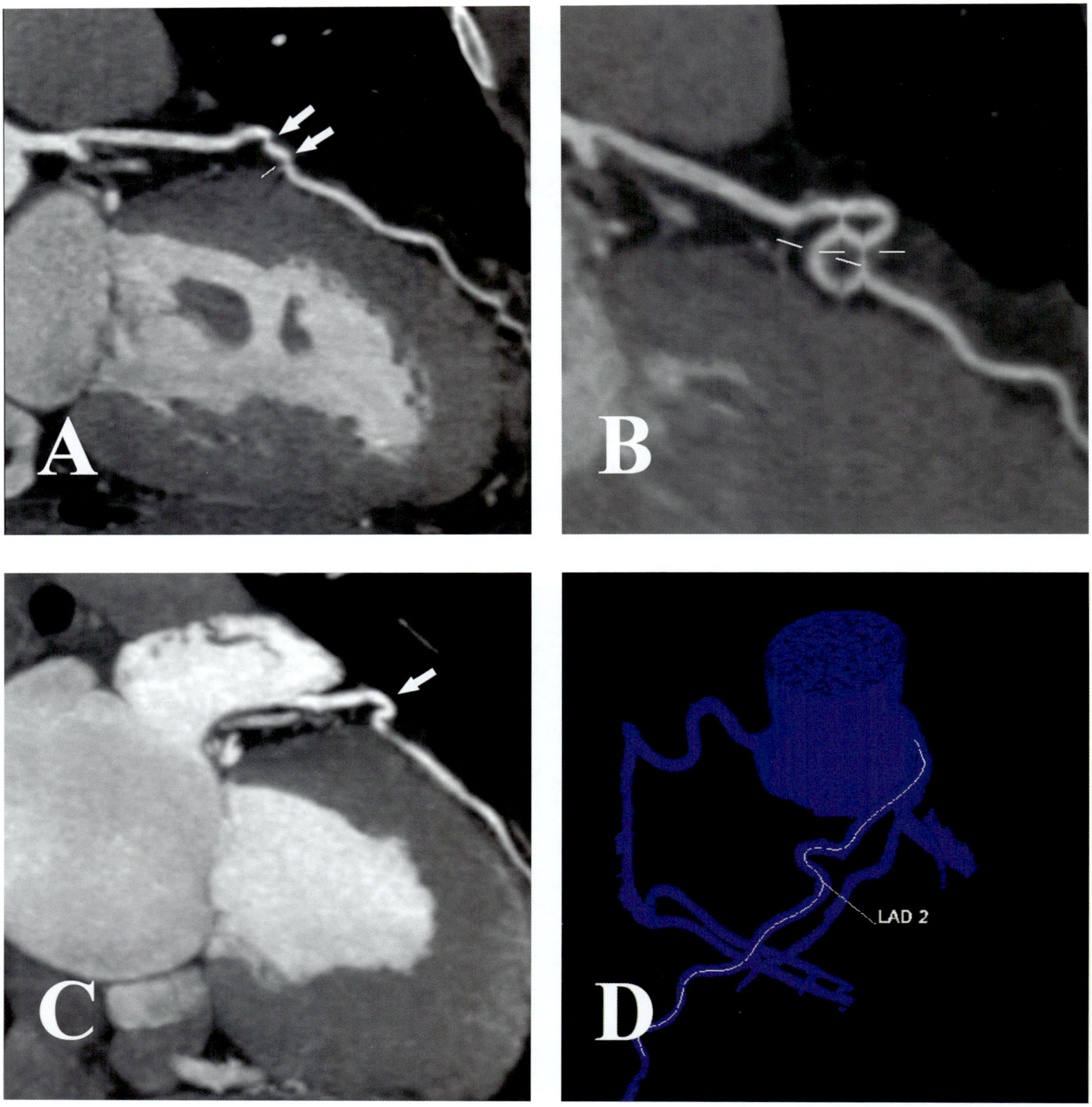

Figure 33.1 **A.** Curved planar reformatted (CPR) image of the left anterior descending coronary artery from a cardiac CT performed in a 44-year-old male with chest pain. There are two focal areas of apparent stenosis in the mid-LAD (arrows). **B.** On CPR images obtained from a different projection, this segment of the coronary artery is displayed incorrectly, with mirror image duplication of the tortuous portion of the vessel. **C.** A sagittal maximum intensity projection (MIP) image created from source images clearly shows the tortuous segment of the coronary artery (arrow), which is entirely free from stenosis. **D.** A volume-rendered image of the segmented coronary arteries shows the path of the centerline used for vessel tracking, which follows the tortuous segment appropriately; however, the software was unable to unfold this section of the vessel to display properly.

CASE 34

Coronary stent visualization

Stefan L. Zimmerman

Imaging description

Evaluation of coronary stents with cardiac CT is challenging due to artifacts associated with the metal stent struts. Several artifacts adversely affect CT imaging of stents, the most important of which are blooming, partial volume averaging, and beam hardening.[1] Both blooming and partial volume effects result in the stent struts appearing larger than reality, obscuring visualization of the lumen, and resulting in underestimation of true lumen diameter (Figure 34.1).[2,3] Beam hardening artifacts occur due to absorption of low-energy photons by the metal stent struts resulting in primarily high-energy photons passing to the detectors. The result is low-attenuation areas adjacent to stent struts that can mimic in-stent restenosis. Stent-related artifacts are most pronounced in smaller stents, and current recommendations suggest that imaging of coronary stents should be restricted to patients with larger stents, at least 3 mm in diameter or more.[4] Stents of similar size from different manufacturers can also have variable artifact severity, due to differences in the type of materials used to create the stent.[2] Widening the window width will reduce the blooming effect of stent struts and improve lumen visualization. (Figure 34.1).[5] Visualization can also be optimized and artifacts reduced through the use of the thinnest possible slices, sharp reconstruction kernels, and iterative reconstruction techniques (Figure 34.2).[5–7]

Importance

Misdiagnosis of in-stent restenosis on cardiac CT can lead to inappropriate cardiac catheterization and the risks and costs associated with the procedure.

Typical clinical scenario

In-stent restenosis, defined as $>$ 50% luminal narrowing, is a common problem in patients with prior percutaneous coronary intervention. Neointimal hyperplasia within the stent is the primary cause of in-stent restenosis. Restenosis rates are approximately 40% with bare metal stents and are reduced to $<$10% with drug-eluting stents.[7]

Differential diagnosis

Stent-related artifacts should be distinguished from true in-stent restenosis or occlusion due to neointimal hyperplasia (Figure 34.3). For stents $<$ 3 mm in size, this may be difficult due to limitations of current scanner technology.

Teaching point

Misdiagnosis of in-stent restenosis can occur in smaller stents due to stent-related reconstruction artifacts. Optimization of coronary CT protocols and reconstruction techniques will improve visualization and reduce the likelihood of incorrect diagnosis.

REFERENCES

1. S. H. Chung, Y. J. Kim, J. Hur, et al. Evaluation of coronary artery in-stent restenosis by 64-section computed tomography: factors affecting assessment and accurate diagnosis. *J Thorac Imaging* 2010; **25**: 57–63.
2. D. Maintz, M. C. Burg, H. Seifarth, et al. Update on multidetector coronary CT angiography of coronary stents: in vitro evaluation of 29 different stent types with dual-source CT. *Eur Radiol* 2009; **19**: 42–9.
3. H. Seifarth, M. Ozgun, R. Raupach, et al. 64-Versus 16-slice CT angiography for coronary artery stent assessment: in vitro experience. *Invest Radiol* 2006; **41**: 22–7.
4. D. B. Mark, D. S. Berman, M. J. Budoff, et al. ACCF/ACR/AHA/NASCI/SAIP/SCAI/SCCT 2010 expert consensus document on coronary computed tomographic angiography: a report of the American College of Cardiology Foundation Task Force on Expert Consensus Documents. *J Am Coll Cardiol* 2010; **55**: 2663–99.
5. A. H. Mahnken. CT Imaging of coronary stents: past, present, and future. *ISRN Cardiol* 2012; **2012**: 139823.
6. U. Ebersberger, F. Tricarico, U. J. Schoepf, et al. CT evaluation of coronary artery stents with iterative image reconstruction: improvements in image quality and potential for radiation dose reduction. *Eur Radiol* 2013; **23**: 125–32.
7. F. Pugliese, F. Cademartiri, C. van Mieghem, et al. Multidetector CT for visualization of coronary stents. *Radiographics* 2006; **26**: 887–904.

Pearls and Pitfalls in Cardiovascular Imaging, ed. Stefan L. Zimmerman and Elliot K. Fishman. Published by Cambridge University Press. © Cambridge University Press 2015.

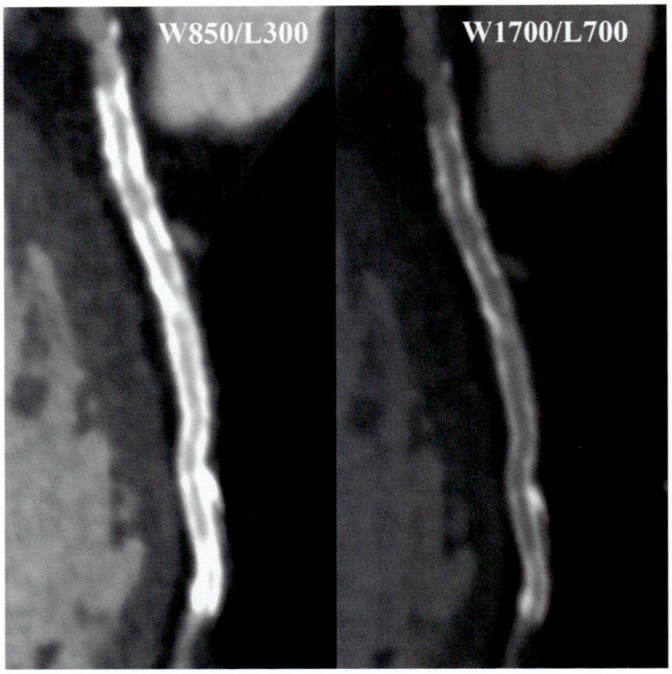

Figure 34.1 Curved planar reformatted (CPR) images of the left anterior descending coronary artery (LAD) in a 63-year-old male being evaluated for a cardiac mass, who had a history of multiple coronary artery stents. The image on the left shows a typical vascular window/level setting, which increases the severity of blooming artifact and obscures visualization of stent lumens. The image on the right shows the advantage of using a wider window/level setting that allows for improved visualization of the stent lumens, which is patent, and reduced blooming artifact.

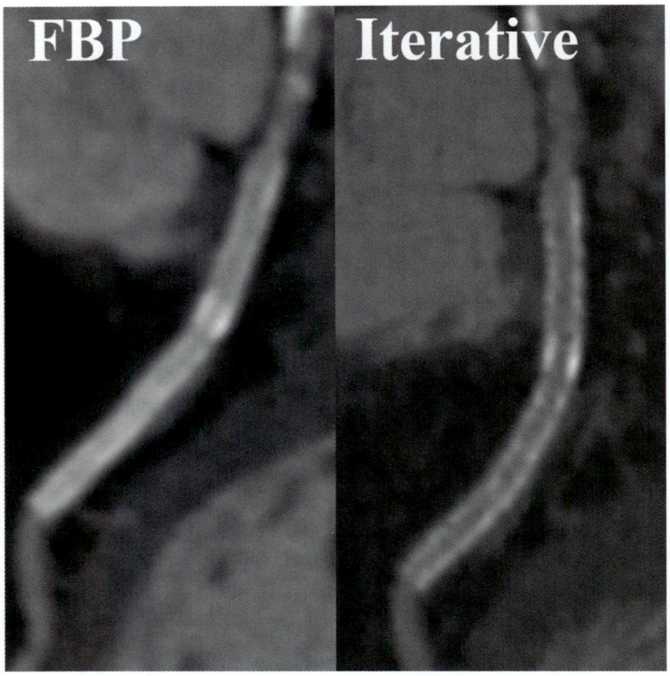

Figure 34.2 CPR images of the LAD from a cardiac CT exam performed in a 74-year-old female with atypical chest pain. On the left, a CPR image was created from filtered back projection images, using a coronary artery specific soft-tissue reconstruction kernel. On the right, the CPR image was created from an iterative reconstruction dataset, using a sharp coronary artery kernel. There is marked improvement in lumen visualization with the use of the sharp iterative reconstruction. Blooming and partial volume artifacts limit evaluation on the filtered back projection dataset.

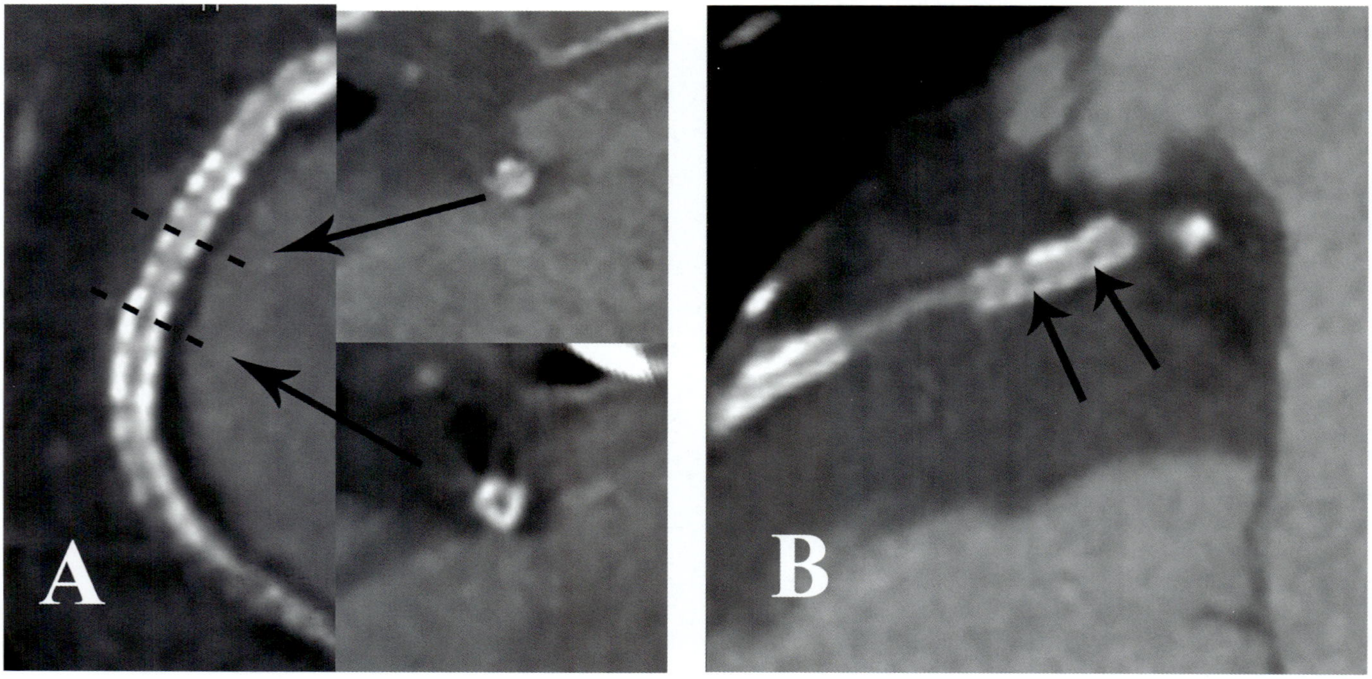

Figure 34.3 A. CPR images of the RCA in oblique sagittal (left) and short-axis (thumbnails, right) views from a cardiac CT obtained in a 66-year-old female with a history of coronary artery disease and multiple stents, who presented with chest pain and an equivocal stress test. There is evidence of in-stent restenosis in the mid-RCA (lower arrow), which can be seen as an area of low attenuation in the stent lumen on the long-axis image, confirmed by the short-axis image in the bottom right. A representative short-axis image from a patent portion of the stent just above the stenosis is shown for comparison in the upper right picture. B. Long-axis image of the proximal LAD from the same patient demonstrates additional areas of in-stent restenosis (arrows), identified by the presence of low attenuation in the stent lumen.

CASE 35

Myocardial bridging

Stefan L. Zimmerman

Imaging description

In myocardial bridging, the epicardial coronary arteries, normally surrounded by fat, dive inferiorly and course through myocardial tissue before exiting distally back into the epicardial fat. Myocardial bridging can range in length from a few millimeters to several centimeters and be of variable depth, typically between 1–4 mm.[1] Bridged segments are recognized on coronary CT when the coronary arteries are circumferentially surrounded by myocardial tissue (Figure 35.1). The left anterior descending coronary artery is the most commonly involved; however, the circumflex and right coronary arteries may also have bridged segments (Figure 35.2). If multiphase images are acquired, narrowing of the intramyocardial segment may be seen during systole as the myocardium contracts. On catheter angiography, this is referred to as the "milking effect" and is the classic finding for the diagnosis of myocardial bridging.[2] In patients with coronary artery disease, atherosclerosis will spare the bridged segment, with plaques typically developing proximal to the segment of bridging (Figure 35.3).[3]

Importance

In the vast majority of cases, myocardial bridging is a benign finding incidentally encountered at cardiac imaging of no clinical consequence. Some studies have associated long and deep myocardial bridges with the presence of ischemia.[1] Intramyocardial segments have been rarely associated with cardiac events such as myocardial infarction or sudden death in small series and case reports.[3] Based upon long-term follow-up studies of patients diagnosed by catheter angiography, the prognosis for patients with myocardial bridging diagnosed with bridging by catheter is very good.[2] Although large cohort studies are lacking, in two studies of patients with bridging identified by coronary CT, 31/74[4] and 117/334[5] had bridged segments; however, there was no association between presence of bridging and adverse cardiac events after several years of follow-up.

Typical clinical scenario

Myocardial bridging is frequently encountered at coronary CT. The prevalence of myocardial bridging at angiography is less than 5%; however, autopsy studies have shown that bridging is much more common, seen in 15–85% of subjects.[6] Rate of identification at coronary CT has more closely matched autopsy studies, ranging from 20% to 60%.[1]

Differential diagnosis

The appearance of myocardial bridging is pathognomonic for the diagnosis and the differential is limited. In patients with infiltrative cardiac tumors, such as lymphoma, the coronary arteries can become encased by tumor which may simulate myocardial bridging. However, the presence of a cardiac mass and aggressive nature of the lesion should allow distinction of the two entities. Prominent intramyocardial coronary arteries may also be seen in congenital heart disease with coronary shunting, such as in anomalous origin of the coronary artery from the pulmonary artery or in fistulas between coronary arteries and the ventricular cavity. These can be distinguished from bridging by the presence of associated anomalies and by the coronary enlargement due to increased blood flow.

Teaching point

Myocardial bridging is commonly encountered at coronary CT, has a very good prognosis, and is usually of no clinical consequence. However, in symptomatic patients with no other explanation for pain, additional testing for ischemia may be warranted.

REFERENCES

1. R. Nakanishi, R. Rajani, Y. Ishikawa, T. Ishii, D. S. Berman. Myocardial bridging on coronary CTA: an innocent bystander or a culprit in myocardial infarction? *J Cardiovasc Comput Tomogr* 2012; **6**: 3–13.

2. S. Mohlenkamp, W. Hort, J. Ge, R. Erbel. Update on myocardial bridging. *Circulation* 2002; **106**: 2616–22.

3. H. Eggebrecht, S. Mohlenkamp. Images in clinical medicine. Myocardial bridging. *N Engl J Med* 2003; **349**: 1047.

4. P. Marcos-Alberca, A. Goncalves, C. F. Golfin, et al. Clinical outcomes of patients with intramyocardial bridging diagnosed by multi-detector cardiac computed tomography. *Int J Cardiol* 2011; **148**: 123–5.

5. R. Rubinshtein, T. Gaspar, B. S. Lewis, A. Prasad, N. Peled, D. A. Halon. Long-term prognosis and outcome in patients with a chest pain syndrome and myocardial bridging: a 64-slice coronary computed tomography angiography study. *Eur Heart J Cardiovasc Imaging* 2013; **14**: 579–85.

6. S. Y. Kim, J. B. Seo, K. H. Do, et al. Coronary artery anomalies: classification and ECG-gated multi-detector row CT findings with angiographic correlation. *Radiographics* 2006; **26**: 317–33; discussion 33–4.

Pearls and Pitfalls in Cardiovascular Imaging, ed. Stefan L. Zimmerman and Elliot K. Fishman. Published by Cambridge University Press. © Cambridge University Press 2015.

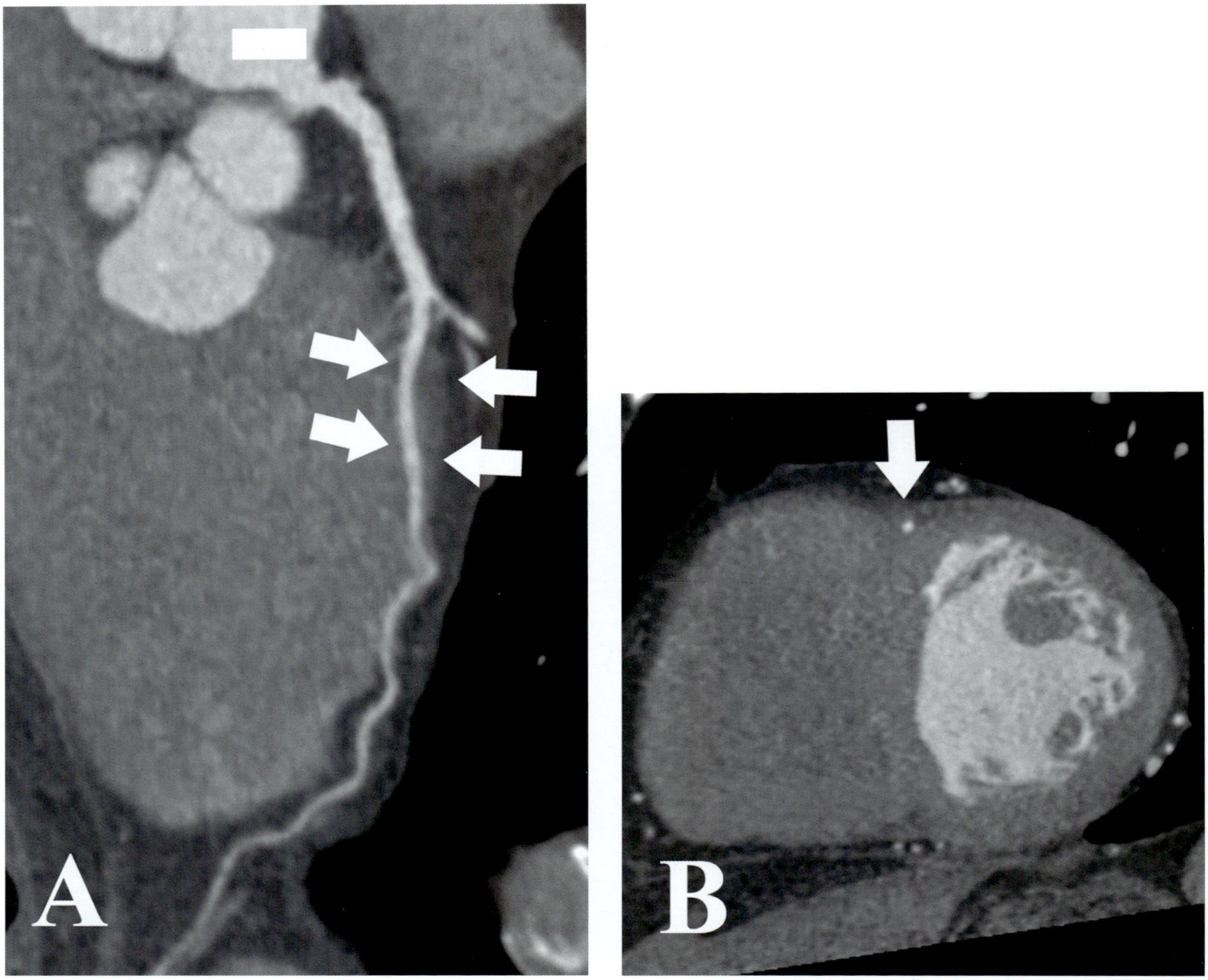

Figure 35.1 **A.** Curved planar reformatted image from a cardiac CT performed in a 70-year-old male with atypical chest pain demonstrates a long segment of intramyocardial bridging in the mid-left anterior descending coronary artery (LAD, arrows). The artery is circumferentially surrounded by myocardium, unlike the non-bridged segments proximal and distally that are surrounded by fat. **B.** Short-axis multiplanar reformatted image from the same study shows the mid-LAD surrounded by myocardial tissue (arrow), diagnostic of intramyocardial bridging.

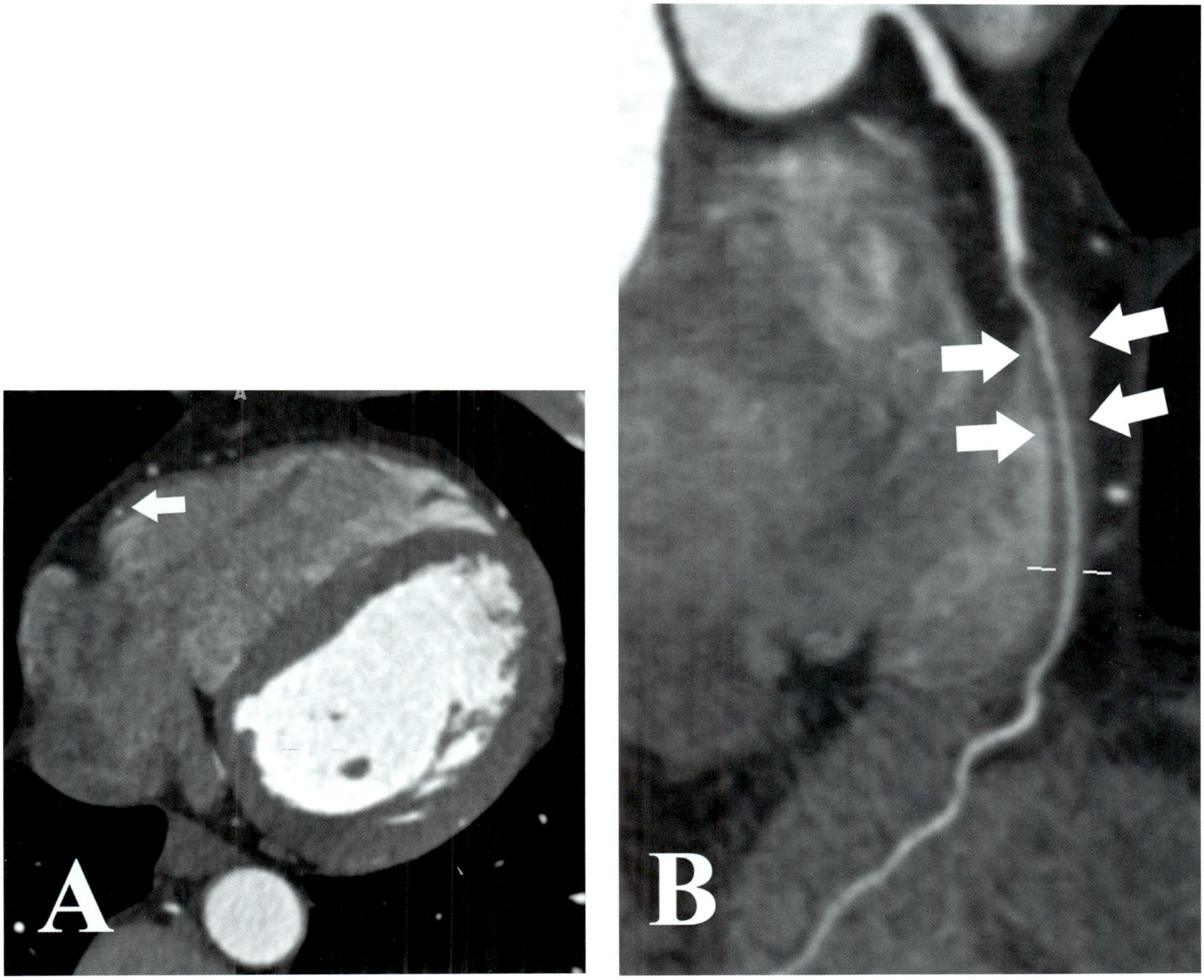

Figure 35.2 A. Axial image from a cardiac CT performed in a 57-year-old male research participant that demonstrates a long segment of right coronary artery (RCA) bridging. The mid-RCA is surrounded by the myocardium of the basilar right ventricular free wall (arrow). B. On a curved planar reformatted image from the same examination, the long bridged segment of the RCA can be easily recognized (arrows) with no significant narrowing relative to the proximal and distal vessel. RCA bridging is less common than bridging of the left anterior descending coronary artery; however, it is occasionally encountered and usually of no clinical significance.

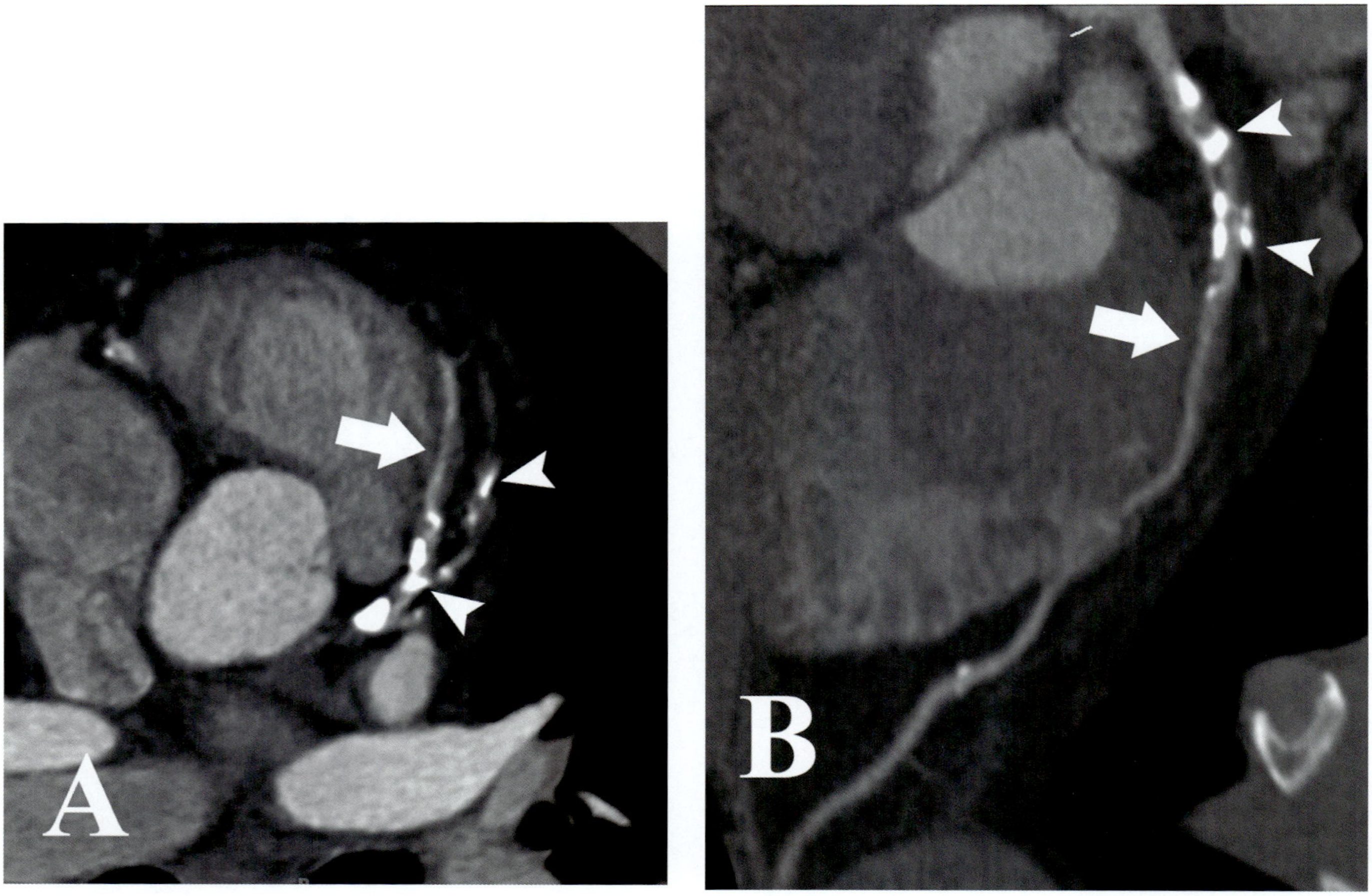

Figure 35.3 Oblique axial multiplanar reformatted image (**A**) and curved planar reformatted image (**B**) from a cardiac CT performed in a 67-year-old male with chest pain shows extensive calcified and mixed atherosclerotic plaque in the proximal and mid-left anterior descending coronary artery (LAD) and the adjacent diagonal branch (arrowheads). Atherosclerotic disease extends up to, but spares, a segment of intramyocardial bridging in the mid-LAD (arrows).

CASE **36**

Intramural versus septal course for anomalous interarterial coronary arteries

Stefan L. Zimmerman

Imaging description

Coronary artery anomalies are important to recognize due to their association with sudden cardiac death. Anomalous coronary arteries originating from the opposite aortic cusp with an interarterial course between the aorta and pulmonary artery are the highest risk,[1] whereas septal, prepulmonic, and retroaortic courses are generally considered benign.[2] Among patients with interarterial course, the presence of intramural coronary artery segments, in which the coronary artery courses within the wall of the aorta between layers of the media, is considered to further increase risk for sudden cardiac death.[3] Intramural segments can be recognized by a slit-like orifice, acute angle of origin from the aorta, and an elliptical shape on sagittal oblique image (Figure 36.1).[3] Interarterial course of the coronary arteries, with or without intramural segments, is important to distinguish from the septal course, which is generally accepted to be a lower-risk lesion.[2,4] In the septal course, the left main coronary artery passes beneath the pulmonary valve, travels intramyocardially through the basilar interventricular septum, and exits in the anterior interventricular groove where it bifurcates into left anterior descending and circumflex coronary arteries (Figure 36.2). In this variant, the coronary artery maintains a uniform round shape throughout its course, unlike the elliptical shape seen in intramural coronary artery segments.

Importance

The distinction of septal and interarterial courses of anomalous coronary arteries is important for patient management, given the elevated risk of sudden cardiac death associated with the latter. In patients with true interarterial course, characterization of intramural segments is important, not only because they confer greater risk, but also because they have a specific surgical management. Intramural segments can be managed through an unroofing procedure, in which the internal aortic wall is excised from the intramural segment, creating a neo-ostium and eliminating the intramural narrowing.[3] Septal anomalies are often managed conservatively.

Typical clinical scenario

Coronary artery anomalies are rare, affecting less than 1% of the population; however, they are the second most common cause of sudden cardiac death in athletes after hypertrophic cardiomyopathy.[4] They may be encountered incidentally in patients with cardiothoracic imaging performed for another purpose or can be identified in patients presenting with sudden cardiac death.

Differential diagnosis

In addition to the interarterial and septal courses, anomalous coronary arteries arising from the opposite cusp can travel posteriorly in the retroaortic subtype or anterior to the pulmonary artery in the prepulmonic subtype. Occasionally, motion artifact in the aortic root can simulate an anomalous interarterial coronary artery; however, this can be verified or excluded by obtaining an ECG-gated CT examination.

Teaching point

When anomalous coronary arteries arising from the opposite cusp are encountered it is important to distinguish interarterial and septal courses, given the increased risk of sudden cardiac death associated with the interarterial course. Careful inspection of the shape and course of the anomalous coronaries will help avoid misdiagnosis.

REFERENCES

1. A. J. Taylor, K. M. Rogan, R. Virmani. Sudden cardiac death associated with isolated congenital coronary artery anomalies. *J Am Coll Cardiol* 1992; **20**: 640–7.
2. J. E. Shriki, J. S. Shinbane, M. A. Rashid, et al. Identifying, characterizing, and classifying congenital anomalies of the coronary arteries. *Radiographics* 2012; **32**: 453–68.
3. J. A. Miller, N. S. Anavekar, M. M. El Yaman, H. M. Burkhart, A. J. Miller, P. R. Julsrud. Computed tomographic angiography identification of intramural segments in anomalous coronary arteries with interarterial course. *Int J Cardiovasc Imaging* 2012; **28**: 1525–32.
4. A. Pursnani, J. E. Jacobs, F. Saremi, et al. Coronary CTA assessment of coronary anomalies. *J Cardiovasc Comput Tomogr* 2012; **6**: 48–59.

Pearls and Pitfalls in Cardiovascular Imaging, ed. Stefan L. Zimmerman and Elliot K. Fishman. Published by Cambridge University Press. © Cambridge University Press 2015.

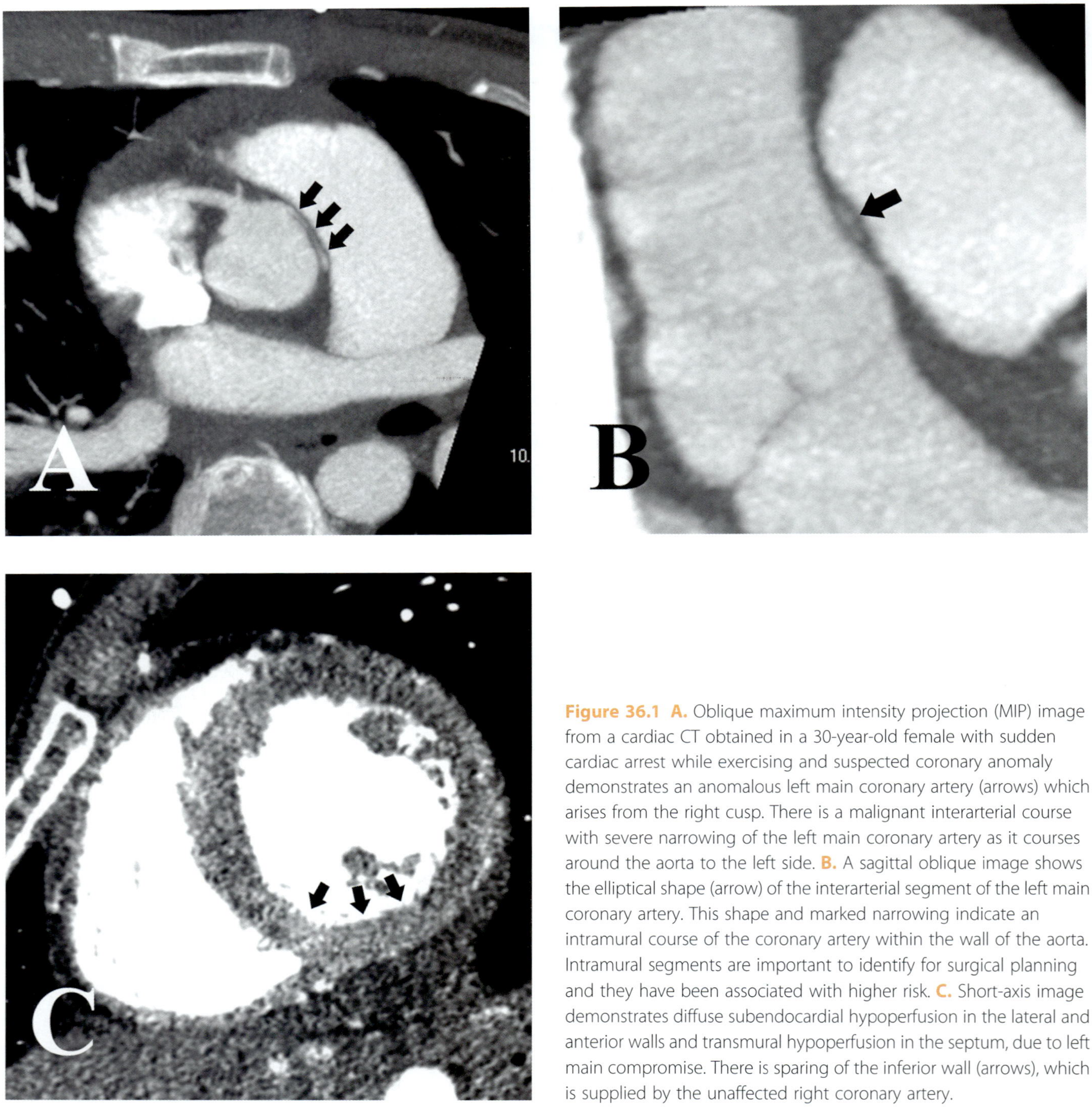

Figure 36.1 **A.** Oblique maximum intensity projection (MIP) image from a cardiac CT obtained in a 30-year-old female with sudden cardiac arrest while exercising and suspected coronary anomaly demonstrates an anomalous left main coronary artery (arrows) which arises from the right cusp. There is a malignant interarterial course with severe narrowing of the left main coronary artery as it courses around the aorta to the left side. **B.** A sagittal oblique image shows the elliptical shape (arrow) of the interarterial segment of the left main coronary artery. This shape and marked narrowing indicate an intramural course of the coronary artery within the wall of the aorta. Intramural segments are important to identify for surgical planning and they have been associated with higher risk. **C.** Short-axis image demonstrates diffuse subendocardial hypoperfusion in the lateral and anterior walls and transmural hypoperfusion in the septum, due to left main compromise. There is sparing of the inferior wall (arrows), which is supplied by the unaffected right coronary artery.

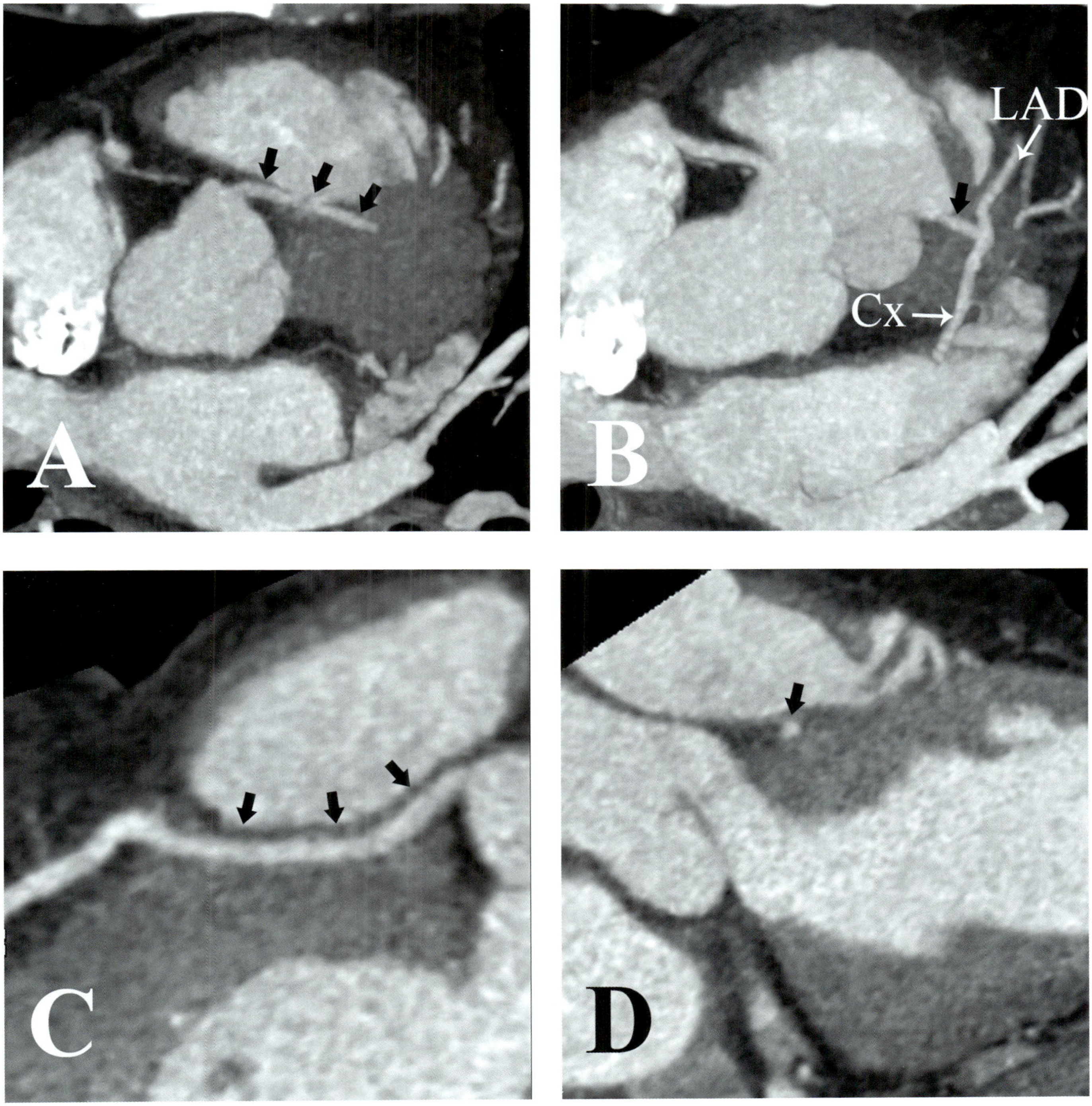

Figure 36.2 A. Axial maximum intensity projection (A,B), curved planar reformatted (C), sagittal oblique (D), and oblique volume rendered (E,F) images from a cardiac CT obtained in a 52-year-old male with chest pain. There is an anomalous left coronary artery from the left cusp with a septal course (arrows). In the septal course, the left main passes anteriorly and inferiorly (A), diving into the basilar portion of the anteroseptum (C,F), coursing below the right ventricular outflow tract (D,E), and emerging onto the epicardial surface then bifurcating into the LAD and circumflex (Cx) (B). Within the intraseptal segment, the anomalous left main artery maintains a rounded configuration with no evidence of narrowing (C,D), unlike the intramural course. The septal course is generally considered a benign variant and treated conservatively.

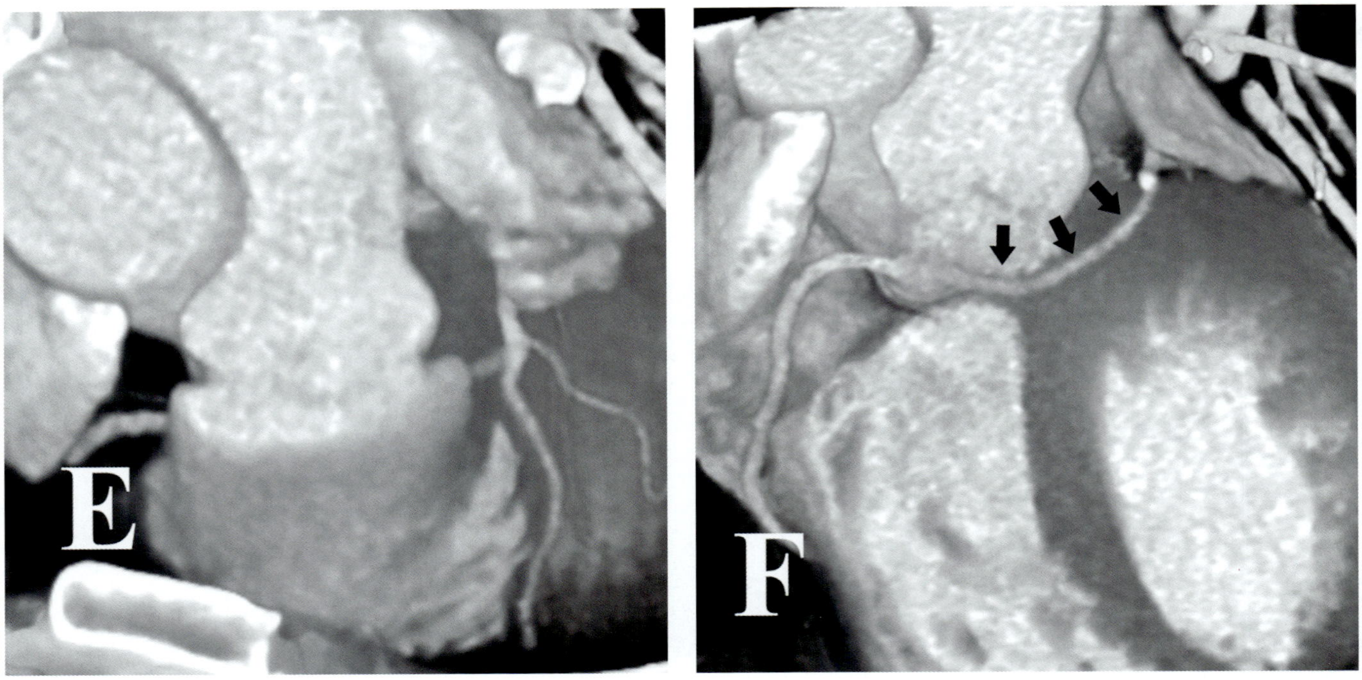

Figure 36.2 *(cont.)*

CASE

37 Coronary artery fistulas and anomalous coronary artery origin

Stefan L. Zimmerman

Imaging description

Coronary artery fistulas are defined by an abnormal connection between a coronary artery and another vessel or cardiac chamber in the absence of an intervening capillary bed.[1] Coronary fistulas are thought to be abnormal remnants of primitive sinusoids and vessels of fetal life that persist into adulthood.[2] At echocardiography, cardiac CT, or cardiac MRI a tortuous and possibly dilated vessel with abnormal drainage will be identified. Fistulas may connect to the cardiac chambers (coronary–cameral fistulas), pulmonary arteries, coronary sinus, pulmonary veins, or superior vena cava (Figures 37.1 and 37.2).[2] Fistulas draining to low pressure right-sided structures are the most common.[2,3]

Anomalous coronary artery origin from the pulmonary artery, also known as Bland-Garland-White syndrome, is an entity distinct from coronary artery fistula. Unlike fistulas, which are anomalies of coronary termination, Bland-Garland-White syndrome is an abnormality of coronary artery origination. The left coronary artery is the most commonly affected, and is also known by the acronym ALCAPA (anomalous left coronary artery from the pulmonary artery). The imaging appearance is similar to coronary fistulas with dilated and tortuous coronary arteries on cross-sectional imaging (Figure 37.3).[1] Unlike fistulas, however, the entire coronary tree is usually involved and the abnormal origin of a coronary artery from the pulmonary artery will be present.

Importance

Although most patients are asymptomatic, large coronary artery fistulas with significant shunting can result in congestive heart failure. Fistulas have also been associated with stroke, arrhythmias, myocardial infarction, and endocarditis.[3] Patients with an anomalous origin of the coronary artery from the pulmonary artery are much more symptomatic, usually presenting in infancy due to significant shunting or myocardial ischemia from a steal phenomenon.[1] However, delayed presentation until adulthood has been reported and can be a cause of sudden cardiac death.[4]

Typical clinical scenario

Coronary artery fistulas are rare, with an incidence estimated at 0.3–0.8% at angiography.[3] Most are congenital; however, post-traumatic and iatrogenic fistulas may occur. Many are asymptomatically discovered at angiography performed for other indications. Symptoms, when present, generally occur in adult patients and manifest as dyspnea and fatigue related to volume overload from shunting.[2] Anomalous origin of the coronary artery from the pulmonary artery is also rare, with an estimated prevalence of 1 in every 300,000 births and 0.25–0.5% of all cases of congenital heart disease.[4] Infants present with heart failure and myocardial infarction, whereas adults tend to present with malignant arrhythmia due to scarring from chronic subclinical ischemia.[4]

Differential diagnosis

Coronary artery aneurysms should be considered in the differential diagnosis for coronary artery fistulas and anomalous coronary artery origin from the pulmonary artery. Coronary artery aneurysms are most often due to atherosclerotic disease or vasculitis, such as Takayasu's or Kawasaki disease. Patients can be differentiated by the presence of multiple focally dilated coronary artery segments rather than diffuse vessel enlargement.[4]

Teaching point

Coronary artery fistulas and anomalous origin of the pulmonary artery from the coronary artery should be considered when encountering a patient with dilated and tortuous coronary arteries. Identification of abnormal coronary artery origination or termination will help make a definitive diagnosis.

REFERENCES

1. J. E. Shriki, J. S. Shinbane, M. A. Rashid, et al. Identifying, characterizing, and classifying congenital anomalies of the coronary arteries. *Radiographics* 2012; **32**: 453–68.

2. C. V. Mangukia. Coronary artery fistula. *Ann Thorac Surg* 2012; **93**: 2084–92.

3. R. M. Gowda, B. C. Vasavada, I. A. Khan. Coronary artery fistulas: clinical and therapeutic considerations. *Int J Cardiol* 2006; **107**: 7–10.

4. E. Pena, E. T. Nguyen, N. Merchant, G. Dennie. ALCAPA syndrome: not just a pediatric disease. *Radiographics* 2009; **29**: 553–65.

Pearls and Pitfalls in Cardiovascular Imaging, ed. Stefan L. Zimmerman and Elliot K. Fishman. Published by Cambridge University Press. © Cambridge University Press 2015.

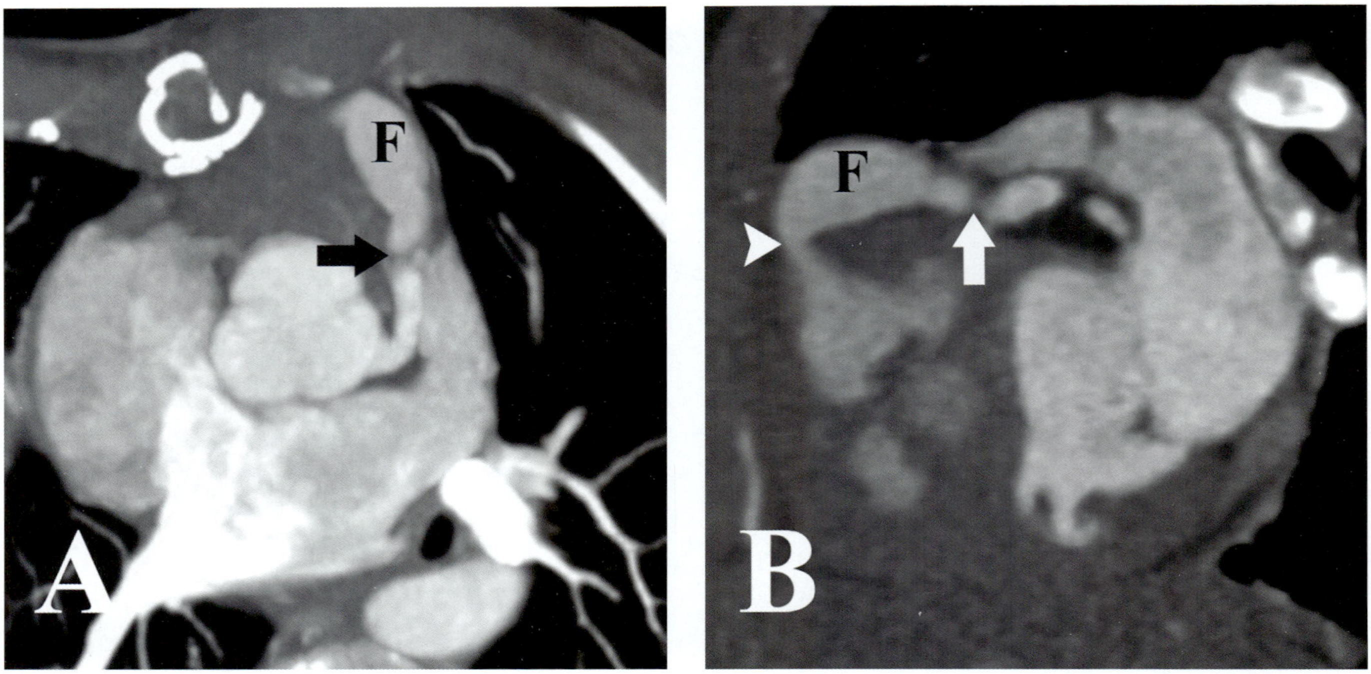

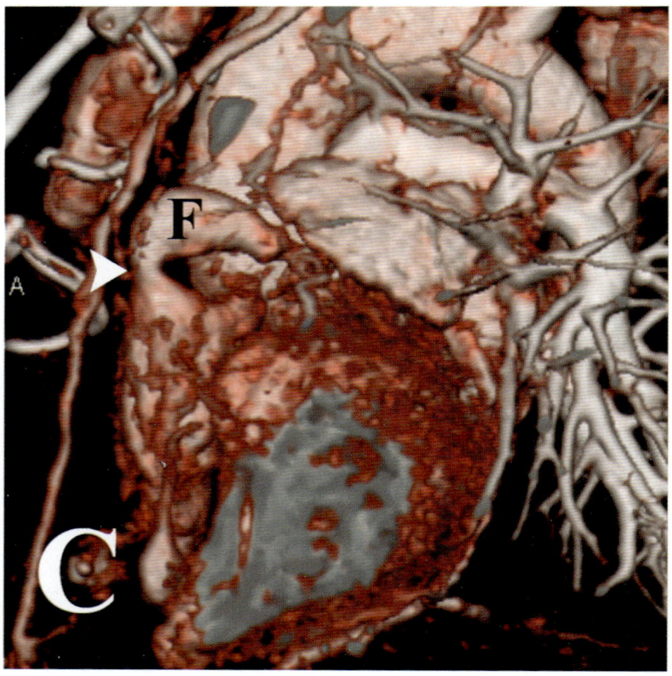

Figure 37.1 **A.** Axial maximum intensity projection (MIP) image from a cardiac CT performed in a 4-year-old male with pulmonary artery atresia and intact ventricular septum and suspicion for coronary–cameral fistulas on echocardiography. There is a large fistula (F) between the left anterior descending coronary artery and the chamber of the right ventricle. A stenosis is seen in the mid-portion of the vessel (black arrow), confirmed at cardiac catheterization. **B.** Sagittal oblique reformatted image demonstrating the connection (arrowhead) between the dilated fistula (F) and the right ventricle. The stenosis is again demonstrated (arrow). **C.** Volume-rendered image clearly demonstrates the fistulous connection (F) between the vessel and the right ventricle.

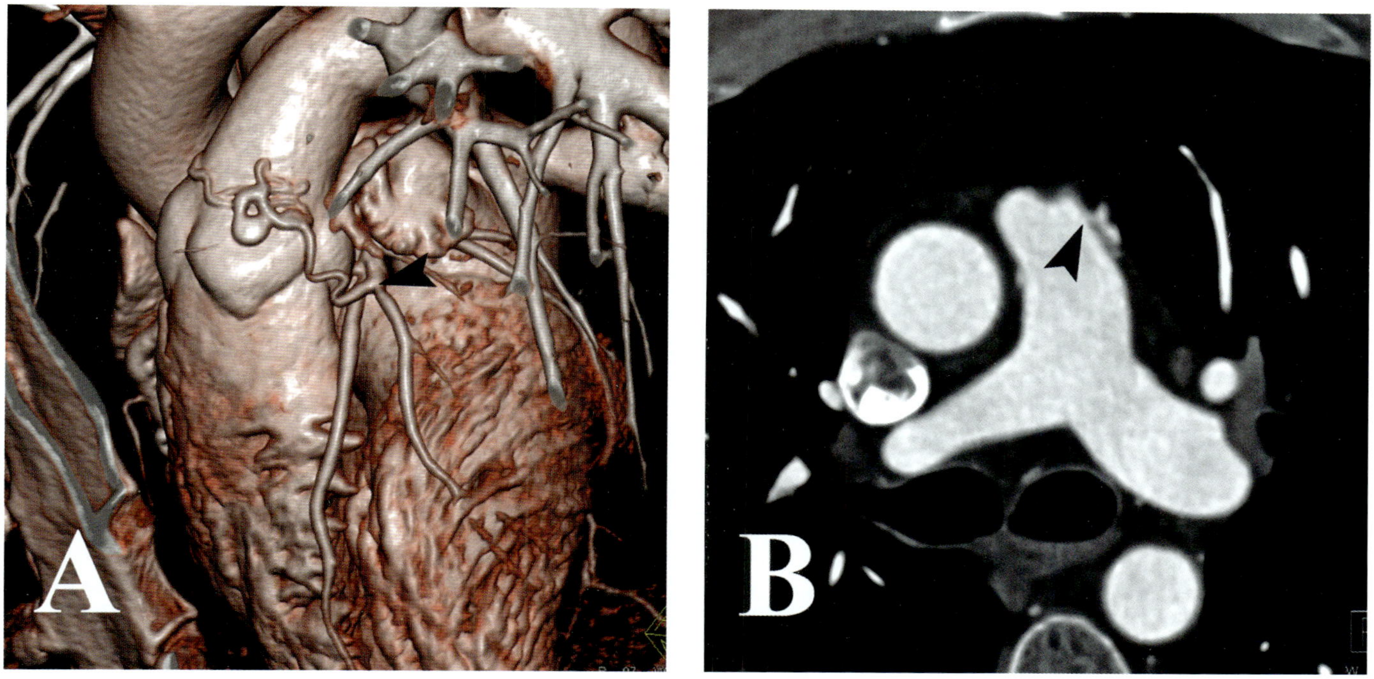

Figure 37.2 **A.** Oblique volume-rendered image from a cardiac CT performed in a 57-year-old male with chest pain and incidentally discovered small coronary artery to pulmonary artery fistula. There is an anomalous vessel that originates from the proximal aspect of a large first diagonal branch (black arrowhead), which is tortuous and aneurysmal, crossing over the proximal main pulmonary artery. **B.** On an axial image from the same study, a small connection between the anomalous vessel and the main pulmonary artery is identified (black arrow).

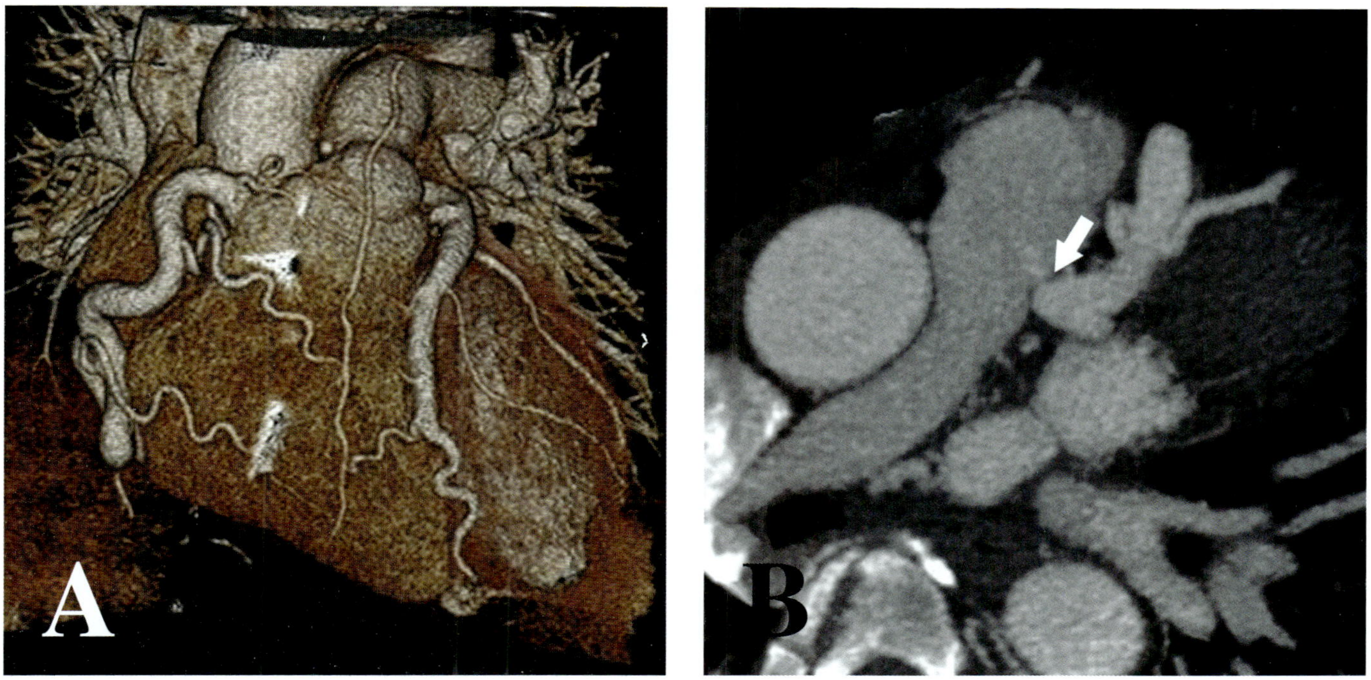

Figure 37.3 **A.** Coronal volume-rendered image from a cardiac CT performed in a 24-year-old female with anomalous origin of the left coronary artery from the pulmonary artery (ALCAPA). The coronary arteries are massively enlarged and tortuous because of chronically increased flow from left-to-right shunting. **B.** An oblique multiplanar reformatted image demonstrates the abnormal connection of the severely dilated left main coronary artery to the proximal pulmonary artery (arrow). There is a tight stenosis at the site of the anomalous left main origin. These ostial stenoses are typical for patients who have a delayed presentation in adulthood.

CASE 38

Giant coronary artery aneurysms

Mark Stellingworth, Saurabh Jha, Koteswara Pothineni, and Stefan L. Zimmerman

Imaging description

Coronary artery aneurysms are defined as localized vessel dilatation exceeding 50% of the adjacent normal coronary artery diameter.[1] A precise definition of the threshold between aneurysm and "giant" aneurysm is not well established, but some authors have suggested that aneurysms > 20 mm meet this criteria.[2] Giant coronary artery aneurysms are identified by the presence of a round or ovoid structure on the epicardial surface of the heart in the typical location for coronary arteries. Often discovered incidentally on echocardiogram, they will appear as a paracardiac mass with varying degrees of flow on Doppler interrogation depending on presence of thrombus. On non-contrast CT, they are low-attenuation, rounded masses that may have peripheral calcifications related to atherosclerosis. After contrast administration, lesions will enhance similar to blood pool, although varying degrees of thrombosis may be present (Figure 38.1). Large aneurysms can erroneously appear thrombosed on cardiac CT due to incomplete filling at the time of arterial phase acquisition (Figure 38.2). Delayed venous images will demonstrate further fill-in of the aneurysm. Cardiovascular magnetic resonance (CMR) imaging will typically show low signal on dark blood images due to flow (Figure 38.1). Steady-state free precession (SSFP) and contrast injections with gadolinium will confirm high signal in the structure due to blood and may show evidence of thrombus (Figures 38.1 and 38.2).

Importance

Patients with giant coronary aneurysms may present with life-threatening tamponade due to rupture. Thrombosis, fistulization to cardiac chambers, and embolization have also been noted in the literature.[3] Giant coronary artery aneurysms can be misinterpreted as cardiac tumors, particularly if only limited imaging is available. The distinction between tumor and aneurysm could have significant impact on treatment.

Typical clinical scenario

Coronary artery aneurysms more commonly affect males and have an incidence between 0.3% and 5%.[4] Coronary aneurysms greater than 20 mm are extremely rare and in one series represented only 0.02% of patients undergoing cardiac surgery.[2] They are more likely to involve the right coronary artery.

The most common cause is atherosclerosis. An additional 20–30% of these lesions are congenital.[4] Kawasaki disease is the most common etiology in Asian countries. Primarily a disease of infants and children, small aneurysms associated with Kawasaki disease most often regress; however, large aneurysms > 8 mm in size will typically persist or develop obstructive stenosis, which can present late in adulthood.[5]

Less common inflammatory disorders associated with coronary aneurysms include Takayasu's arteritis, lupus, and rheumatoid arthritis. Connective tissue disorders such as Marfan and Ehlers–Danlos syndromes, have also been implicated.[4]

Differential diagnosis

Giant coronary aneurysms, particularly those involving the right coronary artery, may be mistaken for a cardiac tumor. Angiosarcoma is the second most common of all primary cardiac neoplasms and has a predilection for the right atrium. It may also extend into the tricuspid valve, right ventricle, and the superior vena cava. These lesions usually enhance very avidly with contrast, which can mimic a vascular lesion.[6]

The presence of thrombus and flow on SSFP images increase the index of suspicion for aneurysm. Tissue characterization on T1-weighted black blood and T2-weighted triple inversion pulse sequences will help distinguish this finding from cardiac lipoma and pericardial cysts, respectively. Location of the tumor is also helpful – lipomatous hyperplasia, for instance, more frequently involves the interatrial septum and has a characteristic "dumbbell" shape whereas atrial myxoma more commonly involves the left atrium.

Coronary fistulas share many of the characteristics of a coronary aneurysm. Coronary CTA is particularly useful in discerning aberrant arteriovenous connections or drainage into a cardiac chamber. This modality can also eliminate anomalous coronary arteries with origin from the pulmonary artery (i.e., right or left coronary artery originating from the pulmonary artery, RCAPA and LCAPA) from the differential.

Teaching point

Giant coronary aneurysms should be suspected when encountering a large, smooth mass on the epicardial surface of the heart and can typically be distinguished from tumor by enhancement characteristics.

REFERENCES

1. P. S. Swaye, L. D. Fisher, P. Litwin, et al. Aneurysmal coronary artery disease. *Circulation* 1983; **67**: 134–8.
2. D. Li, Q. Wu, L. Sun, et al. Surgical treatment of giant coronary artery aneurysm. *J Thorac Cardiovasc Surg* 2005; **130**: 817–21.

Pearls and Pitfalls in Cardiovascular Imaging, ed. Stefan L. Zimmerman and Elliot K. Fishman. Published by Cambridge University Press. © Cambridge University Press 2015.

3. N. K. Jha, H. Z. Ouda, J. A. Khan, G. P. Eising, N. Augustin. Giant right coronary artery aneurysm – case report and literature review. *J Cardiothorac Surg* 2009; **4**: 18.
4. P. Cohen, P. T. O'Gara. Coronary artery aneurysms: a review of the natural history, pathophysiology, and management. *Cardiol Rev* 2008; **16**: 301–4.
5. K. Suda, M. Iemura, H. Nishiono, et al. Long-term prognosis of patients with Kawasaki disease complicated by giant coronary aneurysms: a single-institution experience. *Circulation* 2011; **123**: 1836–42.
6. P. J. Sparrow, J. B. Kurian, T. R. Jones, M. U. Sivananthan. MR imaging of cardiac tumors. *Radiographics* 2005; **25**: 1255–76.

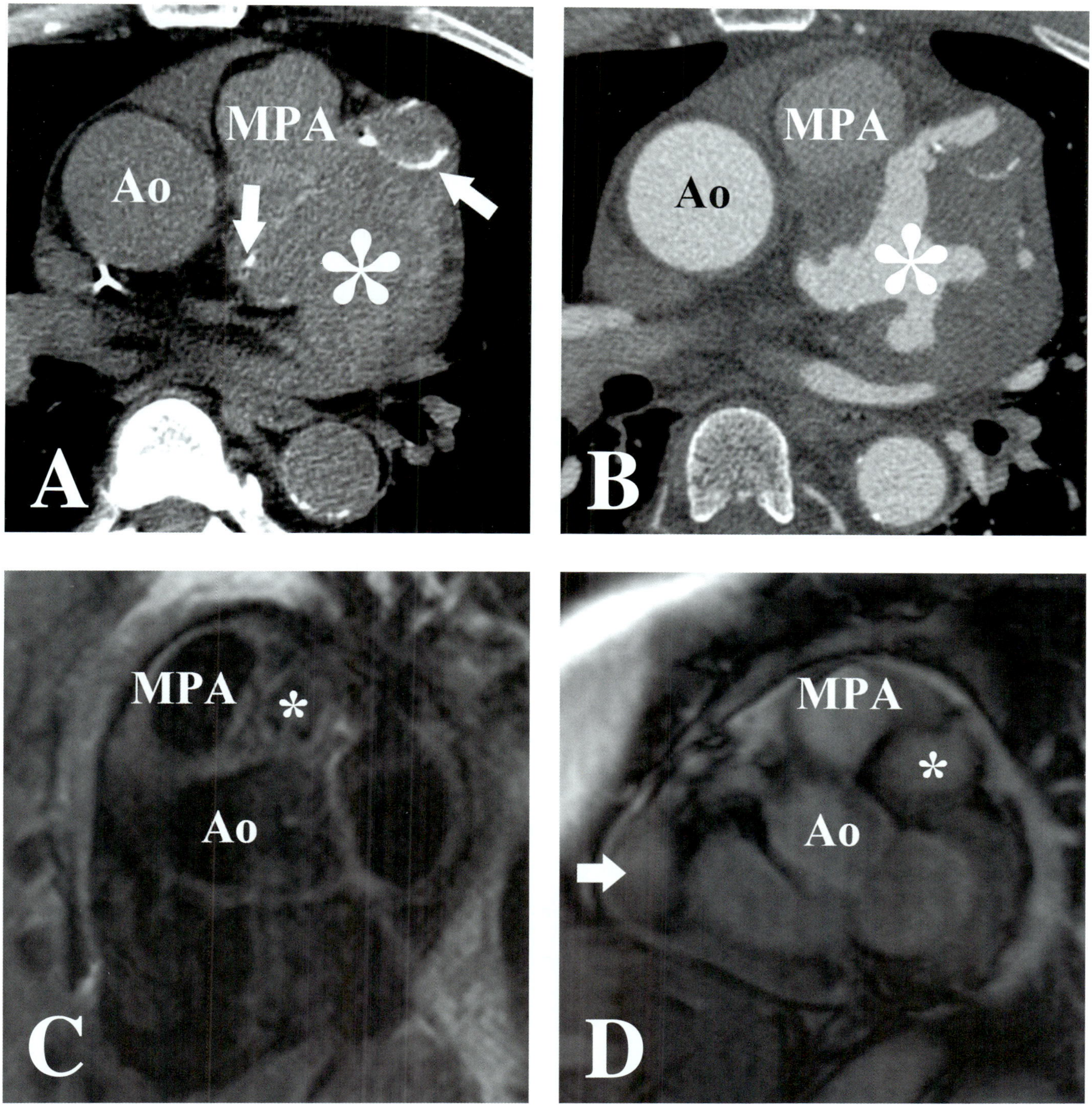

Figure 38.1 Giant complex coronary artery aneurysm in a 55-year-old asymptomatic patient. **A.** Non-contrast ECG-gated axial CT image demonstrates a partially calcified lobulated mass adjacent (asterisk) to the main pulmonary artery (MPA) with some areas of peripheral calcification (arrows) (Ao = ascending aorta). **B.** Post-contrast ECG-gated axial CT image shows central branching enhancement (asterisk) that is identical to blood pool due to a large, complex aneurysm involving the distal left main, proximal left anterior descending coronary artery, and the proximal circumflex coronary artery. **C.** Short-axis dark blood images from cardiac MRI in the same patient show dark signal in the aneurysm due to blood flow (asterisk). **D.** Short-axis bright blood image shows high-signal intensity in the aneurysm matching blood pool (asterisk). A large aneurysm of the mid-RCA is also seen (arrow).

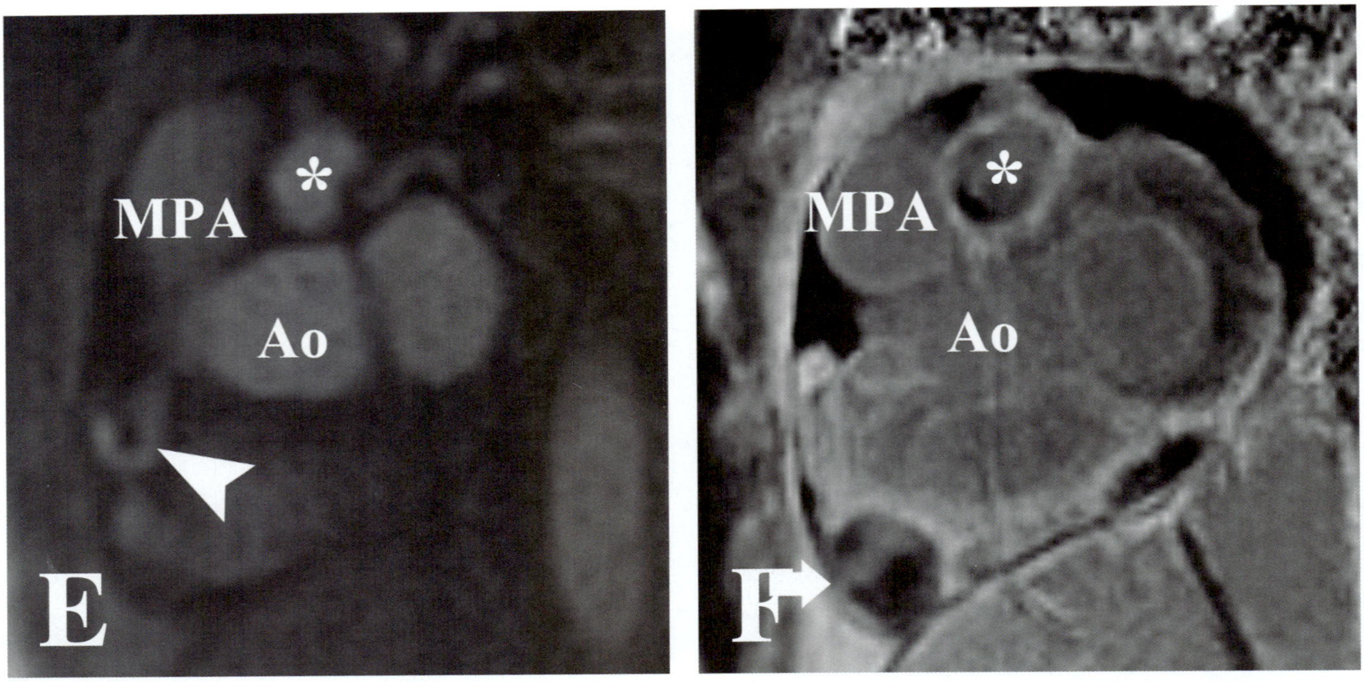

Figure 38.1 (*cont.*) **E.** Perfusion images demonstrate enhancement of the aneurysm that is identical to blood pool and the right coronary artery (arrowhead). **F.** Post-contrast delayed enhancement images show small amounts of low-attenuation non-enhancing thrombus in the aneurysm sac. No definitive diagnosis was available, but the aneurysm was presumed related to Kawasaki disease as a child.

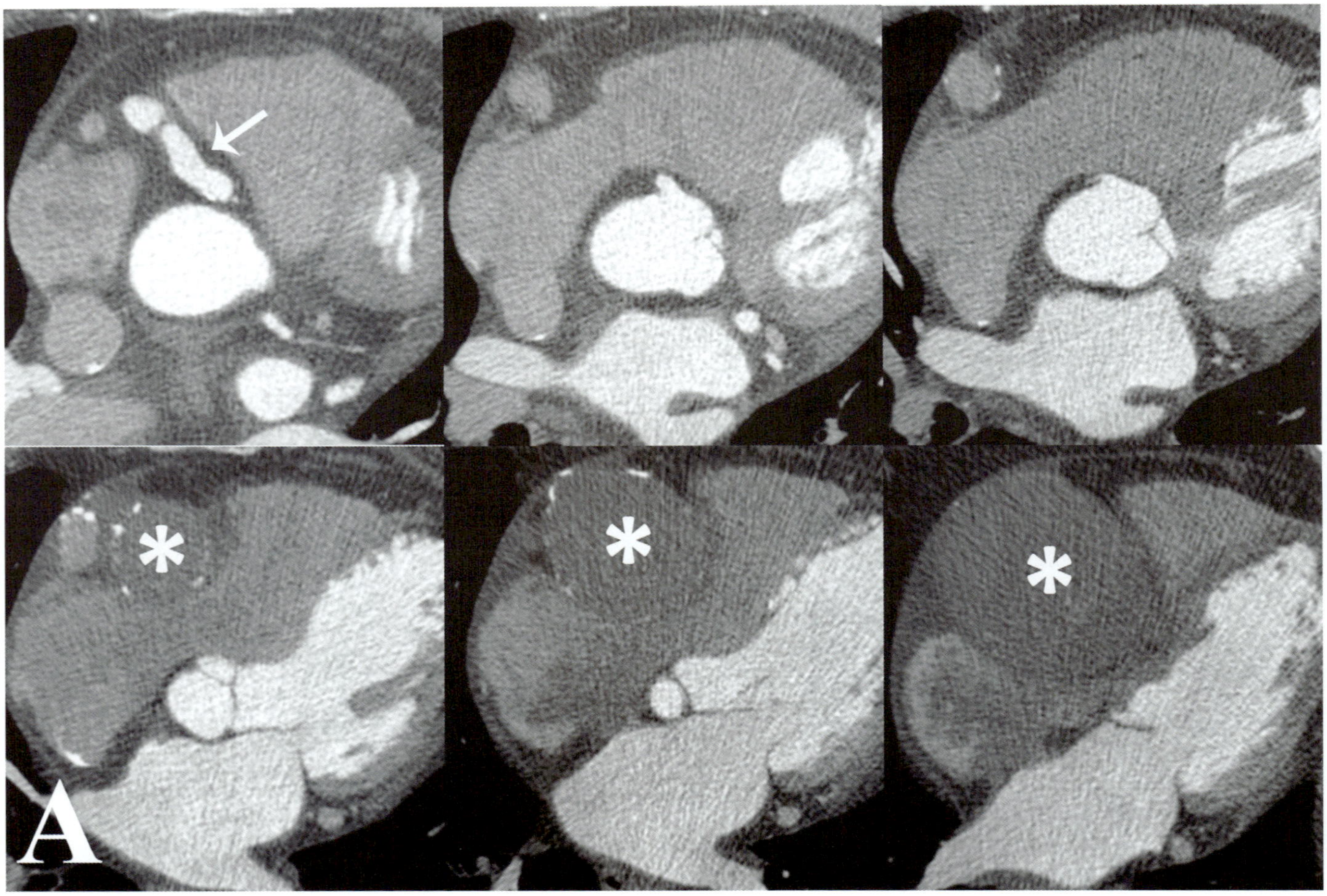

Figure 38.2 Giant coronary aneurysm in a 55-year-old male that was incidentally discovered on a transthoracic echocardiogram and thought to represent a paracardiac tumor. **A.** Contiguous axial images from a cardiac CT examination demonstrate an aneurysmal proximal right coronary

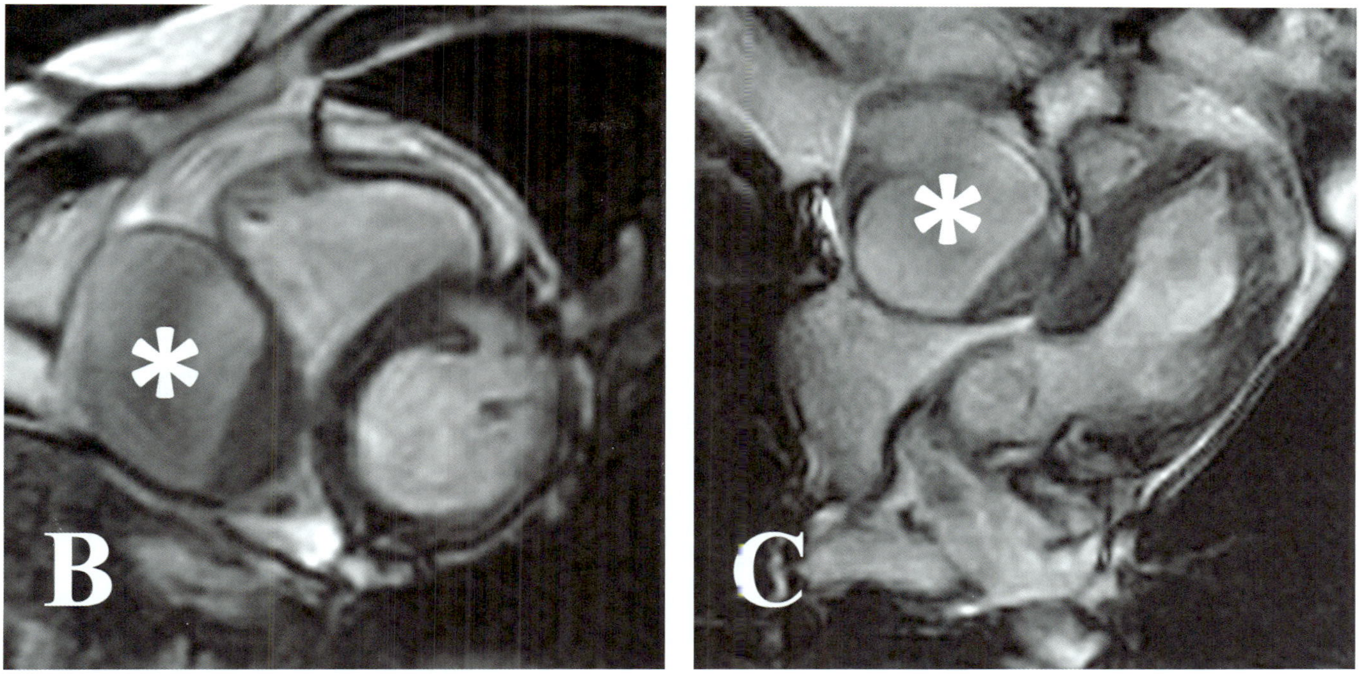

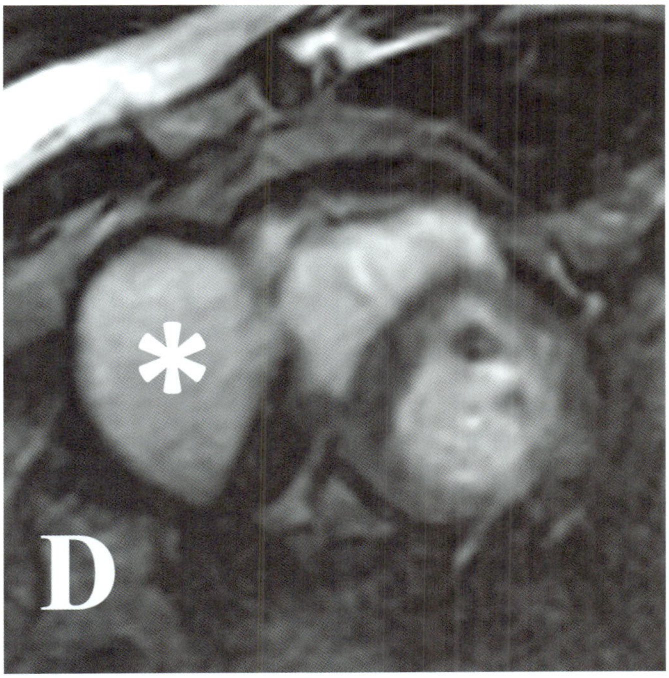

Figure 38.2 (*cont.*) artery (arrow) leading to a large, rim-calcified aneurysm that measured 6 cm in size (asterisk). There is mass effect on the right ventricle. The aneurysm is poorly enhanced due to early arterial phase of scanning, which does not allow enough time for complete mixing of contrast in the aneurysm sac. Short-axis (**B**) and four-chamber (**C**) bright blood steady-state free precession (SSFP) image from a cardiac MR performed in the same patient demonstrates peripheral low signal in the large aneurysm due to mural thrombus. **D.** On dynamic perfusion images obtained after contrast, the aneurysm (asterisk) enhances similar to venricular blood pool. The presumptive diagnosis was childhood Kawasaki disease.

CASE 39

Caseous calcification of the mitral annulus mimicking circumflex coronary artery aneurysm

Stefan L. Zimmerman

Imaging description

Caseous, or liquefactive, calcification of the mitral annulus is a rare variant of mitral annular calcification. In caseous mitral annular calcification, a smooth, ovoid mass is found within the mitral annulus with rim calcification and a homogenous, moderately hyperattenuating center on computed tomography (CT) (Figure 39.1). The liquefactive center of the lesion is not as densely hyperattenuating as vascular or osseous calcifications. In some cases, the center of the lesion may contain low-attenuation components (Figure 39.2). These masses are commonly located in the inferior or lateral aspect of the left atrioventricular groove and may displace mitral valve leaflets from mass effect. In some cases, multiple masses or continuous calcification around the entire mitral valve annulus may be seen (Figure 39.3). Caseous calcification may be initially discovered at echocardiography, where they appear as a rounded echogenic mass with central hypoechogenicity due to a central core of liquefactive necrosis.[1] At pathology, the center of these lesions is composed of a toothpaste-like material that represents a mix of calcium, fatty acids, and cholesterol.[2]

Importance

Rounded masses of caseous mitral annular calcification can be incorrectly diagnosed as circumflex coronary artery aneurysms, given their similar location and attenuation on contrast-enhanced CT (Figure 39.1). This could lead to additional inappropriate diagnostic tests, such as cardiac catheterization, or surgery. Caseous mitral calcification is a benign condition; however, rare complications due to ulceration resulting in distal embolization and/or endocarditis have been reported.[1] Caseous calcifications may also be associated with mitral valve stenosis or regurgitation due to mass effect.

Typical clinical scenario

Caseous mitral annular calcification is an uncommon condition, with a prevalence of $< 0.1\%$ in large echocardiographic studies.[1] Among patients with mitral annular calcification, caseous degeneration is reported in $< 1\%$ of cases.[1] Caseous mitral calcification is typically an incidental finding on CT, MR, or echocardiographic exams performed for other reasons. Occasionally, patients may be referred to cardiac CT or MRI for definitive evaluation if the diagnosis is unclear on echocardiography.

Differential diagnosis

The rounded, smooth appearance of caseous mitral annular calcification and location within the left atrioventricular groove can mimic an aneurysm of the circumflex coronary artery. However, circumflex aneurysms will be contiguous with the circumflex coronary artery, unlike caseous mitral annular calcification. In addition, careful inspection of the location of the lesion on contrast-enhanced images will allow identification of fat in the atrioventricular groove surrounding a circumflex aneurysm. In contrast, caseous mitral annular calcification abuts the mitral valve and the basilar left ventricular myocardium. Non-contrast calcium scoring sequences or non-gated chest CT can easily distinguish these two entities because only caseous mitral annular calcification will be hyperattenuating on these images (Figure 39.1). In addition to a circumflex coronary artery aneurysm, other diagnostic considerations include cardiac tumors or an abscess.[3] However, these will not have the same high attenuation as caseous mitral annular calcification.

Teaching point

Caseous mitral annular calcification may mimic a circumflex coronary artery aneurysm. Careful inspection of lesion location and evaluation of non-contrast images, when available, will allow accurate distinction of these two entities and avoid misdiagnosis.

REFERENCES

1. S. S. Srivatsa, M. D. Taylor, K. Hor, et al. Liquefaction necrosis of mitral annular calcification (LNMAC): review of pathology, prevalence, imaging and management: proposed diagnostic imaging criteria with detailed multi-modality and MRI image characterization. *Int J Cardiovasc Imaging* 2012; **28**: 1161–71.
2. H. Alkadhi, S. Leschka, R. Pretre, A. Perren, B. Marincek, S. Wildermuth. Caseous calcification of the mitral annulus. *J Thorac Cardiovasc Surg* 2005; **129**: 1438–40.
3. A. Gulati, C. Chan, A. Duncan, S. Raza, P. J. Kilner, J. Pepper. Multimodality cardiac imaging in the evaluation of mitral annular caseous calcification. *Circulation* 2011; **123**: e1–2.

Pearls and Pitfalls in Cardiovascular Imaging, ed. Stefan L. Zimmerman and Elliot K. Fishman. Published by Cambridge University Press. © Cambridge University Press 2015.

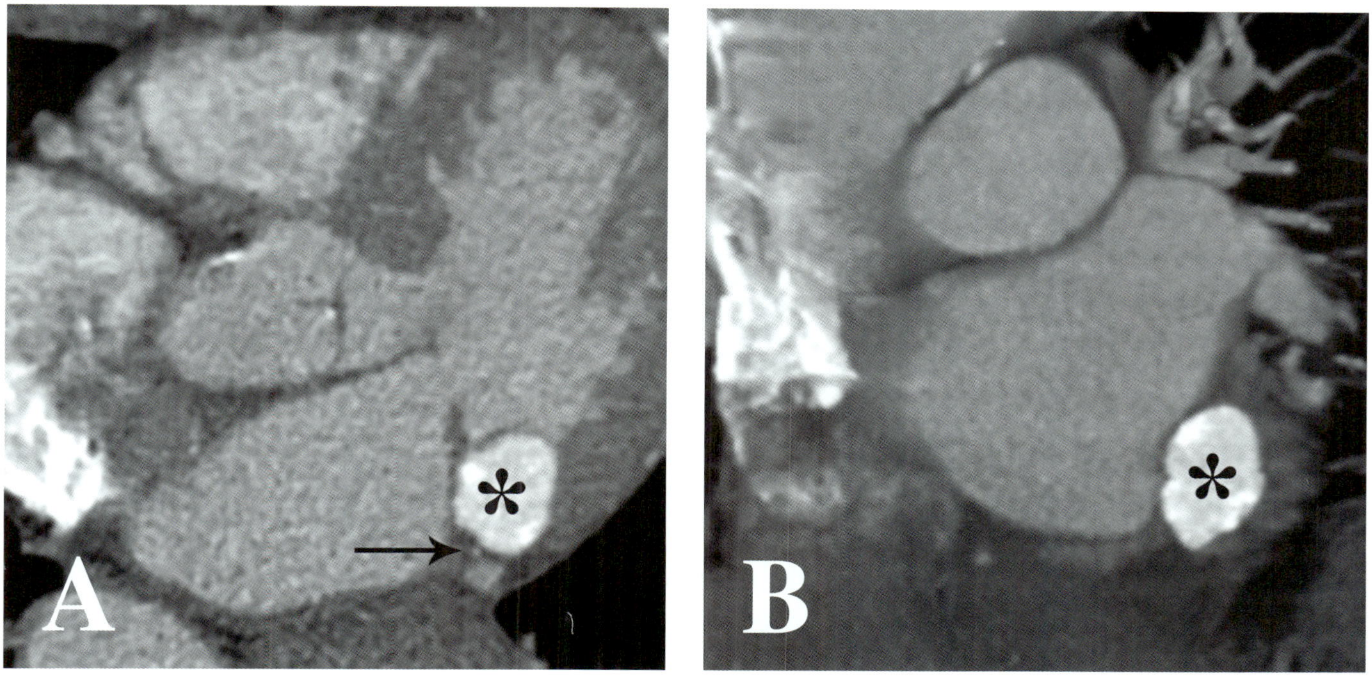

Figure 39.1 **A.** Axial image from cardiac CT performed in a 66-year-old female with chest pain demonstrates an ovoid, homogenously high-attenuation lesion in the region of the left atrioventricular groove (asterisk). The location and high attenuation mimic a circumflex artery aneurysm. However, on close inspection, the circumflex coronary artery can be visualized separate from the lesion (black arrow). The lesion was also hyperattenuating on non-contrast images (not shown), excluding the possibility of circumflex aneurysm. **B.** Coronal oblique volume-rendered image from the same patient again demonstrates the focal ovoid high-attenuation mass in the left atrioventricular groove, the characteristic location of caseous mitral annular calcification (asterisk).

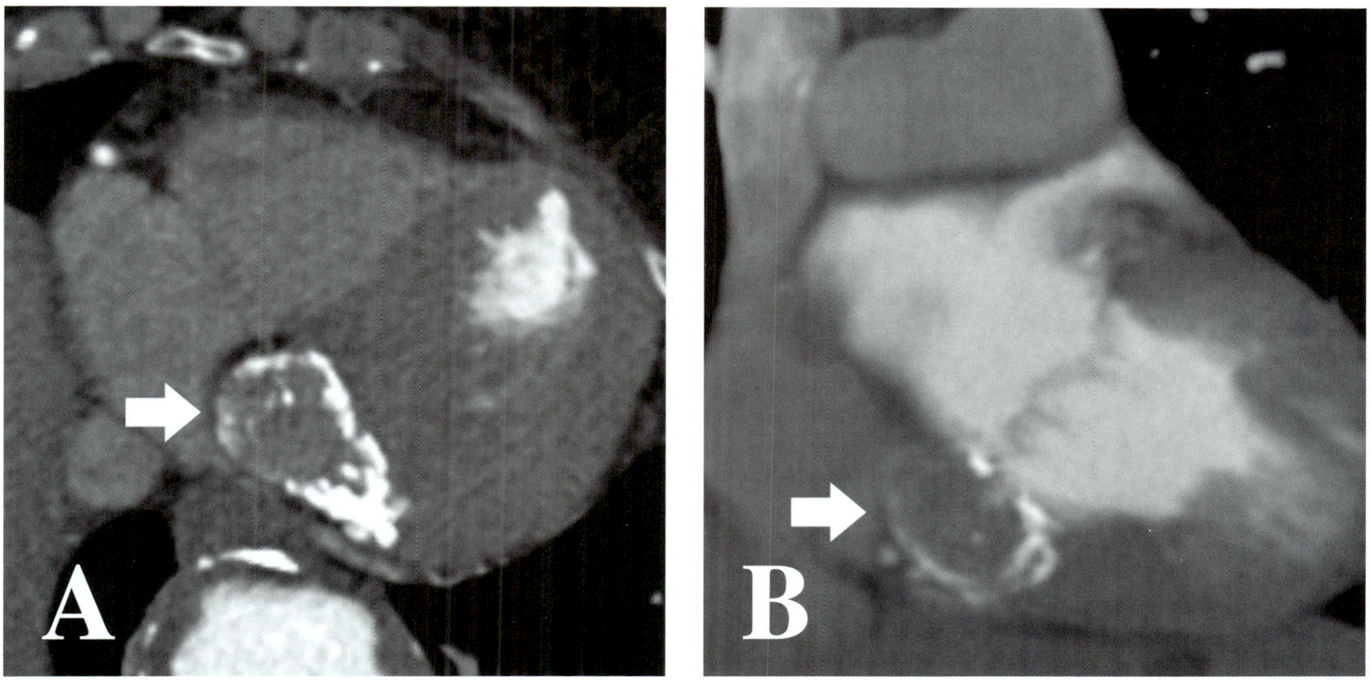

Figure 39.2 **A.** Axial image from an enhanced chest CT performed in a 75-year-old female with prior ascending aortic aneurysm repair demonstrates a low-attenuation, rim-calcified, ovoid mass in the inferior atrioventricular groove (arrow). The location and morphology are characteristic of caseous mitral annular calcification. Although in most patients this entity is homogenously high attenuation, rarely cases may be encountered with a low-attenuation liquefactive core. **B.** Coronal multiplanar reformatted image from the same patient demonstrates the typical relationship of this low-attenuation mass to the mitral valve, characteristic of caseous mitral annular calcification (arrow).

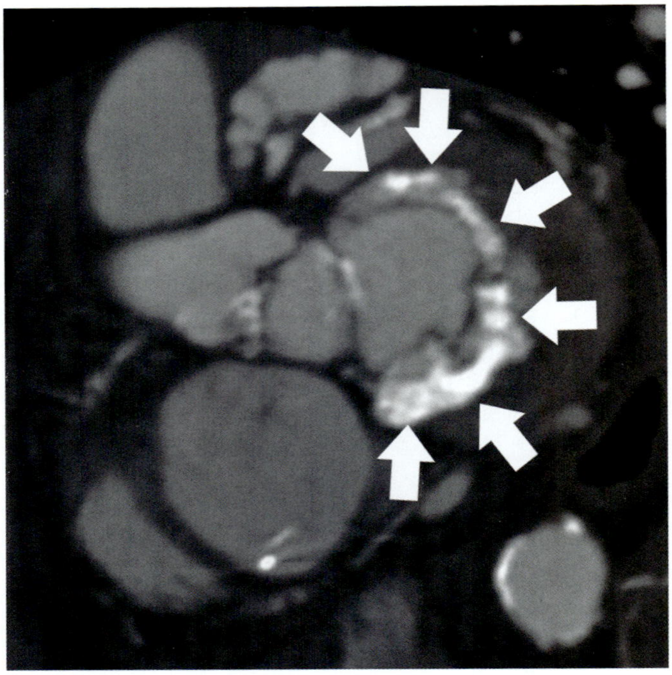

Figure 39.3 Short-axis multiplanar reformatted image from a contrast-enhanced CT examination of the chest performed due to concern for aortic dissection in a 97-year-old female with acute chest pain. There is diffuse circumferential mitral annular calcification (arrows) with a lobulated, mass-like appearance. Extent of mitral annular calcification can vary from patient to patient. When severe, such as in this patient, there is often associated dysfunction of the mitral valve.

CASE 40

Vein graft aneurysms after CABG

Tessa S. Cook

Imaging description

When incidentally detected on radiography, saphenous vein graft aneurysms most commonly present as mediastinal masses (Figure 40.1). This leads to follow-up cross-sectional imaging to narrow the broad differential diagnosis, which will more clearly characterize the "mass" as a large aneurysm (Figure 40.2). Vein graft aneurysms can easily grow to 6 cm or more in greatest diameter, and may be filled with a large amount of thrombus. It is important to identify whether the native coronary artery distal to the aneurysm is patent (Figure 40.3), because this will dictate treatment options (e.g., closure or embolization vs. endovascular stenting).

Importance

Saphenous vein graft aneurysms are an uncommon complication of coronary artery bypass grafting (CABG), thought to occur in less than 1% of patients.[1] However, because of the increased risk of rupture, they are associated with significant morbidity and mortality. If the thrombus within the aneurysm sac is unstable, there is also an increased risk of myocardial infarction in the territory distal to the graft. In addition, as the aneurysm grows, it can exert a mass effect on adjacent structures, such as cardiac chambers or the pulmonary veins, resulting in heart failure.

If the graft and native vessel remain patent, percutaneous repair with a covered stent is the preferred therapy to preserve perfusion.[2] However, if the graft is thrombosed, the aneurysm can be occluded using coil embolization or a closure device.[3] In some cases, such as when the luminal diameter of the coronary arteries is too small to permit passage of the percutaneous repair apparatus, patients may undergo surgical repair involving resection of the aneurysm and replacement of the vein graft.[4]

Typical clinical scenario

Saphenous vein grafts are often used for CABG. In rare cases, aneurysms of the vein grafts can form (as much as a decade or longer after the procedure) due to aggressive atherosclerosis.[5] Such aneurysms are often incidentally detected during follow-up imaging or chest radiography for unrelated reasons. In some cases, they can present with non-specific chest pain, angina, or even myocardial infarction.

Differential diagnosis

As these vein graft aneurysms often present as incidental findings on imaging, the differential diagnosis encompasses all causes of mediastinal or retrocardiac masses, such as lymphadenopathy, aortic aneurysms or pseudoaneurysms and neoplasms of thoracic origin (pulmonary, pleural, etc.). In addition, a ventricular aneurysm should also be included on the differential, given the radiographic appearance of these vein graft aneurysms.

Teaching point

Vein graft aneurysms are a rare long-term complication of CABG and should be addressed expediently after identification to avoid the associated morbidity and mortality.

REFERENCES

1. K. Nishimura, Y. Nakamura, S. Harada, et al. Saphenous vein graft aneurysm after coronary artery bypass grafting. *Ann Thorac Cardiovasc Surg* 2009; **15**: 61–3.
2. C. J. Panetta, W. Schneider, M. A. Boller. Percutaneous management of a long saphenous vein graft aneurysm: a case report and review of literature. *Cardiol Res Pract* 2009; **2009**: 981292.
3. N. L. Cruden, C. Turnbull, I. R. Starkey. Saphenous vein graft aneurysm. *Eur Heart J* 2007; **28**: 1071.
4. S. Kubota, S. Wakasa, T. Ooka, T. Tachibana, S. Sasaki, Y. Matsui. Successful excision of a saphenous vein graft aneurysm with different methods. *Gen Thorac Cardiovasc Surg* 2011; **59**: 426–8.
5. A. A. Frazier, F. Qureshi, K. M. Read, R. C. Gilkeson, R. S. Poston, C. S. White. Coronary artery bypass grafts: assessment with multidetector CT in the early and late postoperative settings. *Radiographics* 2005; **25**: 881–96.

Pearls and Pitfalls in Cardiovascular Imaging, ed. Stefan L. Zimmerman and Elliot K. Fishman. Published by Cambridge University Press. © Cambridge University Press 2015.

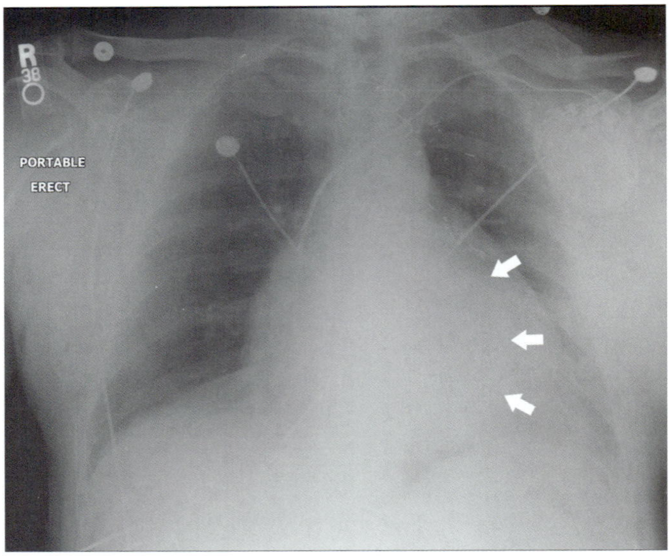

Figure 40.1. Chest radiograph in a 55-year-old male status post-CABG and defibrillator placement showing a retrocardiac opacity resulting in the "double density" sign (arrows). Differential considerations for the mass presented during initial interpretation included a large hiatal hernia but CT was recommended to exclude a pulmonary mass.

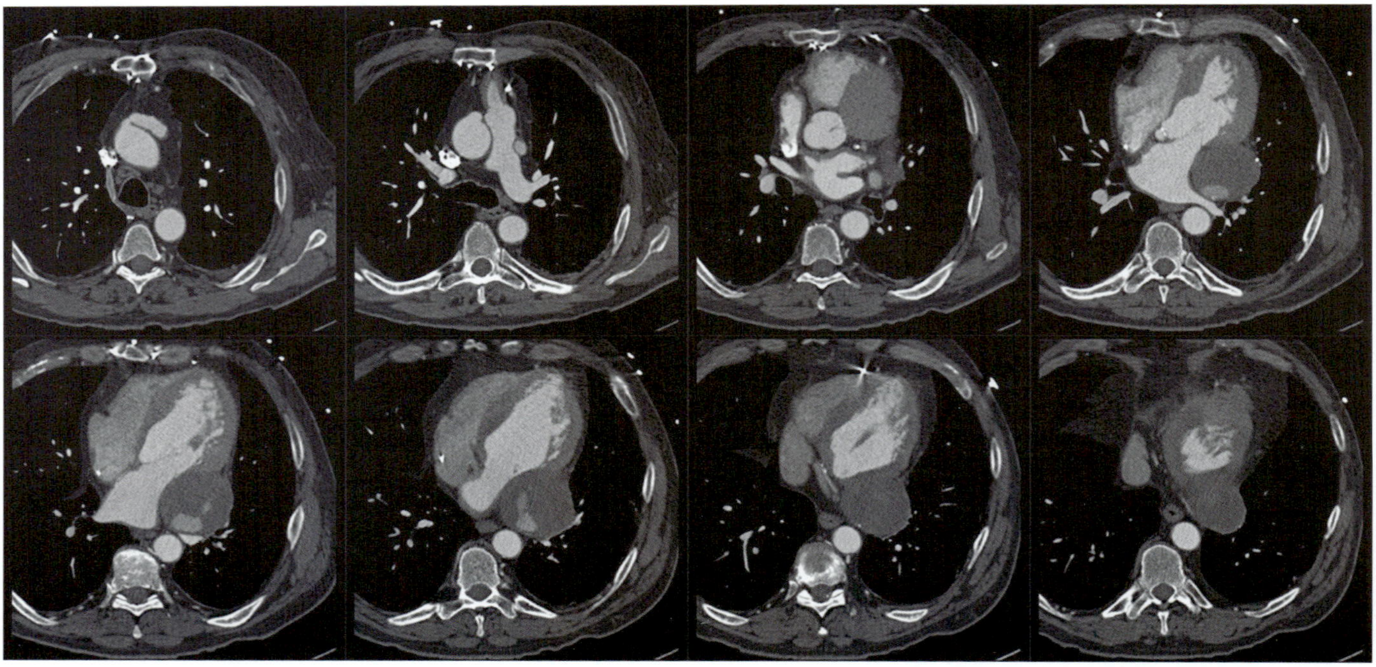

Figure 40.2. Axial images from a cardiac CT exam in the same patient shows the saphenous vein graft extending from the ascending aorta to the left circumflex coronary artery, with a large partially thrombosed aneurysm. Note the mass effect from the aneurysm on the left atrium as well as on the left inferior pulmonary vein (best seen in the top right image).

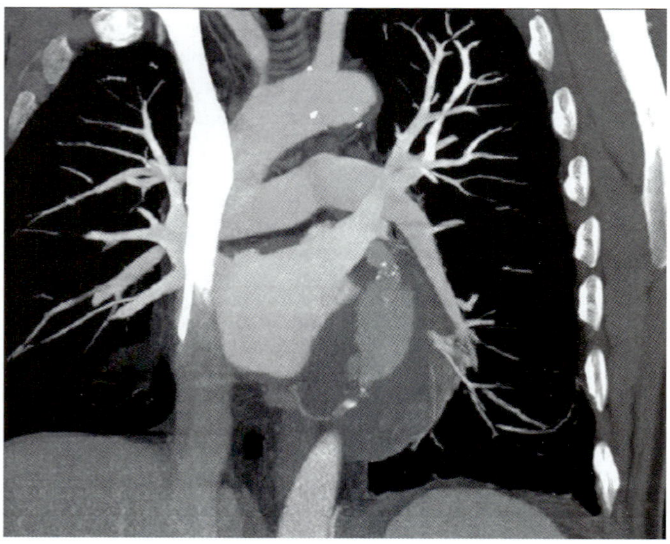

Figure 40.3. Coronal maximum intensity projection image showing that the native circumflex remains patent distal to the partially thrombosed vein graft aneurysm in the same patient.

CASE 41

Hypoattenuating myocardium

Vivek Halappa and Atif Zaheer

Imaging description

Diseases affecting the myocardium, including myocardial infarction (MI), are generally better seen on electrocardiographically gated cardiac CT and cardiac MRI. However, signs of recent or prior MI such as myocardial hypoperfusion, lipomatous metaplasia, wall thinning, aneurysm formation, myocardial calcification, and left ventricular thrombus may be found incidentally on conventional (non-gated) CT performed for non-cardiac indications.

Although the myocardium is usually not well resolved on non-gated studies due to cardiac motion blurring, perfusion abnormalities secondary to myocardial ischemia may be occasionally detected as incidental findings (Figure 41.1). Detection of these abnormalities is dependent on acquisition during the period of optimal myocardial enhancement, which occurs in the late arterial phase.[1] Consequently, these abnormalities may be missed on early arterial phase CT timed for the evaluation of pulmonary embolism.[2] Even in the setting of optimal acquisition timing, care should be taken in diagnosis as false positive results due to beam hardening artifacts from adjacent bones can simulate a perfusion abnormality.[3] In such cases, multiplanar reconstructions may help in assessing if these apparent perfusion defects match vascular territories (Figure 41.1). Subendocardial fat from lipomatous metaplasia, a marker for chronic MI that is frequently identified on non-gated CT examinations, may sometimes mimic an area of perfusion abnormality due to its low attenuation on contrast-enhanced images (Figure 41.2).[4] However, unlike perfusion abnormalities, lipomatous metaplasia will be visible on non-contrast CT examinations. In addition, the presence of fat in the subendocardium can be confirmed by using a region of interest to measure average Hounsfield units, which should be less than zero.

Importance

Myocardial infarction is usually better seen on cardiac gated CT and cardiac MRI. However, conventional CT performed to evaluate non-cardiac causes of chest pain may have important clues suggestive of acute or chronic MI that could suggest a cardiac etiology for the patient's pain

Typical clinical scenario

Patients presenting with acute chest pain with suspicion of pulmonary embolism may get a non-gated chest CT for evaluation. CT may demonstrate presence of subendocardial perfusion abnormality in an anatomic distribution of a coronary artery, highly suggestive of MI. The diagnosis can be confirmed on clinical grounds, EKG, and cardiac enzyme elevation.

Differential diagnosis

The most important differential considerations for perfusion abnormalities include streak artifact from adjacent osseous structures and low-attenuation lipomatous metaplasia. Correlation with cardiac enzymes and EKG may be necessary to make the correct diagnosis.

Teaching point

Detection of subendocardial perfusion abnormality in an anatomic distribution is suggestive of an acute MI in the correct clinical setting. This area should be carefully evaluated on contrast-enhanced CTs, particularly those performed for chest pain. Subendocardial fat attenuation in the left ventricular myocardium indicates prior myocardial infarction that is important to report to ordering clinicians.

REFERENCES

1. R. C. Cury, K. Nieman, M. D. Shapiro, et al. Comprehensive assessment of myocardial perfusion defects, regional wall motion, and left ventricular function by using 64-section multidetector CT. *Radiology* 2008; **248**: 466–75.
2. A. H. Mahnken, M. Katoh, J. E. Wildberger, R. W. Gunther, A. Buecker. Dynamic multisection CT in acute myocardial infarction: preliminary animal experience. *Eur Radiol* 2006; **16**: 746–52.
3. J. E. Shriki, J. Shinbane, C. Lee, et al. Incidental myocardial infarct on conventional nongated CT: a review of the spectrum of findings with gated CT and cardiac MRI correlation. *AJR Am J Roentgenol* 2012; **198**: 496–504.
4. H. M. Zafar, H. I. Litt, D. A. Torigian. CT imaging features and frequency of left ventricular myocardial fat in patients with CT findings of chronic left ventricular myocardial infarction. *Clin Radiol* 2008; **63**: 256–62.

Pearls and Pitfalls in Cardiovascular Imaging, ed. Stefan L. Zimmerman and Elliot K. Fishman. Published by Cambridge University Press. © Cambridge University Press 2015.

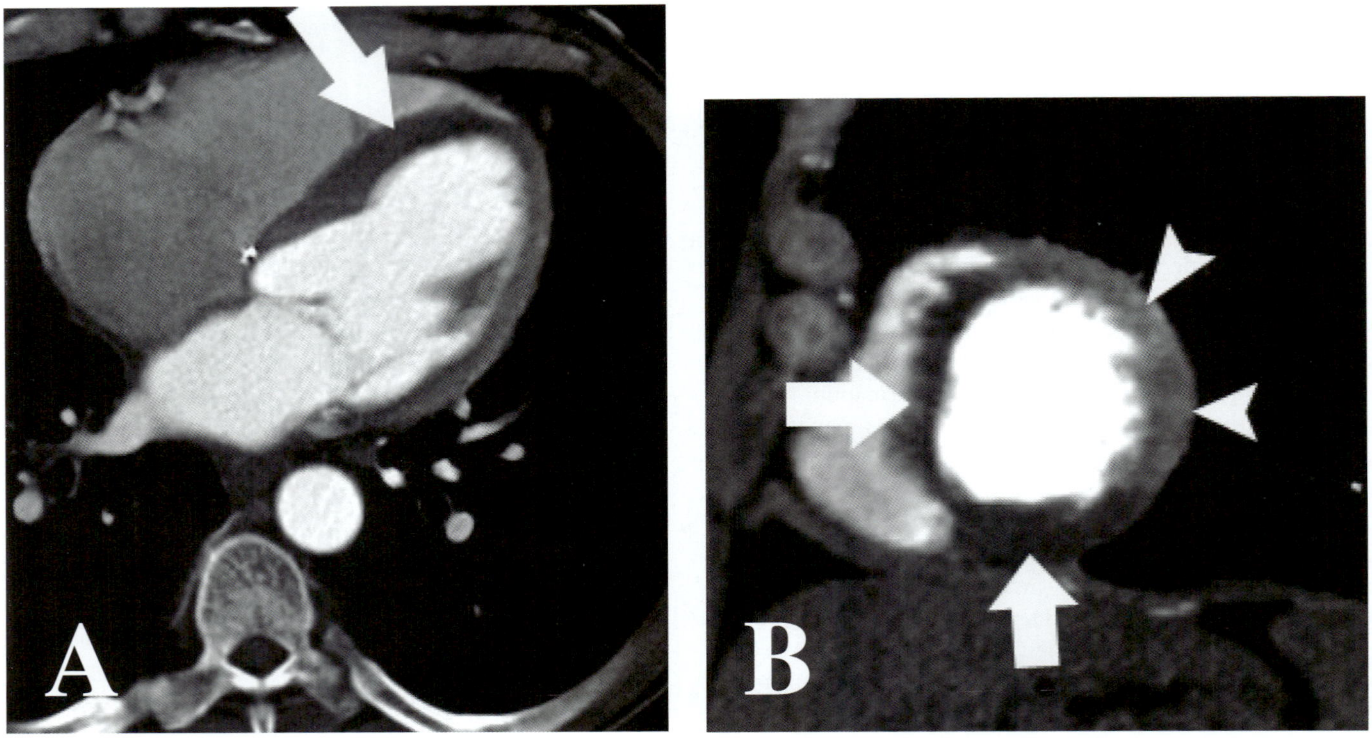

Figure 41.1 A. A 51-year-old man with chest pain. Conventional MDCT performed to evaluate for pulmonary embolism demonstrates hypoperfusion of the subendocardium of the left ventricle in the septum (arrow) on the axial images. Presence of MI was confirmed by elevated troponins and three-vessel disease on cardiac catheterization. **B.** Reconstructed short-axis view of the same patient demonstrates hypoperfusion of the subendocardium of the left ventricle in the septum and the inferior wall (arrows). Please note normal perfusion of the lateral wall for comparison (arrowheads).

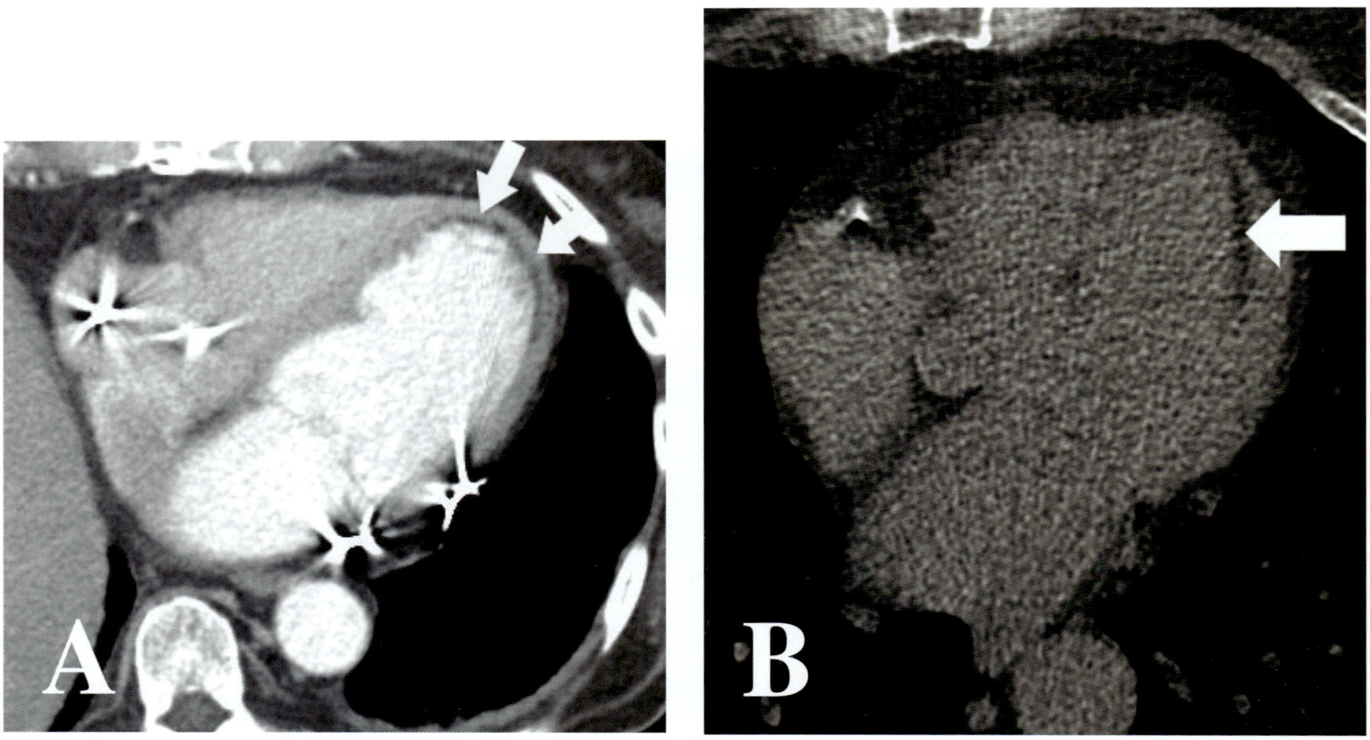

Figure 41.2 A. A 63-year-old woman with chest pain. Axial post-contrast CT of the chest demonstrates an area of low attenuation within the subendocarium of the lateral wall (arrows). **B.** Axial precontrast CT of the chest demonstrates the same area of low attenuation within the subendocarium of the lateral wall (arrow), which measures fat attenuation. Patient has a history of ischemic cardiomyopathy and the findings are consistent with lipomatous metaplasia within an old infarction in this region.

CASE 42

Pitfalls in obtaining optimal vascular contrast for pulmonary embolism examinations

Pamela T. Johnson

Imaging description

The ability to identify pulmonary emboli depends on the quality of the CT scan. Factors that diminish image quality include low contrast enhancement level, noise, motion artifact, and beam hardening artifact from high-density contrast in the SVC. The level of contrast enhancement achieved depends on the rate of contrast infusion and how the scan is timed. Contrast infusion is currently performed with infusion rates of 4–5 ml/second. Volume can be reduced to 100 ml for an average-sized patient, but for larger patients a higher volume may be necessary to ensure adequate contrast-to-noise ratio.

Optimally, the acquisition timing is tailored to the patient's hemodynamics, often performed with the bolus tracking technique. In this method, a region of interest (ROI) positioned on the main pulmonary artery samples the density as contrast is infused. A preset trigger point is applied, and when the contrast level reaches this density, the scan is initiated.

Performing a well-timed exam requires knowledge of the speed of the scanner being used. The new scanners that can perform studies in a few seconds enable the trigger timing to be delayed, so that the very peak of contrast enhancement is captured. For example, using a 64-slice scanner the study is triggered at 120–150 HU. This usually results in a high level of enhancement in the pulmonary arteries (Figure 42.1), prior to aortic enhancement. With a 128-slice dual-source scanner, the trigger point is delayed to 200 HU (Figure 42.2), and very high-quality imaging can result from high pulmonary artery enhancement and absence of motion artifact.

Despite an understanding of how scanner speed dictates scan timing for bolus tracking timing, pitfalls can occur when bolus tracking is used. One pitfall is malpositioning of the ROI cursor due to patient breathing or movement (Figure 42.3). In some cases, although the ROI cursor is well positioned and scan timed properly, the contrast enhancement level is suboptimal (Figure 42.4). This is usually the result of patient Valsalva. Measures to avoid this include coaching the patient on how to take shallow breaths and not asking them to hold their breath, as many will Valsalva if instructed to take a deep breath and hold it. Imaging during expiration can also be used to avoid this pitfall.[1]

Importance

Pulmonary embolism is a life-threatening disorder, and the third most common cardiovascular cause of death.[2] Image quality in pulmonary arterial CT is of paramount importance. Many factors affect image quality, including patient body habitus, cardiac function, quality, and type of IV access, contrast infusion rate, timing of the acquisition, detector configuration used, and reconstruction parameters.[3] Protocols are optimized by use of narrow detectors (submillimeter) and reconstruction sections of 1 mm or less.[4]

The most challenging component of performing these studies is timing the contrast bolus. If contrast administration is not carefully timed, a non-diagnostic study may result. Inconclusive studies occur in 10% of cases.[5] Accordingly, it is essential to understand how these studies are timed and the pitfalls associated with bolus tracking of the pulmonary arteries.

Typical clinical scenario

Pulmonary embolism imaging with CT is a widely utilized diagnostic tool for patients in the emergency department, for inpatients and for outpatients. Patients may present with acute chest pain and dyspnea or more insidious symptoms. Pulmonary embolism may be suspected as the cause of acute onset hypotension or syncope. Those at increased risk include patients with malignancy and clotting disorders, such as lupus anticoagulant, and those who have had prolonged immobilization.

Teaching point

Pulmonary embolism imaging is one of the most critical applications of CT and requires careful scan timing tailored to the scanner speed. Technologists should be cognizant of the challenges associated with bolus tracking and the importance of coaching how the patient breathes, to avoid the pitfalls that may result in suboptimal scan quality.

REFERENCES

1. Chen YH, Velayudhan V, Weltman DI, et al. Waiting to exhale: salvaging the nondiagnostic CT pulmonary angiogram by using expiratory imaging to improve contrast dynamics. *Emerg Radiol* 2008; **15**:161–169.
2. Goldhaber SZ, Bounameaux H. Pulmonary embolism and deep vein thrombosis. *Lancet* 2012; **379**:1835–1846.

Pearls and Pitfalls in Cardiovascular Imaging, ed. Stefan L. Zimmerman and Elliot K. Fishman. Published by Cambridge University Press. © Cambridge University Press 2015.

3. Roggenland D, Peters SA, Lemburg SP, Holland-Letz T, Nicolas V, Heyer CM. CT angiography in suspected pulmonary embolism: impact of patient characteristics and different venous lines on vessel enhancement and image quality. *AJR* 2008; **190**:W351–359.

4. Jung JI, Kim KJ, Ahn MI, et al. Detection of pulmonary embolism using 64-slice multidetector-row computed tomography: accuracy and reproducibility on different image reconstruction parameters. *Acta Radiol* 2011; **52**:417–421.

5. Douma RA, Hofstee HMA, Schaefer-Prokop C, et al. Comparison of 4- and 64-slice CT scanning in the diagnosis of pulmonary embolism. *Thromb Haemost* 2010; **103**:242–246.

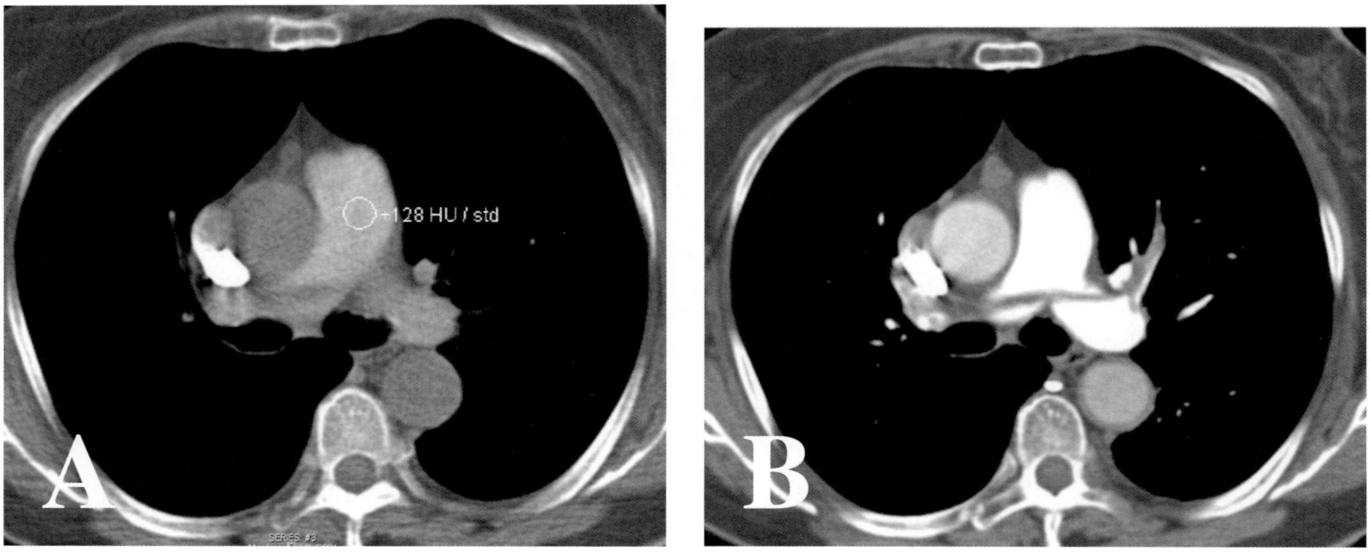

Figure 42.1 Pulmonary embolism detected on 64-slice CT scanner. The ROI cursor is positioned in the main pulmonary artery and the scan was triggered at 128 HU (**A**), resulting in high-quality enhancement of the pulmonary arteries (**B**). Linear thrombus is seen in the bifurcation of the main pulmonary arteries

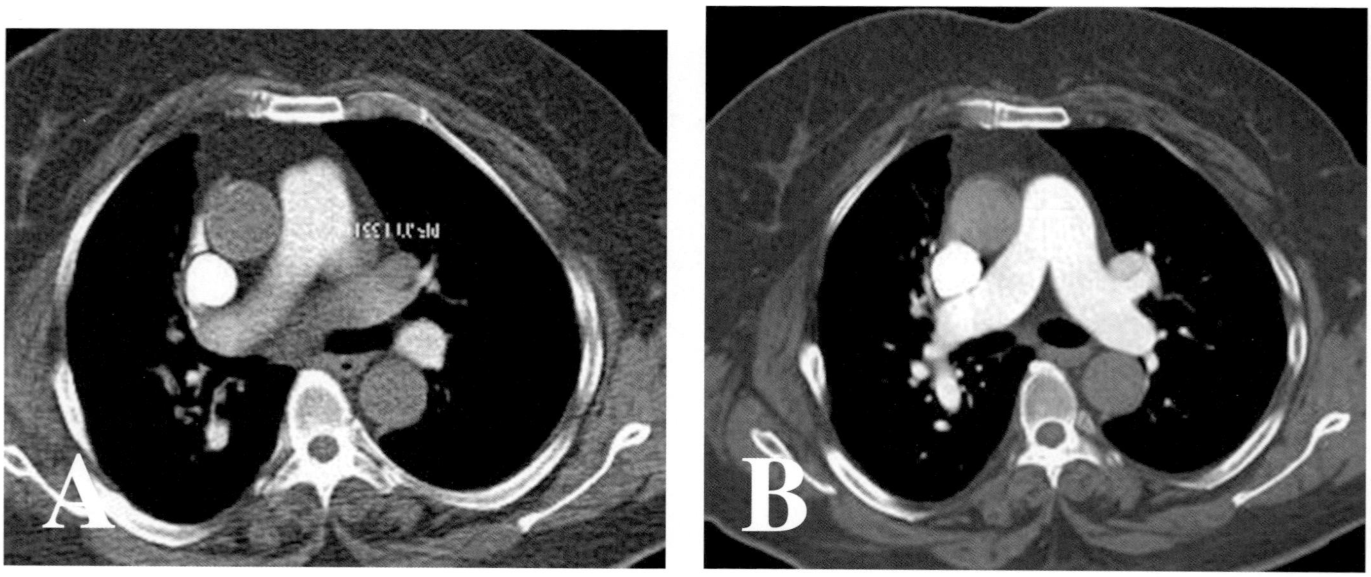

Figure 42.2 A 75-year-old woman with suspected pulmonary embolism: imaging with 128-slice dual-source CT scanner. The ROI cursor is positioned in the main pulmonary artery and the scan was triggered at 199 HU (**A**), resulting in high-quality enhancement of the pulmonary arteries (**B**). Because of scanner speed, trigger timing should be delayed to capture the peak of pulmonary artery enhancement.

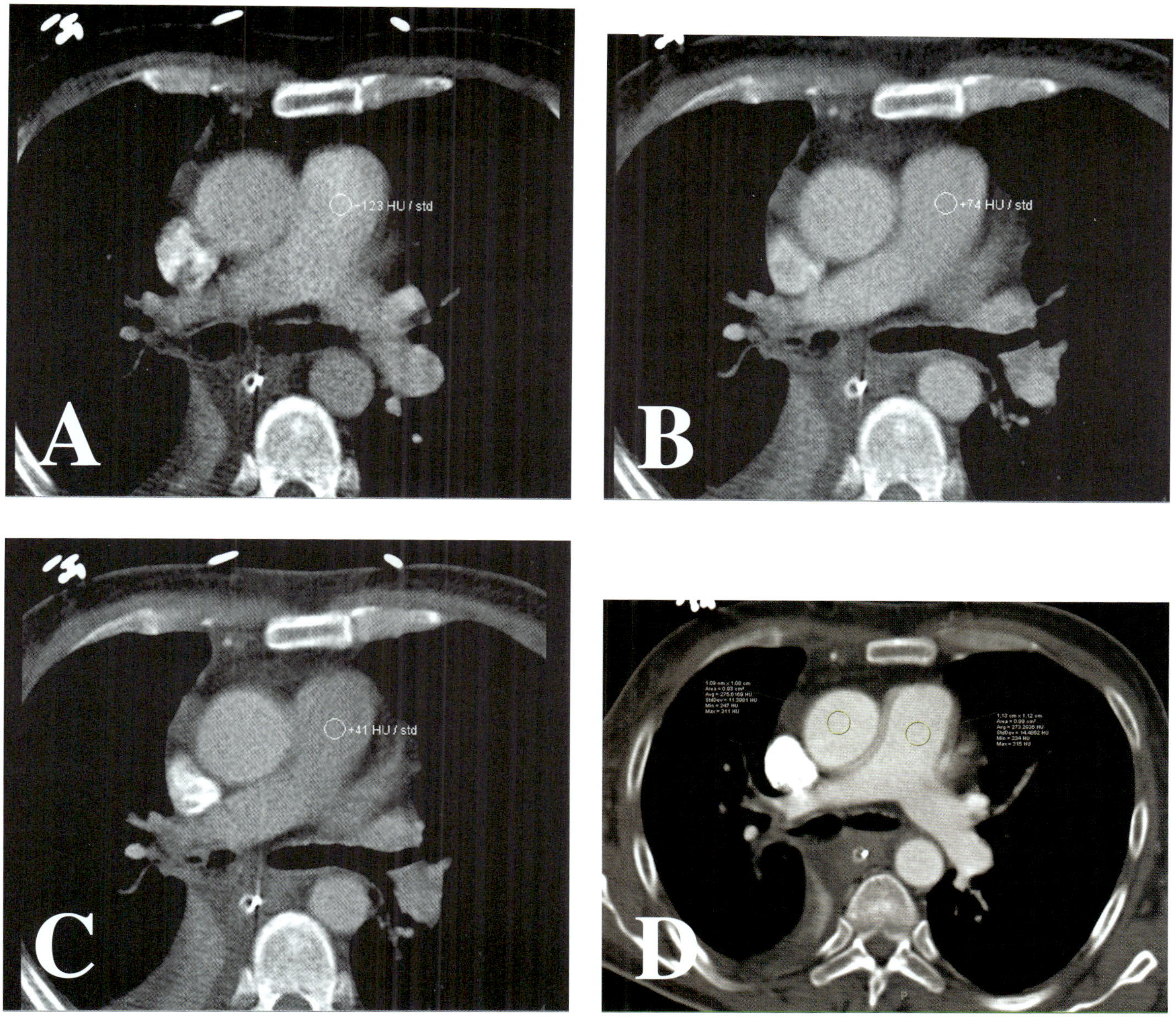

Figure 42.3 Patient breathing causes malpositioning of the ROI cursor. **A.**–**D.** Note how enhancement level of the main pulmonary artery varies with the patient's respiration.

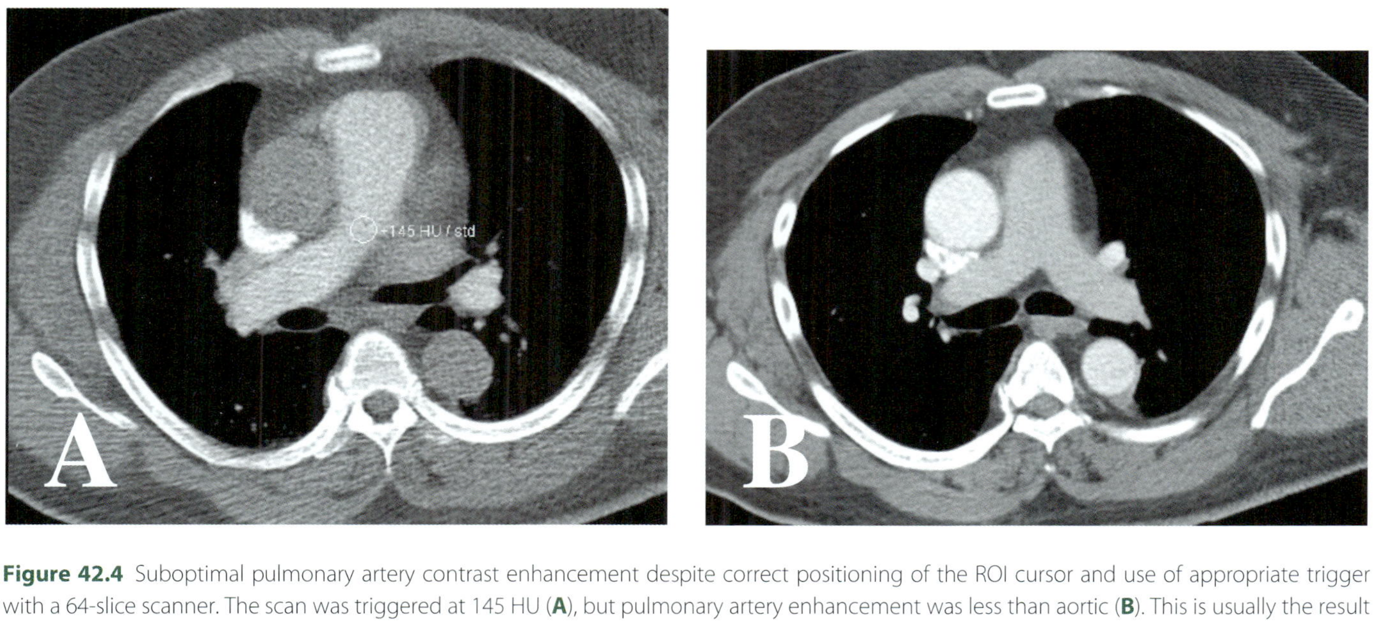

Figure 42.4 Suboptimal pulmonary artery contrast enhancement despite correct positioning of the ROI cursor and use of appropriate trigger with a 64-slice scanner. The scan was triggered at 145 HU (**A**), but pulmonary artery enhancement was less than aortic (**B**). This is usually the result of patient Valsalva, which can be avoided if the patient is not instructed to take a deep breath.

CASE

43 Artifacts mimicking pulmonary embolism

Pamela T. Johnson

Imaging description

Different artifacts that hamper interpretation during pulmonary artery CT include mixing or flow artifact (also called interrupted contrast enhancement) mimicking a pulmonary embolism, respiratory motion artifact resulting in linear decreased enhancement in segmental arteries that also simulates embolism on axial sections, cardiac motion artifact creating pseudodissection, and beam hardening artifact from dense contrast in the SVC obscuring visualization of the right pulmonary arteries. Owing to poor cardiac output, unopacified and opacified contrast mixed in the main and segmental arteries, mimic pulmonary embolism (Figure 43.1). Contrast enhancement is optimized by using bolus tracking software to tailor the scan timing to the patient's cardiopulmonary status, as described in case 42, and by administering contrast at higher infusion rates.[1] Additionally, a number of studies have reported that hyperventilating the patient and imaging in deep inspiration contribute to flow artifacts that mimic emboli.[2,3] Expiratory scanning reduces the incidence of focal diminished contrast enhancement and results in higher pulmonary artery enhancement levels.[4]

A more common cause of pseudothrombus is motion artifact (Figure 43.2). Correlation with coronal MPR reveals linear decreased attenuation parallel to the transverse plane secondary to respiratory motion artifact, which underscores the importance of correlating axial findings with MPRs.

Faster scanners (128 slice and beyond) aid in reduction of both cardiac and respiratory motion artifacts. If pulmonary artery dissection is suspected, identification of linear pulsation artifact within other cardiac structures (i.e., aorta) increases confidence that the finding is due to cardiac motion.[5] Finally, the beam-hardening artifact in the superior vena cava, which sends streaks of high density across the right pulmonary arteries, can be reduced by administering a saline chaser after the contrast bolus.

Importance

Interpretation of pulmonary artery CTA requires protocol optimization to maximize contrast enhancement and minimize artifacts. Ideally, protocol design results in a high-quality dataset with excellent pulmonary artery enhancement and absence of these artifacts. In practice, however, image quality is not always perfect.

Typical clinical scenario

Suspected pulmonary embolism is among the most common CT indications, including inpatient, emergency department and outpatient populations. Patients in the intensive care unit are among the most challenging to image, owing to ventilatory assisted breathing.

Differential diagnosis

As discussed, the differential diagnosis in this case is mixing or motion artifact vs. embolism. Radiologists must recognize the difference in appearance between pseudothrombus and true thrombus and the presence of variables contributing to the artifacts.

Teaching point

Cognizance of protocol optimization to reduce potential artifacts during pulmonary artery CTA is critical for maximizing image quality. When quality is suboptimal, radiologists must be able to distinguish these artifacts from real pathology.

REFERENCES

1. Ozawa Y, Hara M, Shibamoto Y. The frequency of insufficient contrast enhancement of the pulmonary artery in routine contrast-enhanced chest CT and its improvement with an increased injection rate: a prospective study. *J Thorac Imaging* 2011;**26**:42–7.

2. Wittram C. How I do it: CT pulmonary angiography. *AJR Am J Roentgenol* 2007; **188**:1255–61.

3. Gosselin MV, Rassner UA, Thieszen SL, Phillips J, Oki A. Contrast dynamics during CT pulmonary angiogram: analysis of an inspiration associated artifact. *J Thorac Imaging* 2004; **19**:1–7.

4. Chen YH, Velayudhan V, Weltman DI, Balsam D, Patel N, Draves KA, Robinson KA, Vu TH. Waiting to exhale: salvaging the nondiagnostic CT pulmonary angiogram by using expiratory imaging to improve contrast dynamics. *Emerg Radiol* 2008; **15**:161–9.

5. Pua U, Tan CH. CT diagnosis of pulmonary artery dissection – potential pitfall of multidetector CT. *Br J Radiol* 2009;**82**:82–3.

Pearls and Pitfalls in Cardiovascular Imaging, ed. Stefan L. Zimmerman and Elliot K. Fishman. Published by Cambridge University Press. © Cambridge University Press 2015.

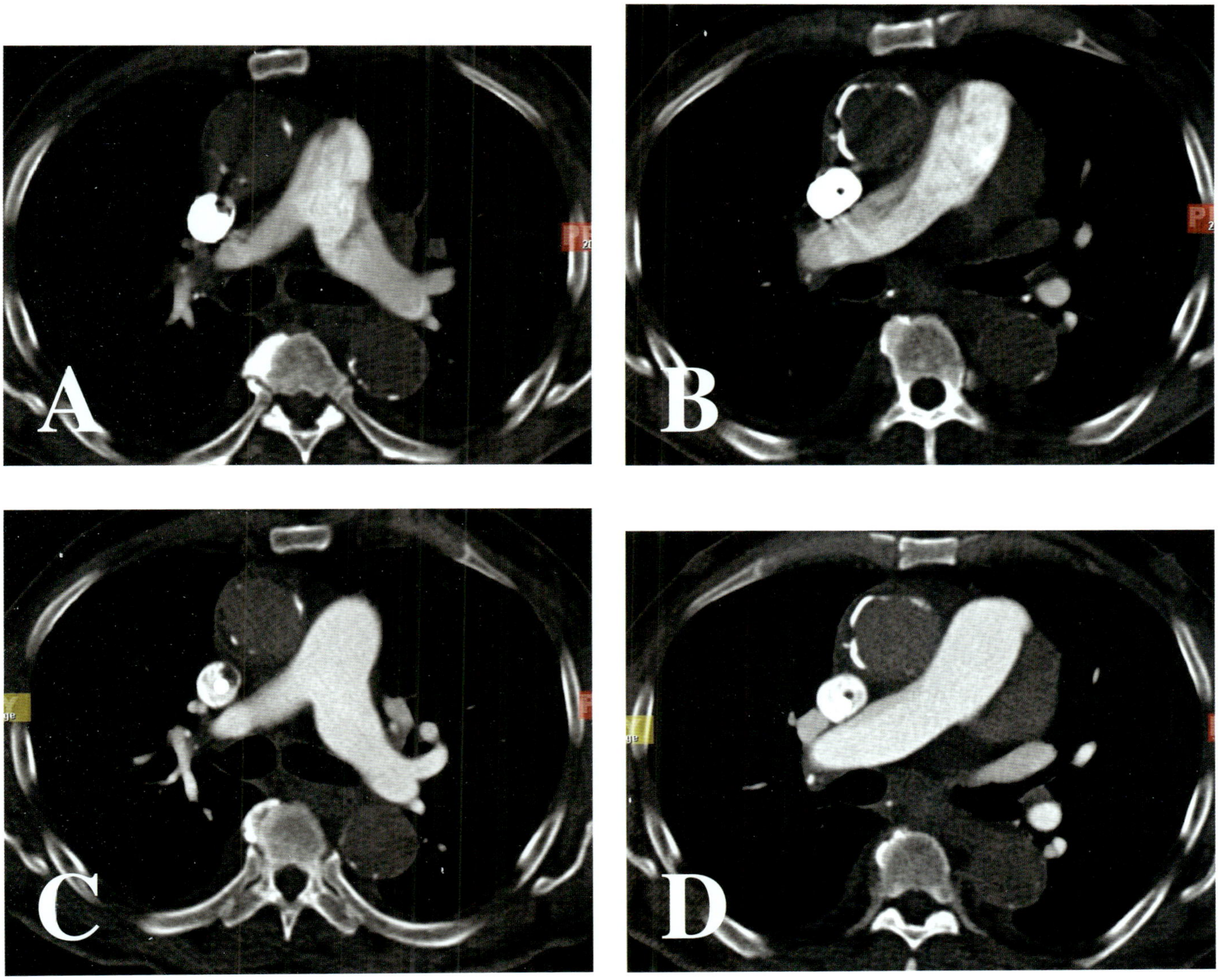

Figure 43.1 An 82-year-old man with suspected pulmonary embolism. Owing to poor cardiac output, unopacified and opacified contrast mixed in the main and pulmonary arteries, mimicking pulmonary embolism (**A,B**). Repeat imaging (**C,D**) with a longer delay and uniform enhancement in the pulmonary arteries confirmed that there was no thrombus in the pulmonary arteries and that the finding was due to flow artifact.

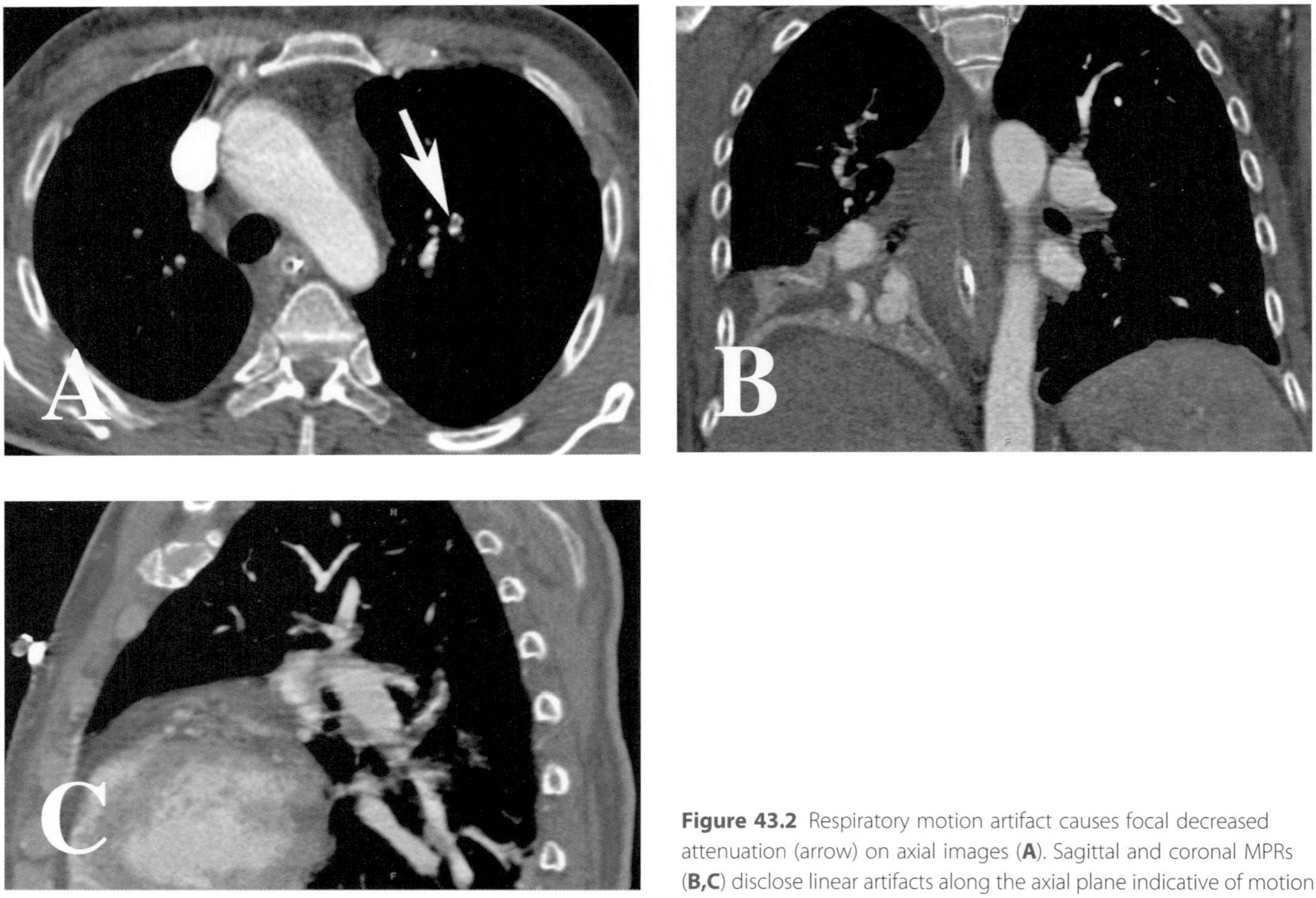

Figure 43.2 Respiratory motion artifact causes focal decreased attenuation (arrow) on axial images (**A**). Sagittal and coronal MPRs (**B,C**) disclose linear artifacts along the axial plane indicative of motion.

CASE **44**

Pulmonary artery imaging for pulmonary embolism in patients with Fontan shunt for congenital heart disease

Pamela T. Johnson

Imaging description

CT imaging for suspected pulmonary embolism is among the most challenging in terms of reproducible high image quality. Even careful timing with bolus tracking does not always guarantee that contrast enhancement levels will be sufficient to image the peripheral pulmonary arteries, as discussed in case 42. In patients with corrected congenital heart disease, the presence of conduits from arteries and veins to cardiac chambers can result in dramatically altered timing of contrast delivery to the right heart, further increasing the complexity of protocol design for imaging of the pulmonary arteries. In the case shown here, the standard timing method of bolus tracking the main pulmonary artery resulted in a non-diagnostic scan because the patient has a Fontan shunt between the inferior vena cava and right pulmonary artery. Markedly dense contrast is seen in the left pulmonary arterial system, with mixing artifact, and complete absence of contrast in the right pulmonary arterial system (Figure 44.1). A longer delay is required to opacify the conduit and pulmonary arterial system (Figure 44.2). Park et al. have reported that the optimal delay to enhance the Fontan conduit and pulmonary arteries is 3 minutes.[1]

An additional pitfall shown in this case is a thrombosed Blalock–Taussig (BT) shunt mimicking acute pulmonary embolism (Figure 44.3). Patients with congenital heart disease may undergo BT shunting in early childhood, followed by other definitive surgical correction, such as a Fontan procedure. Knowledge of their surgical history is critical in recognizing that the thrombosed vessels coursing cranially from the pulmonary arteries are old BT shunts rather than lobar or segmental pulmonary emboli.

Importance

Following surgical repair for congenital heart disease, the standard CT timing for pulmonary artery imaging cannot be used. Timing must be tailored to the altered hemodynamics resulting from indwelling conduits.[1,2]

Typical clinical scenario

In patients with congenital heart disease, multidetector CT (MDCT) may be requested to image the pulmonary arteries for suspected vascular stenoses or atresia as part of the spectrum of their cardiac anomalies or as a secondary complication that develops over time. The pulmonary arteries are not well seen with echocardiography, and MDCT has evolved as a valuable imaging modality for this indication.[3] Additionally, these patients can have respiratory compromise due to various causes, with pulmonary embolism among the potential etiologies. In the latter scenario, high-quality homogeneous enhancement of the pulmonary arteries is critical to assess for the presence of acute thrombus.

Differential diagnosis

The primary differential diagnosis in this case is pseudothrombosis due to inadequate scan timing and suboptimal pulmonary arterial enhancement.

Teaching point

Pulmonary artery CT protocol design and interpretation in patients with a Fontan shunt requires modified timing to image during enhancement of the Fontan conduit, and knowledge of prior surgical shunts, so that thrombosed BT shunts are not confused with pulmonary embolism.

REFERENCES

1. Park EA, Lee W, Chung SY, Yin YH, Chung JW, Park JH. Optimal scan timing and intravenous route for contrast-enhanced computed tomography in patients after Fontan operation. *J Comput Assist Tomogr.* 2010; **34**:75–81.
2. Prabhu SP, Mahmood S, Sena L, Lee EY. MDCT evaluation of pulmonary embolism in children and young adults following a lateral tunnel Fontan procedure: optimizing contrast-enhancement techniques. *Pediatr Radiol.* 2009; **39**:938–944.
3. Spevak PJ, Johnson PT, Fishman EK. Surgically corrected congenital heart disease: utility of 64-MDCT. *Am J Roentgenol.* 2008; **191**:854–861.

Pearls and Pitfalls in Cardiovascular Imaging, ed. Stefan L. Zimmerman and Elliot K. Fishman. Published by Cambridge University Press. © Cambridge University Press 2015.

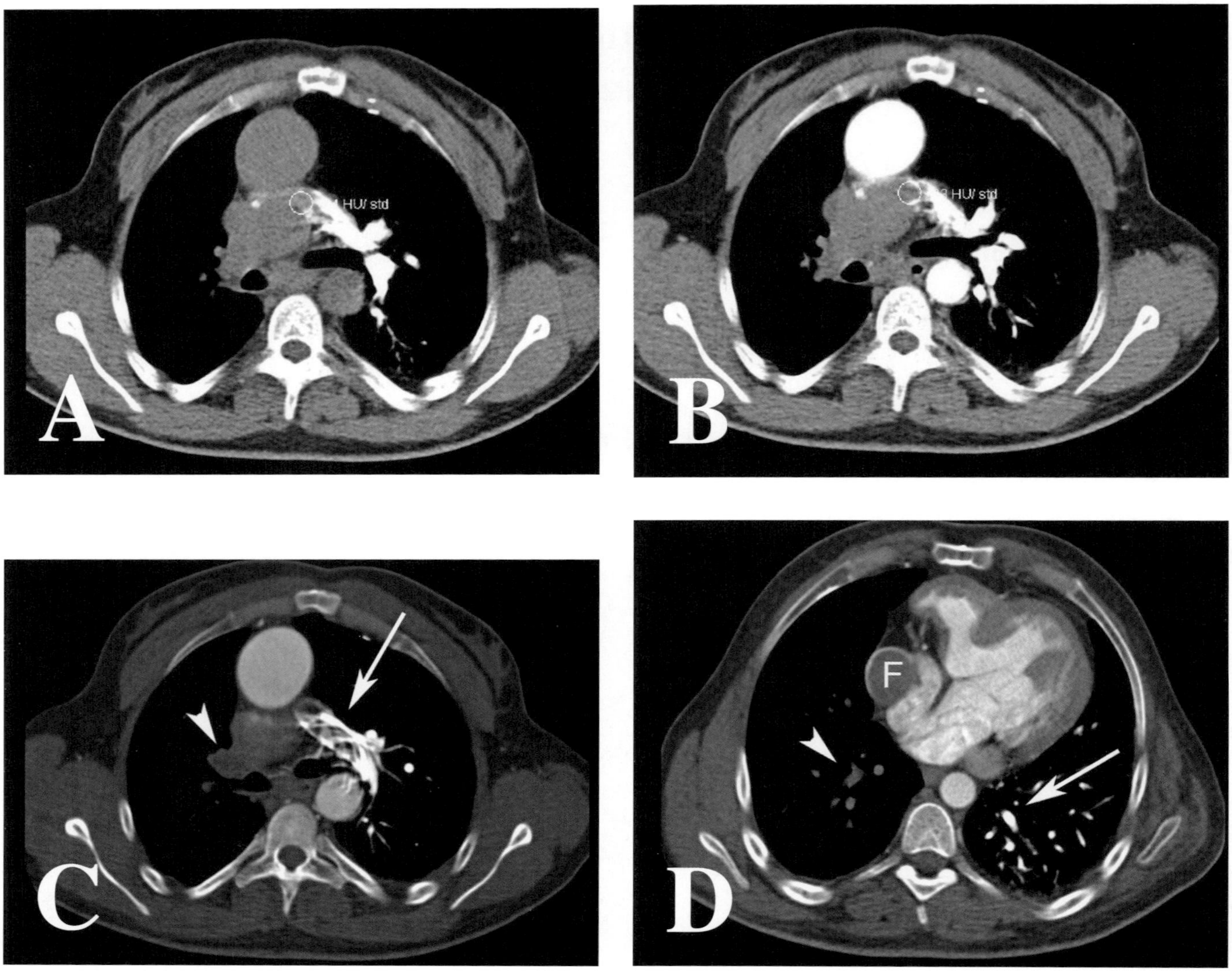

Figure 44.1 A 28-year-old man status post-bilateral BT shunts followed by Fontan procedure for tetrology of Fallot, who presented with acute shortness of breath and concern for pulmonary embolism. IV contrast-enhanced CT was performed with bolus tracking of the main pulmonary artery (**A**,**B**), resulting in dense contrast with mixing artifact in the left pulmonary artery (arrow) and absence of contrast enhancement in the right pulmonary arteries (arrowhead) (**C**), which are perfused by the Fontan shunt (F) from the IVC (**D**). Delayed timing is required to enhance the shunt and right pulmonary artery in these patients.

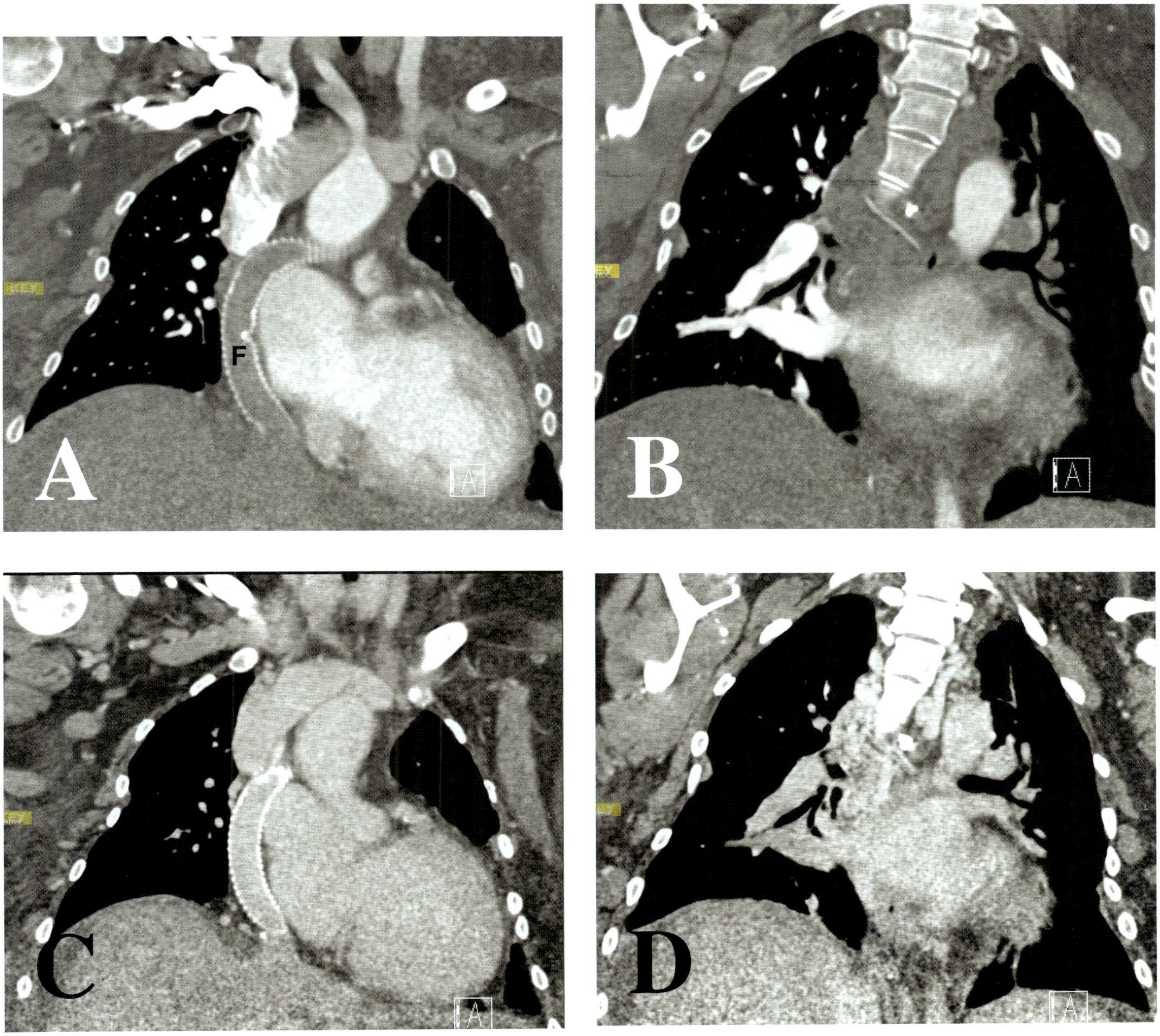

Figure 44.2 A 33-year-old woman with Fontan shunt. **A,B.** Coronal images from arterial phase result in preferential enhancement of the right pulmonary arterial system with non-opacification of the left side, which is supplied by the Fontan conduit (F). **C,D.** Delayed imaging is required to opacify the conduit in both the right and the left pulmonary arterial system.

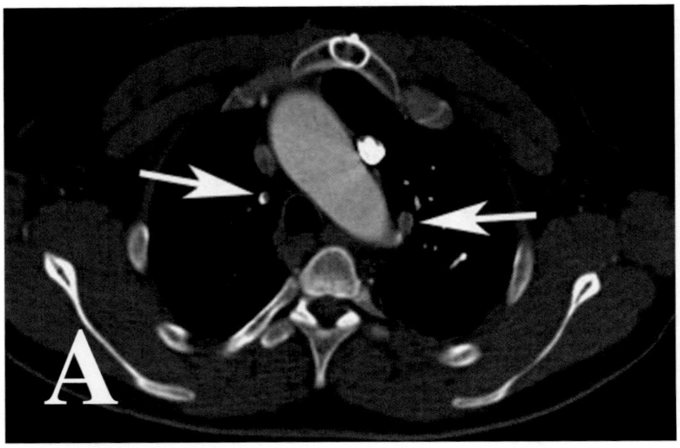

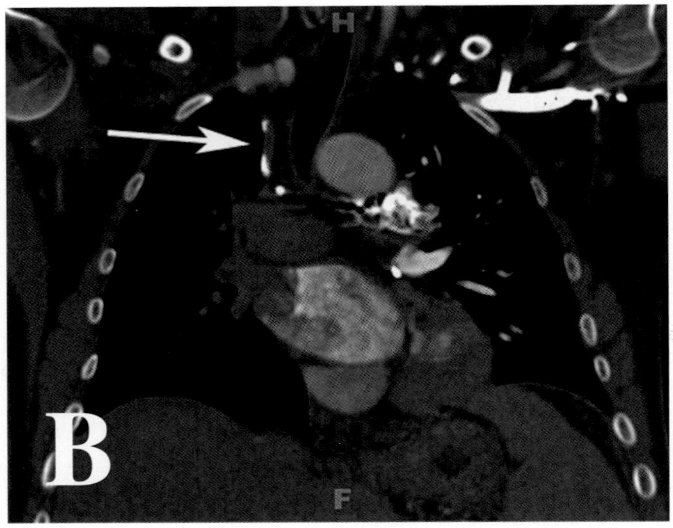

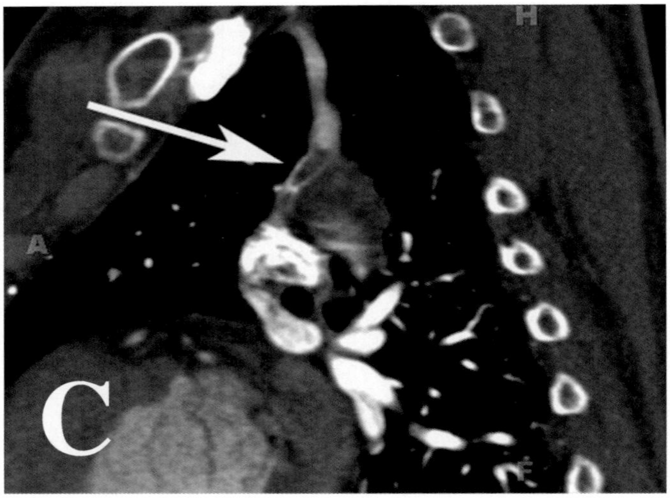

Figure 44.3 Same patient as in Figure 44.1. The patient also had bilateral Blalock–Taussig shunts placed during childhood, which had thrombosed. Axial image (**A**), coronal (**B**) and sagittal (**C**) MPRs show right and left thrombosed BT shunts (arrows) coursing cranially from the pulmonary arteries to the upper extremity veins. These should not be mistaken for upper lobe pulmonary embolism.

CASE

45 Pulmonary arteriovenous malformations

Maera Haider and Atif Zaheer

Imaging description

Pulmonary arteriovenous malformations (AVM) are defined by an abnormal communication between pulmonary arteries and veins. AVMs may be simple or complex depending upon the number of feeding arteries. A simple AVM is fed by one or more arterial branches arising from a single pulmonary segment; a complex AVM is fed by arterial branches from more than one segment. Computed tomography (CT) is a well-established modality for making the diagnosis,[1] as well as for the assessment of size and distribution for preangiographic treatment planning. CT findings include single or multiple smooth, round or lobulated pulmonary nodules or serpiginous masses with feeding and draining vessels mostly in the lower lobes (Figure 45.1A).[2] Multiplanar reformations with thin sections and maximal intensity projection (MIP) images are particularly helpful for confirming the diagnosis (Figures 45.1B, 45.1C, and 45.2). Although morphologic findings are sufficient for making the diagnosis, IV contrast may be administered for confirmation. AVMs follow rapid contrast opacification and washout of the main pulmonary artery. Catheter pulmonary angiography remains the reference standard for diagnosis.

Importance

Correct diagnosis is important, especially when the AVMs are small and may be confused with lung nodules or cancer (Figures 45.1B and 45.1C). This could expose the patient to risks of unnecessary imaging and/or invasive testing such as a biopsy, which may be catastrophic due to severe bleeding. MIP images can increase sensitivity for detection of small lesions.

Typical clinical scenario

The majority of pulmonary AVMs are congenital in etiology. The prevalence of pulmonary AVMs as estimated by low-dose thoracic CT is at 38 per 100,000 individuals.[3]

Among patients with pulmonary AVMs, 70–90% have hereditary hemorrhagic telangiectasia (HHT), an autosomal dominant disorder characterized by AVM in the skin, mucous membranes, and viscera. Conversely, only up to 35% of patients with HHT have pulmonary AVMs,[4] which are more symptomatic when multiple and bilateral.

AVMs result in right-to-left shunting of blood and can lead to cyanosis depending on the size of the shunt. An echocardiographic bubble study can be used to detect the shunt and estimate its severity. Patients with pulmonary AVM usually present with shortness of breath, hemoptysis, or spontaneous hemothorax. However, the first presentation may be of ischemic injury to the brain due to paradoxical embolization or associated polycythemia. Cerebral abscess can also occur.

Differential diagnosis

The most important differential consideration for a small AVM is inflammatory or neoplastic pulmonary nodule, especially when first diagnosed on a chest radiograph. The characteristic morphology with a small feeding artery and a draining vein on CT is helpful to make the diagnosis. The presence of multiple lesions and characteristic contrast enhancement helps confirm the diagnosis. Patients with HHT will often have AVMs of the liver, which if detected, can lend further support to the diagnosis (Figure 45.2).

Teaching point

A nodular or serpiginous opacity with characteristic feeding and draining vessels are features diagnostic of a pulmonary AVM. A large majority of patients with pulmonary AVMs have HHT and may have multisystem manifestation of this disease. Small pulmonary AVMs should not be mistaken for a solitary pulmonary nodule, which could lead to incorrect patient management.

REFERENCES

1. J. Remy, M. Remy-Jardin, F. Giraud, L. Wattinne. Angioarchitecture of pulmonary arteriovenous malformations: clinical utility of three-dimensional helical CT. *Radiology* 1994; **191**: 657–64.
2. J. Jaskolka, L. Wu, R. P. Chan, M. E. Faughnan. Imaging of hereditary hemorrhagic telangiectasia. *AJR Am J Roentgenol* 2004; **183**: 307–14.
3. M. Nakayama, T. Nawa, T. Chonan, et al. Prevalence of pulmonary arteriovenous malformations as estimated by low-dose thoracic CT screening. *Intern Med* 2012; **51**: 1677–81.
4. G. D. Rubin, N. M. Rofsky. *CT and MR angiography: comprehensive vascular assessment.* Lippincott Williams & Wilkins, 2008.

Pearls and Pitfalls in Cardiovascular Imaging, ed. Stefan L. Zimmerman and Elliot K. Fishman. Published by Cambridge University Press. © Cambridge University Press 2015.

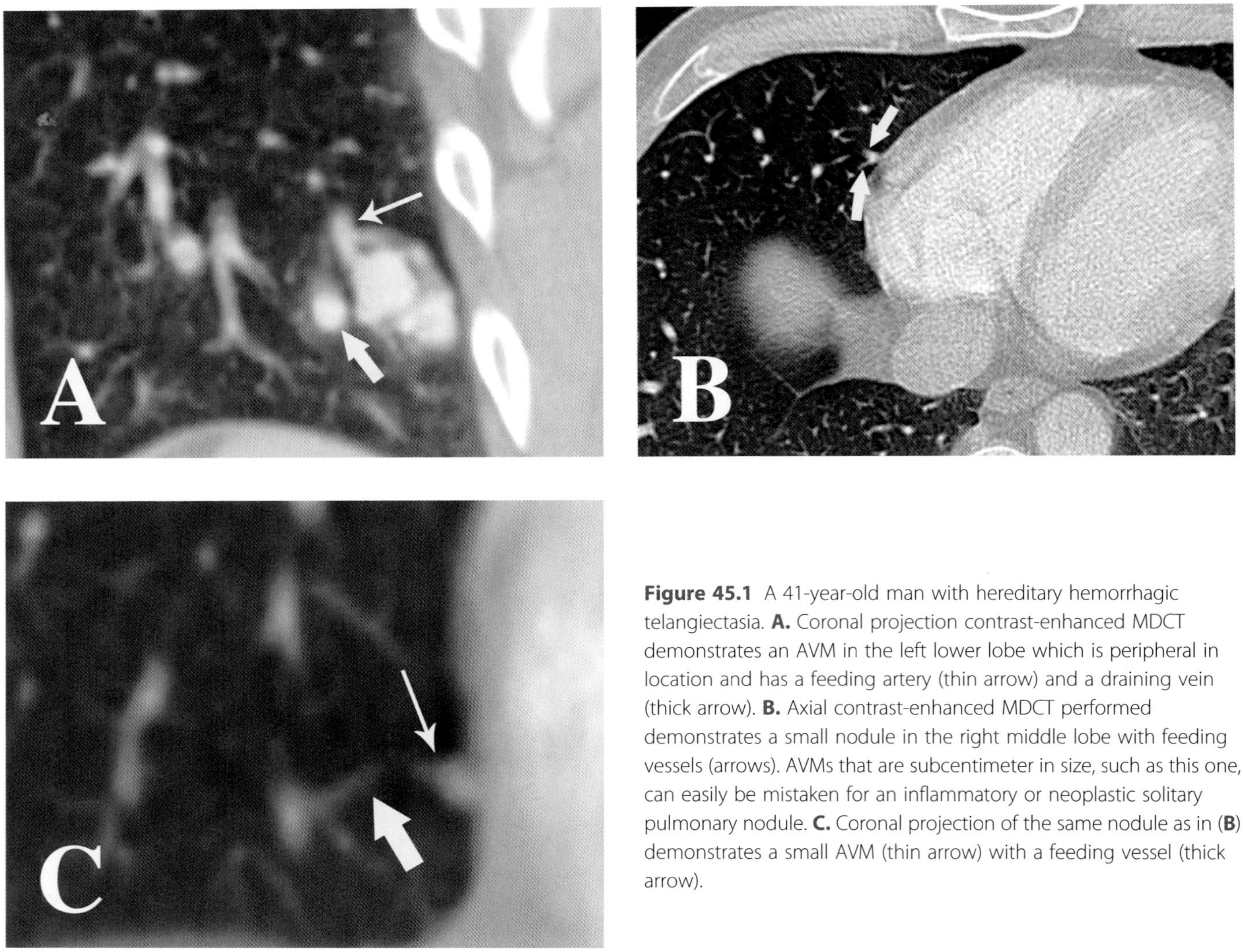

Figure 45.1 A 41-year-old man with hereditary hemorrhagic telangiectasia. **A.** Coronal projection contrast-enhanced MDCT demonstrates an AVM in the left lower lobe which is peripheral in location and has a feeding artery (thin arrow) and a draining vein (thick arrow). **B.** Axial contrast-enhanced MDCT performed demonstrates a small nodule in the right middle lobe with feeding vessels (arrows). AVMs that are subcentimeter in size, such as this one, can easily be mistaken for an inflammatory or neoplastic solitary pulmonary nodule. **C.** Coronal projection of the same nodule as in (**B**) demonstrates a small AVM (thin arrow) with a feeding vessel (thick arrow).

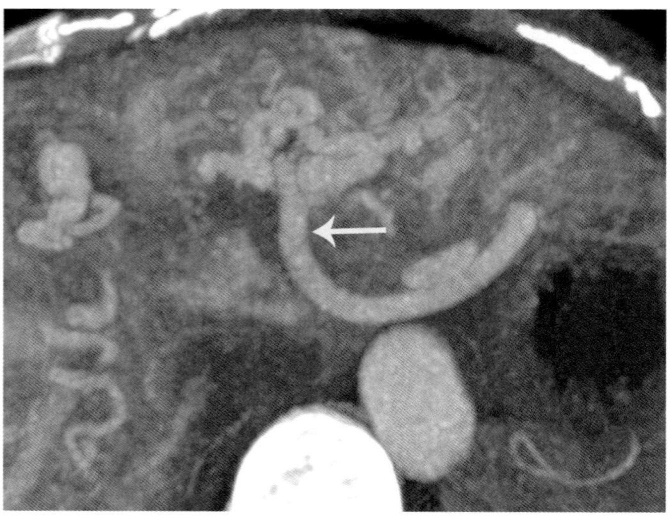

Figure 45.2 A 53-year-old woman with hereditary hemorrhagic telangiectasia and multiple pulmonary AVMs. Axial post-contrast MIP CT image through the liver demonstrates multiple AVMs. A large AVM in the left lobe shows a large feeding left hepatic artery (arrow).

CASE 46

Pulmonary artery sarcoma

Stefan L. Zimmerman

Imaging description

Pulmonary artery (PA) sarcoma is a rare tumor that is difficult to diagnose due to clinical presentation and imaging appearance that mimic pulmonary embolism.[1] On contrast-enhanced CT, pulmonary artery sarcoma can appear nearly identical to a pulmonary embolism, usually appearing as a smooth, low-attenuation intraluminal filling defect (Figure 46.1). Clinically, the absence of risk factors for thrombus formation, progressive worsening of symptoms, and persistence of the pulmonary artery filling defect despite anticoagulation therapy should raise suspicion for pulmonary artery sarcoma (Figure 46.2).[1] CT features that may help distinguish sarcoma from embolus include involvement of the main and proximal pulmonary artery branches, filling and expansion of the entire luminal diameter, and extravascular extension of soft tissue into the adjacent lung parenchyma.[1,2] Contrast enhancement, when identified, is usually heterogenous and will suggest the diagnosis (Figure 46.1). However, enhancement may be difficult to appreciate on CT examinations performed with pulmonary embolism protocol due to early phase of acquisition. Delayed venous phase images or enhanced chest MRI with dynamic post-contrast imaging can be used to confirm the presence of enhancement.[3] PA sarcomas will show increased metabolic activity on FDG-PET examinations, which can be helpful in difficult cases.[4]

Importance

Incorrect interpretation of a PA sarcoma as a pulmonary embolism will lead to a delay in diagnosis and delayed institution of proper treatment.

Typical clinical scenario

Pulmonary artery sarcomas are rare tumors, with only 250 cases reported in the literature to date.[1] Patients are typically middle aged and usually present with symptoms of dyspnea.[5]

Differential diagnosis

The primary differential diagnosis is bland thromboembolism. Metastatic tumor emboli from a non-lung primary can also present with enhancing, expansile pulmonary artery filling defects and should also be considered.

Teaching point

Pulmonary artery sarcoma is a rare tumor that can present with clinical and imaging findings nearly identical to pulmonary embolism. Central filling defects that expand the pulmonary artery and do not respond to anticoagulation should prompt further evaluation. Contrast-enhanced MRI or FDG-PET can help make a definitive diagnosis.

REFERENCES

1. D. Attina, F. Niro, P. Tchouante, et al. Pulmonary artery intimal sarcoma. Problems in the differential diagnosis. *Radiol Med* 2013; **118**: 1259–68.
2. C. A. Yi, K. S. Lee, Y. H. Choe, D. Han, O. J. Kwon, S. Kim. Computed tomography in pulmonary artery sarcoma: distinguishing features from pulmonary embolic disease. *J Comput Assist Tomogr* 2004; **28**: 34–9.
3. G. M. Kacl, E. Bruder, T. Pfammatter, F. Follath, F. Salomon, J. F. Debatin. Primary angiosarcoma of the pulmonary arteries: dynamic contrast-enhanced MRI. *J Comput Assist Tomogr* 1998; **22**: 687–91.
4. K. Ito, K. Kubota, M. Morooka, et al. Diagnostic usefulness of 18F-FDG PET/CT in the differentiation of pulmonary artery sarcoma and pulmonary embolism. *Ann Nucl Med* 2009; **23**: 671–6.
5. J. E. Cox, C. Chiles, S. L. Aquino, P. Savage, T. Oaks. Pulmonary artery sarcomas: a review of clinical and radiologic features. *J Comput Assist Tomogr* 1997; **21**: 750–5.

Pearls and Pitfalls in Cardiovascular Imaging, ed. Stefan L. Zimmerman and Elliot K. Fishman. Published by Cambridge University Press. © Cambridge University Press 2015.

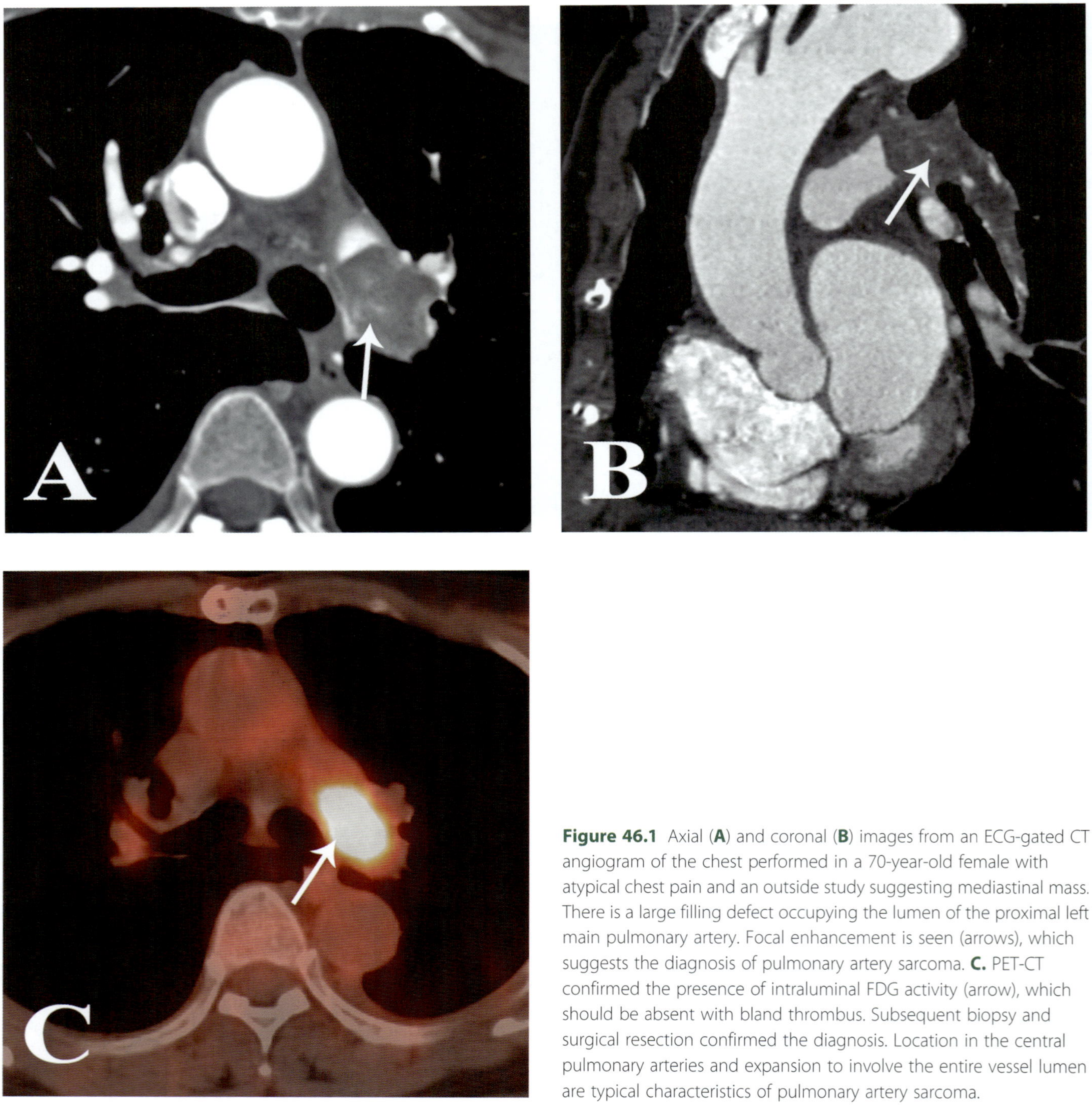

Figure 46.1 Axial (**A**) and coronal (**B**) images from an ECG-gated CT angiogram of the chest performed in a 70-year-old female with atypical chest pain and an outside study suggesting mediastinal mass. There is a large filling defect occupying the lumen of the proximal left main pulmonary artery. Focal enhancement is seen (arrows), which suggests the diagnosis of pulmonary artery sarcoma. **C.** PET-CT confirmed the presence of intraluminal FDG activity (arrow), which should be absent with bland thrombus. Subsequent biopsy and surgical resection confirmed the diagnosis. Location in the central pulmonary arteries and expansion to involve the entire vessel lumen are typical characteristics of pulmonary artery sarcoma.

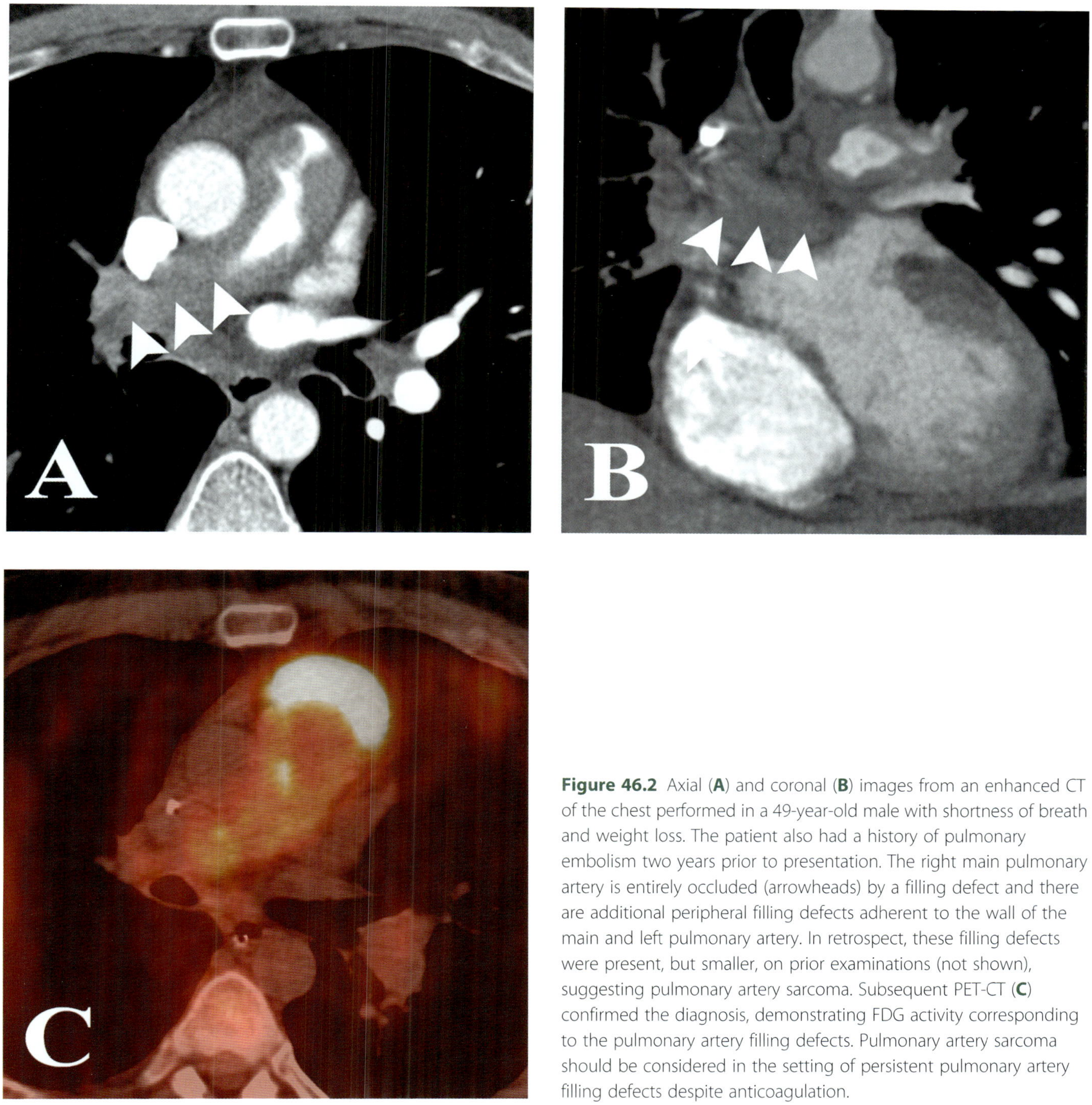

Figure 46.2 Axial (**A**) and coronal (**B**) images from an enhanced CT of the chest performed in a 49-year-old male with shortness of breath and weight loss. The patient also had a history of pulmonary embolism two years prior to presentation. The right main pulmonary artery is entirely occluded (arrowheads) by a filling defect and there are additional peripheral filling defects adherent to the wall of the main and left pulmonary artery. In retrospect, these filling defects were present, but smaller, on prior examinations (not shown), suggesting pulmonary artery sarcoma. Subsequent PET-CT (**C**) confirmed the diagnosis, demonstrating FDG activity corresponding to the pulmonary artery filling defects. Pulmonary artery sarcoma should be considered in the setting of persistent pulmonary artery filling defects despite anticoagulation.

CASE 47

Inappropriate inversion time selection for late gadolinium enhancement imaging

David Bonekamp and Stefan L. Zimmerman

Imaging description

Inappropriate selection of the inversion time (TI) in late gadolinium enhancement (LGE) cardiac MRI (CMR) examinations results in incomplete suppression of the myocardium.[1] Most frequently encountered is the selection of a TI that is slightly too short, resulting in a subendocardial "ring of hypointensity" and a mid-myocardial zone of hyperintensity (Figures 47.1 and 47.2). These artifacts may mimic true mid-myocardial delayed enhancement that can be seen in pathologic conditions such as sarcoidosis or dilated cardiomyopathy (Figure 47.3). In a less commonly encountered clinical scenario, suppression of *abnormal* myocardium (amyloidosis is the prototypical example) will cause hypointensity of *abnormal* myocardium. This will result in the poor quality of delayed enhancement images that is a hallmark of patients with amyloidosis (Figure 47.4).

Importance

Two potential pitfalls result from incorrect inversion time selection. First, incorrect nulling of the myocardium reduces the conspicuity of true myocardial delayed enhancement, potentially hiding underlying pathology, resulting in a false-negative result.[1] Second, incomplete nulling due to a short inversion time, if not recognized as artifact, can be erroneously interpreted as diffuse mid-myocardial LGE, leading to a false-positive result. The interpreting radiologist must be familiar with the appearance of deviations of the TI selection, and be aware of underlying conditions, particularly amyloidosis, that can cause difficulty in selecting the correct TI time.

Typical clinical scenario

TI is selected to provide maximal contrast between normal and abnormal myocardium by completely nulling any signal from normal myocardium. TI selection determines the sensitivity for the detection of myocardial damage.[2] The actual TI time needed for normal myocardial suppression depends on multiple factors, including the time after contrast injection, renal elimination of contrast, patient size, cardiac output, contrast dose and contrast agent.[3,4] A typical approach for TI selection is the use of a "TI scout" sequence, which is typically an ECG-gated post-contrast sequence with images acquired at multiple delay times after an initial 180 degree inversion pulse, resulting in different TI contrasts throughout the cardiac cycle.[1] The range of TI values covers the expected range of T1 values used for myocardial nulling in day-to-day practice, typically between 250 and 350 msec. Slight deviations of TI can lead to significant residual myocardial signal. The typical "dark rim" artifact between myocardium and ventricular blood (Figures 47.1 and 47.2) results from partial volume effects at the interface with mixing of signal from ventricular blood which has already recovered past the null point and of myocardium, which is still below the null point. Slightly too long TI will lead to hyperintense myocardium without a rim artifact (Figure 47.1). These deviations should be recognized and corrected by the MRI technologist; however, the radiologist needs to be aware of the appearance and cause to avoid misinterpretation. The acquisition of phase-sensitive inversion recovery (PSIR) images is a way to avoid these artifacts, as it circumvents the ambiguity of magnitude/modulus reconstruction of the MR data which produces images in which negative and positive MR signal are indistinguishable (Figure 47.3).[5]

Differential diagnosis

Significant deviations in TI suggest diffuse myocardial abnormality.[6,7] Cardiac amyloidosis tends to circumferentially involve the myocardium, beginning in the subendocardium and becoming transmural as the disease progresses. The observation of ventricular blood nulling at longer TI than myocardium should raise additional suspicion, indicating slower contrast washout from abnormal myocardium and leading to abnormal T1 shortening of the myocardium. In cases where TI selection is inappropriately short, artifactual mid-myocardial signal on delayed enhanced images may mimic pathologic conditions with similar delayed enhancement patterns such as myocarditis, sarcoidosis, or dilated cardiomyopathy.

Teaching point

Proper TI selection is critical for the successful acquisition of LGE images, which have high clinical value in the evaluation of a variety of cardiomyopathies. Inappropriate TI selection should be recognized and not mistaken for diffuse mid-myocardial fibrosis. Examination of PSIR images, if available, will eliminate the artifact [5]. Difficulty suppressing the myocardium, strong deviations of TI times, and abnormal nulling of the myocardium before the ventricular blood are indicators that an underlying diffuse infiltrative myocardial disease may be present.

Pearls and Pitfalls in Cardiovascular Imaging, ed. Stefan L. Zimmerman and Elliot K. Fishman. Published by Cambridge University Press. © Cambridge University Press 2015.

REFERENCES

1. Gupta A, Lee VS, Chung YC, Babb JS, Simonetti OP. Myocardial infarction: optimization of inversion times at delayed contrast-enhanced MR imaging. *Radiology*. 2004;**233**:921–6.
2. Nassenstein K, Breuckmann F, Bucher C, Kaiser G, Konorza T, Schafer L, et al. How much myocardial damage is necessary to enable detection of focal late gadolinium enhancement at cardiac MR imaging? *Radiology*. 2008;**249**:829–35.
3. Durmus T, Schilling R, Doeblin P, Huppertz A, Hamm B, Taupitz M, et al. Gadobutrol for magnetic resonance imaging of chronic myocardial infarction: intraindividual comparison with gadopentetate dimeglumine. *Invest Radiol*. 2012;**47**:183–8.
4. Petersen SE, Mohrs OK, Horstick G, Oberholzer K, Abegunewardene N, Ruetzel K, et al. Influence of contrast agent dose and image acquisition timing on the quantitative determination of nonviable myocardial tissue using delayed contrast-enhanced magnetic resonance imaging. *J Cardiovasc Magn Reson*. 2004;**6**: 541–8.
5. Huber A, Hayes C, Spannagl B, Rieber J, Klauss V, Schoenberg SO, et al. Phase-sensitive inversion recovery single-shot balanced steady-state free precession for detection of myocardial infarction during a single breathhold. *Academic Radiol*. 2007;**14**:1500–8.
6. Amano Y, Kumazaki T. Differences in null points between the left and right ventricles in contrast-enhanced inversion recovery MR imaging in patients with cardiac diseases. *Comput Med Imaging Graph*. 2006;**30**:147–51.
7. Desai MY, Gupta S, Bomma C, Tandri H, Foo TK, Lima JA, et al. The apparent inversion time for optimal delayed enhancement magnetic resonance imaging differs between the right and left ventricles. *J Cardiovasc Magn Reson*. 2005;**7**:475–9.

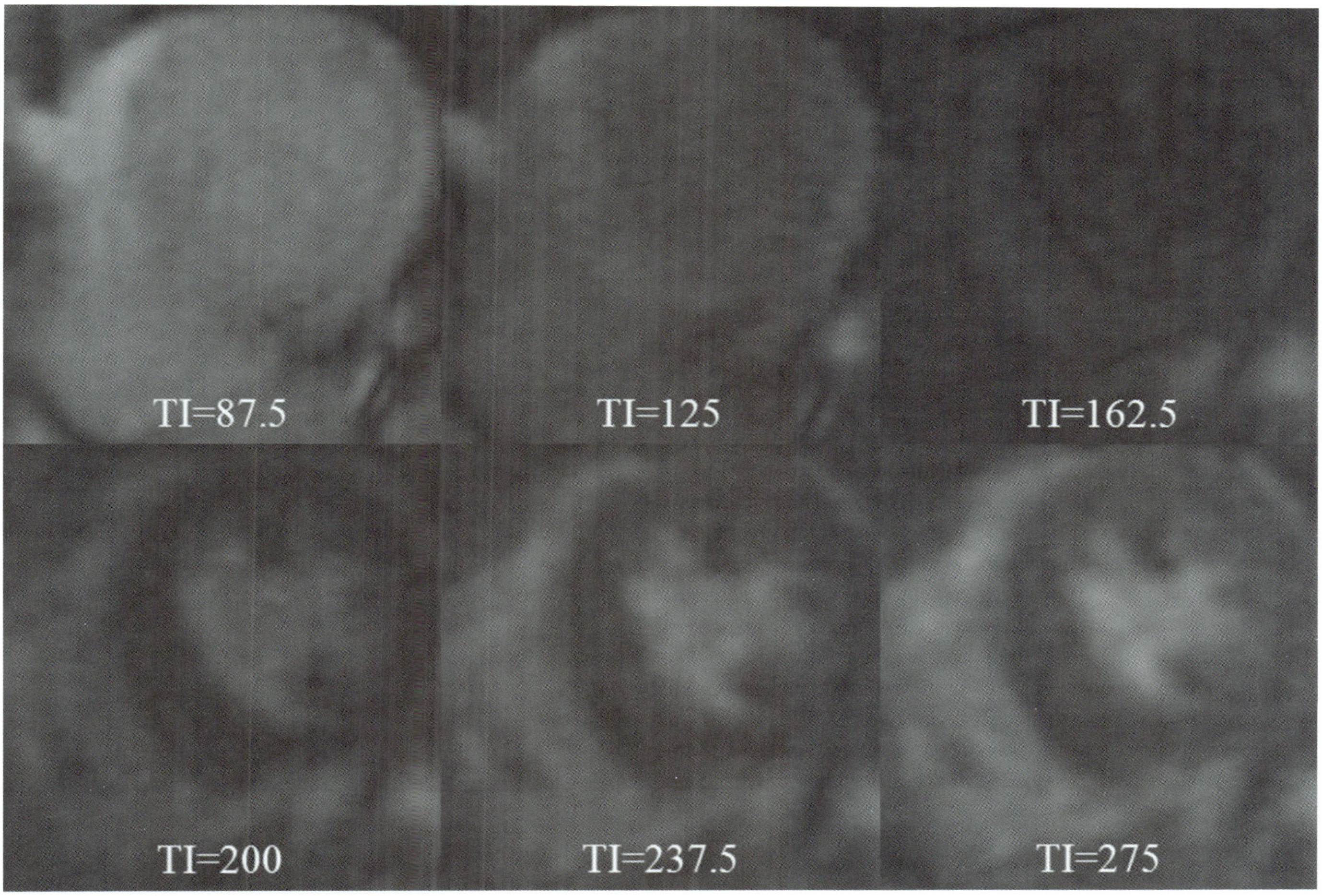

Figure 47.1 Short-axis TI scout images in a 9-year-old female without known myocardial disease. The characteristic "dark rim" artifact is seen at inversion time (TI) 162.5 msec. Note that the blood nulls before the myocardium (TI 162.5 msec). Full myocardial nulling is seen at 200 msec in this normal subject.

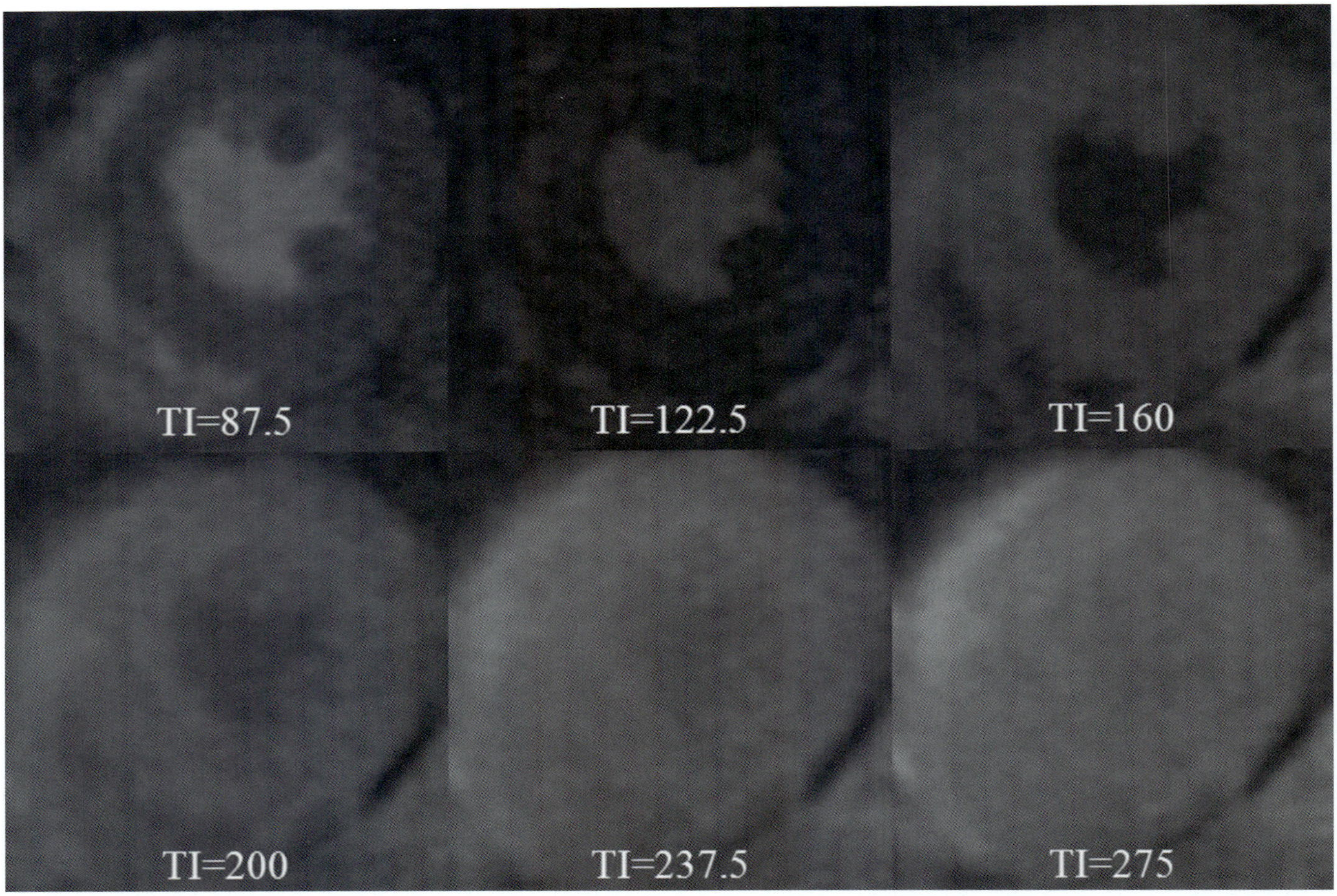

Figure 47.2 Short-axis TI scout images in a 52–year-old female with known myocardial amyloidosis. The characteristic "dark rim" artifact is reduced to 122.5 msec. Note the nulling of blood after the myocardium, the opposite of the normal situation. Note that full myocardial nulling is seen at 200 msec in the normal subject (Figure 47.1), but somewhere between 87.5 and 122.5 msec in this patient with amyloidosis (**B**).

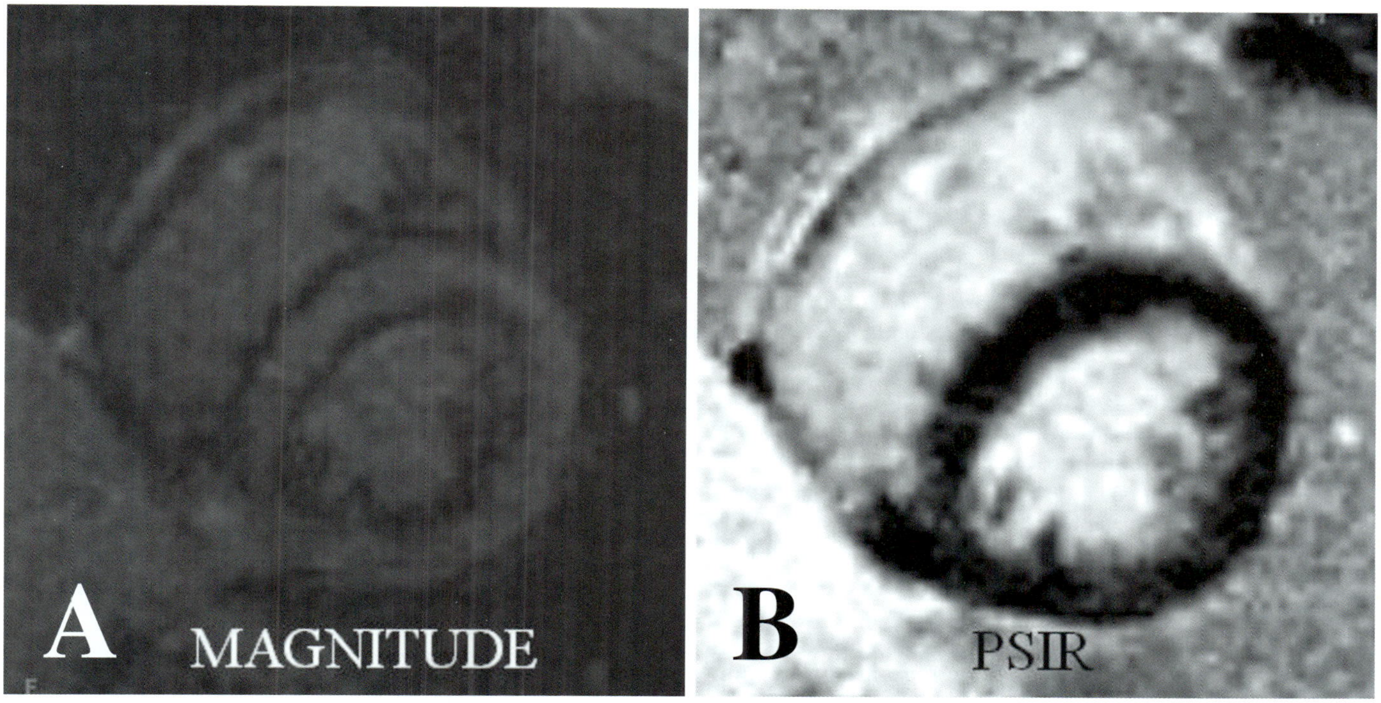

Figure 47.3 Short-axis magnitude (A) and phase-sensitive (B) inversion recovery delayed enhancement images obtained in a 34-year-old male with palpitations and suspected arrhythmogenic right ventricular cardiomyopathy. A characteristic "dark rim" artifact is present in image A due to selection of an inversion time that is too short. This can be mistaken for diffuse mid-myocardial delayed enhancement; however, on phase-sensitive inversion recovery (PSIR) images (B), there is homogenous nulling of the myocardium indicating that the increased signal in A is artifactual.

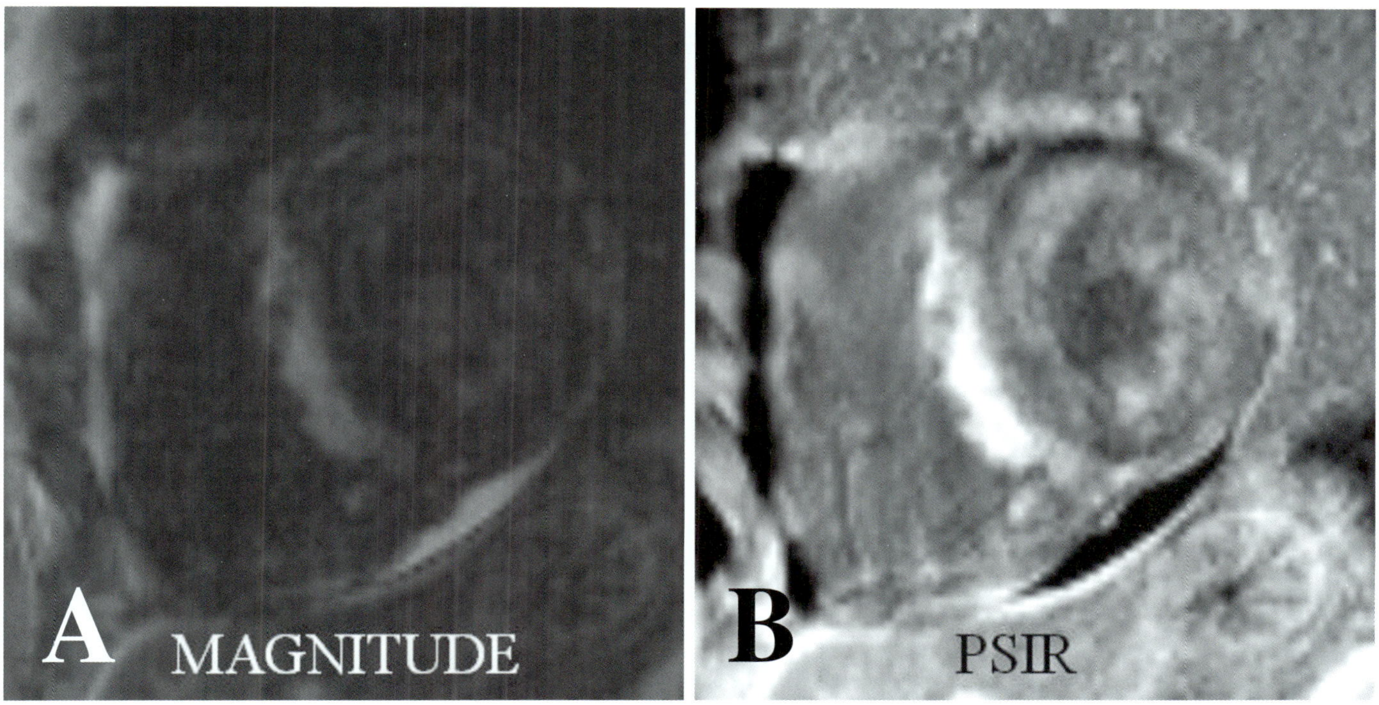

Figure 47.4 Short-axis magnitude (A) and phase-sensitive (B) inversion recovery delayed enhancement images obtained in a 77-year-old male with biopsy proven transthyretin amyloidosis. On magnitude images, A, there is poor contrast between blood pool and myocardium despite attempts at selection of an appropriate inversion time. Difficulty in obtaining optimal contrast in delayed enhancement images is characteristic of amyloidosis and due to binding of gadolinium by amyloid proteins in both the blood and myocardium. Blood–myocardium contrast is slightly improved with PSIR images, B; however, unlike cases of inappropriate inversion time (Figure 47.3), in the setting of diffuse amyloid infiltration even these sequences are limited.

CASE 48

Pseudothrombus on dark blood images

Stefan L. Zimmerman

Imaging description

High-signal mimicking thrombus can occur in cardiac chambers on inversion recovery-based dark blood images due to slow flow. Double inversion recovery dark blood images use an initial non-slice-selective 180 degree inversion pulse followed immediately by a second slice-selective inversion pulse in the plane of interest. The net effect is to invert all protons outside of the imaging plane while leaving protons in the plane unaffected. Image acquisition begins when inverted blood protons cross the null point during T1 recovery, typically corresponding to mid-diastole. The sequence relies on flowing blood to replace non-inverted blood protons in the image plane with nulled blood from outside the plane. If there is slow moving blood in a cardiac chamber, there will be incomplete blood suppression.[1] In patients with localized hypokinetic regions, artifactual high signal in these regions of stasis is common and can mimic thrombus (Figure 48.1). This is also common in the subendocardial region in patients with reduced ejection fraction due to slow flow in trabeculations (Figure 48.2).

Importance

Misdiagnosis of thrombus in cardiac chambers could lead to risks from anticoagulation and additional unnecessary follow-up imaging.

Typical clinical scenario

Artifactual signal from slow flow on dark blood images is common in the left ventricular apex, both in the setting of a global cardiomyopathy or prior apical myocardial infarction. However, artifactual high signal can be seen anywhere there is sluggish flow, including the right ventricle and atria.

Differential diagnosis

Pseudothrombus on dark blood images should be distinguished from a true thrombus. Both of these entities can occur in the setting of blood stasis. However, unlike dark blood artifacts, true thrombus should be present on all pulse sequences both pre- and post-contrast (Figure 48.1).

Teaching point

Slow flow in cardiac chambers results in artifactual signal on dark blood images that may mimic thrombus. Any suspected thrombus should be confirmed on all pulse sequences. Knowledge of this artifact will help avoid misdiagnosis.

REFERENCES

1. F. Saremi, J. D. Grizzard, R. J. Kim. Optimizing cardiac MR imaging: practical remedies for artifacts. *Radiographics* 2008; **28**: 1161–87.

Pearls and Pitfalls in Cardiovascular Imaging, ed. Stefan L. Zimmerman and Elliot K. Fishman. Published by Cambridge University Press. © Cambridge University Press 2015.

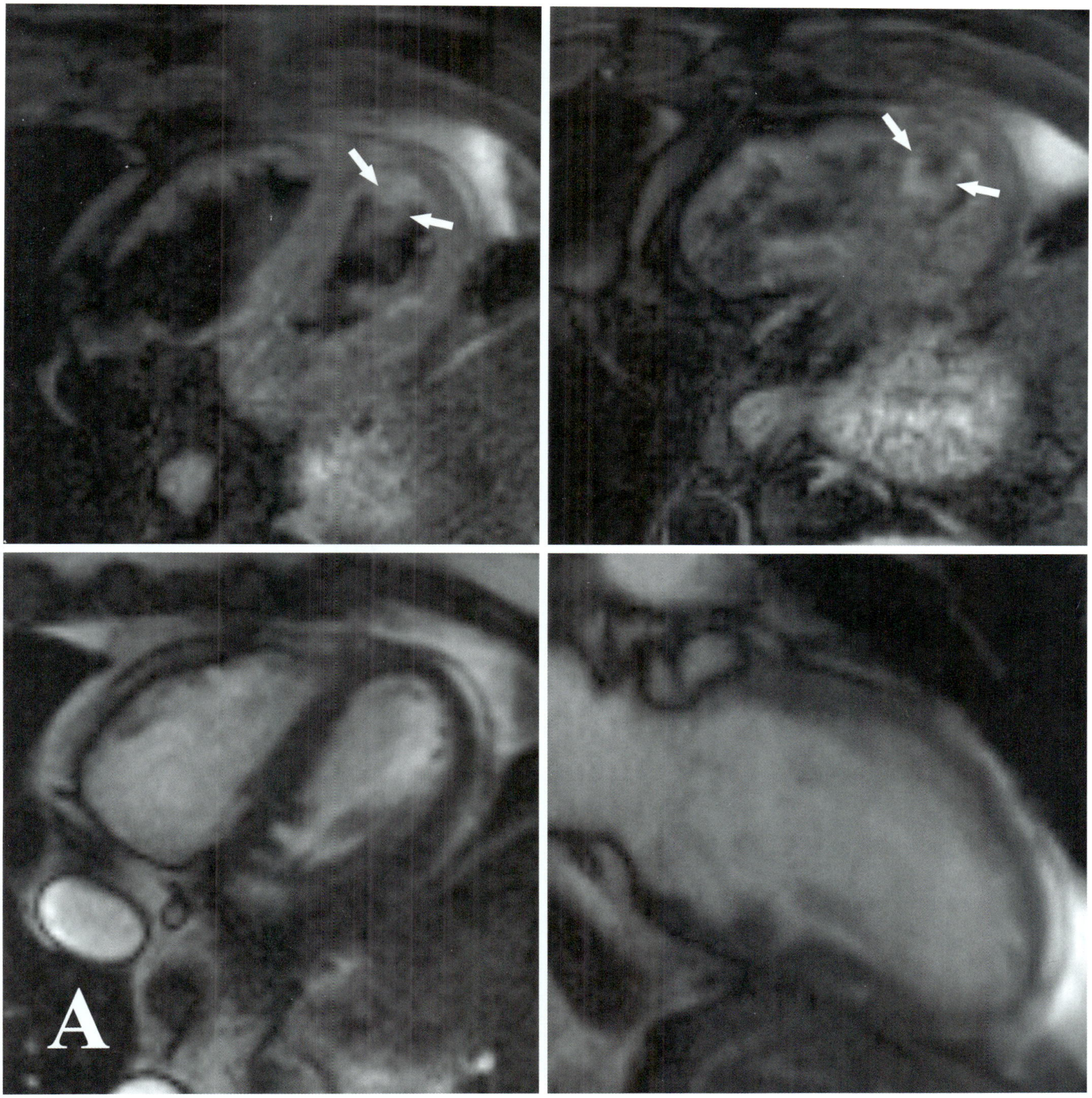

Figure 48.1 A. Axial T2-weighted dark blood images (top row) and axial (bottom left) and vertical long-axis (bottom right) steady-state free precession bright blood images obtained in a 58-year-old male with history of pericardial lymphoma and radiation therapy complicated by LV apical dysfunction and thrombus treated with anticoagulation. There is signal in the apex of the LV on dark blood images (top row) that simulates thrombus (arrows). However, there is no apical filling defect identified on bright blood images (bottom row), confirming this represents an artifact. **B.** Axial T2-weighted dark blood (top row) and axial (bottom left) and vertical long-axis (bottom right) bright blood images obtained in the same patient 6 months earlier, prior to anticoagulation therapy. A filling defect is present in the LV apex (arrows) on the black blood images suggesting thrombus. Unlike (**A**), the presence of thrombus is confirmed on bright blood images. Abnormal signal mimicking thrombus on dark blood images is frequently due to slow flow and any suspected thrombus should be confirmed on additional sequences.

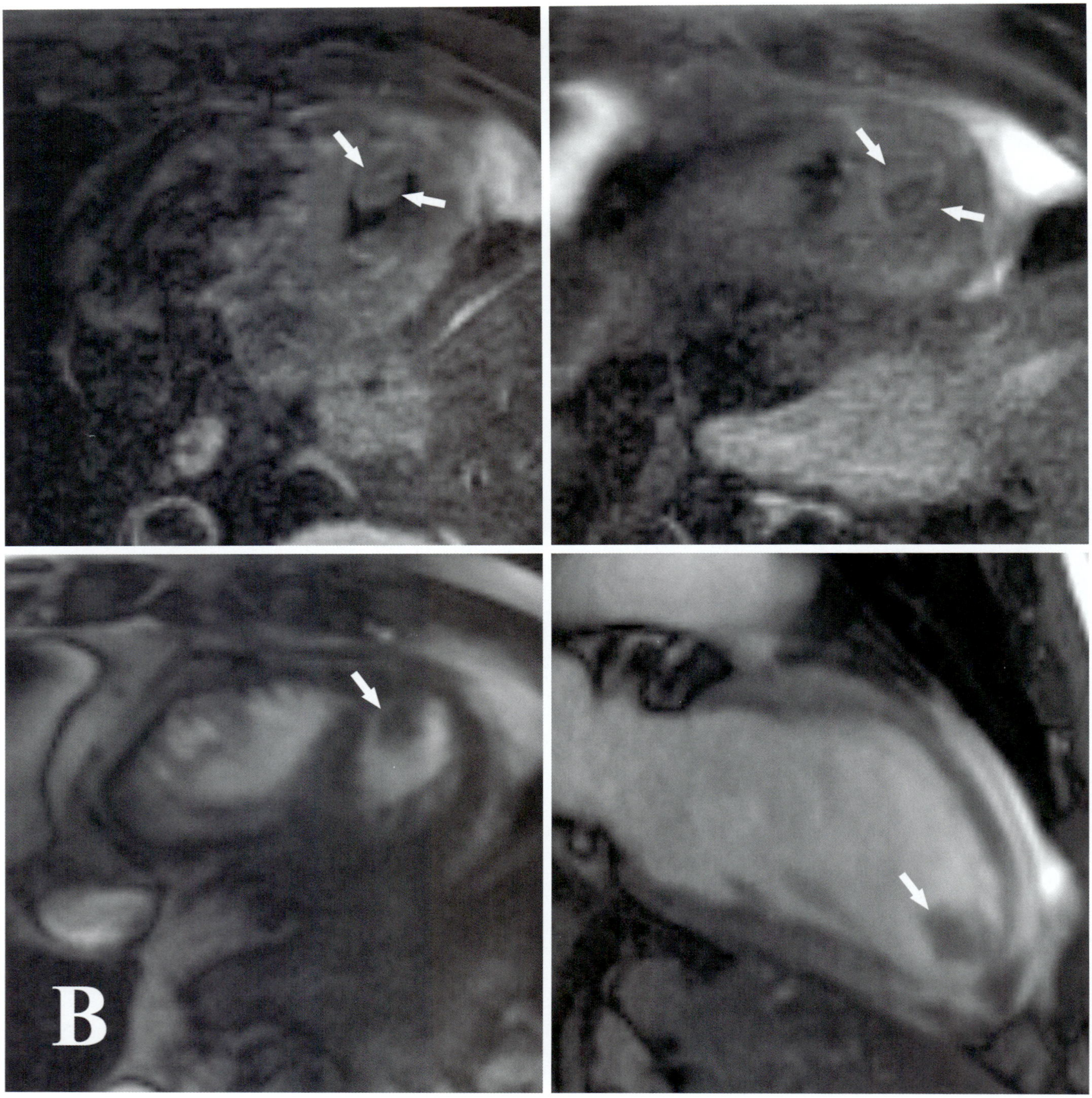

Figure 48.1 *(cont.)*

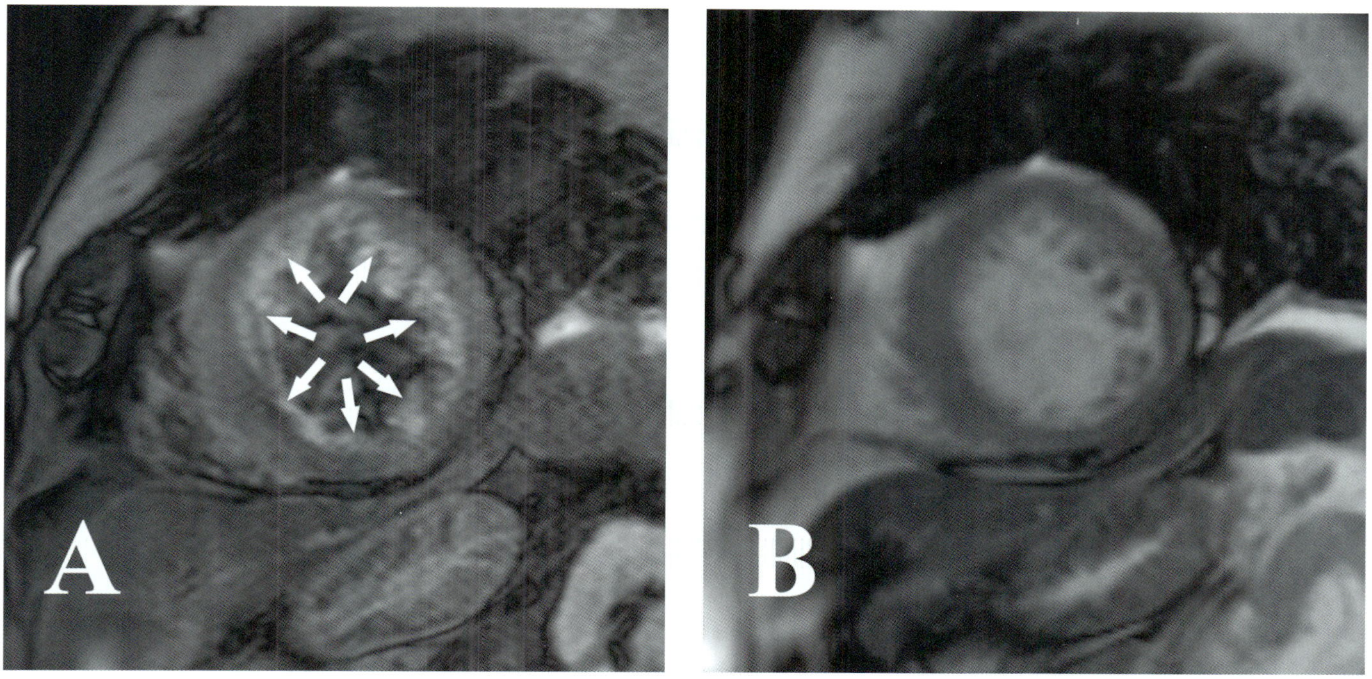

Figure 48.2 A. Short-axis dark blood image from a cardiac MRI obtained in a 65-year-old male with dilated cardiomyopathy demonstrates circumferential high signal in the left ventricular (LV) cavity adjacent to the endocardial surface (arrows). This is caused by incomplete suppression of slowly moving blood in the trabeculae of the LV. **B.** Short-axis steady-state free precession bright blood image from the same examination shows that the high signal on dark blood is artifactual and corresponds to blood within trabeculations.

CASE 49

Gibbs ringing artifact

David Bonekamp and Stefan L. Zimmerman

Imaging description

The Gibbs ringing artifact (truncation artifact) results from the limited fidelity of the superimposition of a finite number of sine and cosine functions to exactly reproduce a sharp border.[1] In cardiac MR, it usually occurs as dark and bright periodic rings with decreasing amplitude at increased distance from the blood–myocardial border. It is the more noticeable the higher the contrast between blood and myocardium, and thus is especially prominent in first-pass perfusion studies during the early frames, where high ventricular contrast concentrations meet essentially unenhanced myocardium (Figure 49.1).[1]

Importance

The Gibbs artifact causes oscillations around the sharp high-contrast blood/myocardial border. It results from the mathematical properties of the representation of MR images as a Fourier series, which can only approximate sharp borders. It can be made arbitrarily small at the cost of imaging time by increasing spatial resolution; however, it can never be fully avoided. The resulting image will show edges with adjacent ringing in the form of a sinc function (sin x/x). The artifact is present in both the frequency and phase directions. Mathematically, it can be shown that the positive and negative side lobes of the Fourier series have approximately 9% deviation from the baseline, thus resulting in a possible 18% deviation of signal in the subendocardium on perfusion studies if pixels are reconstructed exactly in the hills and valleys of these oscillations.[1–3] This is in the range of mild perfusion defects and has important clinical consequences. These artifacts may either mask true underlying early perfusion defects or mimic such defects, leading either to decreased sensitivity for perfusion abnormalities or inappropriate diagnosis of a perfusion defect. Both Gibbs artifact and ischemia affect the subendocardial myocardium preferentially compared to the mid- or subepicardial myocardium (Figure 49.2). Thus, it can be a challenge distinguishing these from each other; and MR sequences should be optimized to minimize Gibbs artifact. By the same mechanism, Gibbs ringing can lead to simulation of a syrinx in the spinal cord or cause ringing artifact around vessels in MR angiographic examinations. In the latter, the diagnostic difficulties arising from the artifact usually play a secondary role compared to other technical and patient factors determining study quality.

Typical clinical scenario

Gibbs artifact typically occurs in myocardial first-pass perfusion studies as one of the important causes of dark rim artifact. This manifests as a transient complete or incomplete dark ring of signal at the subendocardial myocardium. If anisotropic voxel sizes are used, the phase encoding direction is typically more undersampled (larger voxel size in this direction), leading to accentuation of the artifact along the phase-encoding direction. Multiple other factors may contribute to this dark rim artifact, including susceptibility artifacts from highly concentrated gadolinium and myocardial or ventricular blood motion.[4]

Differential diagnosis

Gibbs artifact is often transient, occurring during the early phase of first-pass perfusion studies, and decreases as enhancement of the myocardium and washout of contrast from the ventricular blood pool decrease the contrast gradient between myocardium and blood. Recognizing this transient behavior allows one to distinguish Gibbs artifact from true perfusion defects, which are fixed. However, if the ventricular blood pool washes out slowly, it can be very difficult to distinguish the artifact from true perfusion defects. If post-processing software is used, the presence of Gibbs artifact may lead to erroneous results, as the transient decrease of signal in the subendocardium violates the assumptions of the software that myocardial perfusion under normal circumstances is homogenous. For example, up to 50% differences in the upslope parameter of the perfusion curve have been demonstrated.[4] Persistence of the artifact on both stress and rest images can also help distinguish Gibbs artifact from true stress-induced perfusion defects. True perfusion defects secondary to epicardial coronary artery disease will be best visualized under stress conditions and will correspond to an anatomic coronary artery territory, whereas Gibbs ringing artifact will generally circumferentially involve the entire subendocardium. Circumferential subendocardial perfusion defects thought to be secondary to microvascular disease have been reported in a condition called Syndrome X, characterized by chest pain, abnormal stress electrocardiogram, and normal epicardial coronaries.[5] This diagnosis should be considered in the differential of Gibbs artifact, although this is a controversial topic and others have reported conflicting results.[6]

Pearls and Pitfalls in Cardiovascular Imaging, ed. Stefan L. Zimmerman and Elliot K. Fishman. Published by Cambridge University Press. © Cambridge University Press 2015.

Teaching point

Gibbs ringing artifact is a common and important cause of subendocardial dark band artifacts observed during first-pass perfusion MRI. The artifact should be recognized due to its transient behavior, presence on rest and stress imaging, and accentuation in the most spatially undersampled image axis (phase encoding direction). Raw data should be reviewed for presence of Gibbs artifact before interpreting computer generated perfusion maps, as erroneous parameters may result if this artifact is present in the data used for computer analysis of perfusion data. The artifact can be reduced by using higher resolution and isotropic voxels for first-pass perfusion experiments.

REFERENCES

1. P. Ferreira, P. Gatehouse, P. Kellman, C. Bucciarelli-Ducci, D. Firmin. Variability of myocardial perfusion dark rim Gibbs artifacts due to subpixel shifts. *J Cardiovasc Magn Reson* 2009; **11**: 17.
2. M. L. Wood, R. M. Henkelman. Truncation artifacts in magnetic resonance imaging. *Magn Reson Med* 1985; **2**: 517–26.
3. D. L. Parker, G. T. Gullberg, P. R. Frederick. Gibbs artifact removal in magnetic resonance imaging. *Med Phys* 1987; **14**: 640–5.
4. E. V. Di Bella, D. L. Parker, A. J. Sinusas. On the dark rim artifact in dynamic contrast-enhanced MRI myocardial perfusion studies. *Magn Reson Med* 2005; **54**: 1295–9.
5. J. R. Panting, P. D. Gatehouse, G. Z. Yang, et al. Abnormal subendocardial perfusion in cardiac syndrome X detected by cardiovascular magnetic resonance imaging. *N Engl J Med* 2002; **346**: 1948–53.
6. T. D. Karamitsos, J. R. Arnold, T. J. Pegg, et al. Patients with Syndrome X have normal transmural myocardial perfusion and oxygenation: a 3 tesla cardiovascular magnetic resonance imaging study. *Circ Cardiovasc Imaging* 2012: **5**: 194–200.

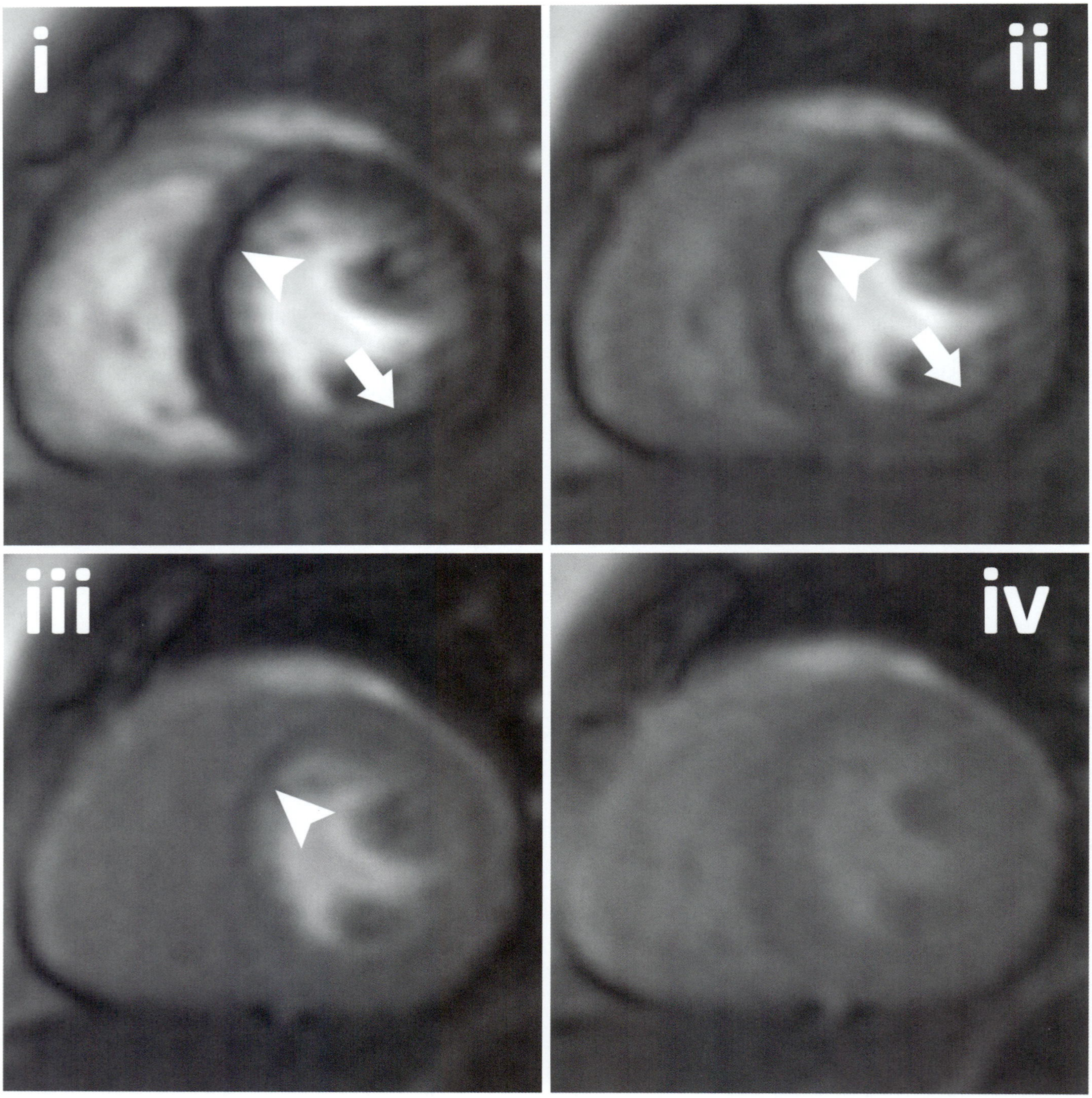

Figure 49.1 Dynamic short-axis resting perfusion images demonstrating Gibbs artifact. Images are shown from multiple time points post-contrast (i-iv). A stripe of subendocardial low signal intensity is most prominent along the phase encoding direction in the septum (arrowhead) and to a lesser extent in the inferolateral wall (arrow) due to undersampling in the anterior–posterior axis. The artifact becomes characteristically less apparent on subsequent dynamic images (iii, iv) as signal intensity in the ventricular cavity decreases. True perfusion defects will persist on all phases.

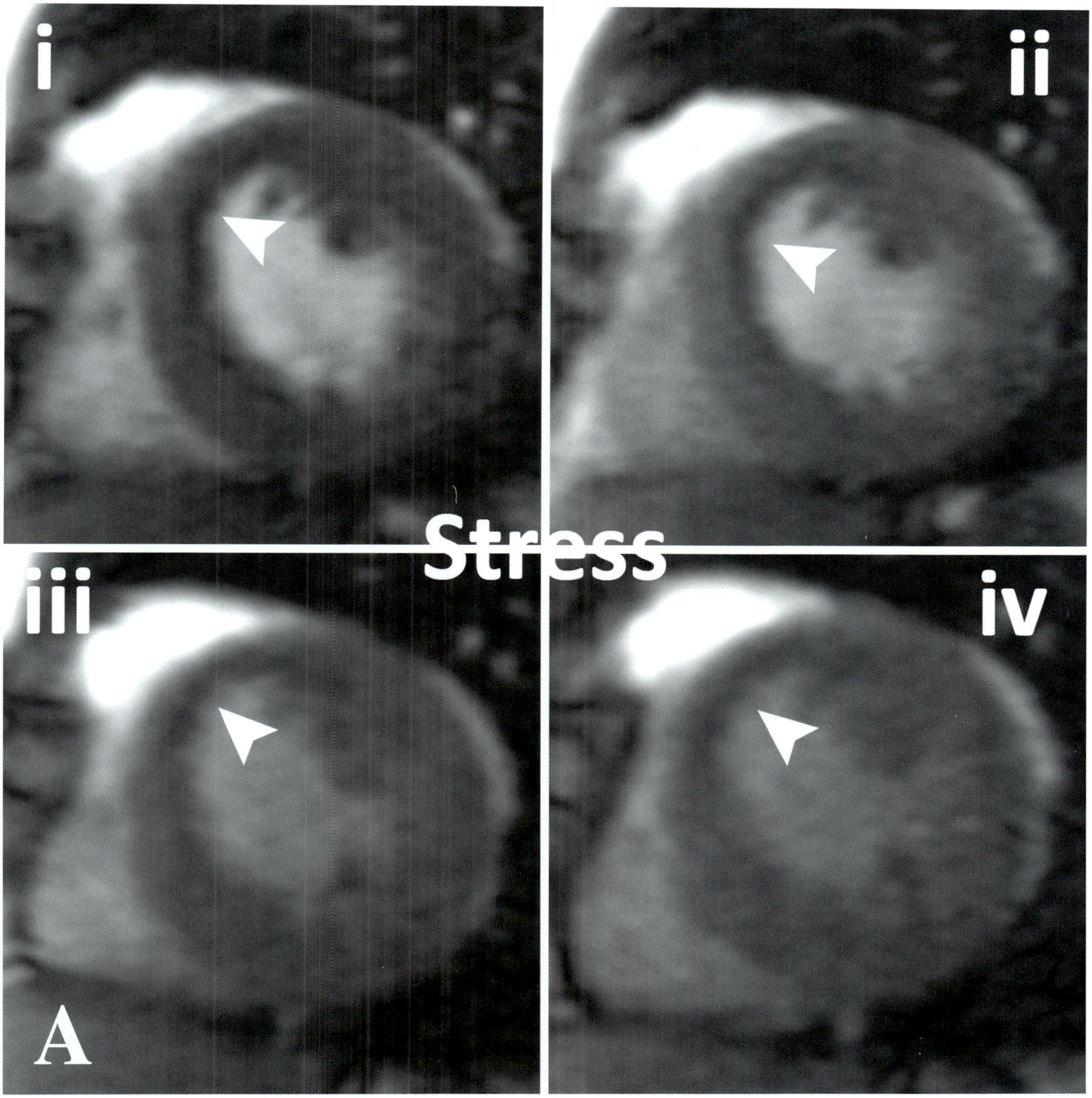

Figure 49.2 A. Dynamic short-axis perfusion images obtained during adenosine stress in a 66-year-old male with suspected coronary artery disease. Images are shown from multiple time points post-contrast (i–iv). A low signal intensity subendocardial perfusion defect is present in the anteroseptum and anterior wall (arrowheads). The abnormality persists on all post-contrast phases (i–iv), becoming more apparent as the signal intensity of the left ventricular blood pool decreases (ii,iii). B. Dynamic resting short-axis perfusion images in the same patient reveal a small Gibbs artifact on the initial first-pass image (i, arrowhead) but normal myocardial signal intensity on subsequent images (ii–iv). Rest-stress findings suggest a reversible perfusion defect due to ischemia. Subsequent coronary catheterization revealed a high-grade lesion in the proximal left anterior descending coronary artery that was treated with angioplasty and stenting.

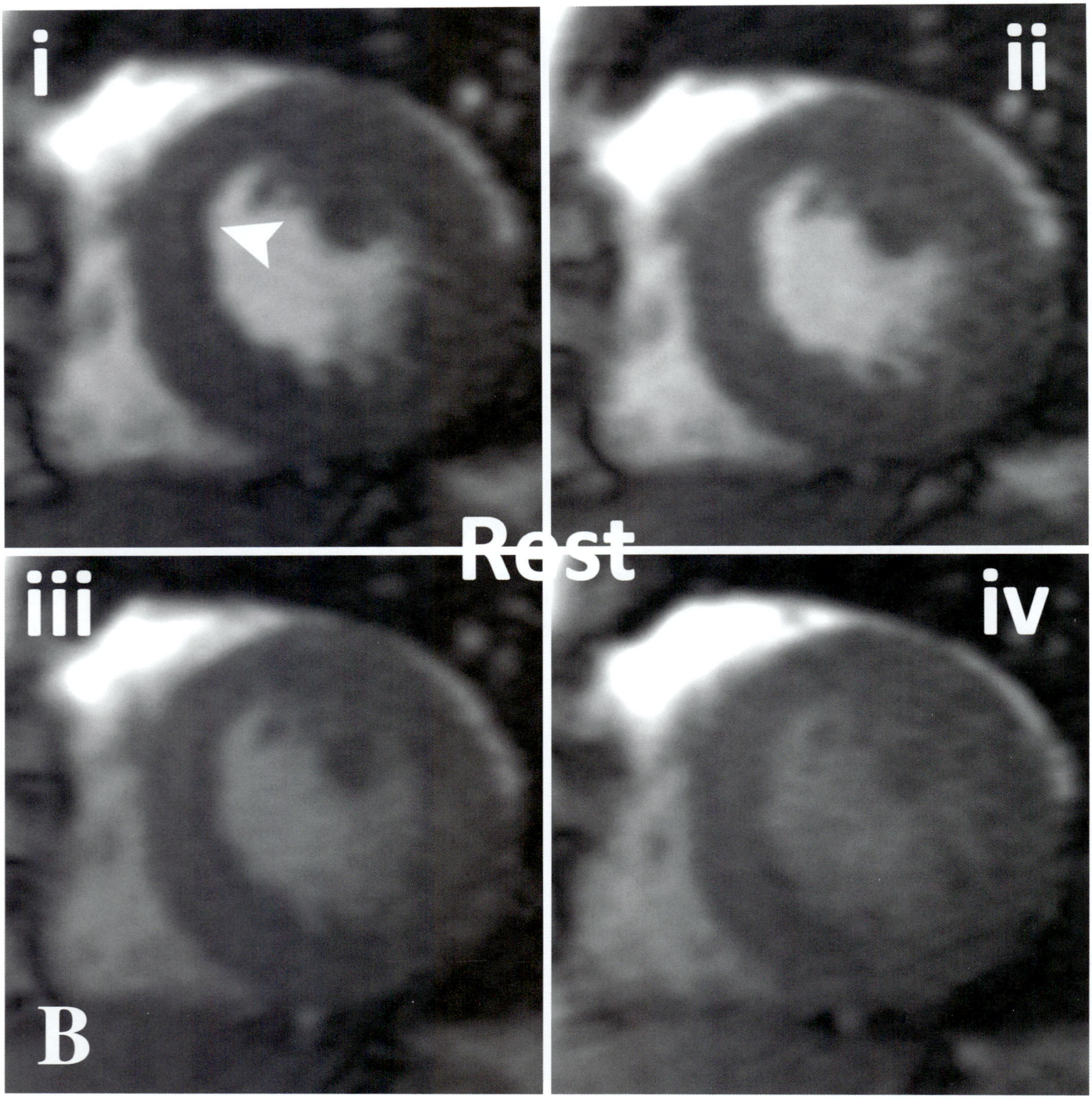

Figure 49.2 (*cont.*)

CASE 50

Aliasing artifact in phase-contrast cardiac MRI

Stefan L. Zimmerman

Imaging description

Aliasing artifact occurs in phase-contrast MRI when the peak velocity of flowing blood being imaged exceeds the encoding velocity, or Venc. In phase-contrast MRI, specialized flow-sensitive gradients are used to encode flow velocity and flow direction information into grayscale pixel values. The Venc is a parameter, expressed in cm/sec, that specifies the maximal velocity that can be measured by a given phase-contrast acquisition. The Venc is adjustable and is set at the MRI scanner before image aquisition. When the vessel being imaged contains flowing blood that is moving faster than the Venc, aliasing will occur. Pixels will become progressively brighter as velocities approach the Venc; however, pixels that represent velocities exceeding the Venc wrap around and are mapped to dark pixels from the opposite end of the grayscale spectrum (Figure 50.1). Depending on the direction of flow, the inverse situation can also occur, where white aliased pixels may be surrounded by dark non-aliased pixels with velocities just below the Venc (Figure 50.1).

Importance

Aliasing will result in inaccurate measurement of peak velocities within a vessel. Peak velocities are used to estimate the pressure gradient across a stenosis which can dictate treatment decisions. Automated flow measurement software can be used to correct for aliasing if peak velocity is less than three times the Venc.[1] However, repeated acquisitions at an increased Venc setting are preferred for maximum measurement reliability.

Typical clinical scenario

Aliasing artifacts are seen whenever the flow velocity is greater than expected when setting the Venc. This is common in the setting of stenotic vessels or valvular stenosis. Elevated velocities may also be seen within the left ventricular outflow tract in the setting of obstructive hypertrophic cardiomyopathy. Typical maximal velocities for ascending aorta, pulmonary artery, and systemic veins are less than 150 cm/sec, less than 100 cm/sec, and less than 50 cm/sec, respectively.[2] In the setting of stenosis, maximal velocities may increase to 500–1000 cm/sec, and repeated acquisitions with incremental increases of Venc may be necessary to find the optimal Venc to prevent aliasing. Empiric use of a high Venc to avoid aliasing is not recommended as this will limit measurement precision by introduction of increased noise. Measurement errors are less than 10% as long as Venc is no more than three times greater than the velocities of interest.[1]

Differential diagnosis

Aliasing on phase-contrast MRI has a characteristic appearance; there is no differential diagnosis.

Teaching point

Aliasing artifacts are critical to recognize when performing phase-contrast imaging for velocity and flow quantification. Increasing the Venc to slightly greater than peak velocity will result in optimal measurement accuracy.

REFERENCES

1. J. Lotz, C. Meier, A. Leppert, M. Galanski. Cardiovascular flow measurement with phase-contrast MR imaging: basic facts and implementation. *Radiographics* 2002; **22**: 651–71.
2. M. B. Srichai, R. P. Lim, S. Wong, V. S. Lee. Cardiovascular applications of phase-contrast MRI. *AJR Am J Roentgenol* 2009; **192**: 662–75.

Pearls and Pitfalls in Cardiovascular Imaging, ed. Stefan L. Zimmerman and Elliot K. Fishman. Published by Cambridge University Press. © Cambridge University Press 2015.

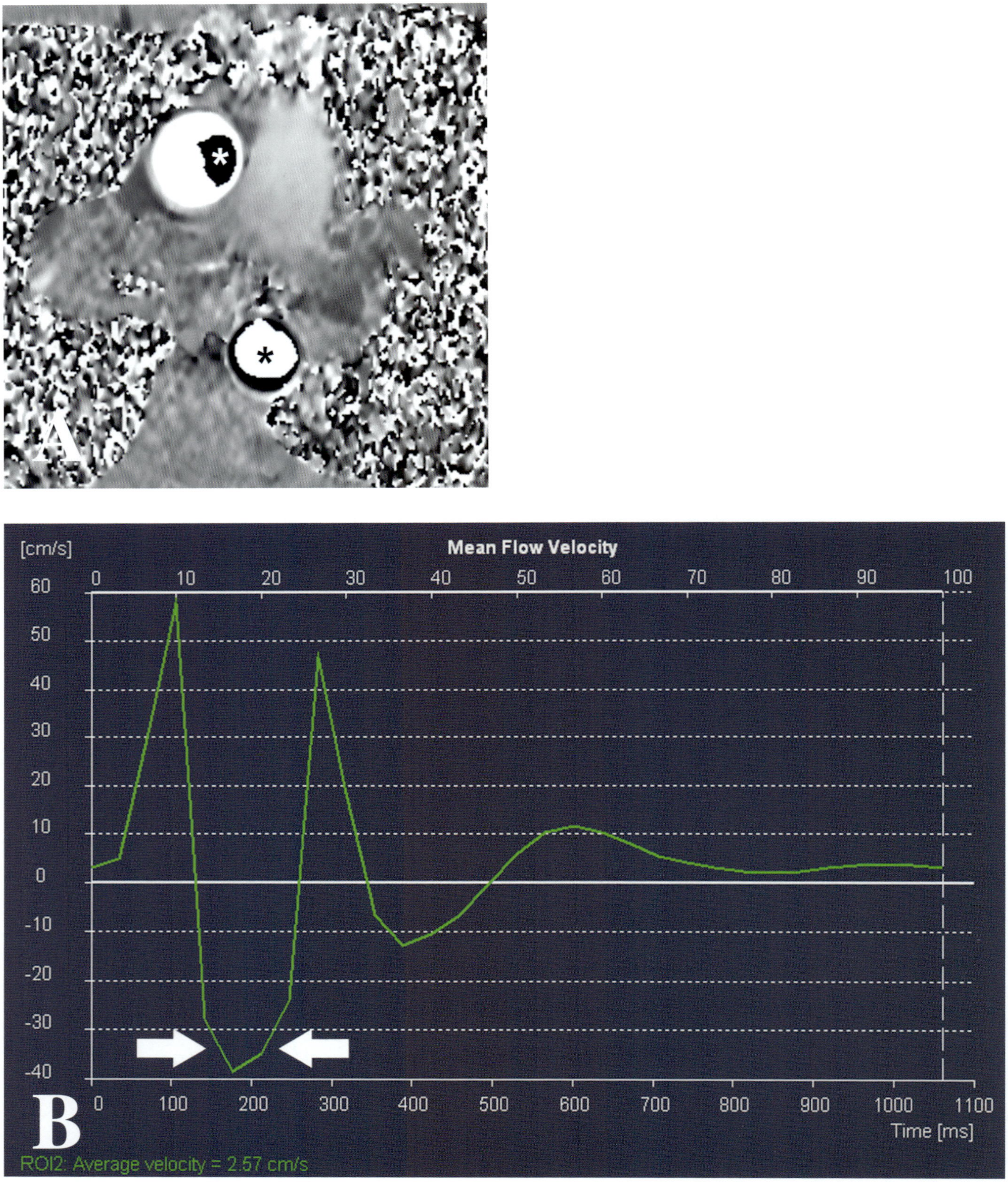

Figure 50.1 **A.** Axial phase-contrast MRI image acquired in a 38-year-old male being evaluated for cardiomyopathy. At a Venc of 75 cm/sec, there is significant aliasing in the ascending and descending thoracic aorta (asterisks), because of velocities encoded by aliased pixels exceed 75 cm/sec and are wrapped to the opposite end of the grayscale. **B.** Graph of mean velocity versus time created from a region of interest placed in the descending thoracic aorta demonstrates truncation of the peak of the velocity curve (arrows), due to aliasing. The aliased velocities are incorrectly mapped to negative values.

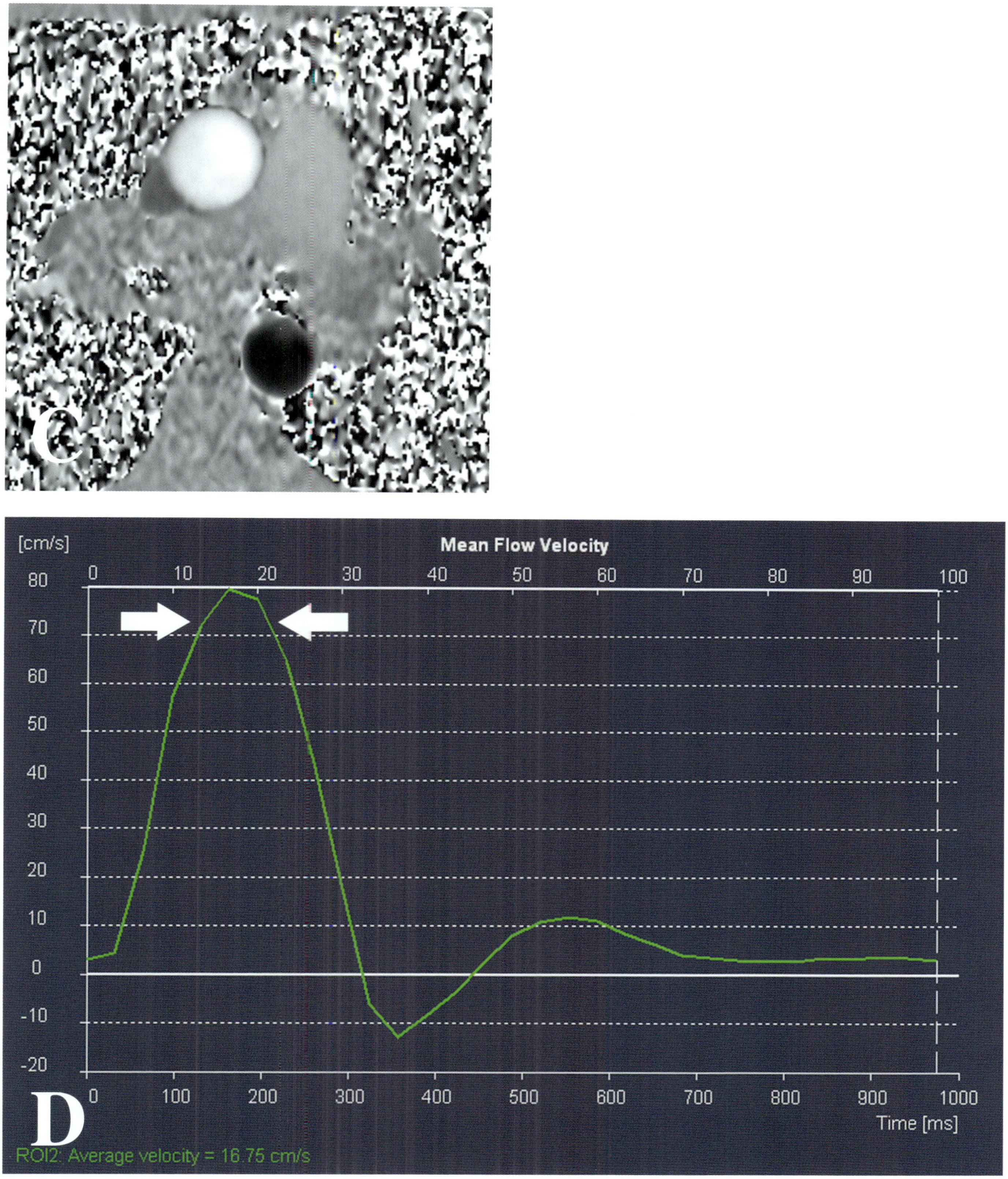

Figure 50.1 *(cont.)* **C.** Phase-contrast image obtained in the same plane with Venc of 150cm/sec demonstrates resolution of aliasing artifact in the aorta. **D.** The velocity–time graph shows the artifactual truncation of peak velocities has now been corrected (arrows) due to lack of aliasing at higher Venc.

CASE 51

Pseudostenoses on MR angiography from susceptibility artifact

Stefan L. Zimmerman

Imaging description

Susceptibility artifacts adjacent to vessels can result in pseudostenoses on MR angiography. Susceptibility artifacts occur when material within the body, usually metal, distorts the local magnetic field in or near the vessel of interest, resulting in a region of low signal intensity on the subsequent MR images. On maximum intensity projection (MIP) subtraction images, this low signal intensity creates the false appearance of a vascular stenosis or occlusion. These artifacts can vary in size depending on the amount of material and the pulse sequence used. For instance, very large artifacts are seen with knee and hip replacements, whereas smaller areas of signal loss are seen around surgical clips. Gradient echo sequences, which are used for gadolinium-enhanced MR angiography, will have more severe artifacts than spin echo-based sequences. Pseudostenoses on MRA due to surgical clips can be seen anywhere in the body, not uncommonly in the superficial femoral artery of the medial thigh due to prior saphenous vein harvesting or in the common femoral artery related to prior groin catheterization.[1] Surgical clips adjacent to lower extremity bypass grafts can also mimic stenosis. Ductus clips can result in large artifacts that obscure the aortic arch (Figure 51.1). Knee prostheses will result in an appearance simulating popliteal artery occlusion, whereas hip prostheses can simulate femoral artery occlusions (Figure 51.2). Susceptibility artifact from metal in vascular stents can obscure the lumen of the stented vessel, giving the false appearance of occlusion or stenosis. One particularly difficult artifact is a pseudostenosis of the subclavian artery due to susceptibility effects of highly concentrated gadolinium in the adjacent subclavian vein (Figure 51.3).[2] These artifacts will be seen only on the side of injection and may resolve on subsequent venous phase images. Occasionally repeat imaging with injection on the contralateral side may be required to exclude the possibility of a true stenosis.

Importance

Susceptibility artifacts can result in misdiagnosis of a significant stenosis in the vessel of interest, potentially leading to inappropriate additional testing or intervention.

Typical clinical scenario

Susceptibility artifacts are common at MR angiography in patients with prior surgery adjacent to the vessel of interest.

Differential diagnosis

Psuedostenoses due to susceptibility must be distinguished from a true stenotic lesion. Source images should be closely evaluated in addition to MIPs in all cases to evaluate for possible susceptibility effects. When susceptibility effects are identified, diagnostic evaluation of the affected vascular segment may not be possible. In these difficult cases, repeat imaging with contrast-enhanced CT angiography or catheter angiography may be necessary if there is a high suspicion for underlying stenotic lesion.

Teaching point

Susceptibility artifacts can result in the artifactual appearance of a stenosis on MR angiography. Close inspection of source images is recommended to allow recognition of these artifacts and avoid potential misdiagnosis.

REFERENCES

1. H. Ersoy, H. Zhang, M. R. Prince. Peripheral MR angiography. *J Cardiovasc Magn Reson* 2006; **8**: 517–28.
2. S. Tatli, M. J. Lipton, B. D. Davison, R. B. Skorstad, E. K. Yucel. From the RSNA refresher courses: MR imaging of aortic and peripheral vascular disease. *Radiographics* 2003; **23** Spec No: S59–78.

Pearls and Pitfalls in Cardiovascular Imaging, ed. Stefan L. Zimmerman and Elliot K. Fishman. Published by Cambridge University Press. © Cambridge University Press 2015.

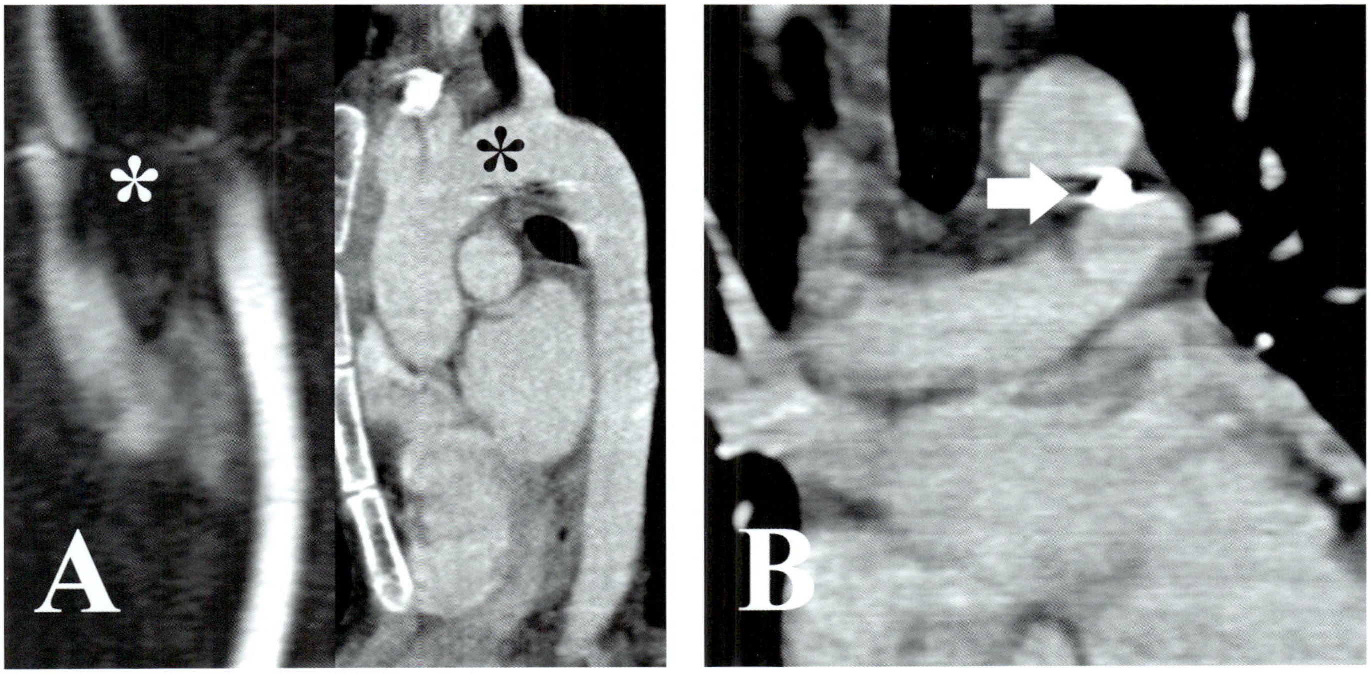

Figure 51.1 **A.** Sagittal oblique images of the aorta from an MR angiogram (left) and a CT angiogram (right) obtained in an 8-year-old male with Marfan syndrome and prior ductus clipping. There is extensive susceptibility artifact on the MRA image that completely obscures visualization of the aortic arch (asterisk). On the CT angiogram, the aortic arch is normal. **B.** A coronal CT image shows the ductus clip (arrow), which creates a relatively small amount of streak artifact on CT but large amounts of susceptibility artifact on MRA.

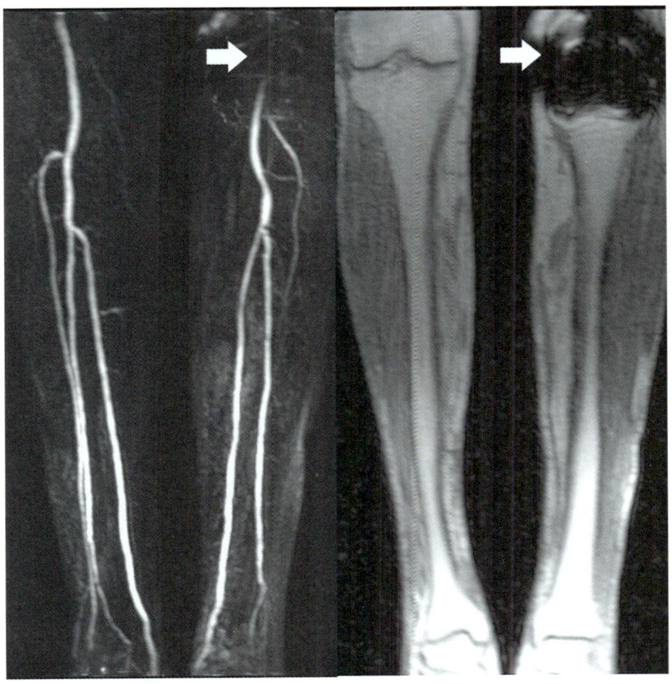

Figure 51.2 Coronal images from an MR angiogram obtained in a 76-year-old male with peripheral vascular disease shows complete loss of signal from the left popliteal artery on coronal post-contrast MIP images (arrow, left). This could be mistaken for occlusion of the popliteal artery. However, on the coronal source images there is susceptibility artifact related to a left knee prosthesis that explains the signal loss (arrow, right).

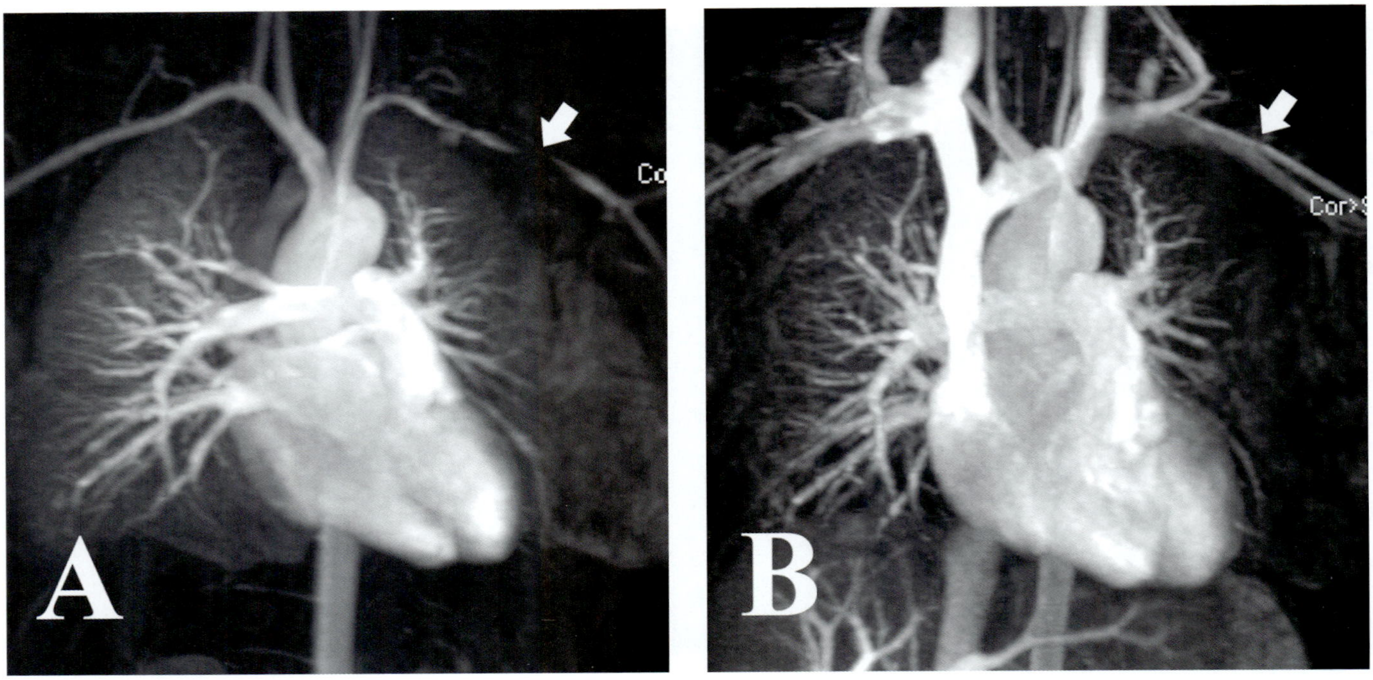

Figure 51.3 **A.** Coronal MIP image from an MR angiogram obtained in a 20-year-old woman with Takayasu's arteritis demonstrates an artifactual stenosis of the left subclavian artery (arrow) that is caused by highly concentrated gadolinium in the adjacent subclavian vein. Susceptibility artifacts can result from retained venous contrast on the side of injection. **B.** On delayed venous images, the artifact resolves, showing a normal left subclavian artery (arrow). Care should be taken in diagnosing subclavian artery stenoses ipsilateral to the side of injection. Delayed venous phase images should always be evaluated to confirm that the stenosis persists. In some cases, a repeat study with right-sided injection may be necessary.

CASE 52

Pseudostenosis on time-of-flight magnetic resonance angiography

David Bonekamp and Stefan L. Zimmerman

Imaging description

Time-of-flight (TOF) magnetic resonance angiography (MRA) images are prone to several artifacts that may suggest stenosis or occlusion of vascular segments. TOF MRA is based on the acquisition of 2D or 3D gradient echo images which are optimized to saturate protons in stationary tissues while maximizing flow-related enhancement from inflowing blood protons that enter the slice during the acquisition. Saturation bands are added to selectively null signal from venous or arterial blood that is flowing in the opposite direction of the vessel of interest. For example, if an image of the abdominal aorta is desired, a saturation band below the plane of interest is used to null inflowing venous blood from the inferior vena cava.[1] Several well-known artifacts occur with TOF imaging. In-plane flow can result in pseudostenosis or artifactual occlusion because blood protons flowing within a vessel parallel to the imaging plane will become saturated during the acquisition (Figure 52.1). Slow-flowing blood may also become saturated before it reaches the end of the TOF slab, such that the distal vessel appears attenuated in luminal diameter and signal. Reversal of flow, which can occur due to retrograde filling with collateral arteries, will be undetectable with TOF techniques due to the use of saturation bands to suppress venous contamination (Figure 52.2). Susceptibility artifacts from surgical clips or adjacent hardware may attenuate the MR signal, and the gradient echo (GRE) sequences used for TOF are especially sensitive for this type of artifact. Finally, dephasing of protons that occurs due to turbulent flow at vessel bifurcations may mimic stenoses, while accelerated and turbulent flow at existing stenoses may lead to overestimation of the degree of stenosis.

Importance

TOF MRA is a widely used unenhanced MRA method.[2] Knowledge of artifacts that may mimic vascular stenosis or occlusion is essential for accurate interpretation. Misinterpretation of the absence or presence of vascular stenosis or occlusion can lead to unnecessary intervention or surgery, or fail to diagnose a treatable cause for the patient's symptoms.

Typical clinical scenario

Classic locations for pseudostenosis or occlusion from in-plane flow artifacts are the renal arteries, common iliac arteries, and the origins of the anterior tibial arteries, where vessels may course horizontally in the body (Figures 52.1 and 52.3). Saturation of retrograde flow has specific importance in patients with arterial occlusions and distal reconstitution by collaterals, such as can occur in focal occlusions of the arteries of the lower extremities. In subclavian steal syndrome, reversed flow through the vertebral artery to the subclavian artery distal to a stenosis will likely be missed by TOF techniques. Finally, in imaging of renal transplants, which often requires non-contrast acquisitions due to renal insufficiency or failure, blood flow in the transplant renal artery flows cranially, in the opposite direction of iliac arteries and aorta, and is prone to pseudostenosis appearance (Figure 52.2).

Differential diagnosis

Whenever a stenosis or occlusion is suggested by TOF MRA, review of the source images is essential to examine if the vessel segment has a long in-plane course or if there is evidence for susceptibility artifact.[3] Knowledge of the expected course of the vessel of interest is critical to prevent misdiagnosis of occlusion due to flow reversal (Figure 52.2). Non-visualization of a vessel on TOF may indicate flow reversal or very slow flow and does not prove occlusion. A signal void distal to a stenosis may indicate dephasing from strongly turbulent flow and has been associated with hemodynamically significant stenosis.[4] If there is persistent doubt, acquisition of contrast-enhanced MRA for confirmation is ideal. However, if not possible due to renal insufficiency or allergy, additional non-contrast MRA techniques such as steady-state free precession (SSFP) bright blood images or 3D partial-Fourier fast spin echo (FSE) MRA [1] may be needed to confirm the presence of stenosis or occlusion.

Teaching point

TOF MRA is a commonly used non-contrast MRA technique of high clinical availability. In-plane flow, slow flow, flow reversal, susceptibility artifact, and turbulent flow are all common causes of pseudostenosis or apparent vascular occlusion. Most of these artifacts can be recognized by analysis of the source images and the anatomical context in which they occur. TOF may be combined with additional non-contrast MRA techniques to complement the angiographic information and for problem solving.

REFERENCES

1. M. Miyazaki, V. S. Lee. Nonenhanced MR angiography. *Radiology* 2008; **248**: 20–43.

Pearls and Pitfalls in Cardiovascular Imaging, ed. Stefan L. Zimmerman and Elliot K. Fishman. Published by Cambridge University Press. © Cambridge University Press 2015.

2. S. Morita, A. Masukawa, K. Suzuki, M. Hirata, S. Kojima, E. Ueno. Unenhanced MR angiography: techniques and clinical applications in patients with chronic kidney disease. *Radiographics* 2011; **31**: E13–33.

3. J. A. Kaufman, D. McCarter, S. C. Geller, A. C. Waltman. Two-dimensional time-of-flight MR angiography of the lower extremities: artifacts and pitfalls. *AJR Am J Roentgenol* 1998; **171**: 129–35.

4. H. Zhang, M. R. Prince. Renal MR angiography. *Magn Reson Imaging Clin N Am* 2004; **12**: 487–503, vi.

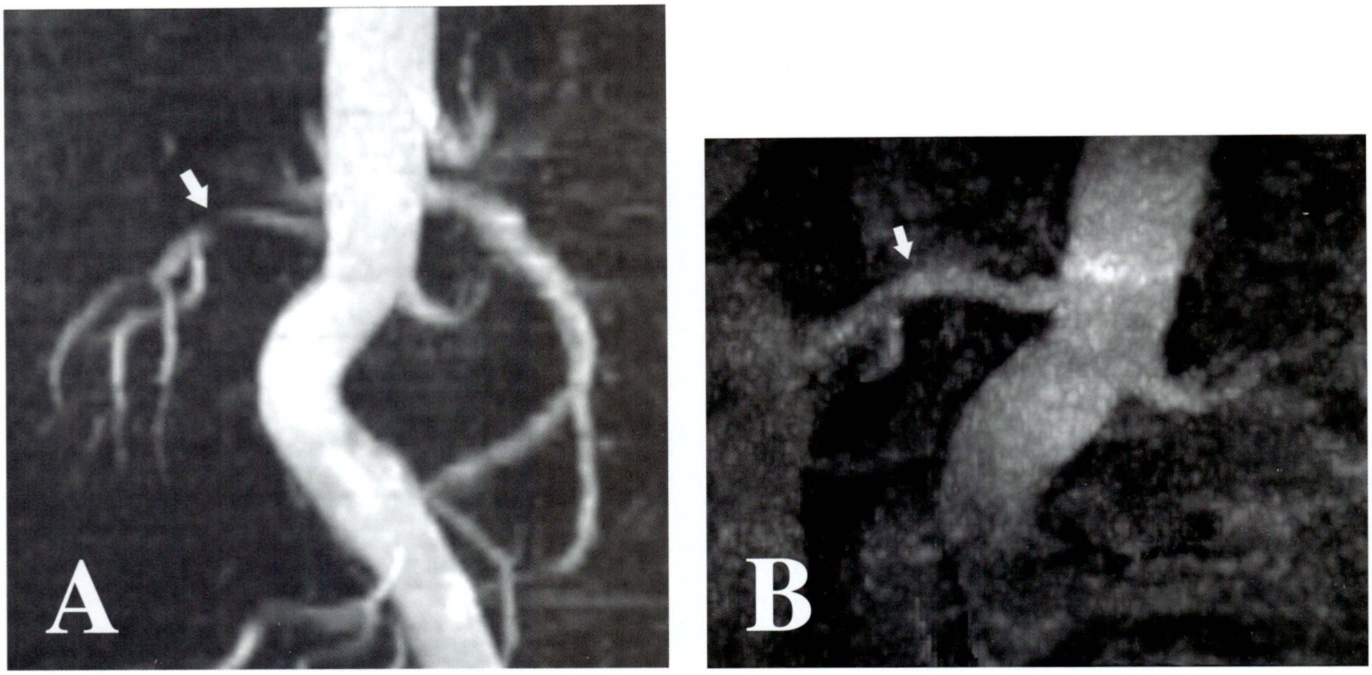

Figure 52.1 A 68-year-old male with chronic renal failure and hypertension; non-contrast MRA was requested to evaluate for renal artery stenosis. **A.** Coronal maximum intensity projection time-of-flight image shows loss of signal in the distal main right renal artery, suggesting stenosis (arrow). **B.** Coronal maximum intensity projection from ECG-gated balanced steady-state free precession sequence shows no stenosis in this region, indicating that the abnormality on time-of-flight images was an artifact due to in-plane flow saturation.

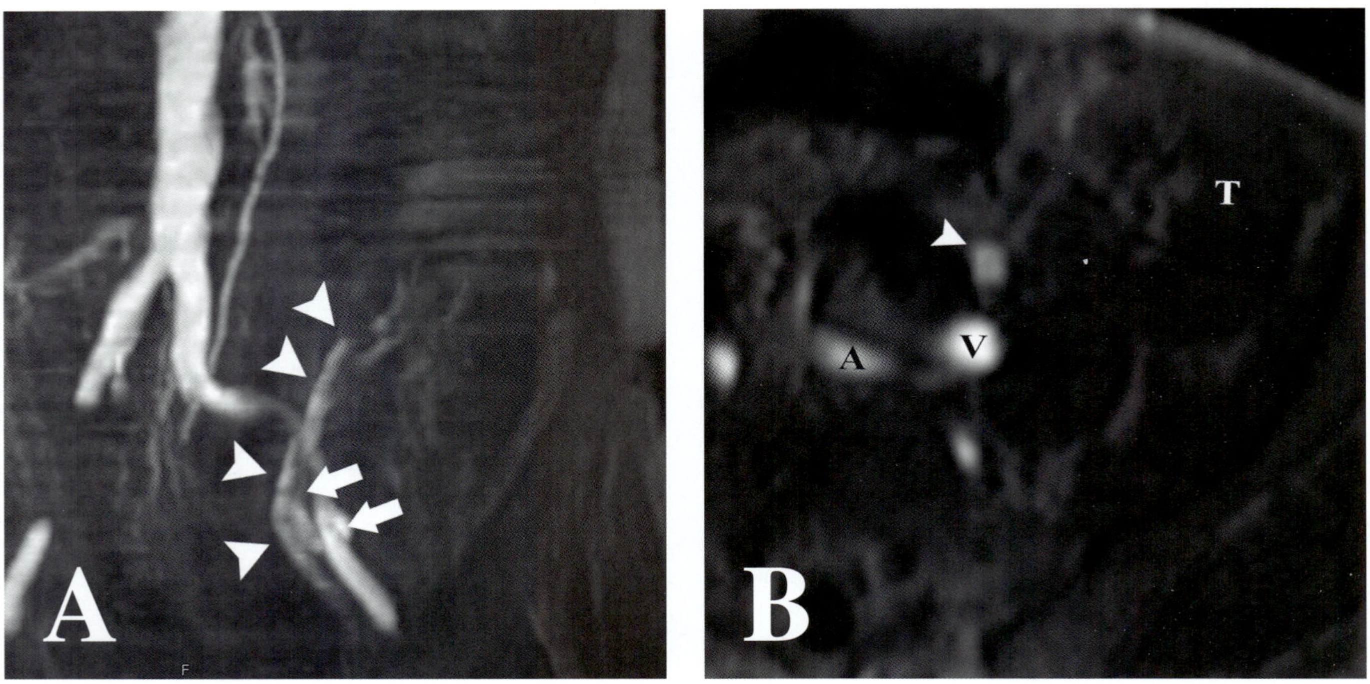

Figure 52.2 A 70-year-old male with history of left lower quadrant renal transplant and increased creatinine with clinical concern for stenosis of the transplant renal artery. **A.** Coronal MIP from time-of-flight (TOF) non-contrast MRA shows the patent transplant renal vein (arrowheads) but

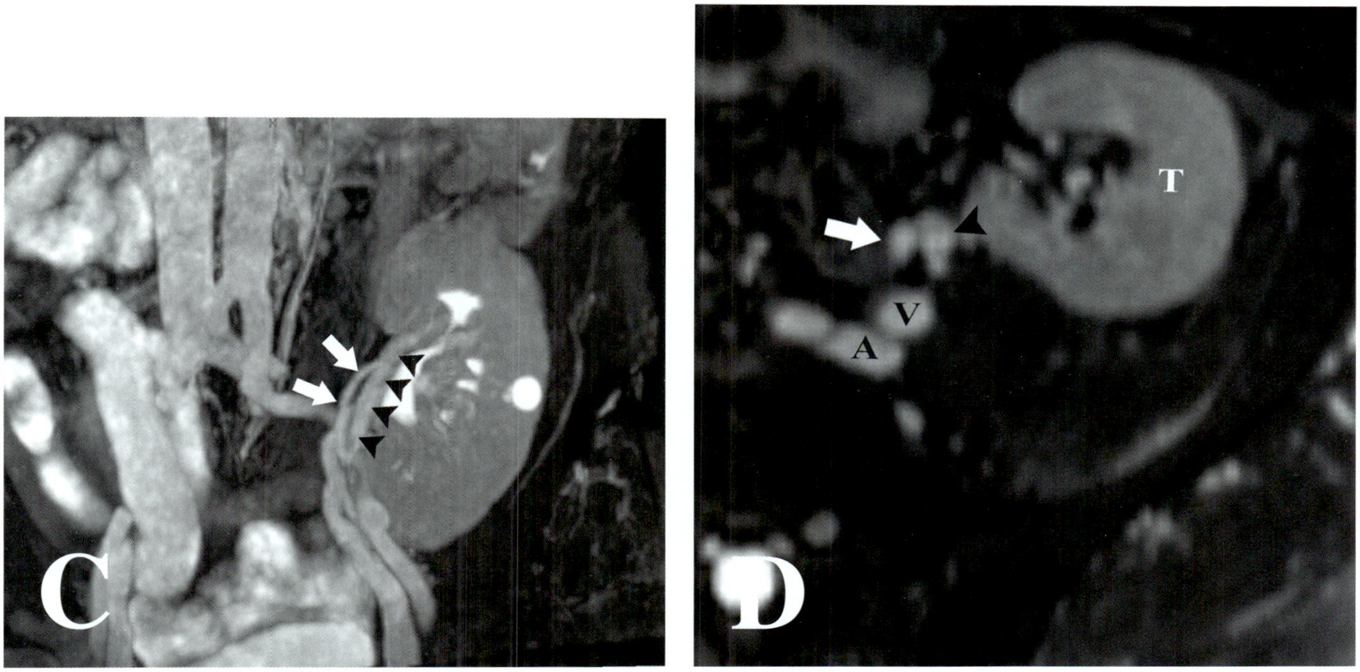

Figure 52.2 (*cont.*) only the proximal portion of the transplant artery is visible (arrows) suggesting stenosis. **B.** Axial TOF image showing the transplant renal vein (arrowhead) arising from the external iliac vein (V), but no visible transplant artery (A = external iliac artery, T = transplant kidney). Coronal MIP (**C**) and reformatted axial image (**D**) from an ECG-gated balanced steady-state free precession sequence shows patent transplant renal artery (arrows) and vein (black arrowheads). The artifactual transplant artery stenosis and visualization of the transplant vein on the TOF images are due to saturation effects from the inferior saturation band that was placed to select for aortic flow. Because flow is retrograde in the renal artery, opposite the direction of the aorta, it becomes saturated. Antegrade flow in the renal vein is visualized because it flows in the same direction of the aorta.

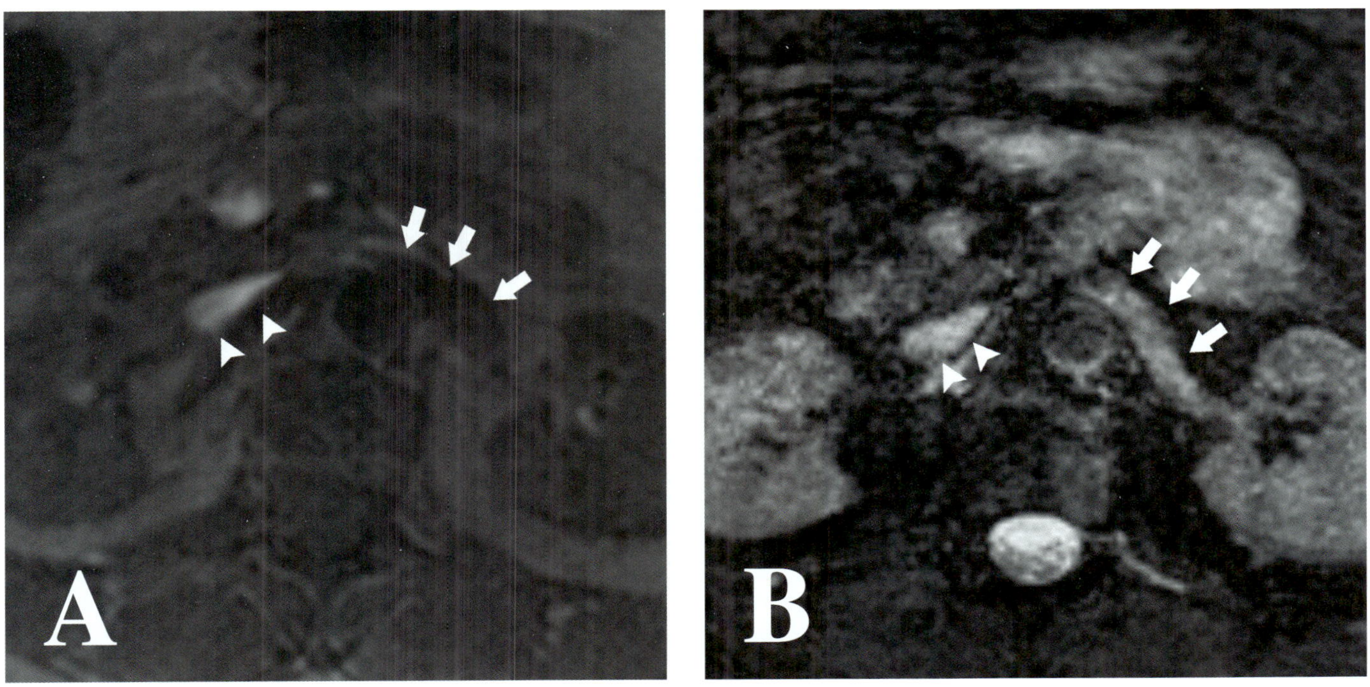

Figure 52.3 A 49-year-old female with nephrotic syndrome, renal failure, and concern for renal vein thrombosis. Non-contrast MRA was requested. **A.** Axial TOF image. A superior saturation band was placed to selectively visualize venous flow. Bright signal is visualized in the inferior vena cava (arrowheads) but not in the left renal vein (arrows), suggesting the possibility of thrombosis. **B.** Axial image from ECG-gated balanced steady-state free precession sequence showing bright signal in both the inferior vena cava (arrowheads) and the left renal vein (arrows), indicating that the absence of signal in the left renal vein on the TOF image is an artifact, related to in-plane flow in the horizontally oriented left renal vein.

CASE 53

Maki effect

David Bonekamp and Stefan L. Zimmerman

Imaging description

"Maki" artifact or effect is named after Jeffrey H. Maki, MD, PhD, who first comprehensively described this as a "ringing" or "banding" artifact occurring in MRA studies (Figure 53.1).[1,2] It manifests as lack of central arterial enhancement with parallel bands of decreasing hyperintensity in the location of the arterial walls. The proximal margin and the transition to normal arterial enhancement are gradual, without a sharply defined border. The effect is often most pronounced on subtracted images.

Importance

"Maki" artifact may be incorrectly diagnosed as arterial thrombosis, leading to inappropriate referral to invasive angiography. The artery exhibiting the artifact is not adequately imaged and underlying pathology such as thrombosis or dissection is not evaluated. Recognition of the artifact is important to adjust the clinical protocol to avoid too early acquisition of MRA images after bolus injection.[1,3]

Typical clinical scenario

This artifact is observed in MR angiography studies if the center of k-space is acquired before the peak arterial contrast concentration has been reached. The leading edge of the bolus is typically narrow and enhancement is brisk, while the exact delay between injection and bolus arrival is influenced by multiple factors. These include cardiac output, the distance of the artery from the heart, vascular shunts, and stenoses. Optimal arterial enhancement is only achieved if the acquisition of the center of k-space occurs at the time of maximal arterial enhancement. Imaging too early will result in the Maki artifact, whereas imaging after the peak will decrease the signal-to-noise ratio and venous contamination will be more pronounced. The challenge of correct bolus timing is increased when a shorter contrast bolus is used to minimize the amount of contrast. Centric k-space encoding acquires the center of k-space first, allowing for the most precise bolus timing; however, it renders the MRA technique more prone to artifacts.[4,5]

Differential diagnosis

The artifact has a pathognomonic appearance of a high-pass filtered image, in which edges are accentuated. Gibbs ringing artifact, manifesting itself as side-lobes of decreasing intensity but constant spacing, is typically juxtaposed to the arterial walls. The hypointense signal in the arterial lumen raises the primary differential diagnostic consideration of arterial thrombosis. However, these can typically be distinguished from artifact by finding sharply demarcated proximal and distal margins, a meniscus between the hypointense thrombus and the arterial wall, and hyperintense vascular walls due to thrombus-related inflammation. By contrast, the Maki artifact will be long in extent without a sharp transition from enhanced to unenhanced lumen. Other causes for arterial filling defects can be signal loss due to vascular stents or adjacent susceptible material such as surgical clips or highly concentrated venous contrast.

Teaching point

Bolus timing in MRA can be challenging due to the required balance between minimal contrast material use, optimal arterial signal, and lack of venous contamination. The pathognomonic appearance of the Maki artifact should be recognized as resulting from acquisition of the MRA images prior to contrast bolus arrival. Given the sometimes unpredictable nature of bolus timing, it is good practice to routinely include a second MRA acquisition immediately after the arterial acquisition to have a fallback in case this artifact occurs (Figure 53.1).

REFERENCES

1. Maki JH, Prince MR, Londy FJ, Chenevert TL. The effects of time varying intravascular signal intensity and k-space acquisition order on three-dimensional MR angiography image quality. *J Magn Reson Imaging.* 1996;**6**:642–51.
2. Zhang H, Maki JH, Prince MR. 3D contrast-enhanced MR angiography. *J Magn Reson Imaging.* 2007;**25**:13–25.
3. Lee VS, Martin DJ, Krinsky GA, Rofsky NM. Gadolinium-enhanced MR angiography: artifacts and pitfalls. *AJR Am J Roentgenol.* 2000;**175**:197–205.
4. Riederer SJ, Fain SB, Kruger DG, Busse RF. Real-time imaging and triggering of 3D contrast-enhanced MR angiograms using MR fluoroscopy. *Magma.* 1999;**8**:196–206.
5. Wilman AH, Yep TC, Al-Kwifi O. Quantitative evaluation of nonrepetitive phase-encoding orders for first-pass, 3D contrast-enhanced MR angiography. *Magn Reson Med.* 2001;**46**:541–7.

Pearls and Pitfalls in Cardiovascular Imaging, ed. Stefan L. Zimmerman and Elliot K. Fishman. Published by Cambridge University Press. © Cambridge University Press 2015.

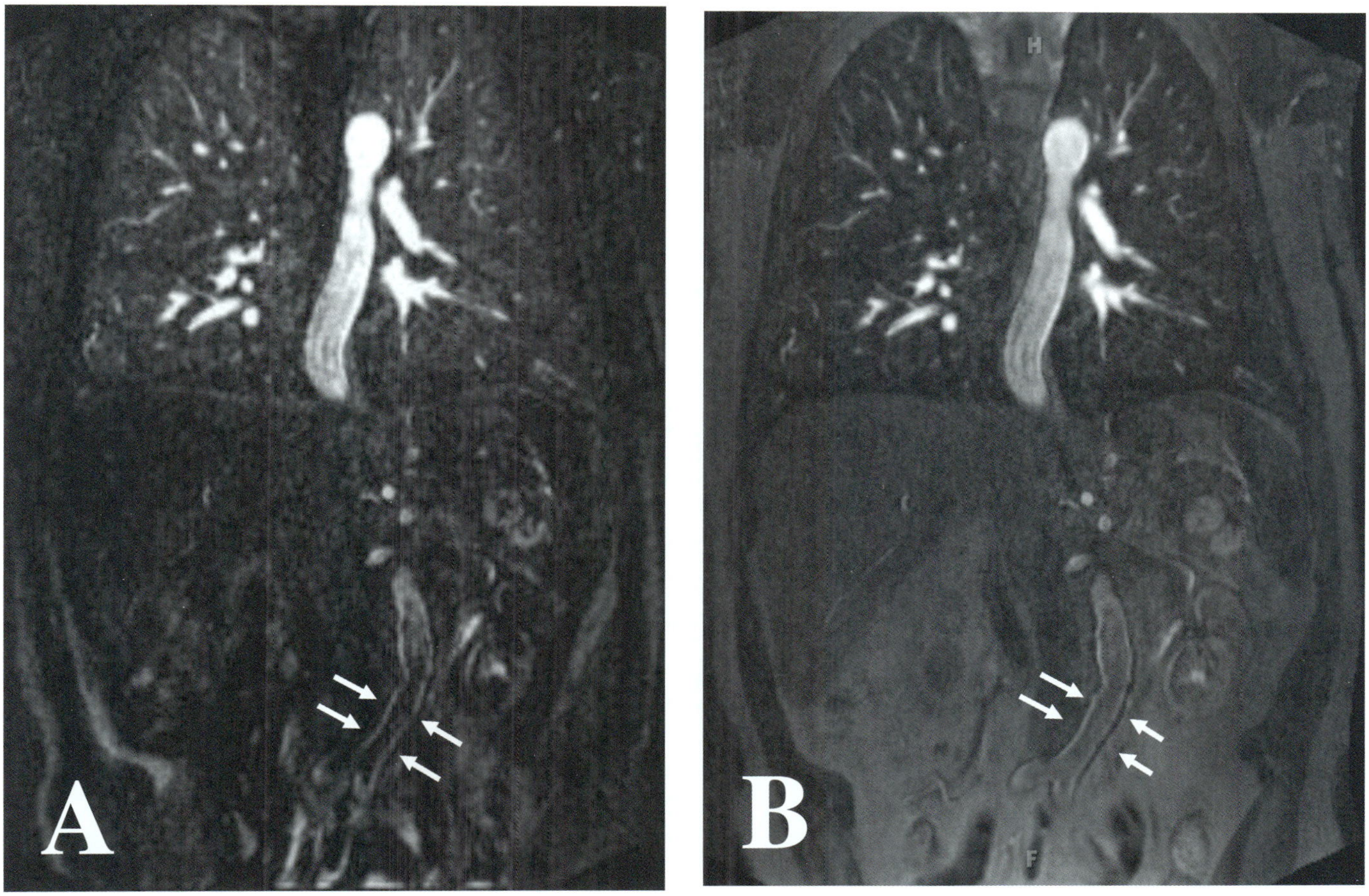

Figure 53.1 A. Subtracted coronal image of a contrast-enhanced MRA of the chest and abdomen performed in a 64-year-old male with Marfan syndrome. The typical hyperintense bands of the Maki artifact are present in the abdominal aorta surrounding the hypointense arterial lumen (arrows). B. Non-subtracted coronal image of a contrast-enhanced MRA of the chest and abdomen performed in a 64-year-old male with Marfan syndrome. The hyperintense bands of the Maki artifact are less prominent compared to the subtracted image. C. Coronal MIP from contrast-enhanced MRA of the chest and abdomen performed in a 64-year-old male with Marfan syndrome. There is a gradual change in signal intensity from enhanced to hypoenhanced lumen (arrows), which helps differentiate this finding from thrombus. D. Subtracted venous phase coronal image from contrast-enhanced MRA of the chest and abdomen performed in a 64-year-old male with Marfan syndrome. On the delayed images, there is resolution of the arterial hypoenhancement present on the initial acquisition (arrows).

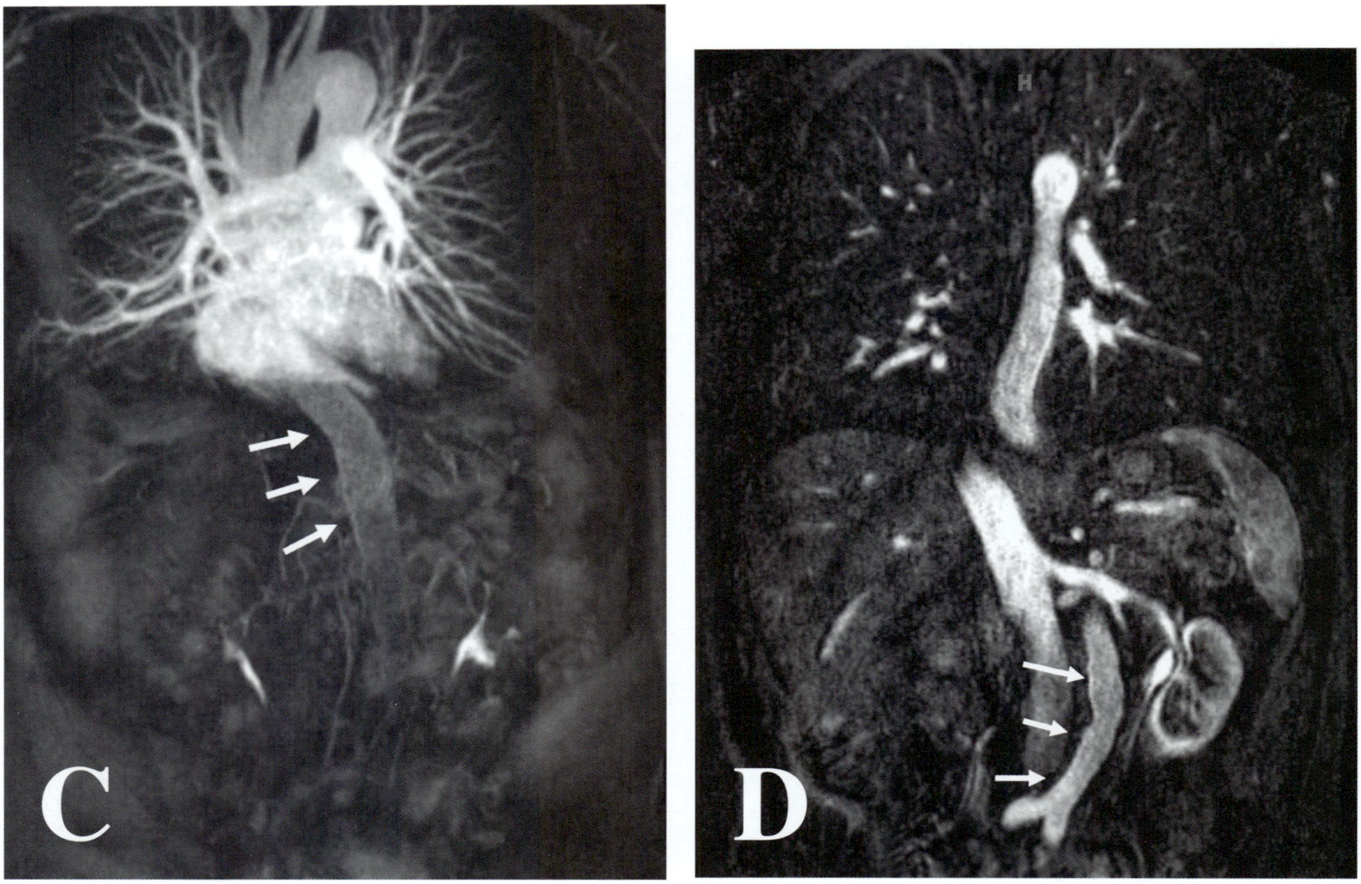

Figure 53.1 *(cont.)*

CASE 54

Pitfalls in arterial enhancement timing

Pamela T. Johnson and Spencer T. Lake

Imaging description

Early arterial phase imaging is critical for high-quality CT angiography examinations; however, accurate imaging can be problematic in patients with large aneurysms or aortic dissections. In some cases, an early arterial acquisition may not allow enough time for complete filling of the aneurysm sac or false lumen with contrast (Figures 54.1–54.3). The incompletely opacified aneurysm sac or false lumen may appear thrombosed, when in actuality it is merely filled with unopacified blood. Swirling of contrast within the aneurysm sac is often present and can be a clue that incomplete contrast filling has occurred (Figure 54.3).

Importance

In the patient with acute pain, large aneurysms must be evaluated for signs of instability or rupture. One of the most critical findings is contrast extravasation reflective of active hemorrhage, which requires immediate repair. The case shown here (Figure 54.1) demonstrates how this important finding could be missed if the arterial timing did not allow for complete aneurysm filling.

Patients with aortic dissection may have very slow flow in the false lumen, resulting in the appearance of pseudothrombosis of both the false lumen and the branches that arise from this lumen. As shown by the second case (Figure 54.2), a longer imaging delay will elucidate that the false lumen, arterial branch and end organ are actually perfused. The distinction is important because in the setting of arterial thrombosis intervention is necessary, whereas uncomplicated type B dissections do not require endovascular or surgical repair.

Although much less common, proper characterization of a coronary artery aneurysm (Figure 54.3) as patent or thrombosed is critical to determine whether repair is indicated to avert rupture.

Typical clinical scenario

Aortic aneurysms and dissections are two of the most common forms of aortic pathology. Patients may present acutely with pain, or may undergo serial imaging to guide management of previously diagnosed aneurysm or partially repaired dissection. Coronary aneurysms are much less common, particularly larger aneurysms.[1–5] In adults, atherosclerosis is the most common cause, whereas in children it is Kawasaki disease.[1]

Differential diagnosis

The differential diagnosis in these cases primarily relates to whether or not the aneurysm, false lumen, and aortic branches are thrombosed. Imaging during both early arterial and late arterial or venous phases is necessary to determine if there is slow, progressive perfusion. In the setting of actual thrombosis, there will be no change in luminal density on delayed acquisitions.

Teaching point

The teaching point of these cases is that large aneurysms and aortic dissections may appear thrombosed on an early arterial phase acquisition. This distinction is essential to guide patient management. These cases underscore the importance of delayed imaging in such patients.

REFERENCES

1. Nichols L, Lagana S, Parwani A. Coronary artery aneurysm: a review and hypothesis regarding etiology. *Arch Pathol Lab Med* 2008; **132**:823–828.
2. Ebina T, Ishikawa Y, Uchida K, et al. A case of giant coronary artery aneurysm and literature review. *J Cardiol* 2009; **53**:293–300.
3. Jha NK, Ouda HZ, Khan JA, Eising GP, Augustin N. Giant right coronary artery aneurysm – case report and literature review. *J Cardiothorac Surg* 2009; **4**:18.
4. Ríos Gómez E, Martín M, Lozano I, Luyando LH. A giant right coronary artery aneurysm as an incidental finding. *Eur J Echocardiogr* 2011; **12**:371.
5. Kanamitsu H, Yoshitaka H, Kuinose M, Tsushima Y. Giant right coronary artery aneurysm complicated by acute myocardial infarction. *Gen Thorac Cardiovasc Surg* 2010; **58**:186–189.

Pearls and Pitfalls in Cardiovascular Imaging, ed. Stefan L. Zimmerman and Elliot K. Fishman. Published by Cambridge University Press. © Cambridge University Press 2015.

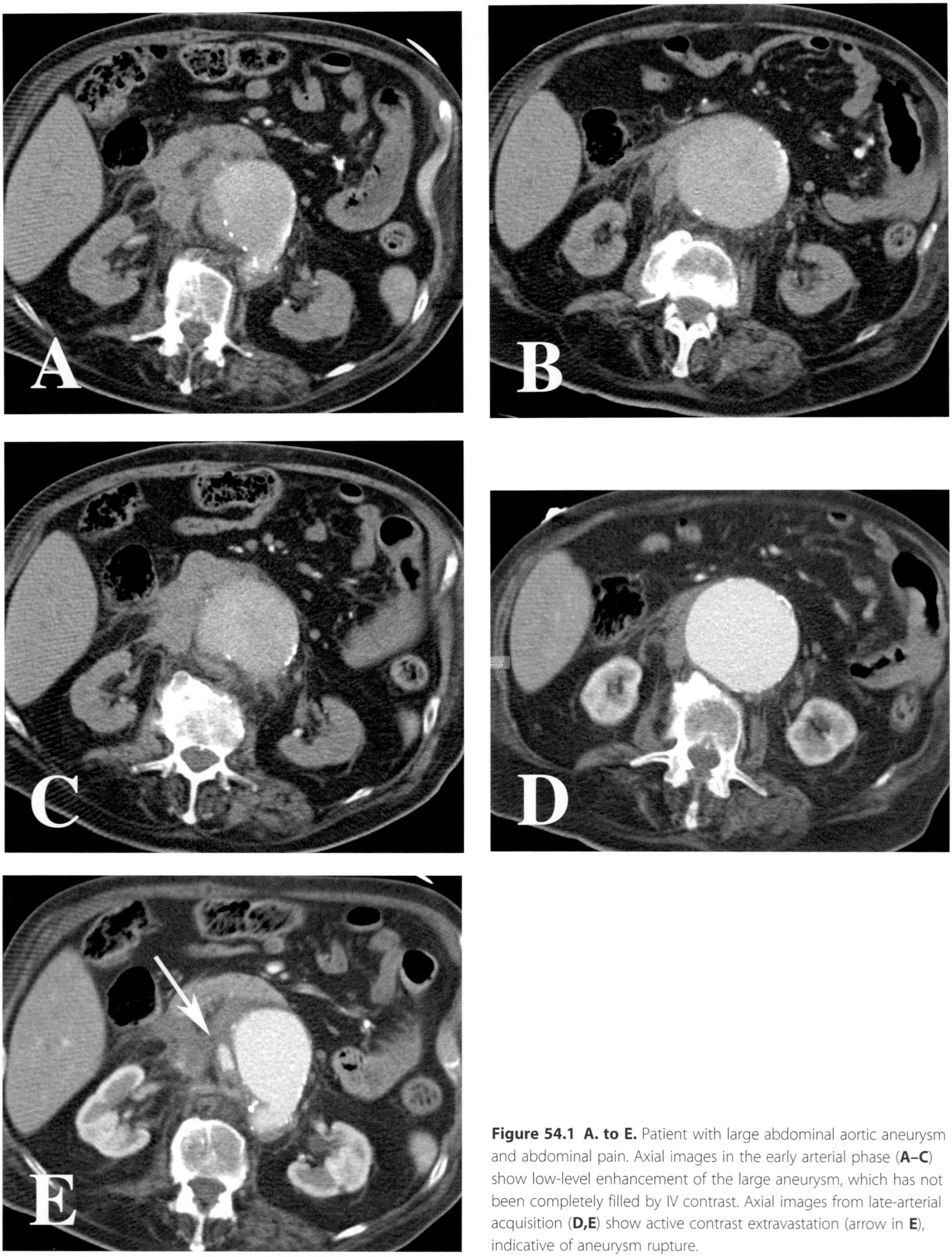

Figure 54.1 A. to E. Patient with large abdominal aortic aneurysm and abdominal pain. Axial images in the early arterial phase (**A–C**) show low-level enhancement of the large aneurysm, which has not been completely filled by IV contrast. Axial images from late-arterial acquisition (**D,E**) show active contrast extravastation (arrow in **E**), indicative of aneurysm rupture.

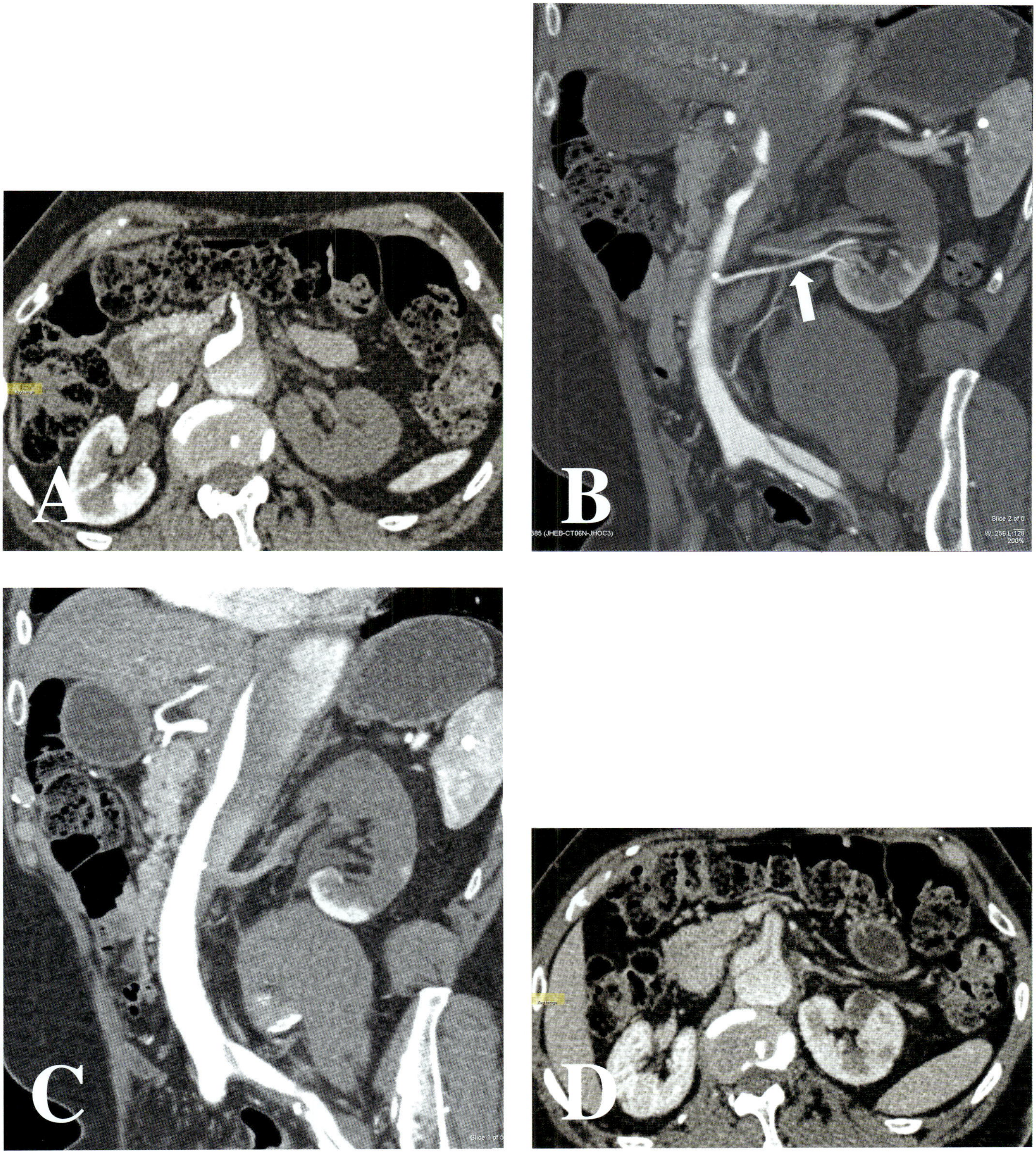

Figure 54.2 A. to E. A 75-year-old man with acute aortic dissection. On the early arterial phase (**A–C**), the false lumen does not enhance, and neither does the main left renal artery arising from the false lumen. The lower pole of the left kidney is supplied by an accessory renal artery (arrow) arising from the true lumen. On delayed acquisition (**D,E**), both false lumen and main left renal artery are enhanced, indicative of slow flow.

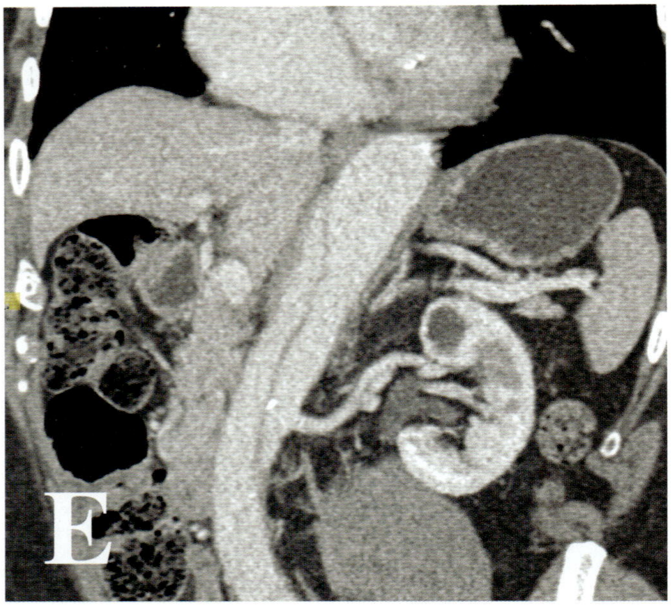

Figure 54.2 *(cont.)*

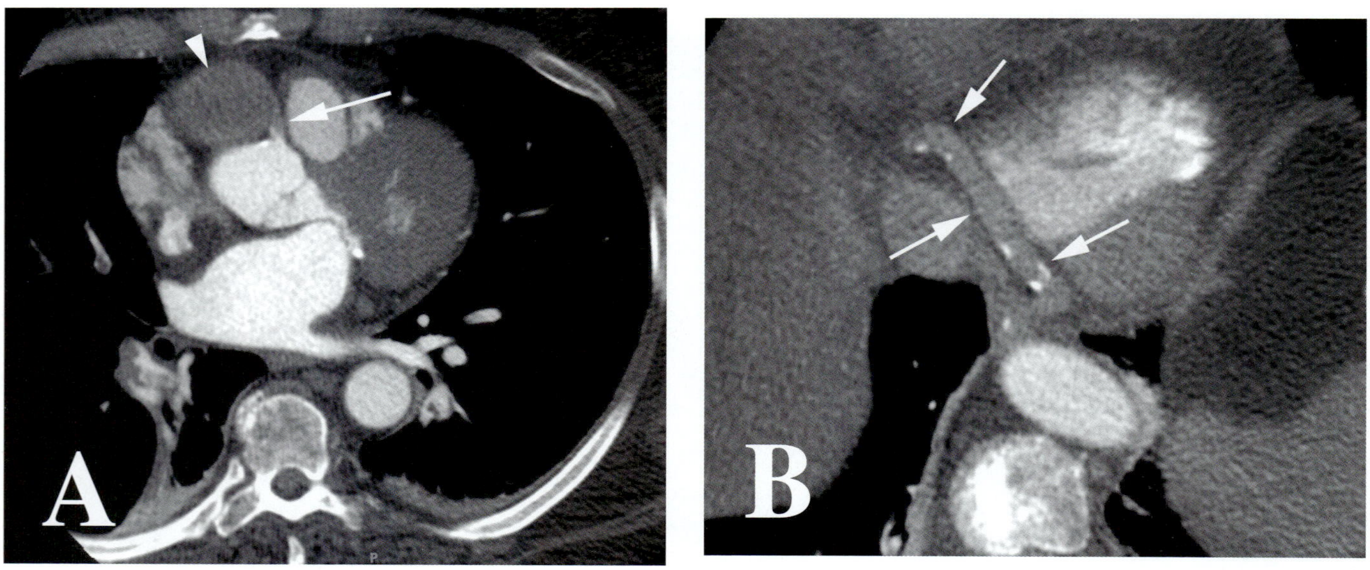

Figure 54.3 A. to H. A 73-year-old woman with incidental giant coronary artery aneurysm. **A,B.** Axial images from gated IV contrast-enhanced coronary artery CT angiography show nonenhancement of the origin of the right coronary artery (arrow in **A**), just proximal to a large coronary artery aneurysm (arrowhead), with thrombosis of the right distal coronary artery (arrows in **B**). **C,D.** The left coronary artery is shown to be patent on axial images from gated IV contrast-enhanced coronary artery CT angiography, and the patient has bilateral pulmonary emboli (PE). **E,F.** Adrenal protocol CT performed to evaluate adrenal masses preoperatively confirms that the aneurysm is completely perfused, enhancing homogeneously on the venous phase axial image (**F**) in comparison to the precontrast scan (**E**). **G,H.** Axial images from gated IV contrast-enhanced coronary artery CT angiography demonstrate heterogeneous attenuation within the low-density aneurysm, (75 HU centrally, 147 HU peripherally). These attenuation levels are higher than even acute thrombus, which is typically in the range of 50–70 HU, and reflect admixing of contrast and blood.

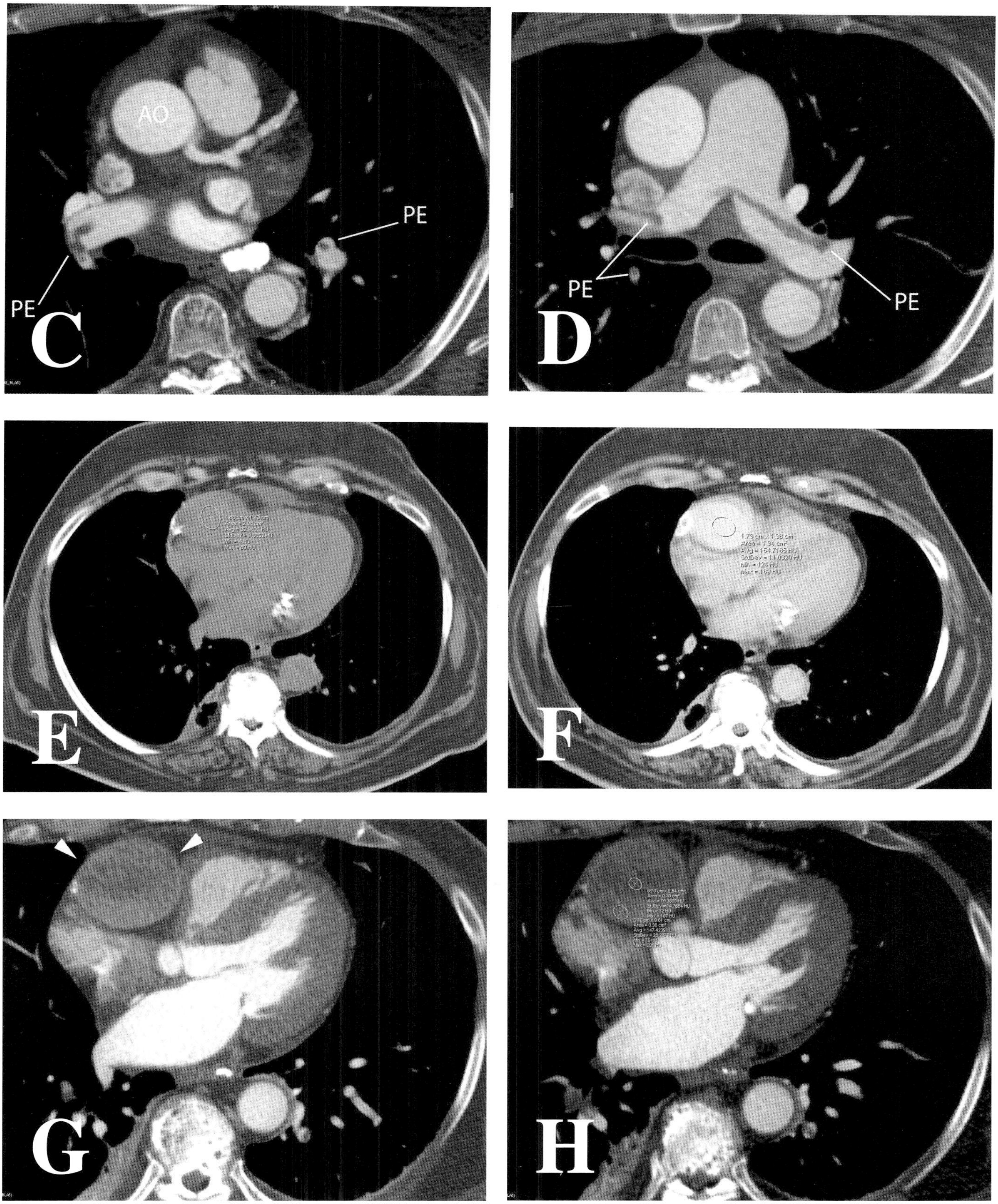

Figure 54.3 *(cont.)*

CASE

55 Misdiagnosis of acute aortic syndrome in the ascending aorta due to cardiac motion

Nathan Johnson and Stefan L. Zimmerman

Imaging description

Acute aortic syndrome is a term describing a group of emergent conditions of the aorta with similar clinical presentations. There are three types of acute aortic syndrome: aortic dissection, intramural hematoma, and penetrating atherosclerotic ulcer. In each of these entities, blood accumulates in the medial layer of the aortic wall. In aortic dissection, blood flows within a false lumen in the medial layer created by proximal and distal entry tears in the aortic intima. In intramural hematoma, high sheer forces result in bleeding of small vessels in the aortic media. Finally, penetrating ulcers result when atherosclerotic disease erodes through the intima into the media of the aortic wall. Contrast-enhanced CT is generally considered the test of choice for diagnosis of acute aortic syndrome. However, these screening exams are typically performed without electrocardiographic gating and the resultant images of the ascending aorta are limited by pulsatile motion during the cardiac cycle. This motion can produce images that mimic dissection or intramural hematoma, resulting in false-positive diagnosis.[1,2] Motion blurring can be recognized by an indistinct aortic wall, irregular outer contour of the aorta, a doubled appearance of the aorta, and blurring of adjacent cardiac structures. The appearance of a false intimal flap is common, and is most often seen in the left anterior or right posterior wall of the aortic root.[3] Partially imaged aortic valve leaflets may also contribute to the false appearance of an intimal flap in this location.[3] Motion blurring can also result in volume averaging of portions of the aortic wall with adjacent mediastinal fat, giving the false appearance of aortic wall thickening that can be mistaken for intramural hematoma (Figure 55.1). In most cases, these findings can be easily dismissed as motion artifacts; however, if there is uncertainty, ECG-gated CT angiogram or MR angiogram should be obtained for definitive evaluation (Figure 55.1). Additionally, acute aortic syndrome protocols should include precontrast images to evaluate for high-attenuation aortic wall thickening that is present in intramural hematoma.

Importance

Motion-related artifacts in the proximal aorta that simulate dissection are commonly encountered in practice. In an early study performed with single-slice scanning, artifacts simulating dissection were seen in 18% of cases.[4] The prevalence with current technology is not known; however, it is probably lower given improvements in speed of scanning with advent of multidetector CT.

Accurate and timely diagnosis of acute aortic syndrome is critical given the significant morbidity and mortality associated with both the disease process and treatment. Standard treatment for dissection or intramural hematoma of the ascending aorta is open repair, and a false positive diagnosis could lead to unnecessary performance of cardiothoracic surgery, which carries a relatively high morbidity. A false negative diagnosis, which can occur if a true dissection is incorrectly attributed to motion artifact, will have severe consequences. Without surgical treatment, patients with dissections and intramural hematomas of the ascending aorta have very high mortality rates of 62% and 40%, respectively, based upon a study from the International Registry of Acute Aortic Dissection.[5] It is therefore of utmost importance that a timely and accurate diagnosis is made in these patients.

Typical clinical scenario

Patients with acute aortic syndrome are generally older patients with hypertension, with males slightly outnumbering females. The mean age of patients with dissection of the ascending aorta is 61 years, whereas patients with intramural hematoma of the ascending aorta are slightly older at a mean age of 70 years.[5] Over 80% of patients present with acute chest pain and most will be initially evaluated by CT.[5]

Differential diagnosis

In addition to cardiac motion, streak artifacts from high-attenuation contrast in the central veins can create linear low-attenuation bands that can mimic dissection if passing through the aorta.[3,6] For cases of aortic wall thickening due to intramural hematoma, alternative diagnoses can be considered. Aortitis, either due to inflammatory vasculitis or infection, can result in circumferential aortic wall thickening. Intramural hematoma can be distinguished from these entities by the presence of wall thickening that is crescentic in shape and high-attenuation blood products in the aortic wall. Fluid within the superior pericardial recess that abuts the ascending aorta can sometimes be mistaken for aortic wall thickening; however, this can be recognized by fluid attenuation and shape that conforms to a pericardial recess, often best appreciated on sagittal or coronal images.[6]

Pearls and Pitfalls in Cardiovascular Imaging, ed. Stefan L. Zimmerman and Elliot K. Fishman. Published by Cambridge University Press. © Cambridge University Press 2015.

Teaching point

Motion-related artifacts may mimic acute aortic syndrome in the ascending aorta. Knowledge of the typical appearance of these artifacts will help avoid the potentially significant morbidity associated with misdiagnosis. Electrocardiographically gated CT angiography should be considered for definitive diagnosis in uncertain cases.

REFERENCES

1. M. C. Hamilton, A. K. Nightingale, S. Masey, et al. A case report of a normal aorta misdiagnosed as type A dissection by modern multidetector computed tomography. *Eur Radiol* 2010; **20**: 1856–8.

2. W. C. Chiang, P. C. Kao, C. P. Su, J. Hsu. Image pitfall of computed tomography in diagnosis of aortic dissection. *Am J Emerg Med* 2007; **25**: 127–9.

3. P. Batra, B. Bigoni, J. Manning, et al. Pitfalls in the diagnosis of thoracic aortic dissection at CT angiography. *Radiographics* 2000; **20**: 309–20.

4. M. A. Burns, P. L. Molina, F. R. Gutierrez, S. S. Sagel. Motion artifact simulating aortic dissection on CT. *AJR Am J Roentgenol* 1991; **157**: 465–7.

5. K. M. Harris, A. C. Braverman, K. A. Eagle, et al. Acute aortic intramural hematoma: an analysis from the International Registry of Acute Aortic Dissection. *Circulation* 2012; **126**: S91–6.

6. D. Souza, S. Ledbetter. Diagnostic errors in the evaluation of nontraumatic aortic emergencies. *Semin Ultrasound CT MR* 2012; **33**: 318–36.

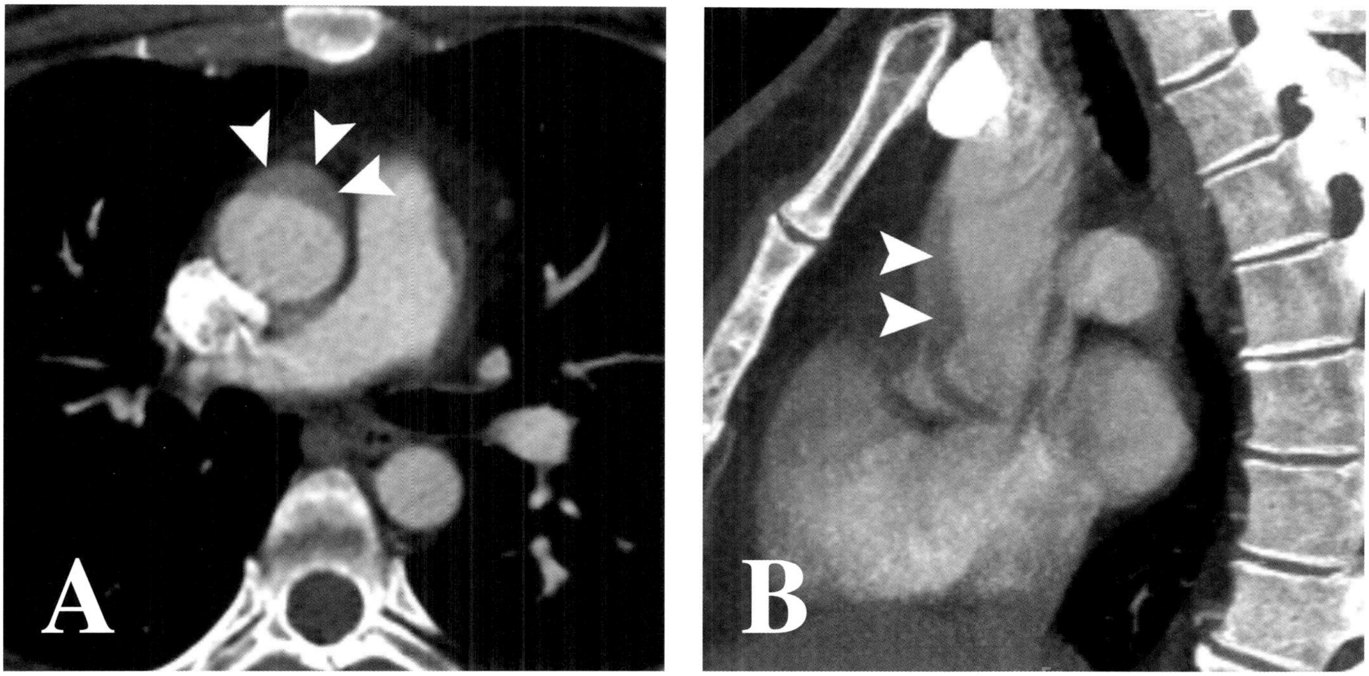

Figure 55.1 A. Axial image from contrast-enhanced non-gated chest CT performed in a 41-year-old woman with acute chest pain and hypertension demonstrates apparent wall thickening of the ascending aorta anteriorly suggesting intramural hematoma (arrowheads). The patient was transferred from an outside hospital after this CT was read as suspicious for ascending aortic intramural hematoma. **B.** Sagittal MIP reconstruction through the ascending aorta demonstrates the apparent intramural hematoma of the ascending aorta anteriorly (arrowheads). **C.** Axial post-contrast CT images from an ECG-gated scan obtained through the ascending aorta obtained after transfer from outside hospital. Images were obtained to confirm the presence of intramural hematoma. The exam was normal, with no intramural hematoma identified to correspond to the abnormality on the initial scans (arrowheads). **D.** Sagittal post-contrast CT images from the ECG-gated scan again demonstrate a normal ascending aorta with no evidence of intramural hematoma suggested on non-gated scans (arrowheads). **E.** Axial dark blood cardiac MRI images through the ascending aorta in the same patient demonstrate no evidence of intramural hematoma (arrowheads). The patient was having persistent chest pain, therefore MRA was obtained hours after the ECG-gated chest CT to repeat evaluation for intramural hematoma or dissection. If present, an intramural hematoma would appear as an intermediate to a high signal intensity crescent of aortic wall thickening.

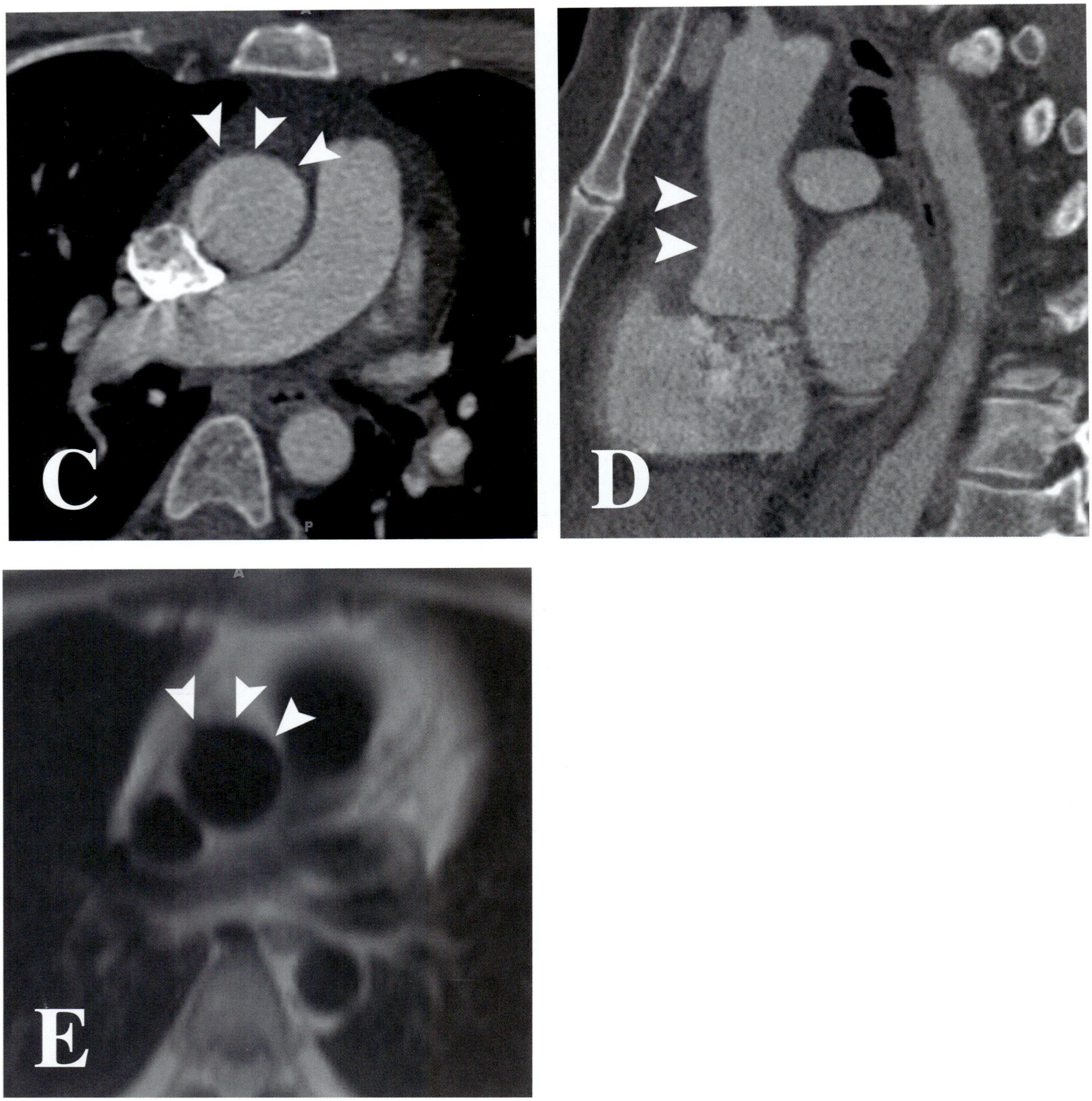

Figure 55.1 *(cont.)*

CASE 56 Aortic pseudodissection from penetrating atherosclerotic ulcer

Tessa S. Cook

Imaging description

Axial images of the aorta that are perpendicular to a penetrating atherosclerotic ulcer may demonstrate a displaced intimal flap (Figure 56.1), suggestive of a dissection. However, upon inspection of the coronal oblique multiplanar reformats, penetrating atherosclerotic ulcers (PAUs) are easily distinguished from dissection (Figure 56.2). Penetrating atherosclerotic ulcers will communicate with the aortic lumen via a single, narrow-necked intimal defect. Dissections communicate with the aorta through at least two separate intimal defects at the proximal entry point and the distal exit point with an intervening false lumen. The appearance of a pseudodissection from large PAUs occurs when the PAU is viewed in a plane perpendicular to its long axis. At the levels near the proximal and distal neck of the ulcer where the PAU projects along the long axis of the aorta, the wall of the ulcer compressed against the wall of the aorta can simulate a displaced intimal flap.

Importance

Distinguishing between a large PAU and an aortic dissection is important for the immediate management of the patient. A type B dissection is typically managed without surgical intervention. However, an enlarging PAU, such as in this patient, may lead more expediently to surgical repair, particularly if the patient is acutely symptomatic.

Typical clinical scenario

Penetrating atherosclerotic ulcers and aortic dissection lie on the spectrum of acute aortic syndrome.[1] When symptomatic, PAUs can have a similar clinical presentation to acute aortic dissection, consisting of a sudden onset of chest pain and discomfort. There is debate as to whether penetrating atherosclerotic ulcers can progress to aortic dissection.[2] PAUs are often discovered incidentally during CT angiography.[3]

Differential diagnosis

Differential considerations for an apparent displaced intimal flap commonly include aortic dissection or traumatic aortic injury, as well as artifacts from beam hardening or cardiac motion.[4] However, this case illustrates that in patients with severe atherosclerosis and hypertension, a large PAU resulting in a pseudodissection should also be considered. Multiplanar reformats are valuable in cases such as these to distinguish between true dissections and large PAUs imitating dissection.

Teaching point

Pseudodissection from PAU commonly results from large PAUs that parallel the long axis of the aorta. Careful distinction must be made between a large PAU and a true aortic dissection, as the management of these two conditions can be considerably different.

REFERENCES

1. K. Patatas, V. Shrivastava, D. F. Ettles. Penetrating atherosclerotic ulcer of the aorta: a continuing debate. *Clin Radiol* 2013; **68**: 753–9.

2. H. Hayashi, Y. Matsuoka, I. Sakamoto, et al. Penetrating atherosclerotic ulcer of the aorta: imaging features and disease concept. *Radiographics* 2000; **20**: 995–1005.

3. D. P. Nathan, W. Boonn, E. Lai, et al. Presentation, complications, and natural history of penetrating atherosclerotic ulcer disease. *J Vasc Surg* 2012; **55**: 10–5.

4. M. A. Burns, P. L. Molina, F. R. Gutierrez, S. S. Sagel. Motion artifact simulating aortic dissection on CT. *AJR Am J Roentgenol* 1991; **157**: 465–7.

Pearls and Pitfalls in Cardiovascular Imaging, ed. Stefan L. Zimmerman and Elliot K. Fishman. Published by Cambridge University Press. © Cambridge University Press 2015.

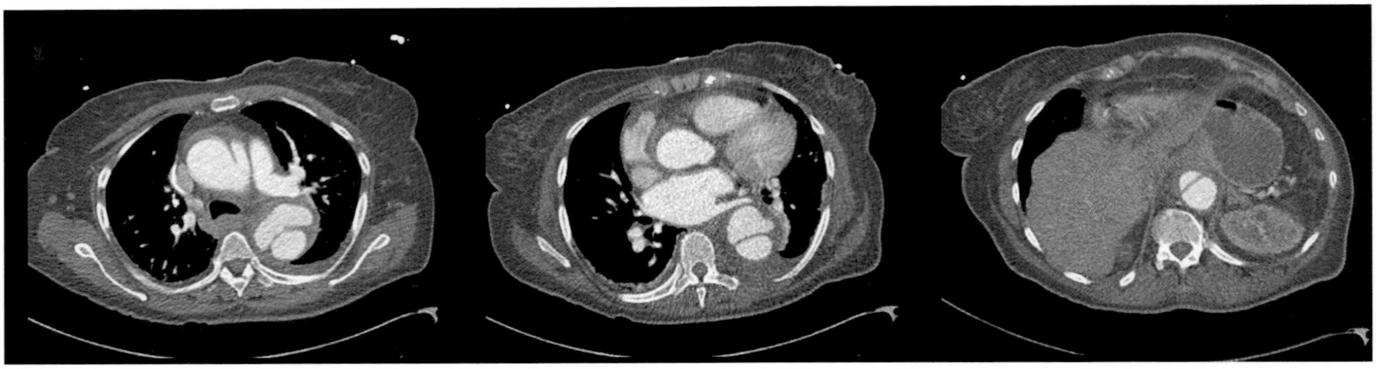

Figure 56.1 Multiple axial images from a 68-year-old female with hypertension and atherosclerosis who presented for evaluation of multiple enlarging penetrating atherosclerotic ulcers. When viewed in the axial plane at multiple levels, these PAUs give the appearance of displaced intimal flaps within the descending aorta.

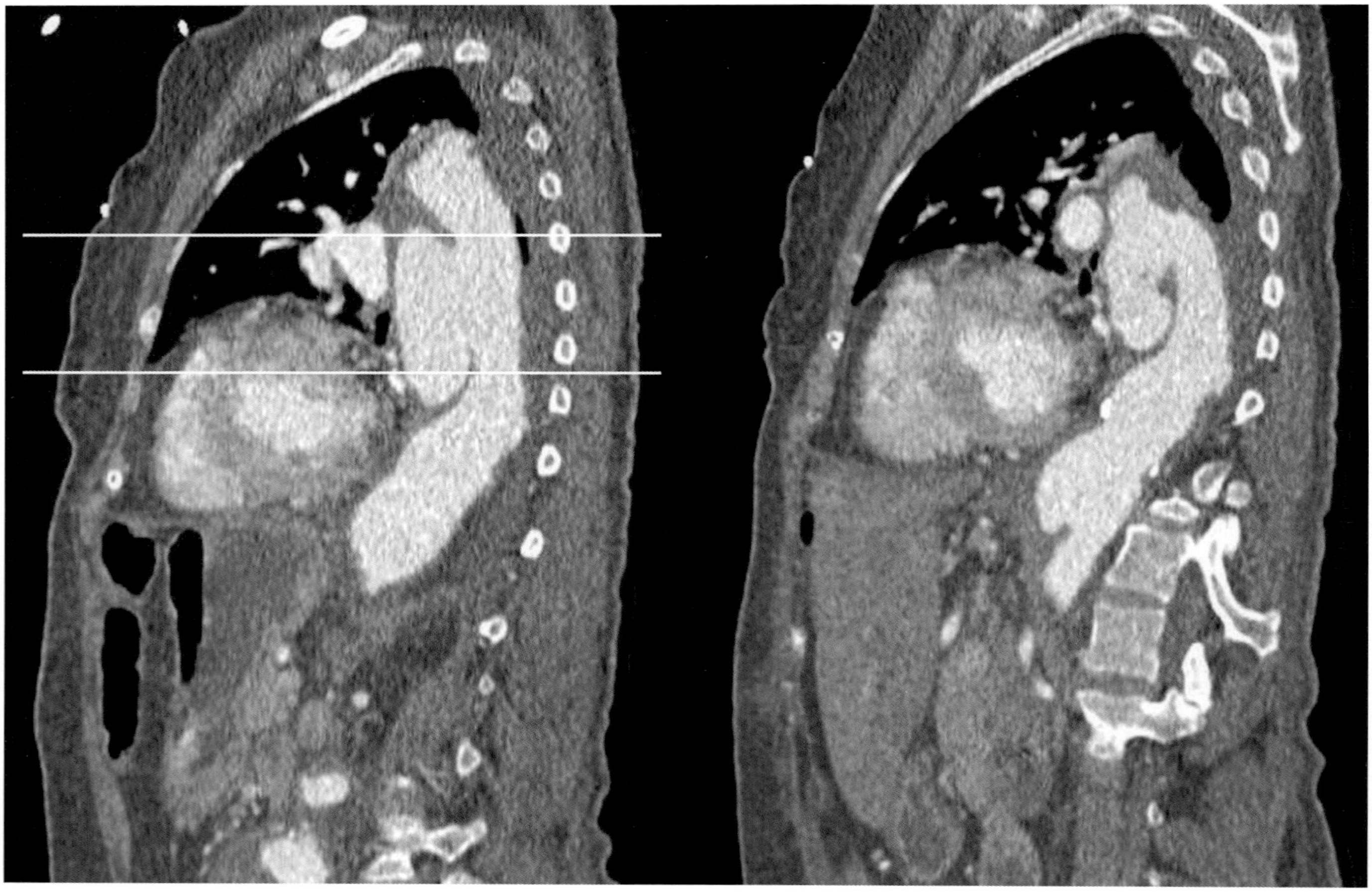

Figure 56.2 Coronal oblique multiplanar reformats from the same patient demonstrate two large left-sided PAUs projecting anteriorly from the mid-descending aorta (left) and the proximal abdominal aorta (right). On these sagittal oblique images, the pseudodissection appearance seen on the axial images can be explained by the planes that intersect the neck of each PAU proximally and distally (lines), falsely giving the impression of a displaced intimal flap at these levels.

CASE 57

Ductus diverticulum mimicking ductus arteriosus aneurysm

Pejman Motarjem and Stefan L. Zimmerman

Imaging description

Ductus diverticulum (DD) is an anatomic variant incidentally found at cardiovascular imaging characterized by a smooth bulge of the anterior wall of the aorta at the aortic isthmus, just distal to the origin of the left subclavian artery.[1]

DD is best visualized on sagittal oblique reconstructions on CT, MRI, or digital subtraction angiography (DSA) (Figures 57.1 and 57.2). DD may be difficult to appreciate on standard axial images. On reconstructions, it is recognized as an anteriorly directed bulge of the undersurface of the aortic arch that extends to the proximal descending thoracic aorta. DD has smooth, gentle margins, and obtuse shoulders.

Importance

DD must not be confused with traumatic aortic transection or ductus arteriosus aneurysm, both of which can occur at the same location and have a greater risk of morbidity and mortality.

Typical clinical case scenario

DD is typically encountered as an incidental finding on CT, MR or DSA and is of no clinical significance. It occurs in approximately 26% of adults and requires no follow-up or treatment.[2]

Differential diagnosis

Traumatic aortic transection, also known as post-traumatic pseudoaneurysm, is found in patients with a history of high-velocity trauma. At cross-sectional imaging, aortic transections arise from the anterior wall of the aorta at the isthmus, similar to DD. However, aortic transections have acute angles with the aortic wall, are irregular in shape and size, and often have a visible intimal flap (Figure 57.3). There may be a narrow neck that communicates with the aorta. Associated periaortic and mediastinal hematoma are typically present with traumatic aortic transection.[3]

Aneurysm of the ductus arteriosus is a rare entity characterized by a saccular aneurysm of the undersurface of the aortic arch in the region of the ductus arteriosus (Figure 57.4). Wall calcifications and partial thrombosis are frequently present. Some believe this entity is due to incomplete obliteration of the patent ductus arteriosus during early development that results in a blind-ending stump communicating with the aortic lumen. Progressive enlargement occurs over years. Ductus aneurysms have a high complication rate, including rupture, thromboembolism, erosion into the adjacent bronchus or esophagus, infection, and mass effect on the recurrent laryngeal nerve.[4] Repair is recommended when the aneurysm size is greater than 3 cm.[4] Ductus aneurysm can be distinguished from DD by its saccular appearance with acute margins at the interface with the aortic wall.

Teaching point

Ductus diverticulum is an anatomic variant characterized by smooth, focal bulging of the anterior aorta that has obtuse angles relative to the aortic wall. It is located at the aortic isthmus and must not be confused with high-risk aortic syndromes that can occur in the same location.

1. P. Batra, B. Bigoni, J. Manning, D. R. Aberle, K. Brown, E. Hart, J. Goldin. Pitfalls in the diagnosis of thoracic aortic dissection at CT angiography. *Radiographics* 2000; **20**:309–20.
2. S. S. Morse, M. G. Glickman, L. H. Greenwood, D. F. Denny Jr., E. B. Strauss, B. R. Stavens, M. Yoselevitz. Traumatic aortic rupture: false positive aortographic diagnosis due to atypical ductus diverticulum. *AJR Am J Roentgenol* 1988; **4**:793–6.
3. K. J. Macura, F. M. Corl, E. K. Fishman, D. A. Bluemke. Pathogenesis in acute aortic syndromes: aortic aneurysm leak and rupture and traumatic aortic transection. *AJR Am J Roentgenol* 2003; **181**:303–7.
4. P. Pastuszko, J. A. Eisenberg, J. A. Diehl. Ductus arteriosus aneurysm in an adult patient presenting with hoarseness. *J Card Surg* 2005; **20**:386–8.

Pearls and Pitfalls in Cardiovascular Imaging, ed. Stefan L. Zimmerman and Elliot K. Fishman. Published by Cambridge University Press. © Cambridge University Press 2015.

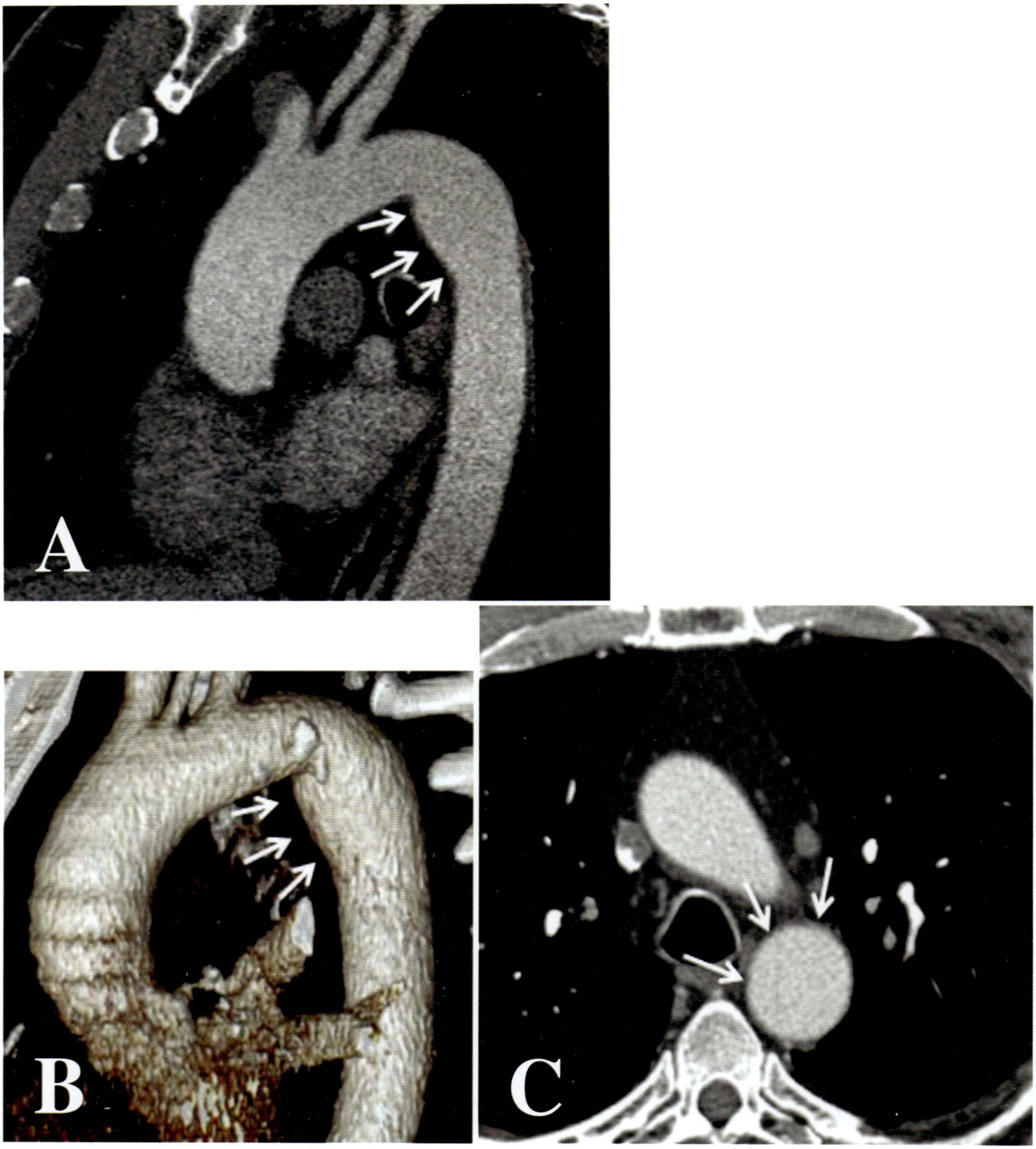

Figure 57.1 Typical appearance of a ductus diverticulum. Sagittal oblique multiplanar reformatted image (**A**) and volume-rendered image (**B**) of the thoracic aorta in a CT angiogram performed in a 61-year-old male with chest pain shows a smooth bulge of the anterior wall of the descending thoracic aorta with obtuse margins (arrows). Ductus diveriticulum is not easily appreciated on axial images (**C**) obtained through the same region (arrows).

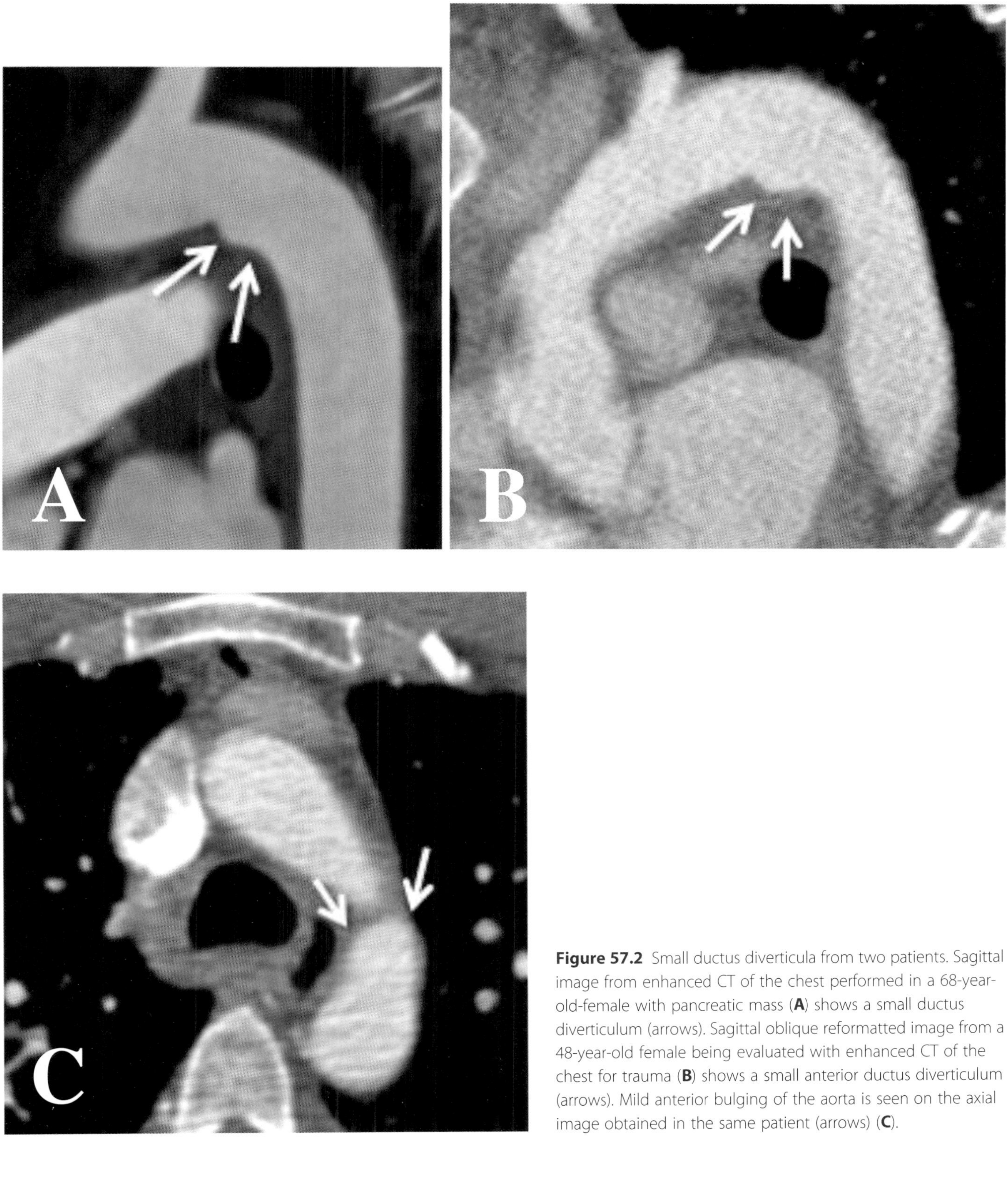

Figure 57.2 Small ductus diverticula from two patients. Sagittal image from enhanced CT of the chest performed in a 68-year-old-female with pancreatic mass (**A**) shows a small ductus diverticulum (arrows). Sagittal oblique reformatted image from a 48-year-old female being evaluated with enhanced CT of the chest for trauma (**B**) shows a small anterior ductus diverticulum (arrows). Mild anterior bulging of the aorta is seen on the axial image obtained in the same patient (arrows) (**C**).

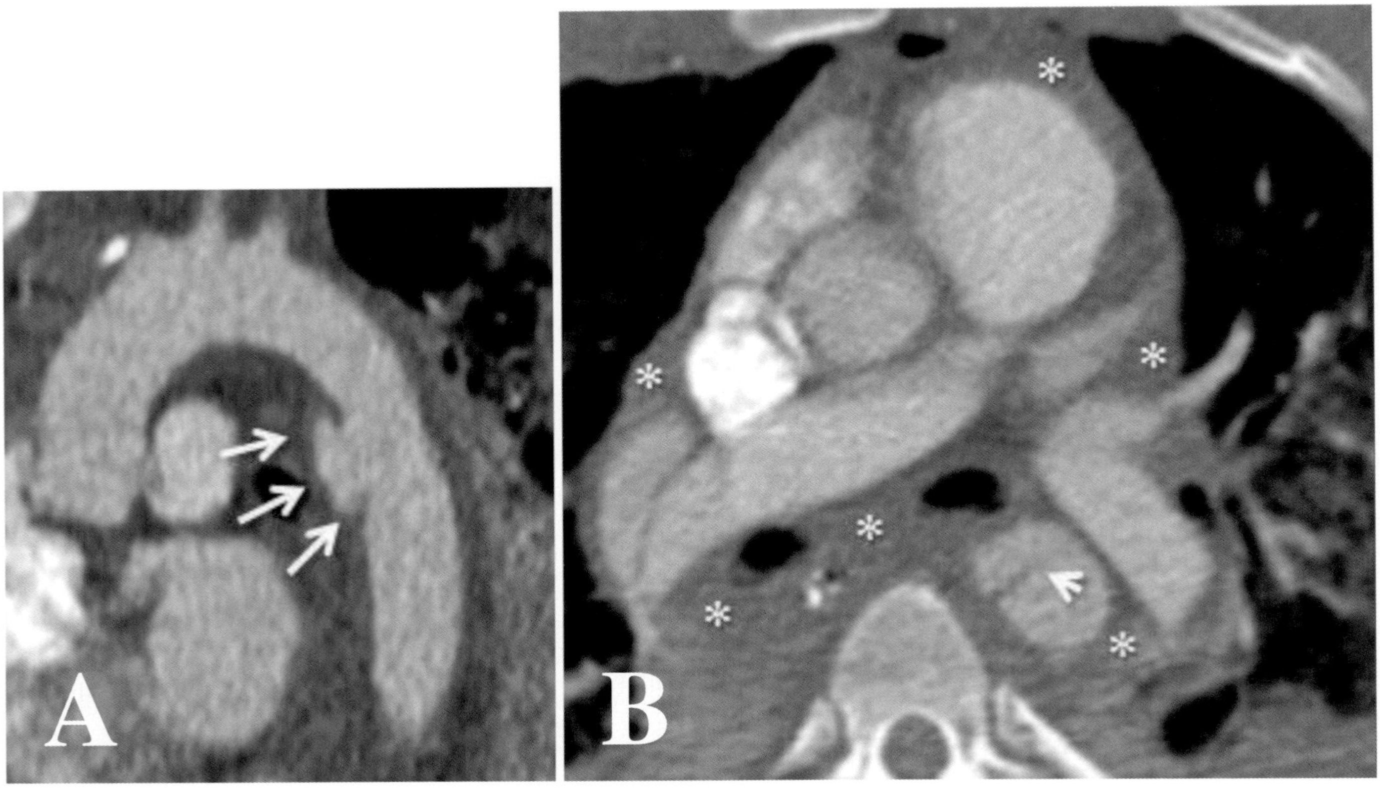

Figure 57.3 Traumatic aortic transection occurring at the same location as ductus diverticulum. **A.** Sagittal oblique reformatted image obtained from contrast-enhanced CT performed in a 19-year-old-male with trauma shows a saccular outpouching of contrast arising from the anterior descending thoracic aorta (arrows), typical for traumatic aortic transection. Unlike ductus diverticulum, there are sharp, acute margins between the wall of the aorta and the pseudoaneurysm. **B.** Axial image obtained in the same patient shows a small intimal flap in the aorta due to traumatic laceration (arrow) and extensive high-attenuation mediastinal hematoma (asterisk).

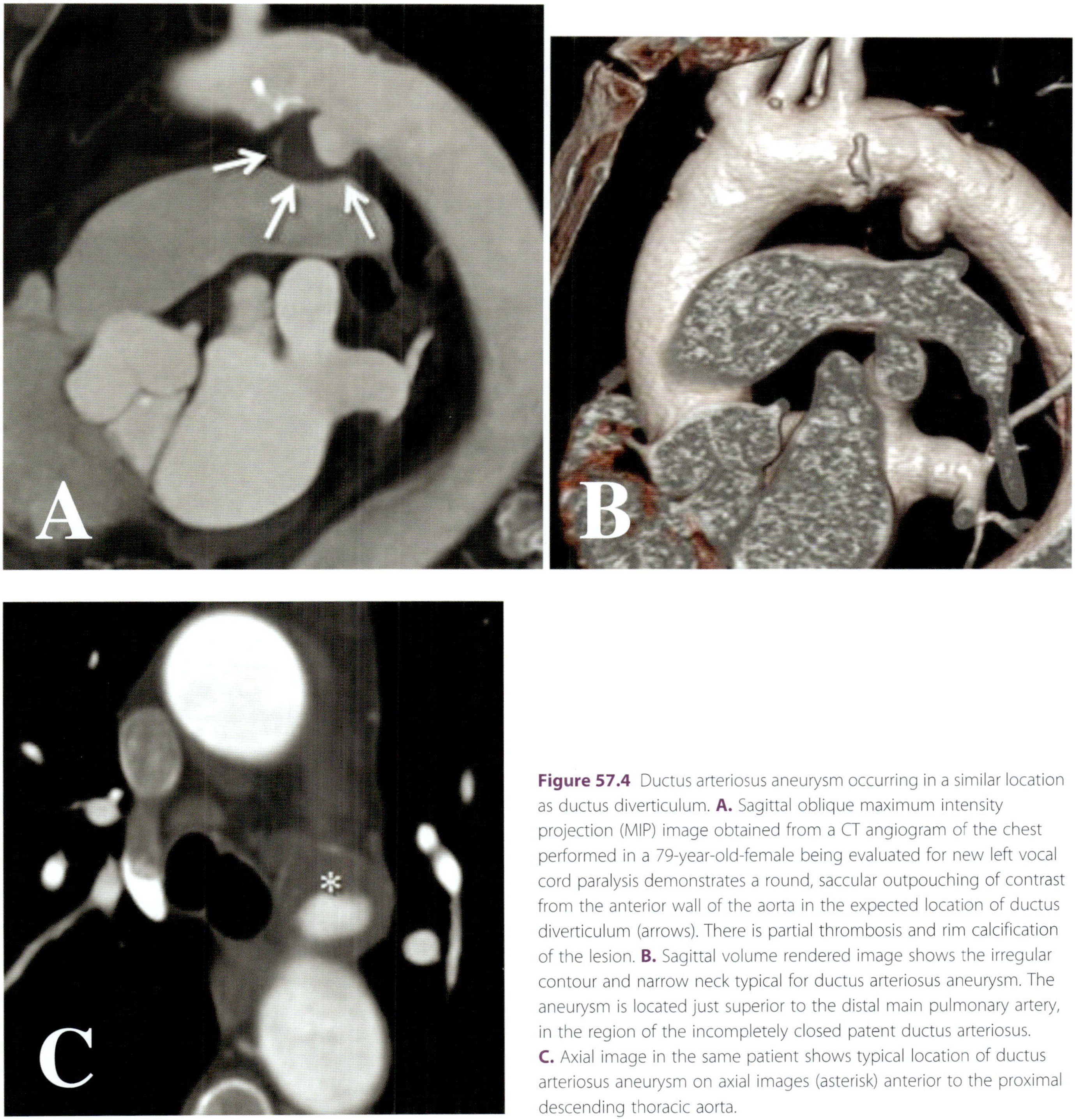

Figure 57.4 Ductus arteriosus aneurysm occurring in a similar location as ductus diverticulum. **A.** Sagittal oblique maximum intensity projection (MIP) image obtained from a CT angiogram of the chest performed in a 79-year-old-female being evaluated for new left vocal cord paralysis demonstrates a round, saccular outpouching of contrast from the anterior wall of the aorta in the expected location of ductus diverticulum (arrows). There is partial thrombosis and rim calcification of the lesion. **B.** Sagittal volume rendered image shows the irregular contour and narrow neck typical for ductus arteriosus aneurysm. The aneurysm is located just superior to the distal main pulmonary artery, in the region of the incompletely closed patent ductus arteriosus. **C.** Axial image in the same patient shows typical location of ductus arteriosus aneurysm on axial images (asterisk) anterior to the proximal descending thoracic aorta.

CASE

58 Pericardial recess mimicking traumatic aortic injury

Stefan L. Zimmerman

Imaging description

In some patients, fluid in the anterior portion of the superior aortic recess of the pericardium can extend cranially and abut the aortic arch and the arch branch vessel origins. In patients being evaluated for trauma with multidetector CT, this fluid may be mistaken for periaortic hematoma (Figure 58.1). However, unlike hemorrhage, fluid in a pericardial recess will measure simple fluid attenuation and will have sharp, well-defined borders. Pericardial fluid abuts the aorta and great vessels without an intervening fat plane. Patients with acute aortic injury and hematoma will have high-attenuation fluid next to the aorta and a contour abnormality or intimal flap within the aorta itself.

Importance

Misdiagnosis of traumatic aortic injury could lead to inappropriate invasive catheter angiography or surgery.

Typical clinical scenario

Fluid in the superior aortic recess is common and may be encountered in patients with or without an associated pericardial effusion.

Differential diagnosis

In the setting of trauma, fluid in the superior pericardial recess can mimic periaortic hemorrhage; however, these entities can usually be distinguished by attenuation measurements (Figure 58.2). Fluid collections in the superior aortic recess simulating lymphadenopathy or aortic dissection have also been described.[1,2]

Teaching point

Fluid in the anterior portion of the superior aortic recess abutting the aortic arch can mimic periaortic hematoma. Measurement of fluid attenuation values and close inspection of the aorta for contour abnormalities or intimal injury will help avoid misdiagnosis.

REFERENCES

1. Y. W. Choi, H. P. McAdams, S. C. Jeon, H. S. Seo, C. K. Hahm. The "High-Riding" superior pericardial recess: CT findings. *AJR Am J Roentgenol* 2000; **175**: 1025–8.
2. L. S. Broderick, G. N. Brooks, J. E. Kuhlman. Anatomic pitfalls of the heart and pericardium. *Radiographics* 2005; **25**: 441–53.

Pearls and Pitfalls in Cardiovascular Imaging, ed. Stefan L. Zimmerman and Elliot K. Fishman. Published by Cambridge University Press. © Cambridge University Press 2015.

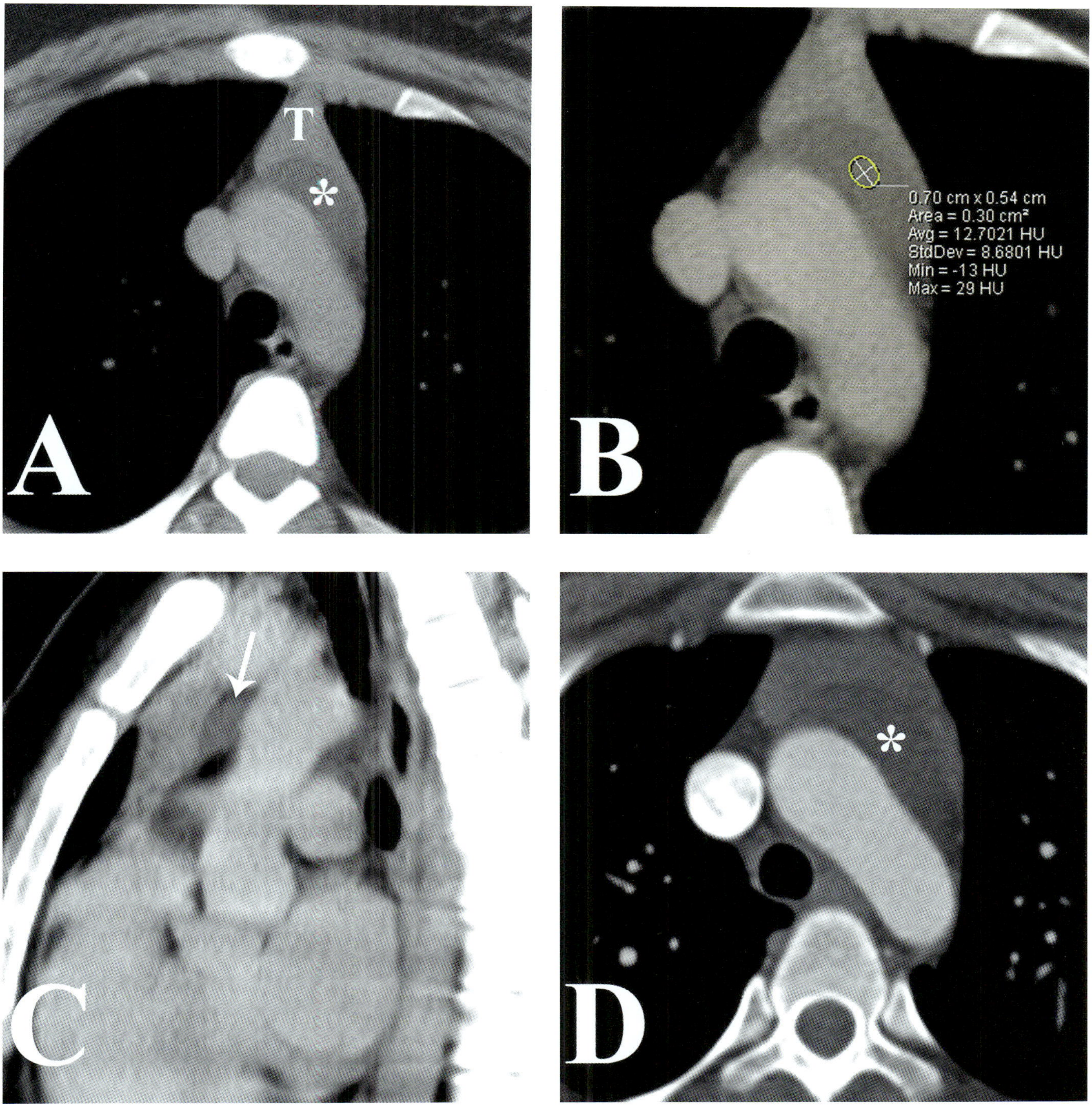

Figure 58.1 High pericardial recess mistaken for periaortic hematoma on a contrast-enhanced CT exam of the chest performed in a 19-year-old female involved in a high-speed motor vehicle collision. On the axial image (**A**), there is a collection of fluid (asterisk) adjacent to the aorta anteriorly and posterior to the thymus (T). This was mistaken for a periaortic hematoma on the initial read at an outside hospital. However, the collection measures simple fluid density (**B**), has well-defined margins, and a somewhat angulated shape on the sagittal images (arrow, **C**), that is typical for a pericardial recess. A follow-up CT angiogram was performed 24 hours later and no change was seen (**D**). The remainder of the aorta was entirely normal.

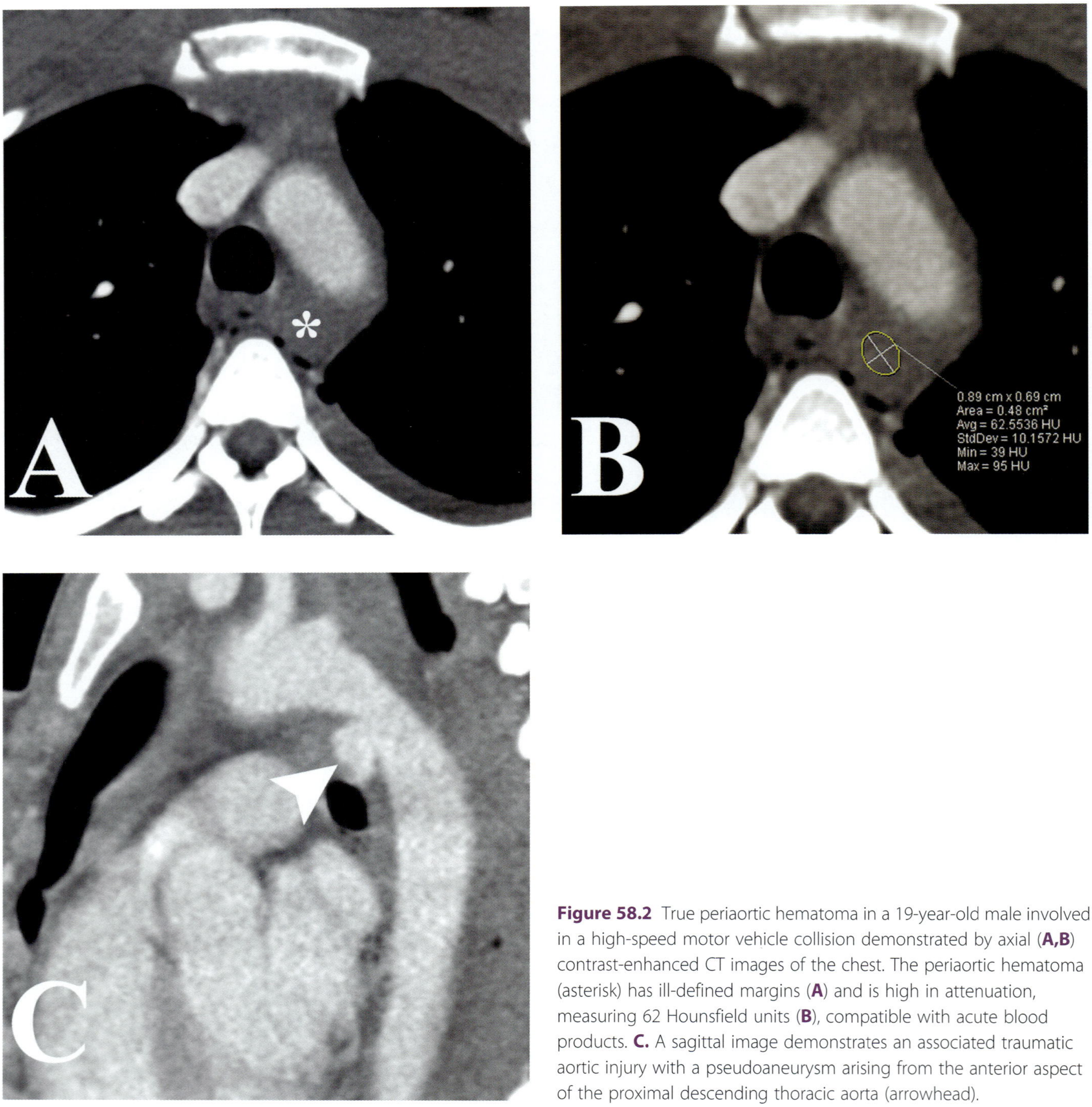

Figure 58.2 True periaortic hematoma in a 19-year-old male involved in a high-speed motor vehicle collision demonstrated by axial (**A,B**) contrast-enhanced CT images of the chest. The periaortic hematoma (asterisk) has ill-defined margins (**A**) and is high in attenuation, measuring 62 Hounsfield units (**B**), compatible with acute blood products. **C.** A sagittal image demonstrates an associated traumatic aortic injury with a pseudoaneurysm arising from the anterior aspect of the proximal descending thoracic aorta (arrowhead).

CASE 59

Neointimal calcifications mimicking displaced intimal calcifications on unenhanced CT

Saurabh Jha

Imaging description

The aortic wall comprises three layers: intima, media, and adventitia. The wall is imperceptible and inferred on contrast-enhanced CT by a boundary separating two tissues of contrasting attenuations: arterial lumen and the periarterial soft tissue. Processes such as intramural hematoma (IMH) that thicken the media expand the wall and displace the intimal layer inwards toward the lumen.[1]

Aortic calcifications are usually centered on the intima and are, therefore, peripherally located (Figure 59.1). A process in the media that displaces the intima renders the calcifications non-peripheral (Figures 59.2A and 59.3).

However, non-peripheral calcifications can also be dystrophic calcifications of the mural thrombus, also known as neointimal calcifications (Figures 59.2B, 59.4, and 59.5).

How can the distinction be made on unenhanced CT?

1. Neointimal calcifications are chunky and random, since any part of the thrombus can calcify (Figure 59.2B). Intimal calcifications are thin, linear, and circumferentially configured (Figure 59.2A).
2. Neointimal calcifications may co-exist with intimal calcifications, in which case there are calcifications peripheral to neointimal calcifications (Figure 59.4).
3. Mural thrombus is of a lower attenuation (< 30 HU) than acute intramural hematoma (50–80 HU) and blood pool (40–50 HU).

Importance

Distinguishing between neointimal calcifications and displaced intimal calcifications is important because the latter reflects acute aortic pathology such as IMH and dissection. Dystrophic calcifications of the mural thrombus reflect an indolent process. The pitfall can result in incorrect diagnosis of acute aortic syndrome.

Similarity in terminology aggravates the confusion. Mural thrombus is thrombus *adherent to* the wall of the aorta. Intramural hematoma is hematoma *within* the aortic wall.

Typical clinical scenario

Unenhanced CT in patients with chest or abdominal pain, or who have follow-up of a known aneurysm, and who cannot receive iodinated contrast because of renal impairment.

Differential diagnosis

Non-peripheral calcifications are either displaced intimal calcifications or dystrophic calcifications of the mural thrombus.

Displaced intimal calcifications represent a process in the media such as intramural hematoma (bleeding within the media because of rupture of the vasa vasorum), aortitis (inflammation leading to an edematous medial layer) and dissection (split of the media).

> **Teaching point**
>
> An important sign of acute aortic pathology on unenhanced CT is the presence of non-peripheral calcifications. However, dystrophic calcifications of the mural thrombus also lead to non-peripheral calcifications. It is important to be aware of this mimic.

REFERENCE

1. Macura KJ, Corl FM, Fishman EK, et al. Pathogenesis in acute aortic syndrome: aortic dissection, intramural hematoma and penetrating atherosclerotic ulcer. *AJR Am J Roentgenol* 2003; **181**: 309–316

Pearls and Pitfalls in Cardiovascular Imaging, ed. Stefan L. Zimmerman and Elliot K. Fishman. Published by Cambridge University Press. © Cambridge University Press 2015.

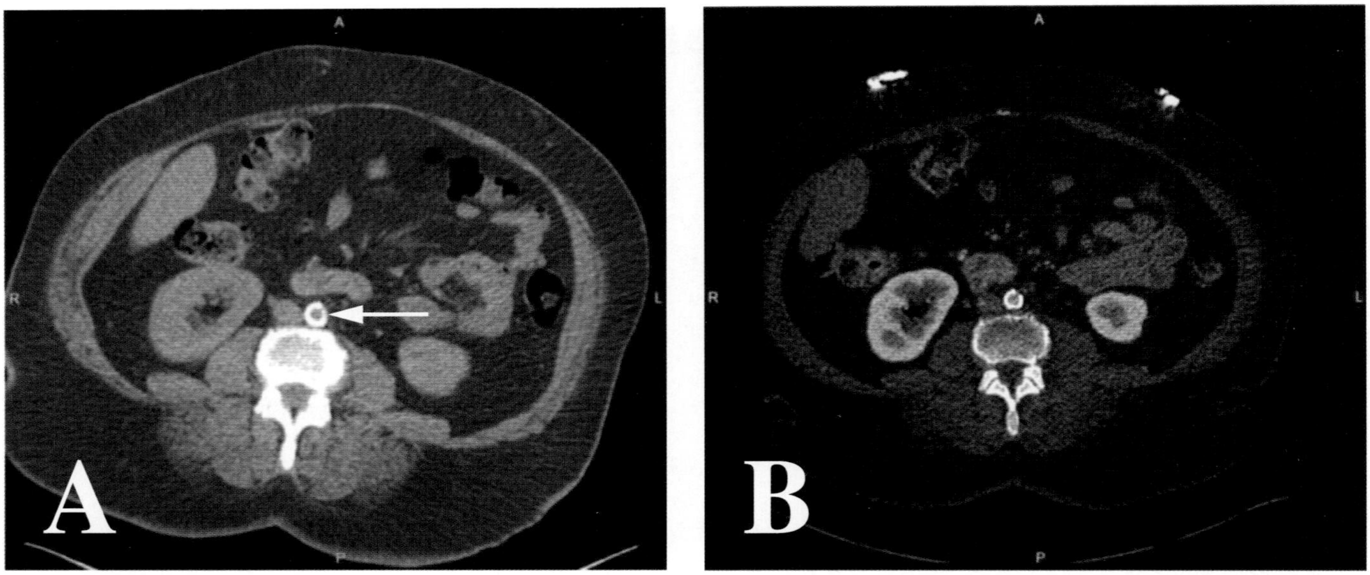

Figure 59.1. Axial unenhanced (**A**) and contrast-enhanced (**B**) CT in a 64-year-old female with follow-up of renal artery aneurysms show thick circumferential calcification of the abdominal aorta (white arrow in **A**), which is peripheral in location. This is the normal configuration of dystrophic calcification when there is neither a process in the aortic wall nor mural thrombus.

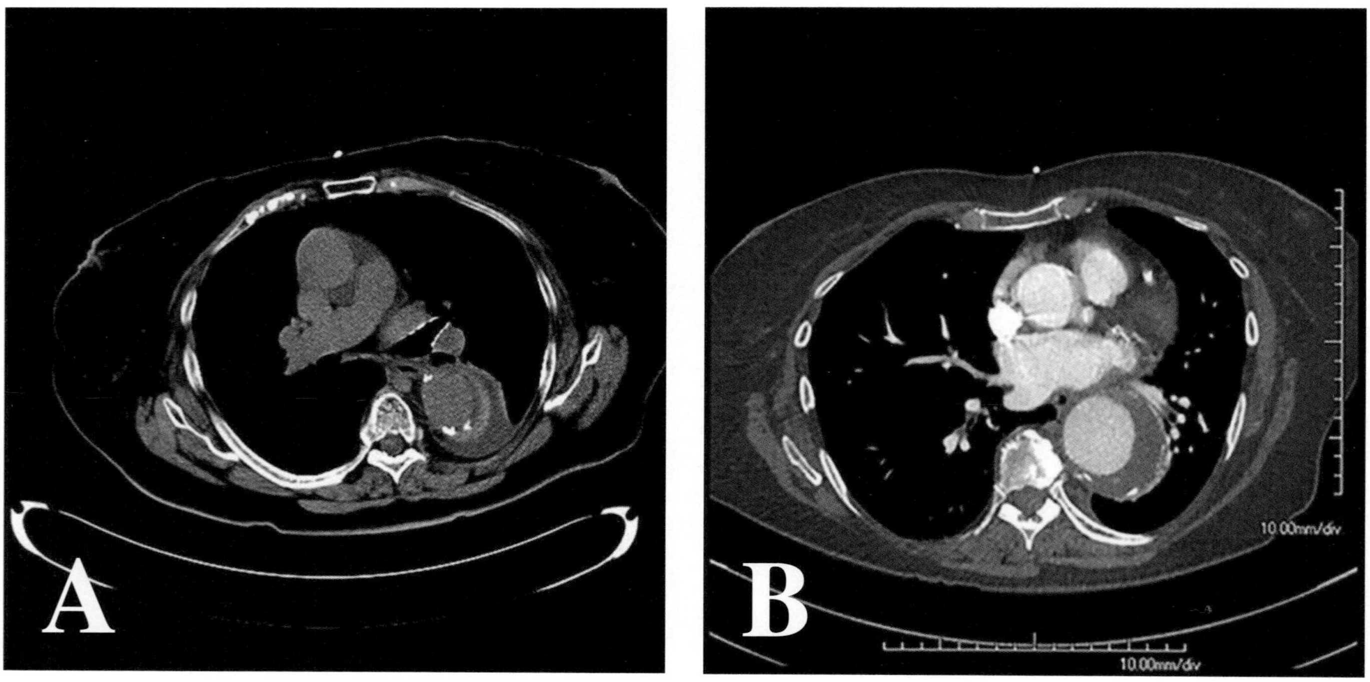

Figure 59.2 A. Axial unenhanced CT in a 76-year-old male with back pain. **B.** Axial contrast-enhanced CT in a 67-year-old male with a known thoracic aortic aneurysm. Intimal calcifications, when displaced, are useful in distinguishing between intramural hematoma (**A**) and mural thrombus (**B**). The two entities share the term "mural", which can be confusing. In the former, the term indicates that the bleeding is within the wall. In the latter, the term indicates that the thrombus is adherent to the wall. Note in (**A**) that there is a crescenteric high attenuation area in the aortic wall peripheral to the displaced calcification representing the subacute hematoma. Note that in (**B**) the intimal calcifications are peripheral to the neointimal calcifications.

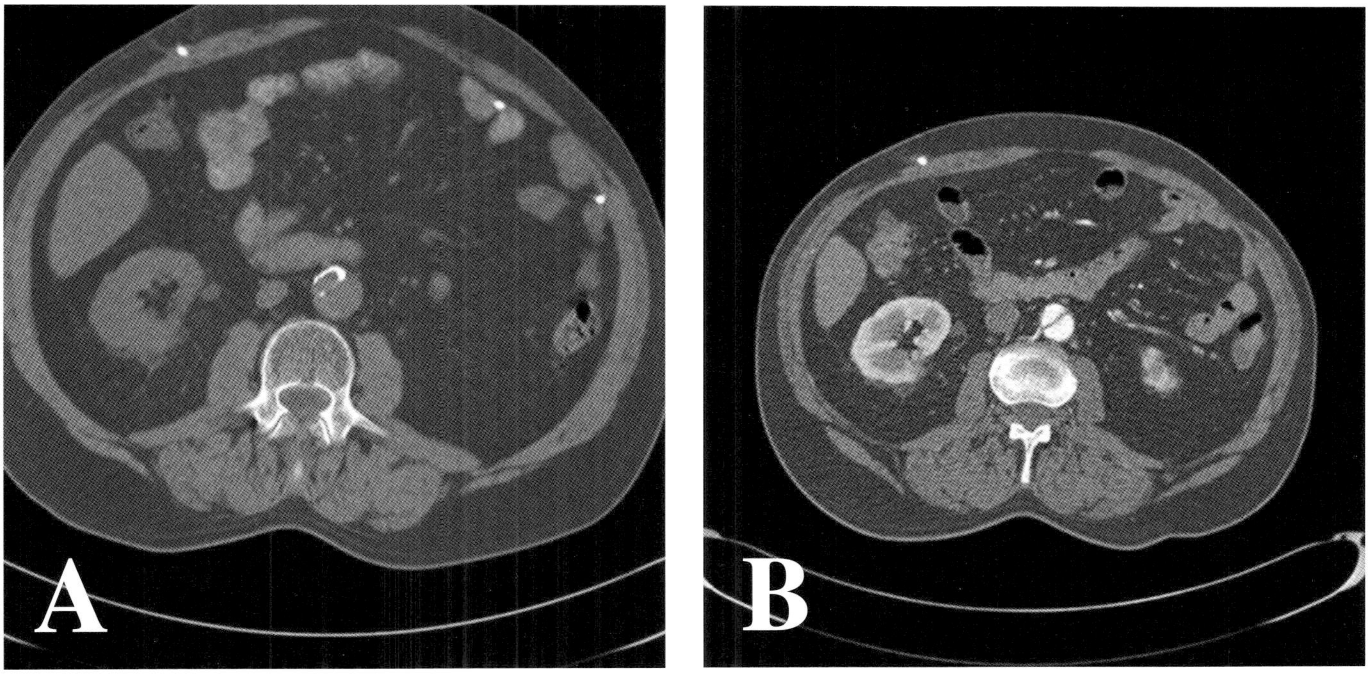

Figure 59.3 A 62-year-old female with back pain. Unenhanced CT of the abdominal aorta (**A**) shows calcifications displaced from the posterior wall of the aorta indicating a dissection, which is confirmed on the post-contrast (**B**) images. Note that the displacement of the calcifications not only signify a process in the media, in this case a dissection, but also point to the true lumen, which is the lumen bound by the intima marked by the presence of intimal calcifications.

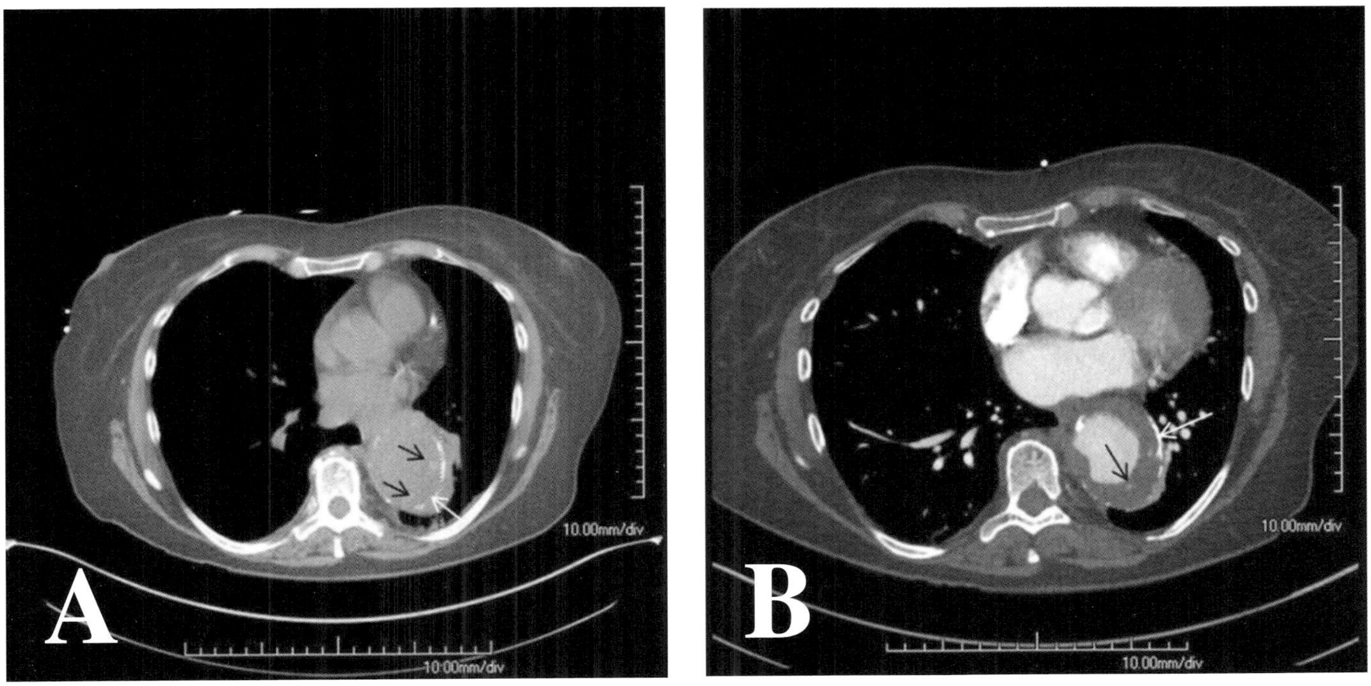

Figure 59.4 A 72-year-old female with known thoracic aortic aneurysm. Axial unenhanced CT (**A**) and contrast-enhanced (**B**) CT through the thoracic aorta shows foci of calcification (black arrows) that are non-peripheral and appear displaced but are, in fact, calcifications within the mural thrombus. This is confirmed on the contrast-enhanced CT (**B**). Note that there is linear calcification peripheral to this (white arrow), which marks the position of the intima.

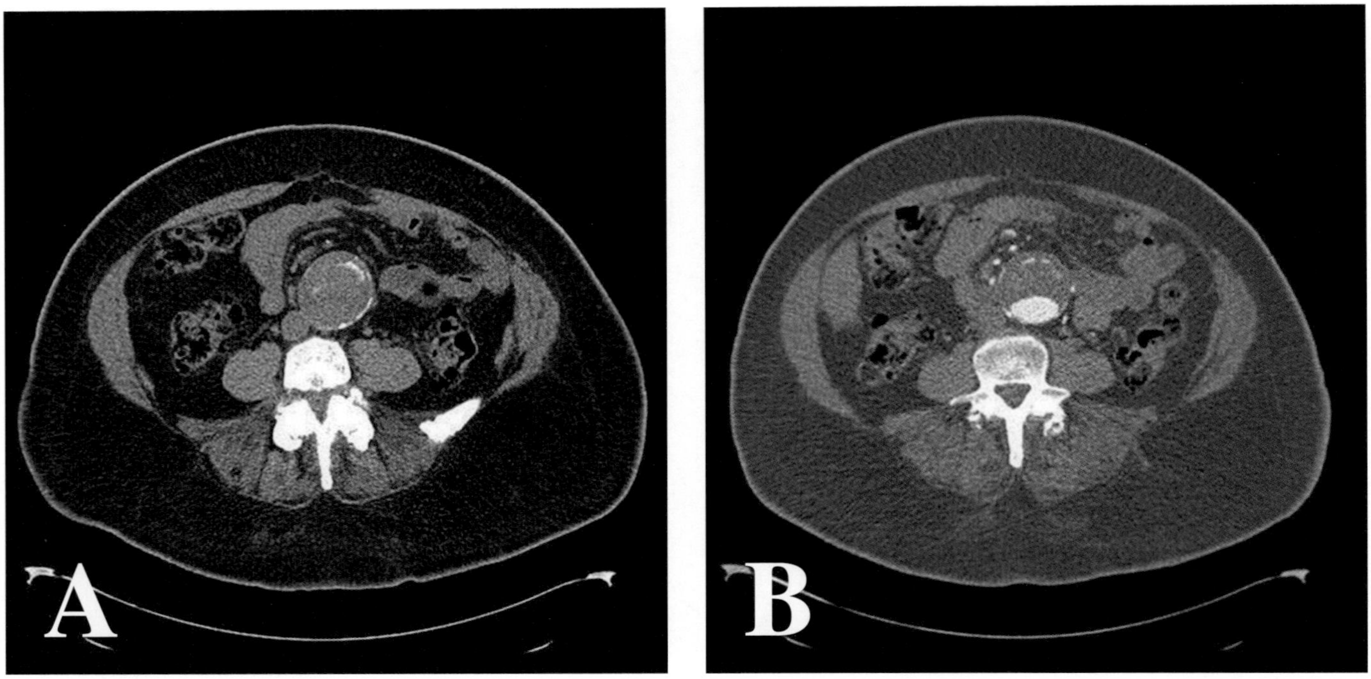

Figure 59.5 A 78-year-old female for pre-stent evaluation. Unenhanced CT of the abdominal aorta (**A**) shows non-peripheral calcifications in an aneurysmal abdominal aorta, which are actually calcifications within the mural thrombus, or neointimal calcifications. Note that there are calcifications peripheral to these supposedly displaced calcifications that represent the true intimal calcifications. Note also the somewhat haphazard pattern of calcifications, since any part of the mural thrombus can undergo dystrophic calcifications. Contrast-enhanced CT (**B**) at the same level show the large amount of mural thrombus.

CASE 60

The value of non-contrast CT in vascular imaging

Saurabh Jha and Benoit Desjardins

Imaging description

The attenuation of blood depends on the hematocrit but is usually 20–35 HU. Subacute blood has a higher attenuation (50–80 HU) than flowing blood. This is because of a reduction of water content, which raises the concentration of hemoglobin. This property makes it possible to identify a vascular process such as an aortic rupture (Figure 60.1), aortic injury (Figure 60.2), acute thrombus (Figure 60.3), intramural hematoma or instability of aneurysm on non-contrast CT, by the "hyperattenuating sign."[1]

Hyperattenuating sign can be unmasked by using narrow windows and comparing diseased vessel to normal vessel.

Importance

Understanding the value of non-contrast CT in vascular imaging is important because sometimes iodinated contrast cannot be administered.

Typical clinical scenario

Unenhanced CT is almost routinely obtained in vascular imaging. This is to prevent mistaking inherently high-attenuation material for iodinated contrast (Figure 60.4). Additionally, after the administration of iodinated contrast the subacute hematoma in the vessel wall or thrombus becomes less apparent.

In certain circumstances iodinated contrast cannot be administered, such as impaired renal function, allergy to iodinated contrast or difficult venous access. The vascular imager, in these situations, should not write off the study because no contrast is in the arteries, as much information can still be gleaned.

Unenhanced CT may be obtained for a suspected non-vascular medical emergency such as renal stone or pancreatitis. It is important to look for an acute vascular process, which is in the differential diagnosis for renal colic and back pain.

Differential diagnosis

Aortic rupture, intramural hematoma, unstable thrombus, calcification, and periaortic hypercellular tumor.

Teaching point

Sometimes only non-contrast CT is available. The imagers should be aware that valuable information about the acuity of a vascular process can still be obtained without iodinated contrast.

REFERENCE

1. Mortia S, Ueno E, Masukawa A, *et al.* Hyperattenuating signs at unenhanced CT indicating acute vascular disease. *Radiographics* 2010; **30**: 111–125.

Pearls and Pitfalls in Cardiovascular Imaging, ed. Stefan L. Zimmerman and Elliot K. Fishman. Published by Cambridge University Press. © Cambridge University Press 2015.

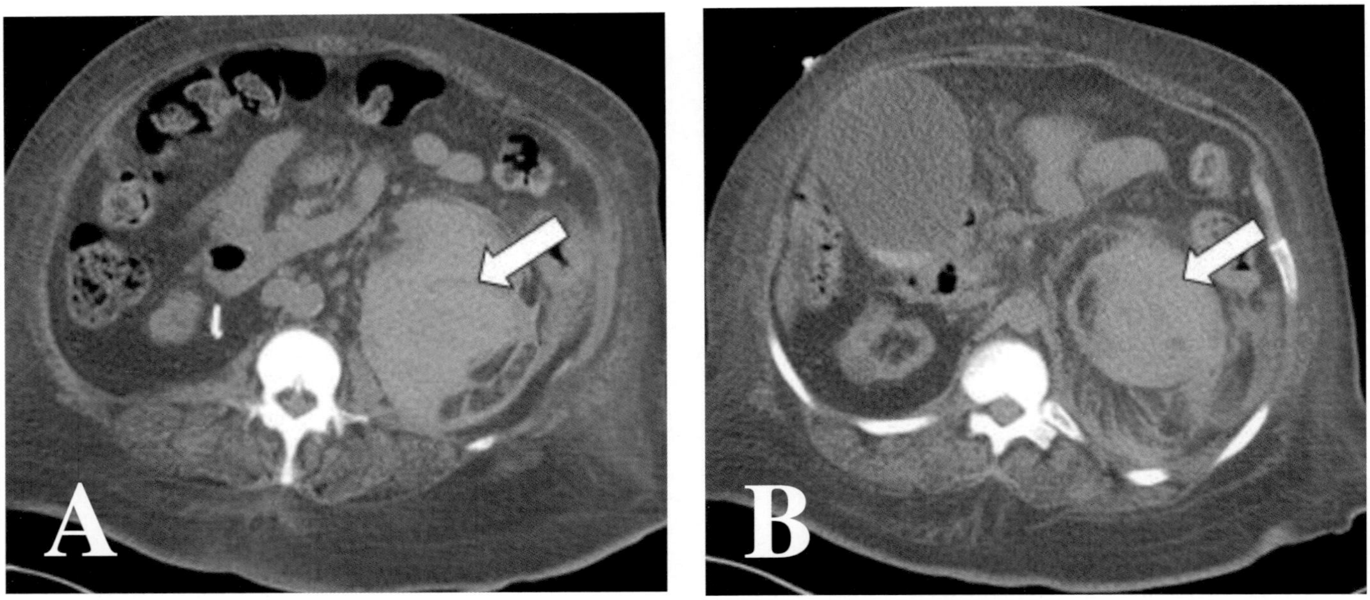

Figure 60.1 A 64-year-old male with chronic renal impairment had a drop in hematocrit post-renal biopsy. Unenhanced CT through the mid-abdomen (**A** and **B**) shows a retroperitoneal and perinephric hematoma. The diagnosis was made without administration of intravenous contrast, which was relatively contraindicated because of renal impairment.

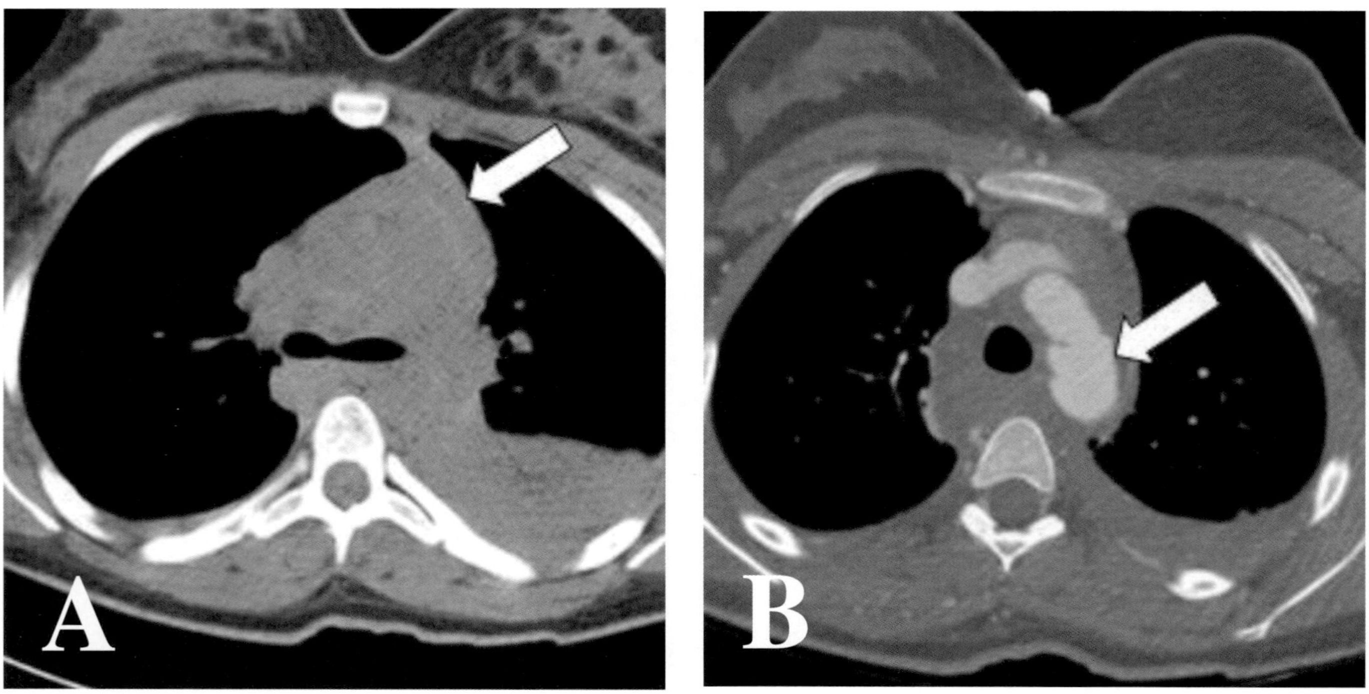

Figure 60.2 A 24-year-old female in a motor vehicle accident. CT was initially obtained without intravenous contrast (**A**). This showed high attenuation in the anterior mediastinum raising suspicion for acute traumatic aortic injury, which was confirmed on CT angiogram. There is contour irregularity in the proximal descending aorta (**B** and **C**).

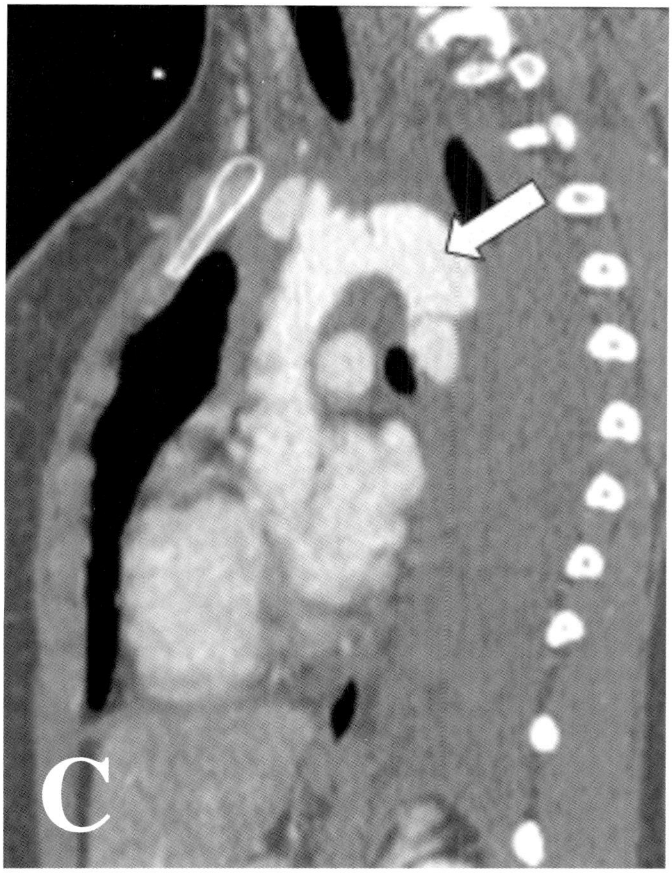

Figure 60.2 *(cont.)*

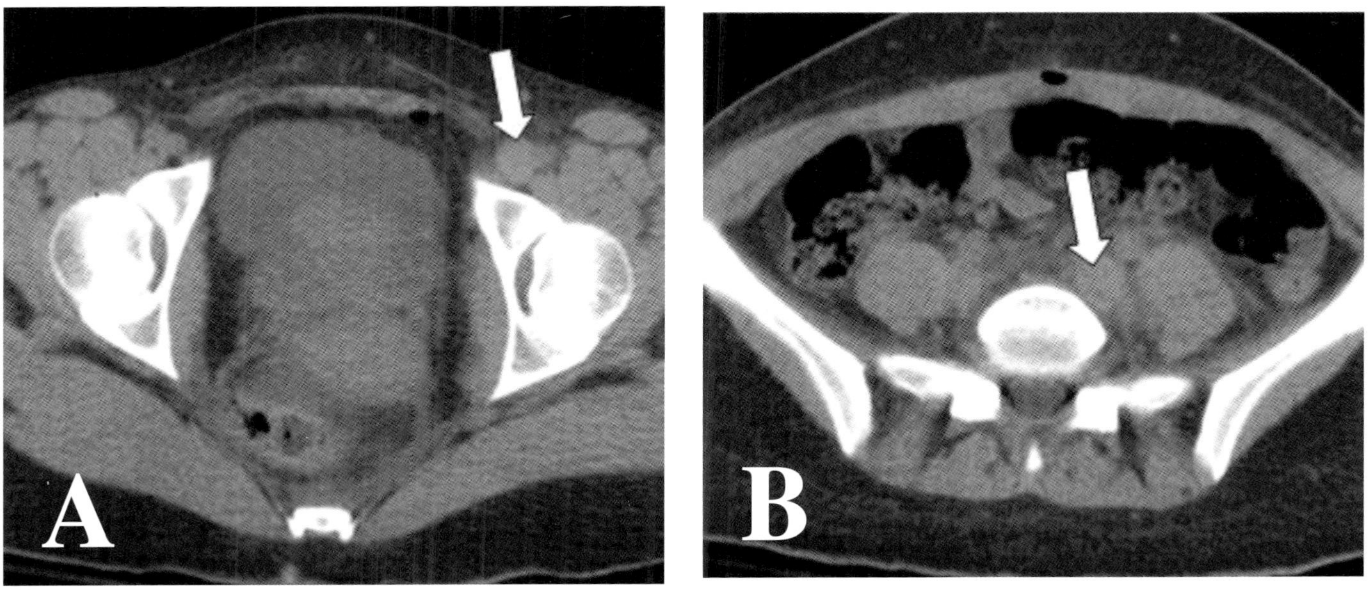

Figure 60.3 A 28-year-old female presents with pelvic and thigh pain. Unenhanced CT of the pelvis shows expanded left common femoral vein which is of high attenuation (arrow, **A**) as is the left common iliac vein (arrow, **B**). There is surrounding perivenular soft tissue stranding. A diagnosis of acute thrombus of the left iliofemoral venous system was made. Venous thrombosis was not in the original differential diagnosis.

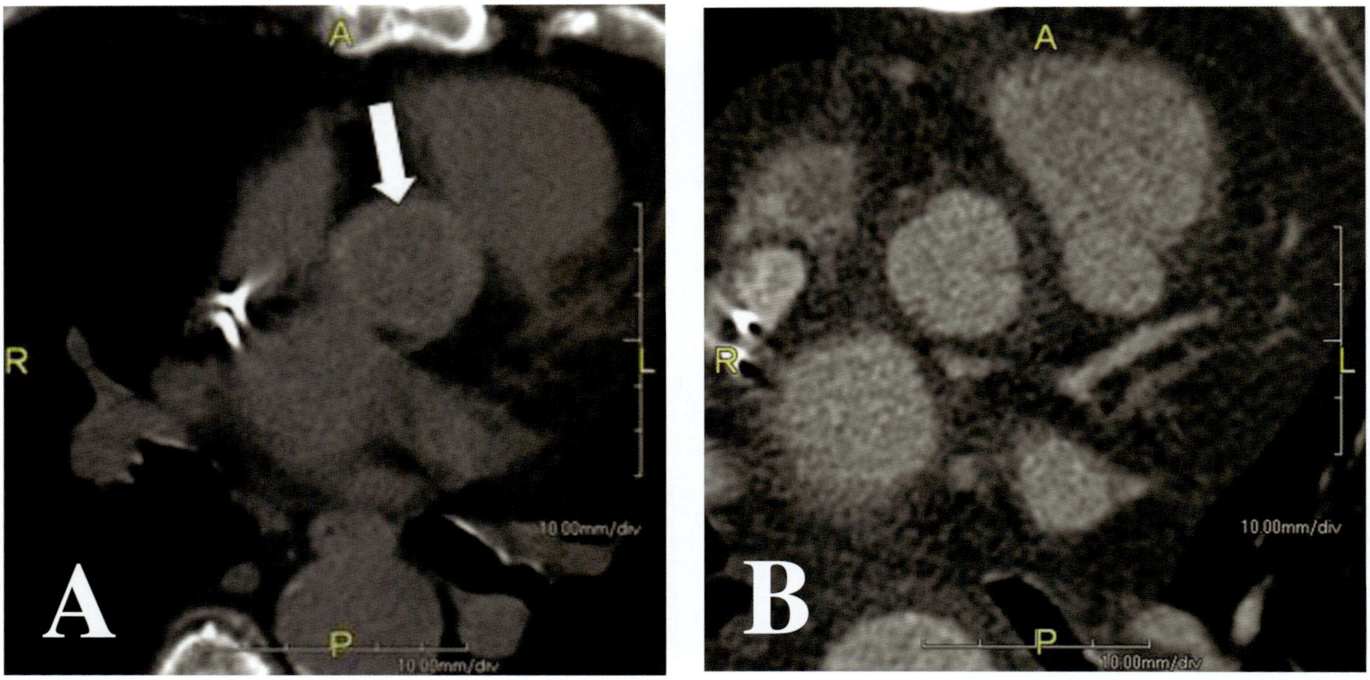

Figure 60.4 A 45-year-old male presents for post-operative surveillance. Unenhanced CT (**A**) shows a high-attenuation ring surrounding the ascending aorta (arrow), which simulates intramural hematoma but is an expected finding post-graft repair (**B**).

CASE

61 Shearing of branch arteries in intramural hematoma: a mimic of active extravasation

Saurabh Jha

Imaging description

The medial layer of the aorta expands in intramural hematoma (IMH) due to the accumulation of subacute blood products. The expansion can shear the wall of exiting arteries such as the intercostal and lumbar arteries.[1]

Contrast collects between the sheared wall of the intercostal artery and the medial layer of the aorta. The contrast collection is beyond the confines of the arterial lumen but the pooled contrast is well localized (Figures 61.1 and 61. 2).

The shearing of the intercostal arteries is also called the "Chinese Ring Sword Sign".[1]

Importance

This entity can be confused for active extravasation.

In vascular imaging, active extravasation of contrast has important connotations. It means that there is active bleeding. The use of the present participle (bleeding) as opposed to the past tense (bled) elevates the clinical severity and urgency of the vascular process and the promptness with which corrective action is required. Both inappropriate usage and inappropriate non-usage of this term by imagers can have negative consequences.

Typical clinical scenario

Patient presents with chest or back pain with suspicion of an acute aortic syndrome.

Differential diagnosis

Active extravasation is inferred when there is contrast outside the confines of a vascular structure; the contrast outline does not conform to the shape of an arterial branch of venous tributary. Typically the contrast progressively pools in the arterial and venous phases of acquisition.

The pooled contrast can mimic false lumen of a dissection. It can also mimic a penetrating atherosclerotic ulcer.

Teaching point

Mistaking the pooled contrast from sheared vessels for active bleeding can lead to inappropriate operative intervention. IMH of the descending aorta is typically managed medically.

REFERENCE

1. Wu M-T, Wu T-H, Lee D. Multislice computed tomography of aortic intramural hematoma with progressive intercostal artery tears. *Circulation* 2005; **111**: e92–93.

Pearls and Pitfalls in Cardiovascular Imaging, ed. Stefan L. Zimmerman and Elliot K. Fishman. Published by Cambridge University Press. © Cambridge University Press 2015.

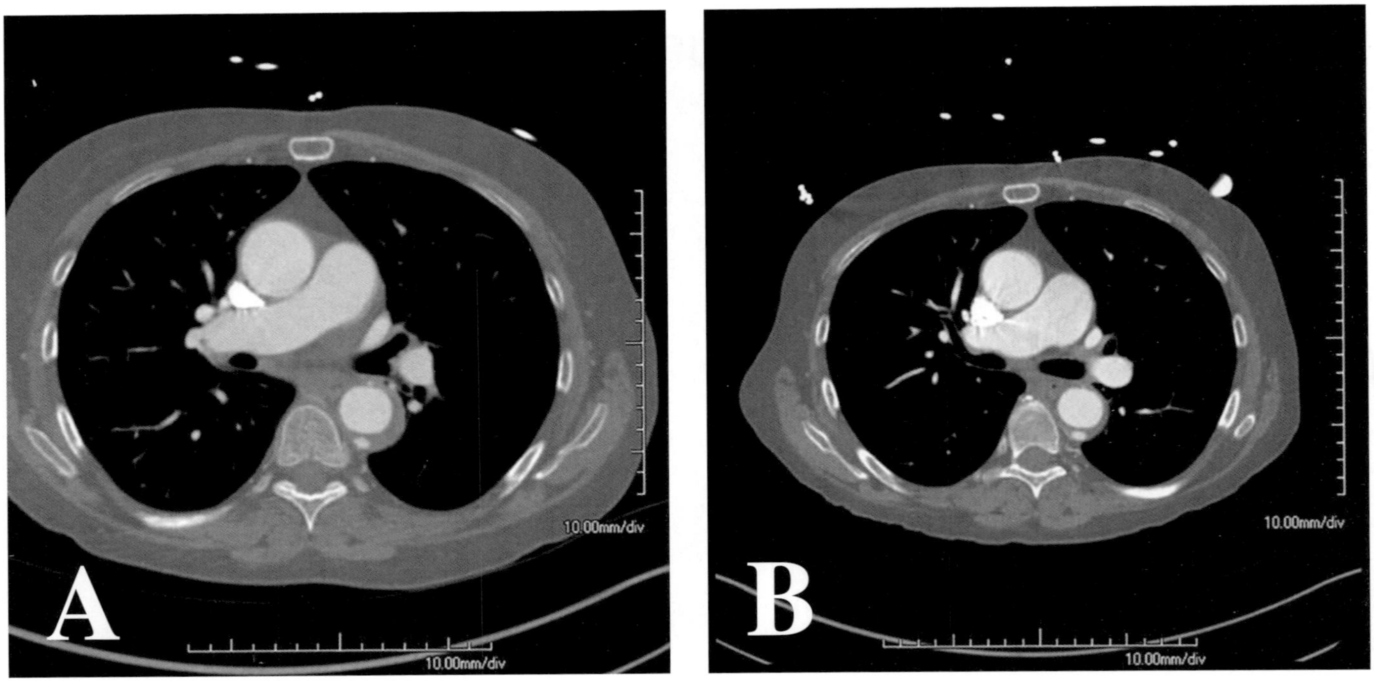

Figure 61.1 A 53-year-old female with hypertension presents with chest pain. Axial contrast-enhanced CT in the arterial phase of acquisition (**A**) shows a focus of contrast at the 6 o'clock position. This represents pooled contrast from shearing of the intercostal artery. Note the thickening of the left lateral and posterior walls of the aorta representing an IMH. Representative image from a repeat CT (**B**) shows that the pooled contrast collection has not changed. Note that the IMH has reduced along the left lateral wall but persists along the posterior wall.

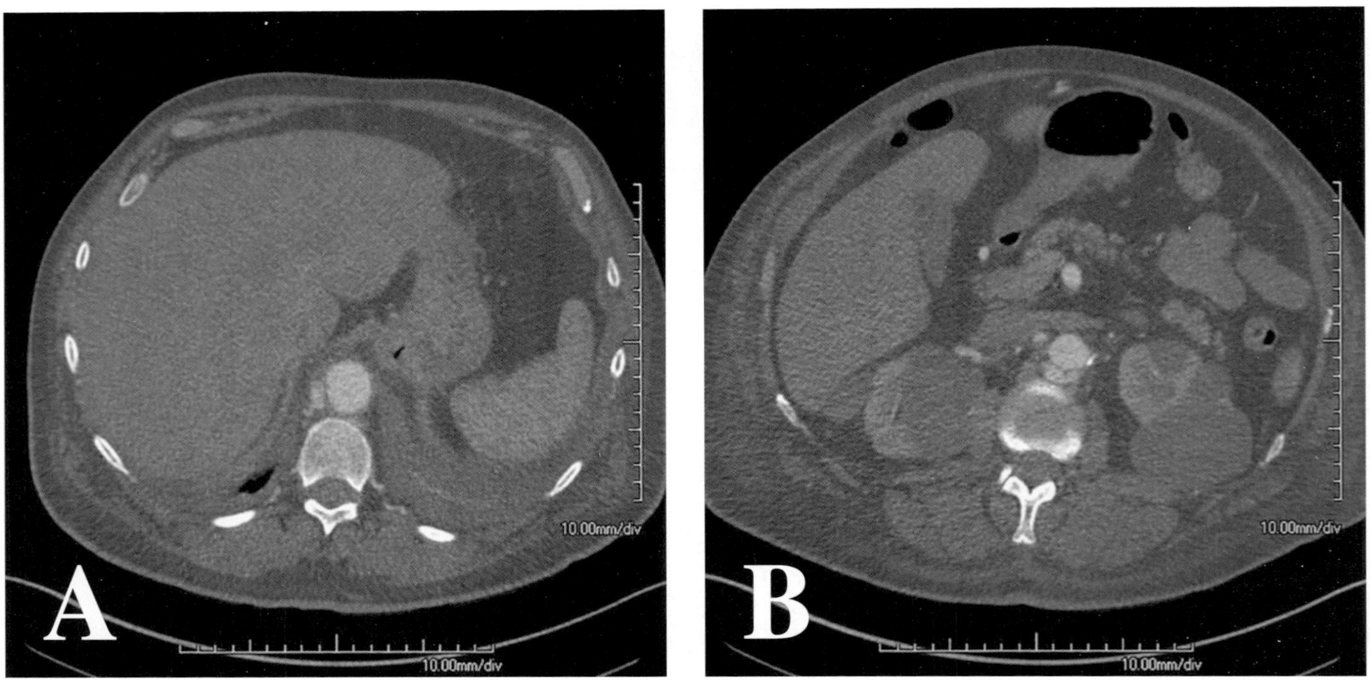

Figure 61.2 A 61-year-old male presented with chest pain and was diagnosed with IMH. Axial contrast-enhanced CT (**A–C**) shows foci of pooled contrast along the right lateral and posterior aspects of the aorta due to shearing of the exiting lumbar arteries. The pooled contrast mimics a dissection flap. The IMH is shown to better advantage on the unenhanced image (**D**).

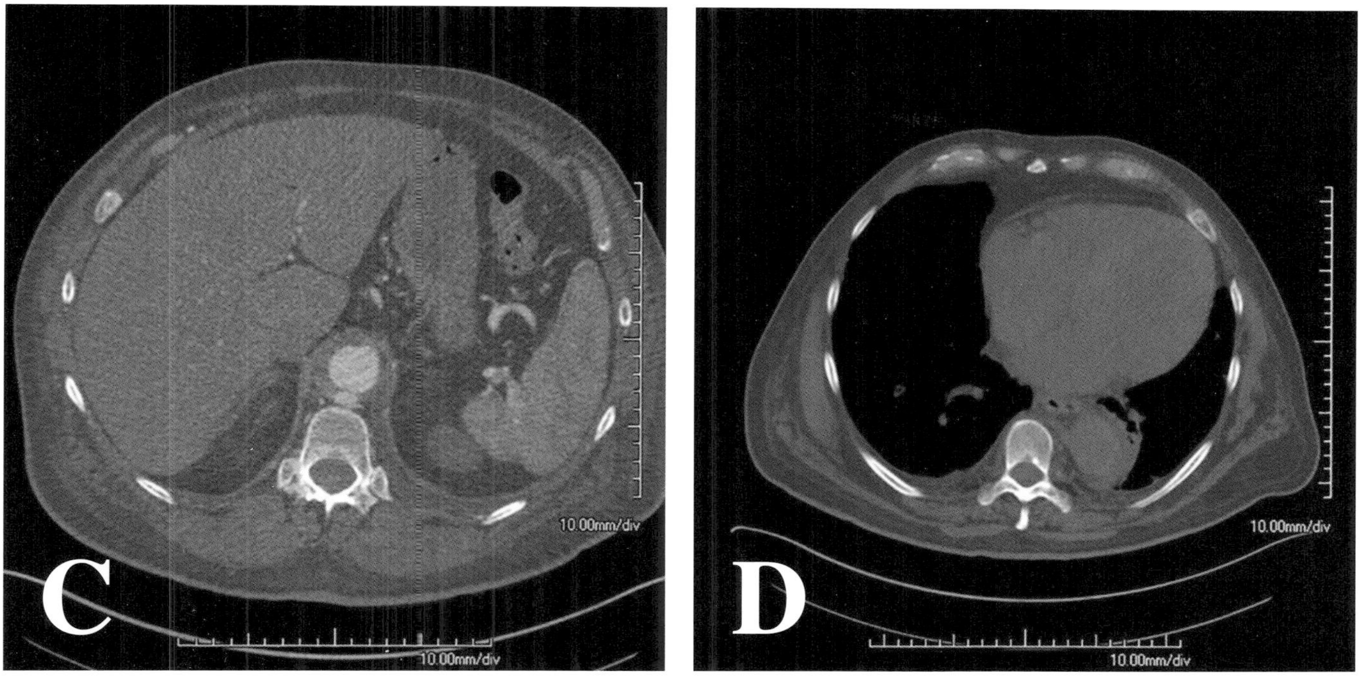

Figure 61.2 *(cont.)*

CASE 62

Imaging features of aortic aneurysm instability

Pamela T. Johnson

Imaging description

The diagnosis of aortic aneurysm rupture is straightforward on CT. Both precontrast and post-contrast acquisitions will demonstrate disruption of the aneurysm wall with perianeurysm hemorrhage extending into the retroperitoneum and possibly the peritoneal cavity. Prior to frank rupture, certain findings on CT may reflect instability of an intact abdominal aortic aneurysm or contained rupture.[1–3] Instability indicators include intramural or intrathrombus hemorrhage ("hyperattenuating crescent" sign), perianeurysmal hemorrhage, and disruption of previously continuous aortic wall calcification.[1–3] The hyperattenuating crescent sign indicates hemorrhage within aneurysm thrombus or the aneurysm wall, and can be recognized by high-attenuation material within the plaque or the wall (Figure 62.1). A small perianeurysm hematoma may be identified prior to frank rupture, suggesting contained rupture (Figure 62.2).

Contained rupture may also manifest as a new focal outpouching of the aortic wall or the "draped aorta" sign (Figures 62.3, 62.4). The latter appears as loss of the fat plane between the posterior wall of the aortic aneurysm and the adjacent vertebral body, and psoas muscle on axial images, and a focal posterior outpouching on sagittal MPRs.[3] Cognizance of these findings is essential so that the interpreting radiologist can alert the vascular surgeon to guide intervention.

Careful assessment for aneurysm enlargement is equally important. A size threshold of 5.5 cm has been defined for repair of an abdominal aortic aneurysm. The typical rate of aneurysm enlargement is 1–4 mm/year. Rapid aneurysm enlargement is defined as > 6 mm in 6 months or >1 cm in one year.[3–5] Measurement should be tailored to the configuration of the aneurysm and performed on current and prior CT examinations for optimal reproducibility. If available, comparison to older studies is recommended, because changes in size may be more apparent than comparison to recent studies alone.

Importance

Imaging signs that suggest a high risk of rupture are important to recognize to prompt treatment before the occurrence of acute aortic rupture, which has a very high mortality rate.

Typical clinical scenario

Serial imaging with CT is the primary diagnostic method used to evaluate abdominal aortic aneurysms and guide management. Interpretation should include careful measurement with comparison to older studies for interval increase in size or development of CT indicators of instability.

Differential diagnosis

Specific differentials exist for some of these CT findings. The intramural crescent should not be confused with uncomplicated mural plaque, which is not as dense as hemorrhage. Unopacified venous structures or bowel may abut the aortic aneurysm wall and should not be mistaken for perianeurysmal hematoma. Perianeurysmal fibrosis can appear the same as the soft tissue surrounding the aorta; however, identifying a rapid rate of enlargement suggests the presence of an active leak precipitating the periaortic infiltration. Focal outpouchings can be seen with mycotic pseudoaneurysms (Figure 62.5), which are surgical emergencies and also have a high risk of rupture. These patients generally present with pain. In these studies, the CT should be inspected for other findings that indicate the presence of infection (e.g., vertebral body osteomyelitis, retrocrural or psoas abscess).

Teaching point

Radiologists must be aware of these important findings on CT that indicate aneurysm instability and may prompt emergent or semiemergent intervention.

REFERENCES

1. Rakita D, Newatia A, Hines JJ, Siegel DN, Friedman B. Spectrum of CT findings in rupture and impending rupture of abdominal aortic aneurysms. *Radiographics* 2007; **27**:497–507.
2. Schwartz SA, Taljanovic MS, Smyth S, O'Brien MJ, Rogers LF. CT findings of rupture, impending rupture, and contained rupture of abdominal aortic aneurysms. *AJR Am J Roentgenol* 2007; **188**:W57–62.
3. Wadgaonkar A, Black JH, Weihe E, Zimmerman SL, Fishman EK, Johnson PT. Abdominal aortic aneurysms revisited: MDCT with multiplanar reconstructions for identifying indicators of instability in the pre- and postoperative patient. *Radiographics* 2015; **35**:254–68.
4. Chaikof EL, Brewster DC, Dalman RL, et al. The care of patients with an abdominal aortic aneurysm: the Society for Vascular Surgery practice guidelines. *J Vasc Surg* 2009; **50**:S2–49.
5. Brady AR, Thompson SG, Fowkes FG, Greenhalgh RM, Powell JT; UK Small Aneurysm Trial Participants. Abdominal aortic aneurysm expansion: risk factors and time intervals for surveillance. *Circulation* 2004; **110**:16–21.

Pearls and Pitfalls in Cardiovascular Imaging, ed. Stefan L. Zimmerman and Elliot K. Fishman. Published by Cambridge University Press. © Cambridge University Press 2015.

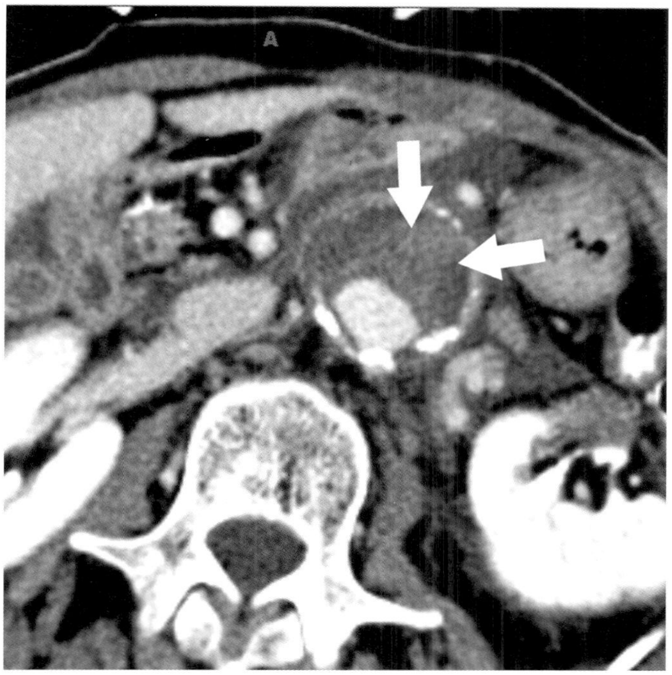

Figure 62.1 A. Axial image from a contrast-enhanced CT obtained in a 60-year-old female with metastatic esophageal cancer and acute abdominal pain demonstrates an aneurysm of the abdominal aorta with high-attenuation material within mural thrombus of the aneurysm sac (arrows). This finding was new from the prior examination, suggesting instability.

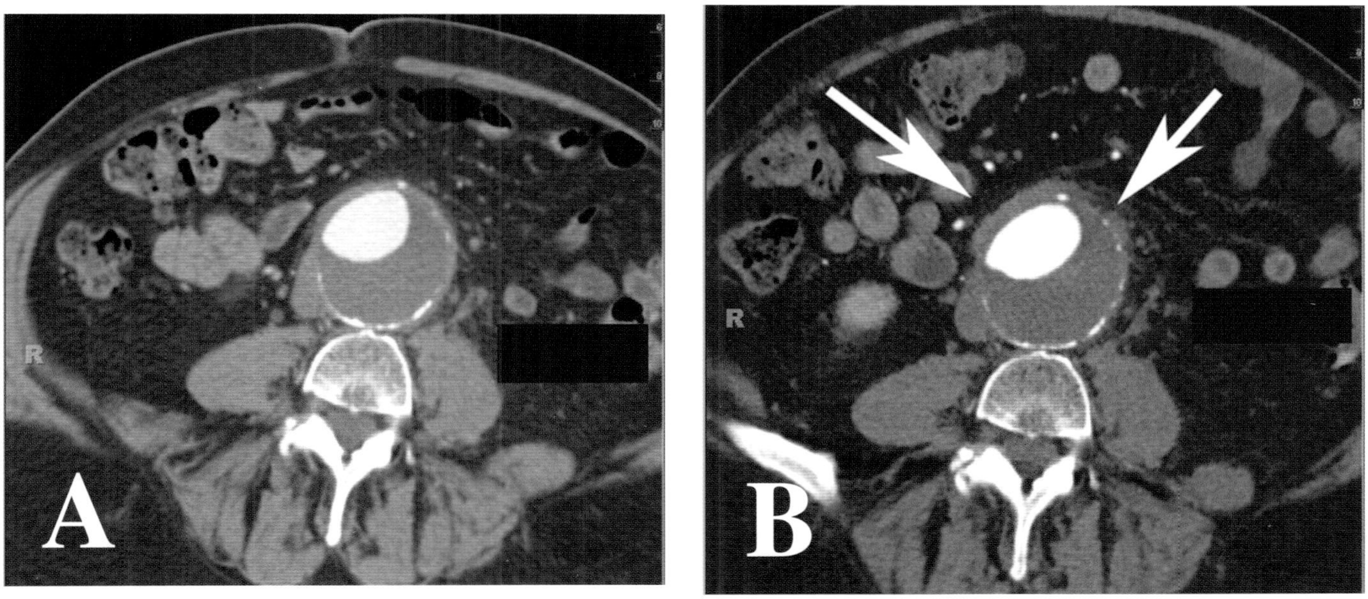

Figure 62.2 An 85-year-old man with abdominal aortic aneurysm. Baseline IV contrast-enhanced axial CT (**A**). Follow-up images at 6 months (**B**) and 12 months (**C**) after baseline showed progressively increasing perianeurysmal soft tissue, consistent with the presence of a slow leak.

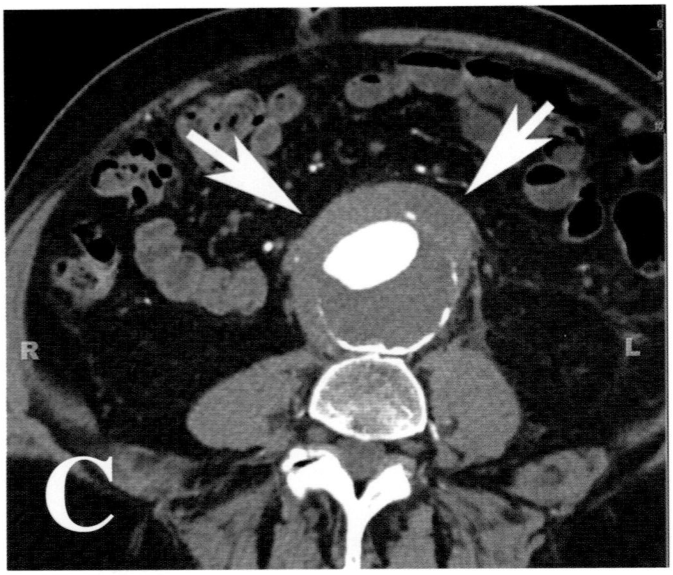

Figure 62.2 *(cont.)*

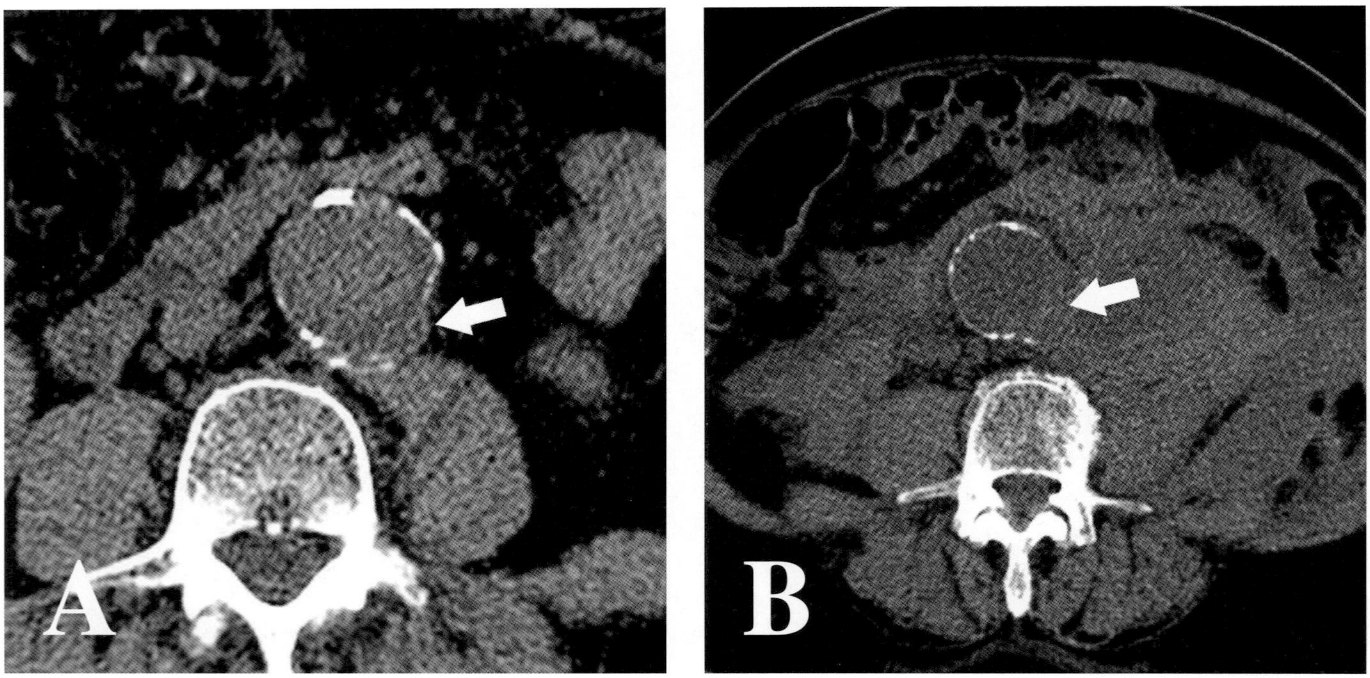

Figure 62.3 Axial CT imaging from a non-contrast CT examination obtained in a 55-year-old male with aortic aneurysm and abdominal pain demonstrates focal outward bulging of the aortic wall contour posterolaterally with disruption of intimal calcification continuity (arrow) (**A**). Follow-up CT examination performed 9 days later demonstrates aortic rupture arising from the location of previously seen aortic wall disruption (arrow) (**B**).

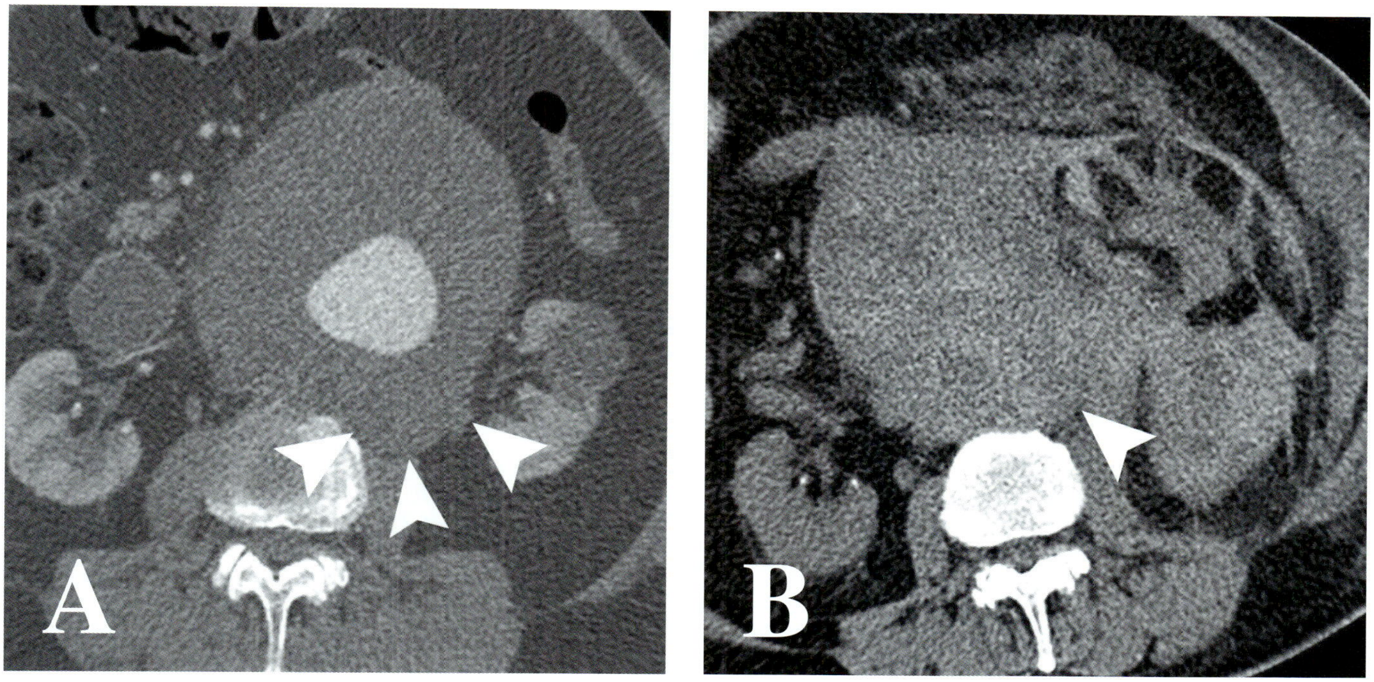

Figure 62.4 Axial contrast-enhanced CT examination performed in a 78-year-old male with abdominal aortic aneurysm demonstrates the "draped aorta" sign, with loss of fat plane between the vertebral body and aorta (arrowheads) (**A**). Follow-up CT examination performed emergently 15 days later when the same patient presented with acute abdominal pain demonstrates aortic rupture into the left retroperitoneum, likely arising from the site of previous "draped aorta" sign (arrowhead) (**B**).

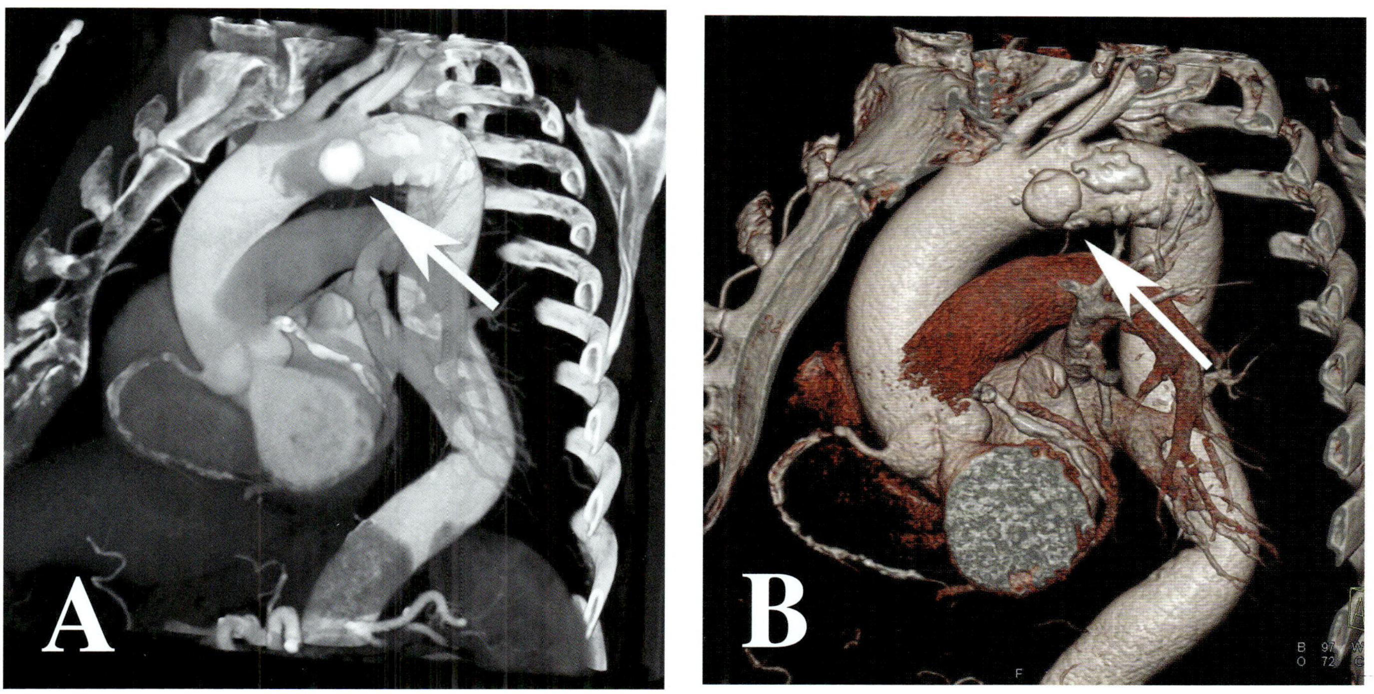

Figure 62.5 A. and **B.** A 76-year-old man with salmonella bacteremia and mycotic pseudoaneurysm of the aortic arch status post-homograft repair. Coronal oblique 3D volume renderings show a 2 x 1 cm exophytic pseudoaneurysm (arrow) arising from the aortic arch.

CASE

63 Aortoenteric fistula

Siva P. Raman

Imaging description

The most important finding in an aortoenteric fistula is ectopic gas either within the aortic lumen or adjacent to the aorta (Figure 63.1). Direct extravasation of intravenous contrast from the aortic lumen into the adjacent bowel, or extension of enteric contrast from the bowel into the aorta are extraordinarily rare, but highly specific signs. A number of less specific findings can also be identified, including effacement of the fat plane between the aorta and adjacent bowel, focal bowel wall thickening adjacent to the aorta, periaortic soft tissue thickening and fluid, or intramural hematoma with an adjacent thickened loop of bowel.[1–2]

Importance

Although aortoenteric fistulas are quite rare, the development of a fistula is incredibly life-threatening, with a mortality rate of almost 100% in the absence of treatment.[1]

Typical clinical scenario

Aortoenteric fistulas can be divided into primary and secondary forms. The secondary form is the most common, occurring in the setting of prior aortic surgery or graft placement, while the primary form is rarer, occurring in patients without a history of prior surgery or intervention (Figure 63.2). While the classic clinical presentation of patients with an aortoenteric fistula has been described with the triad of abdominal pain, massive gastrointestinal hemorrhage, and a pulsatile abdominal mass, many patients demonstrate only vague abdominal pain on initial presentation. While nearly all patients will eventually experience gastrointestinal bleeding, this may not be apparent on initial presentation.[3] Unfortunately, endoscopy is of limited value in the diagnosis of a fistula, and conventional angiography can often struggle to make the diagnosis in cases of intermittent bleeding through the fistula.[1] Nuclear medicine tagged red blood cell (RBC) scans are limited by poor spatial resolution and a lack of specificity. As a result, the diagnosis is often ultimately dependent on CT.[1,3–5] The treatment for aortoenteric fistulas has gradually moved away from surgical intervention, and toward the use of endovascular techniques.[1]

Differential diagnosis

The primary differential diagnosis is perigraft infection, which can share many of the imaging features of an aortoenteric fistula. However, the clinical history can often suggest one diagnosis over the other, and ectopic gas is more common with a fistula than with a perigraft infection (Figure 63.3).[1] Other mimics of a fistula include aortitis, infected aneurysms, retroperitoneal fibrosis, and the immediate post-operative state (where gas and fluid surrounding the aorta can be normal findings).[1–2]

Teaching point

The diagnosis of an aortoenteric fistula is critically dependent upon CT, and a missed diagnosis can have disastrous consequences with regard to patient mortality. The diagnosis should be considered when confronted with ectopic gas, free fluid, and soft tissue thickening around the aorta, particularly when the patient has undergone prior aortic surgery or intervention.

REFERENCES

1. Raman SP, Kamaya A, Federle M, and Fishman EK. Aortoenteric fistulas: spectrum of CT findings. *Abdom Imaging* 2013; **38**: 367–375.
2. Hagspiel KD, Turba UC, Bozlar U, et al. Diagnosis of aortoenteric fistulas with CT angiography. *J Vasc Interv Radiol* 2007; **19**: 497–504.
3. Perks FJ, Gillespie I, and Patel D. Multidetector computed tomography imaging of aortoenteric fistula. *J Comput Assis Tomogr* 2004; **28**: 343–347.
4. Senadhi V, Brown JC, Arora D, Shaffer R, Shetty D, and Mackrell P. A mysterious cause of gastrointestinal bleeding disguising itself as diverticulosis and peptic ulcer disease: a review of diagnostic modalities for aortoenteric fistula. *Case Rep Gastroenterol* 2010; **4**: 510–517.
5. Ranasinghe W, Loa J, Allaf N, Lewis K, and Sebastian MG. Primary aortoenteric fistulae: the challenges in diagnosis and review of treatment. *Ann Vasc Surg* 2011; **25**: 386. e1–5.

Pearls and Pitfalls in Cardiovascular Imaging, ed. Stefan L. Zimmerman and Elliot K. Fishman. Published by Cambridge University Press. © Cambridge University Press 2015.

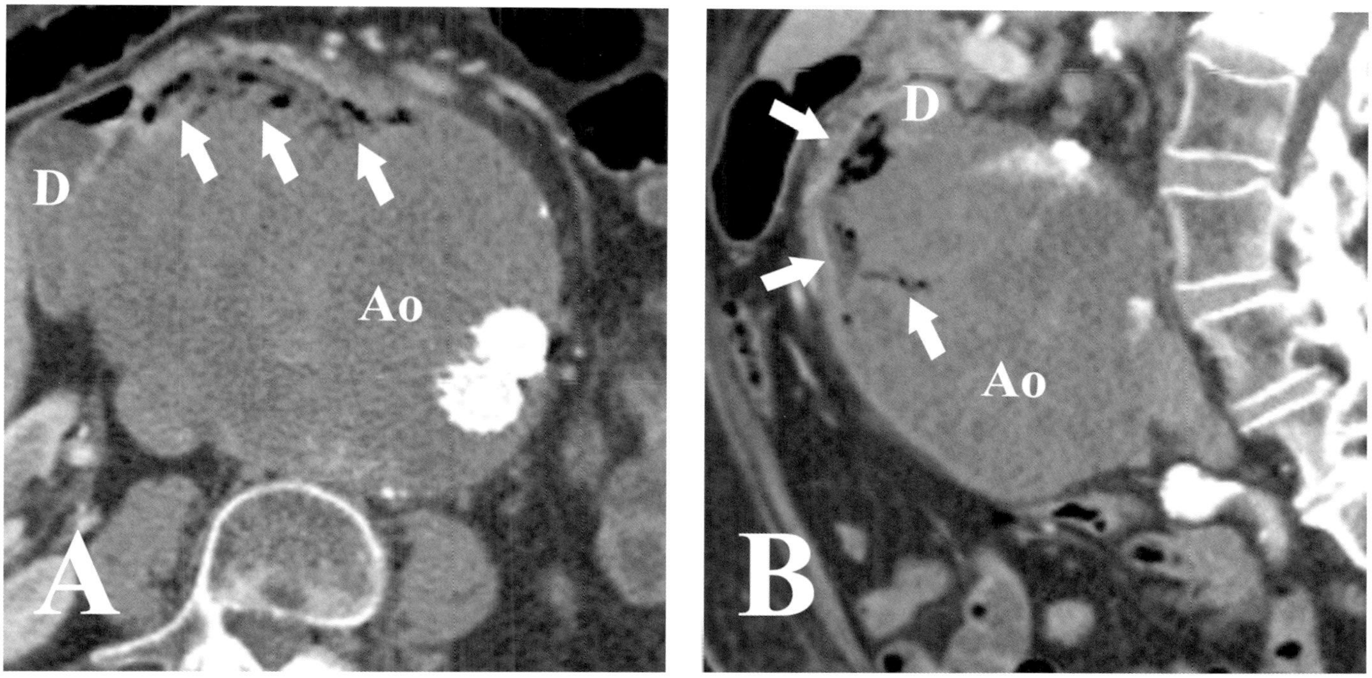

Figure 63.1 A. Axial contrast-enhanced CT image in an 87-year-old female patient status post-prior aortic endograft repair demonstrates a large amount of gas (arrows) in direct contiguity between the aorta (Ao) and adjacent duodenum (D). This was presumed to represent a large aortoenteric fistula, but the patient died shortly after the scan. **B.** Sagittal image demonstrates the same findings with gas (arrows) tracking toward the duodenum (D) from the aortic aneurysm sac (Ao).

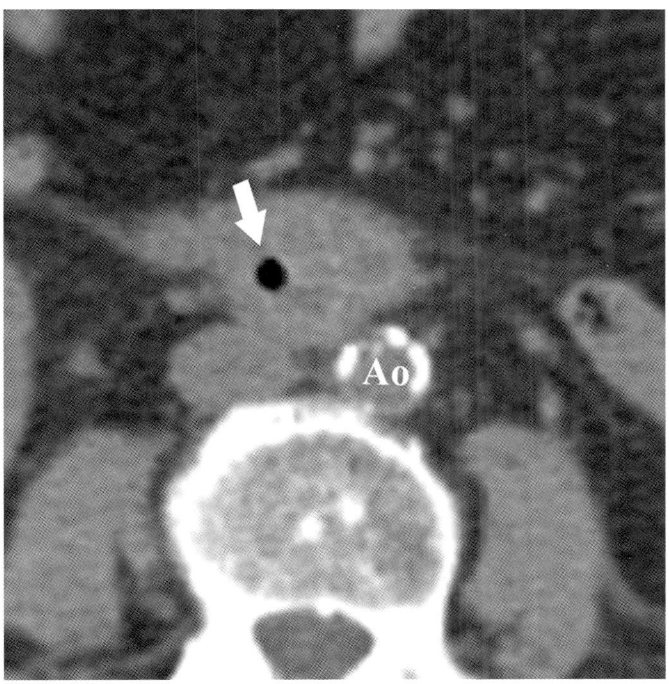

Figure 63.2 Axial non-contrast image in a 71-year-old female with a surgically proven aortoenteric fistula demonstrates ectopic gas (arrow) immediately adjacent to the aortic lumen (Ao).

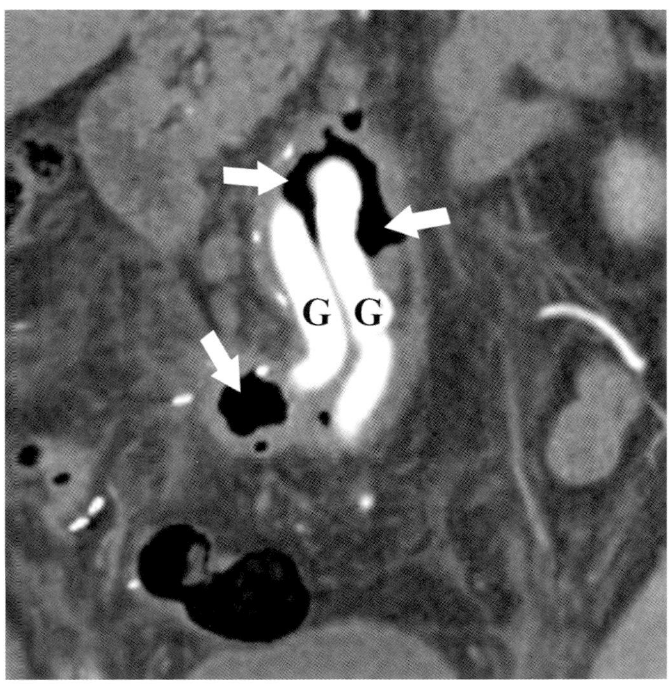

Figure 63.3 Coronal contrast-enhanced image in a 73-year-old male with a surgically proven aortoenteric fistula demonstrates significant ectopic gas (arrows) surrounding two iliac limbs of an aortic graft (G).

CASE

64 Inflammatory aortic aneurysm

Atif Zaheer

Imaging description

Soft tissue thickening in the periaortic region due to inflammatory aortic aneurysm is well visualized with cross-sectional imaging. CT demonstrates a low-attenuation soft tissue mass representing the fibrotic plaque surrounding a calcified aortic wall. The soft tissue is most prominent anterior and laterally and demonstrates mild enhancement after contrast administration, which has high sensitivity and almost 100% specificity for this diagnosis (Figure 64.1.A).[1] The soft tissue thickening appears slightly T2 hyperintense on MRI indicative of active inflammation. Ultrasound has lower accuracy in diagnosing inflammatory aneurysms and demonstrates the soft tissue thickening as a hypoechoic area surrounding the aorta.[2] Involvement of adjacent retroperitoneal structures including the psoas muscles and medial displacement of the ureters may also occur (Figures 64.1.B and 64.1.C).

Importance

Inflammatory aneurysms of the aorta constitute 3–10% of aortic aneurysms and mostly occur in men.[3] The etiology may be due to chronic inflammation, slow leakage of blood cells or an autoallergic reaction.[2] Although mostly contained, rupture may occur with a higher operative mortality than an ordinary aneurysm.[2] Additionally, due to the frequent extension of inflammation to the ureters leading to hydronephrosis and subsequent renal failure, operative management remains optimum treatment. Endovascular treatments have demonstrated decreased mortality rates; however, problems with residual hydronephrosis remain in a significant number of patients.[4]

Typical clinical scenario

Symptoms of abdominal or back pain, fatigue, and weight loss with an elevated sedimentation rate in a patient with a history of an abdominal aortic aneurysm is highly suggestive of an inflammatory aneurysm.

Differential diagnosis

Soft tissue thickening in other infectious and non-infectious causes of aortitis as well as in idiopathic retroperitoneal fibrosis may occur in the absence of an aortic aneurysm (Figures 64.2A, 64.2B and 64.2C). Similar to inflammatory aneurysm, retroperitoneal fibrosis can result in medial displacement of the ureters (Figure 64.2C). Lymphadenopathy due to lymphoma or metastatic disease is usually differentiated by the presence of discrete nodal masses, elevation of the aorta from the spine, and the lateral displacement of the ureters (Figure 64.3). Plaque due to atherosclerotic disease is surrounded by a calcified rim. Aortic rupture shows hyperdense hematoma extending into the retroperitoneum and possibly the peritoneal space. Soft tissue thickening in the periaortic region may also be seen as an extrapancreatic manifestation of autoimmune pancreatitis. Again, the absence of an aortic aneurysm, presence of characteristic pancreatic changes such as a sausage-shaped appearance and a peripancreatic rim along with the possible elevation of serum IgG4 may be the key differentiating features.

Teaching point

Inflammatory aortic aneurysms have a significantly high operative mortality than ordinary aneurysms due to their involvement of the adjacent organs, particularly the ureters. Imaging findings of an enhancing soft tissue rim surrounding a calcified aneurysm wall may be the key imaging finding.

REFERENCES

1. M. Iino, S. Kuribayashi, S. Imakita, et al. Sensitivity and specificity of CT in the diagnosis of inflammatory abdominal aortic aneurysms. *J Comput Assist Tomogr* 2002; **26**: 1006–12.

2. R. C. Pennell, L. H. Hollier, J. T. Lie, et al. Inflammatory abdominal aortic aneurysms: a thirty-year review. *J Vasc Surg* 1985; **2**: 859–69.

3. L. Arrive, J. M. Correas, G. Leseche, L. Ghebontni, J. M. Tubiana. Inflammatory aneurysms of the abdominal aorta: CT findings. *AJR Am J Roentgenol* 1995; **165**: 1481–4.

4. H. Maeda, H. Umezawa, T. Hattori, et al. Early and late outcomes of inflammatory abdominal aortic aneurysms: comparison with the outcomes after open surgical and endovascular aneurysm repair in literature reviews. *Int Angiol* 2013; **32**: 67–73.

Pearls and Pitfalls in Cardiovascular Imaging, ed. Stefan L. Zimmerman and Elliot K. Fishman. Published by Cambridge University Press. © Cambridge University Press 2015.

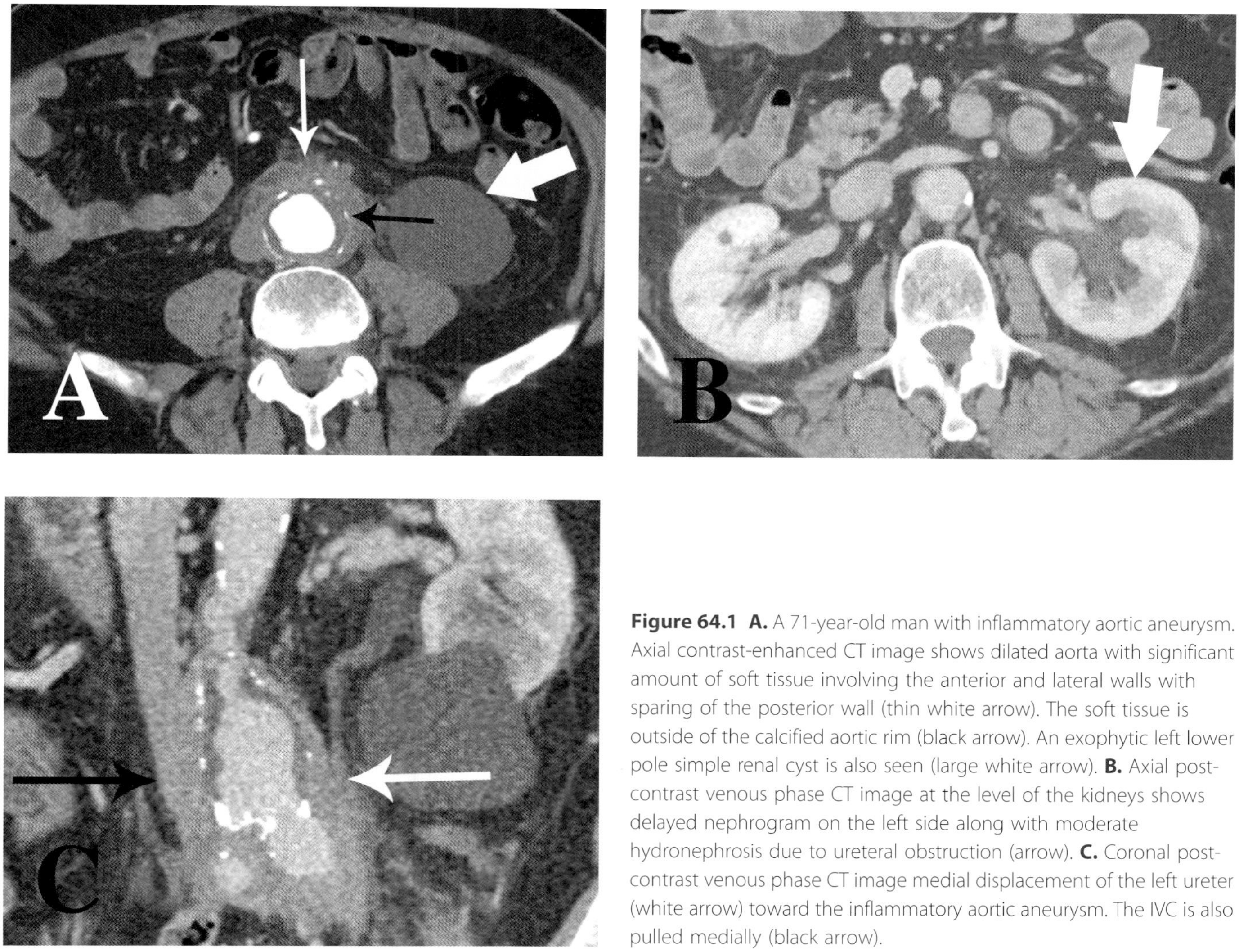

Figure 64.1 A. A 71-year-old man with inflammatory aortic aneurysm. Axial contrast-enhanced CT image shows dilated aorta with significant amount of soft tissue involving the anterior and lateral walls with sparing of the posterior wall (thin white arrow). The soft tissue is outside of the calcified aortic rim (black arrow). An exophytic left lower pole simple renal cyst is also seen (large white arrow). **B.** Axial post-contrast venous phase CT image at the level of the kidneys shows delayed nephrogram on the left side along with moderate hydronephrosis due to ureteral obstruction (arrow). **C.** Coronal post-contrast venous phase CT image medial displacement of the left ureter (white arrow) toward the inflammatory aortic aneurysm. The IVC is also pulled medially (black arrow).

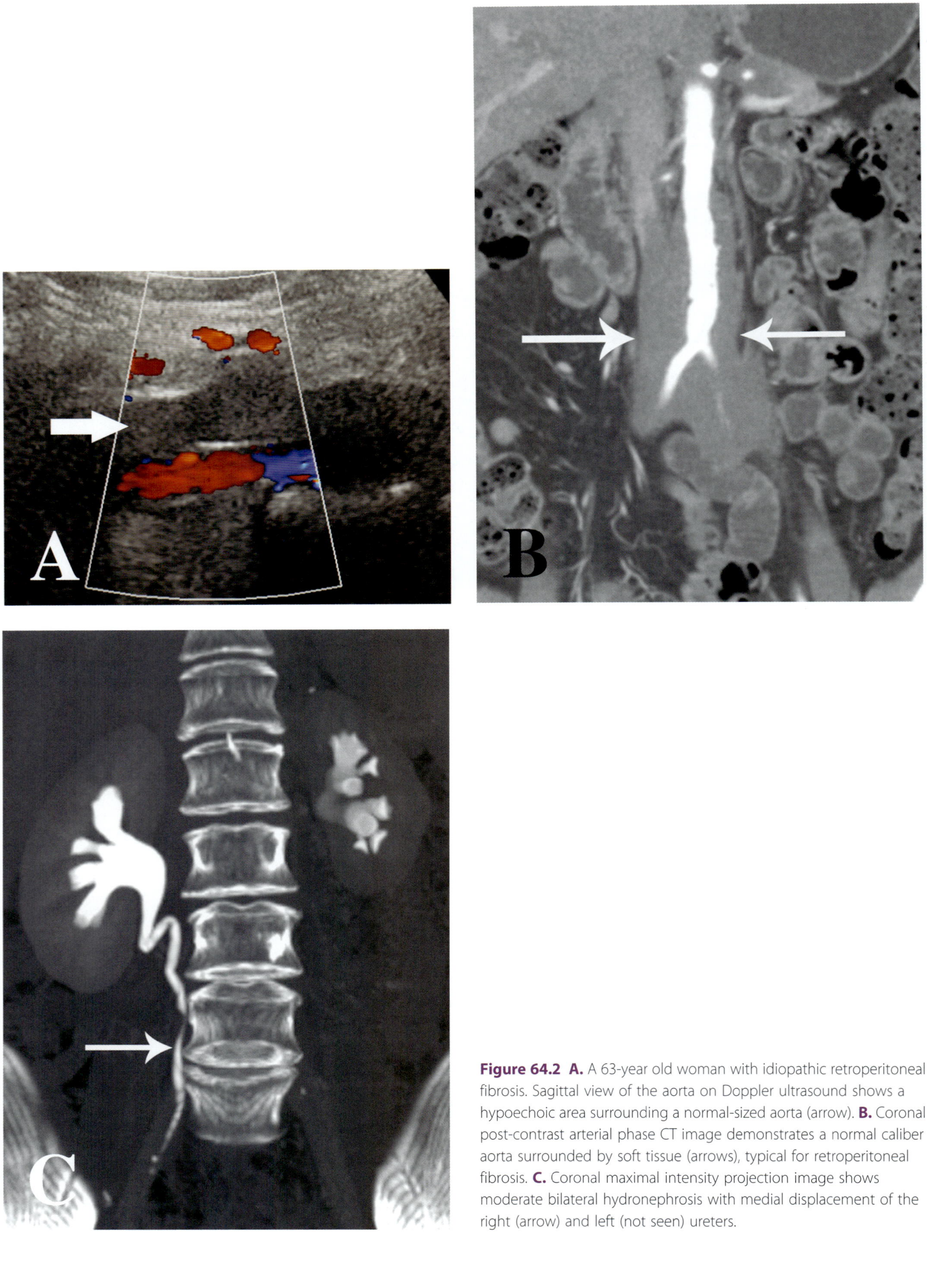

Figure 64.2 A. A 63-year old woman with idiopathic retroperitoneal fibrosis. Sagittal view of the aorta on Doppler ultrasound shows a hypoechoic area surrounding a normal-sized aorta (arrow). **B.** Coronal post-contrast arterial phase CT image demonstrates a normal caliber aorta surrounded by soft tissue (arrows), typical for retroperitoneal fibrosis. **C.** Coronal maximal intensity projection image shows moderate bilateral hydronephrosis with medial displacement of the right (arrow) and left (not seen) ureters.

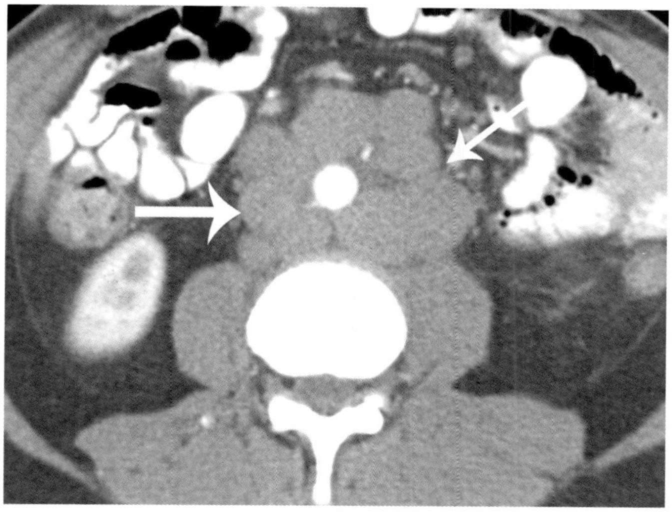

Figure 64.3 A 59-year old man with lymphoma. Axial contrast-enhanced CT shows soft tissue thickening around the aorta (arrows). Note the presence of discrete nodal masses with anterior displacement of the aorta due to circumferential encasement of the aorta including the posterior surface.

CASE 65

Incorrect aneurysm measurement due to aortic tortuosity

Pamela T. Johnson

Imaging description

In patients with tortuous aortas due to aging or atherosclerotic disease, measurements of aneurysm on axial images can lead to falsely elevated aneurysm diameters. Figure 65.1 shows an axial CT image of the ascending thoracic aorta in a 64-year-old woman, which measured 3.9 cm. However, when the aneurysm is evaluated on double oblique, sagittal, and coronal multiplanar reformatted images (MPRs), it becomes apparent that the actual size is 3.5 cm. The thoracic aorta has a candy-cane configuration, which may necessitate measurements using MPRs to accurately determine the cross-sectional diameter. Similarly, Figure 65.2 shows a 64-year-old man with an abdominal aortic aneurysm, the course of which is not entirely perpendicular to the z-axis of the scan. Accordingly, to accurately determine the diameter, the measurements must be made on MPRs tailored to reflect the actual cross-sectional diameter perpendicular to the aortic centerline.

Importance

One of the primary roles of CT in the patient with aortic aneurysm is aneurysm measurement, as the risk of rupture directly correlates with aneurysm size. Surgical thresholds have been defined based on anatomic segment. For the ascending thoracic aorta it is 5.5 cm, for descending thoracic aorta 6.5 cm, and for abdominal aorta 5.5 cm.[1] Serial imaging is critical to evaluate for rate of growth, an additional risk factor that reflects an increased risk of rupture. Aneurysms that grow more than 5–7 mm in 6 months or 1 cm in one year are considered rapidly enlarging and may warrant repair.[2] Accordingly, accurate methods of measurement are critical to patient management.

As shown in this case, axial CT images should not be relied upon for thoracic aortic and abdominal aortic aneurysm measurements. Tortuosity of the aorta results in a course that is no longer directly perpendicular to the axial plane. In these cases, MPRs or 3D renderings are required to generate accurate bi-dimensional aneurysm measurements orthogonal to the aortic lumen centerline.[3–5] Either manual double oblique MPRs or short-axis images generated from software-based automated centerline tracking are recommended for the most reliable aneurysm measurement.[6,7] This avoids overestimation of aortic diameter, which could lead to unnecessary surgery.[6] Serial measurements should be made by the reading radiologist, rather than relying on the prior radiologists' interpretation.

Typical clinical scenario

Aneurysm measurement is performed at baseline and on serial follow-up imaging, for which CT is the primary imaging modality.

> **Teaching point**
>
> Radiologists must recognize the limitations of axial sections for aortic measurements and should tailor measurements to the configuration of the aorta or aortic aneurysm using oblique multiplanar reformatted images.

REFERENCES

1. H. J. Patel, G. M. Deeb. Ascending and arch aorta: pathology, natural history, and treatment. *Circulation* 2008; **118**: 188–95.
2. E. L. Chaikof, D. C. Brewster, R. L. Dalman, et al. The care of patients with an abdominal aortic aneurysm: the Society for Vascular Surgery practice guidelines. *J Vasc Surg* 2009; **50**: S2–49.
3. A. R. Brady, S. G. Thompson, F. G. Fowkes, R. M. Greenhalgh, J. T. Powell. Abdominal aortic aneurysm expansion: risk factors and time intervals for surveillance. *Circulation* 2004; **110**: 16–21.
4. L. R. Sprouse, 2nd, G. H. Meier, 3rd, F. N. Parent, et al. Is three-dimensional computed tomography reconstruction justified before endovascular aortic aneurysm repair? *J Vasc Surg* 2004; **40**: 443–7.
5. G. A. Pitoulias, K. P. Donas, S. Schulte, E. A. Aslanidou, D. K. Papadimitriou. Two-dimensional versus three-dimensional CT angiography in analysis of anatomical suitability for stentgraft repair of abdominal aortic aneurysms. *Acta Radiol* 2011; **52**: 317–23.
6. D. D. Mendoza, M. Kochar, R. B. Devereux, et al. Impact of image analysis methodology on diagnostic and surgical classification of patients with thoracic aortic aneurysms. *Ann Thorac Surg* 2011; **92**: 904–12.
7. S. Ahmed, S. L. Zimmerman, P. T. Johnson, et al. MDCT interpretation of the ascending aorta with semiautomated measurement software: improved reproducibility compared with manual techniques. *J Cardiovasc Comput Tomogr* 2014; **8**: 108–14.

Pearls and Pitfalls in Cardiovascular Imaging, ed. Stefan L. Zimmerman and Elliot K. Fishman. Published by Cambridge University Press. © Cambridge University Press 2015.

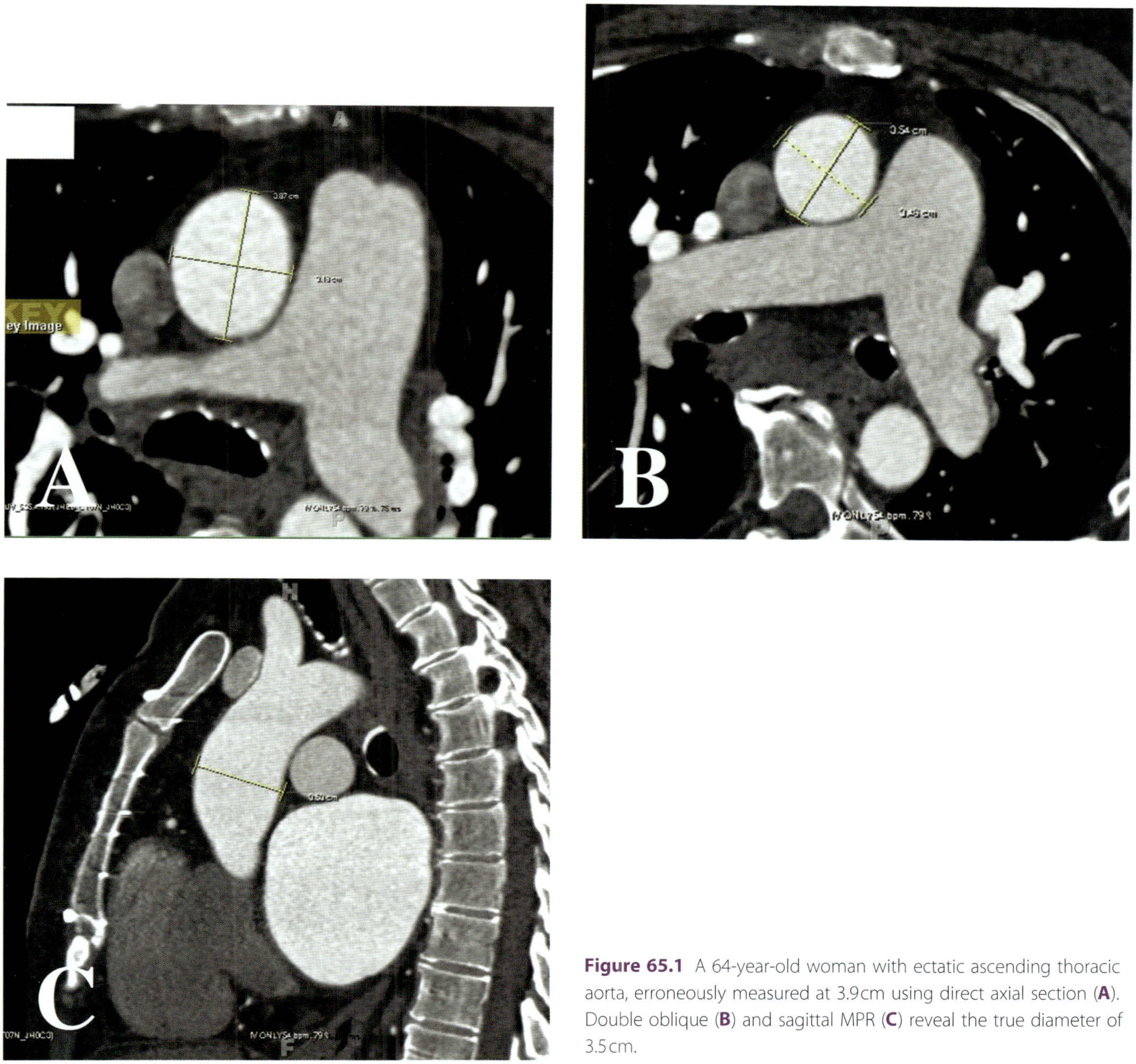

Figure 65.1 A 64-year-old woman with ectatic ascending thoracic aorta, erroneously measured at 3.9cm using direct axial section (**A**). Double oblique (**B**) and sagittal MPR (**C**) reveal the true diameter of 3.5cm.

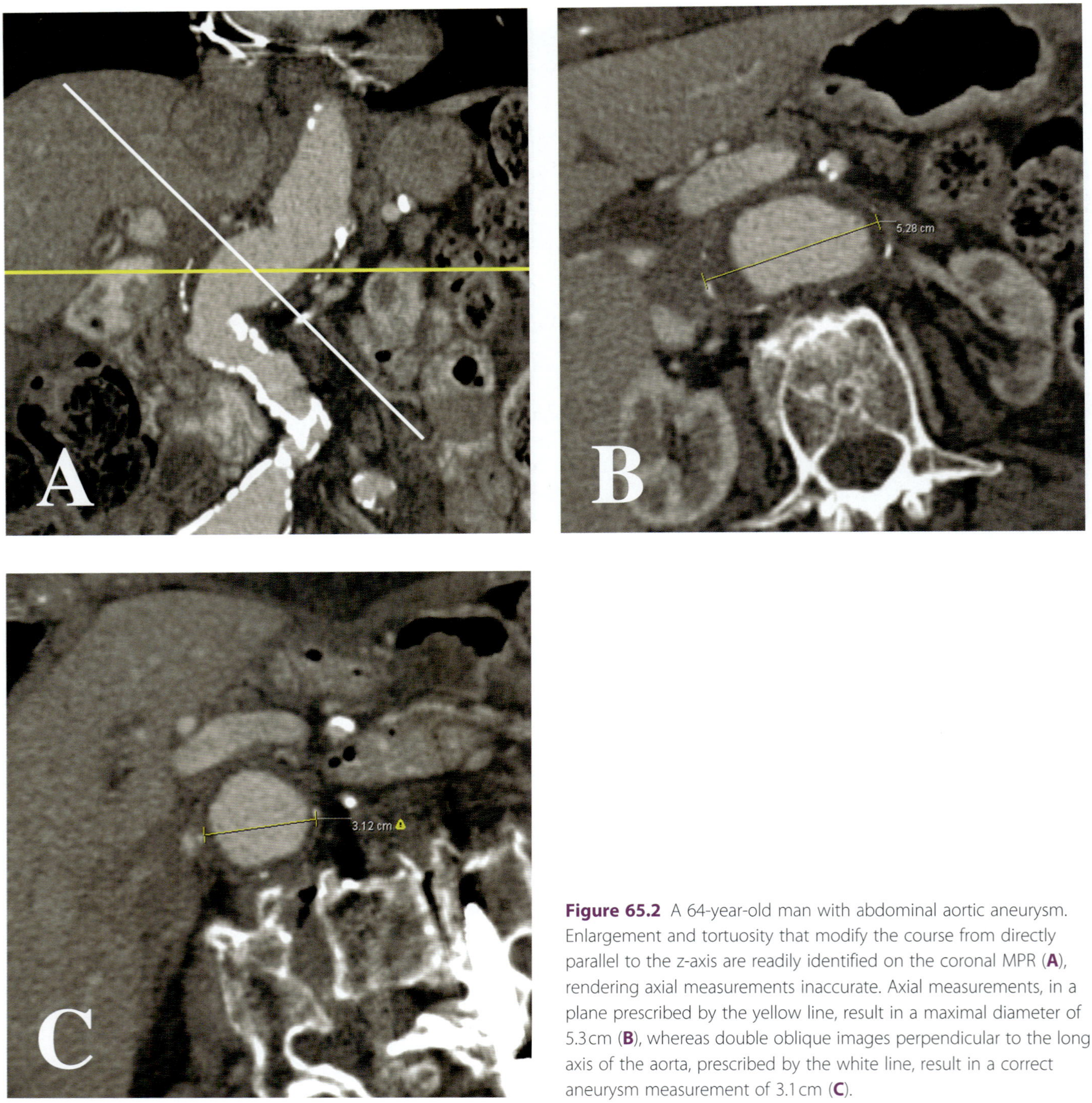

Figure 65.2 A 64-year-old man with abdominal aortic aneurysm. Enlargement and tortuosity that modify the course from directly parallel to the z-axis are readily identified on the coronal MPR (**A**), rendering axial measurements inaccurate. Axial measurements, in a plane prescribed by the yellow line, result in a maximal diameter of 5.3 cm (**B**), whereas double oblique images perpendicular to the long axis of the aorta, prescribed by the white line, result in a correct aneurysm measurement of 3.1 cm (**C**).

CASE 66

Surgical pledget mimicking aortic pseudoaneurysm

Stefan L. Zimmerman

Imaging description

In patients with prior cardiothoracic surgery requiring cardiopulmonary bypass, felt pledgets are used to ensure hemostasis during closure of cannula sites in the ascending aorta. On imaging, these pledgets are high attenuation and are located immediately adjacent to the aortic wall in the high ascending aorta (Figure 66.1).[1] Sometimes on axial source images these high-attenuation foci can mimic small pseudoaneurysms. Correct diagnosis of surgical material can be made by inspection of volume-rendered images, which will often show a rectangular shape (Figures 66.1 and 66.2). Non-contrast images, if available, will also be helpful for showing pledgets as high-attenuation precontrast (Figure 66.1).

Importance

Misdiagnosis of pseudoaneurysm of the ascending aorta can lead to inappropriate additional follow-up scans or, in the worst case scenario, repeat surgery.

Typical clinical scenario

Felt pledgets are used for suturing of cannula sites when cardiopulmonary bypass is used, such as for cardiac surgery or thoracic aortic repair.

Differential diagnosis

Surgical material should be distinguished from true aortic pseudoaneurysms, which can occur at cannula sites or anastomoses due to suture break down after thoracic surgery.[2] These will be recognized by a narrow-necked connection to the aortic lumen and attenuation that is similar to blood pool on both pre- and post-contrast imaging.

Teaching point

Felt pledgets adjacent to the ascending aorta in patients with prior cardiothoracic surgery should not be mistaken for pseudoaneurysms. High attenuation on precontrast scans and characteristic shape on volume-rendered reconstructions will allow definitive diagnosis.

REFERENCES

1. B. Sundaram, L. E. Quint, H. J. Patel, G. M. Deeb. CT findings following thoracic aortic surgery. *Radiographics* 2007; **27**: 1583–94.
2. L. C. Chu, D. E. Cameron, P. T. Johnson, E. K. Fishman. MDCT evaluation of postoperative aortic root pseudoaneurysms: imaging pearls and pitfalls. *AJR Am J Roentgenol* 2012; **199**: W84–90.

Pearls and Pitfalls in Cardiovascular Imaging, ed. Stefan L. Zimmerman and Elliot K. Fishman. Published by Cambridge University Press. © Cambridge University Press 2015.

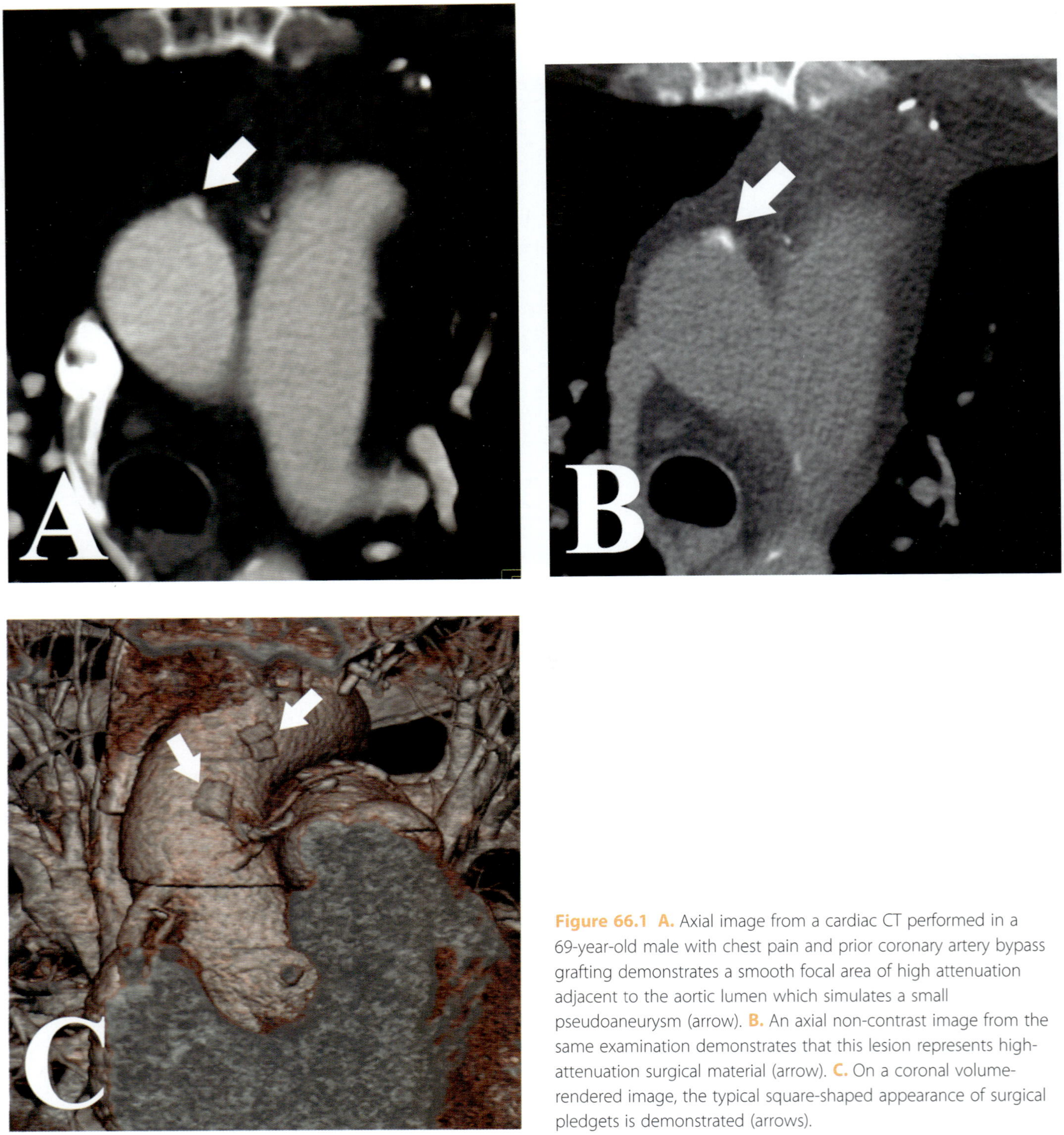

Figure 66.1 **A.** Axial image from a cardiac CT performed in a 69-year-old male with chest pain and prior coronary artery bypass grafting demonstrates a smooth focal area of high attenuation adjacent to the aortic lumen which simulates a small pseudoaneurysm (arrow). **B.** An axial non-contrast image from the same examination demonstrates that this lesion represents high-attenuation surgical material (arrow). **C.** On a coronal volume-rendered image, the typical square-shaped appearance of surgical pledgets is demonstrated (arrows).

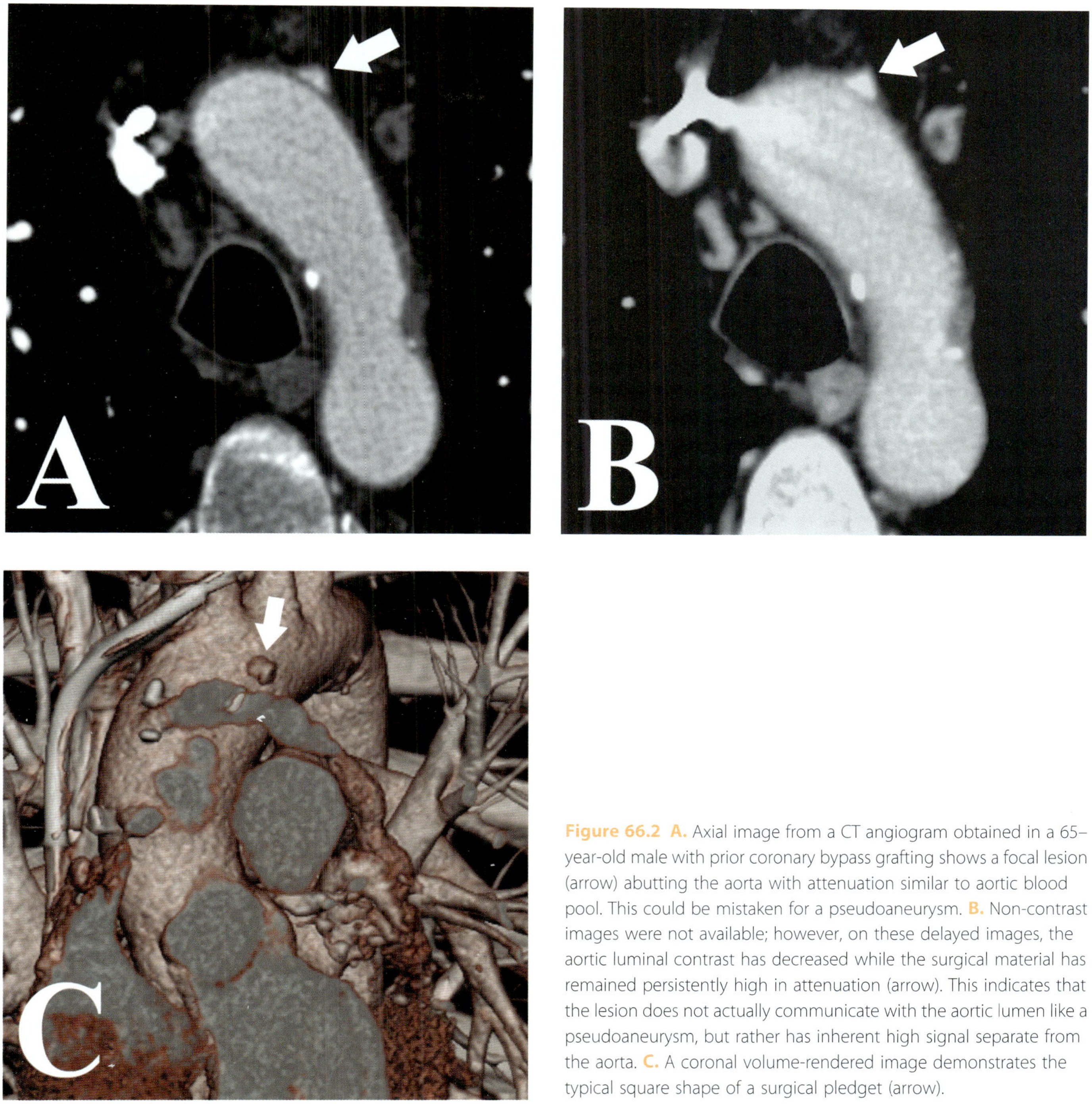

Figure 66.2 **A.** Axial image from a CT angiogram obtained in a 65-year-old male with prior coronary bypass grafting shows a focal lesion (arrow) abutting the aorta with attenuation similar to aortic blood pool. This could be mistaken for a pseudoaneurysm. **B.** Non-contrast images were not available; however, on these delayed images, the aortic luminal contrast has decreased while the surgical material has remained persistently high in attenuation (arrow). This indicates that the lesion does not actually communicate with the aortic lumen like a pseudoaneurysm, but rather has inherent high signal separate from the aorta. **C.** A coronal volume-rendered image demonstrates the typical square shape of a surgical pledget (arrow).

CASE 67

Pseudoendoleak post-endovascular stent graft placement due to calcified material in the aneurysm sac

Pamela T. Johnson

Imaging description

CT is the primary imaging modality used to evaluate patients after endoluminal stent placement. The role of CT is to confirm that the aortic pathology (aneurysm and/or dissection) has been excluded, demonstrate that the aortic branches remain patent, and to identify complications, most commonly the presence of an endoleak. An endoleak occurs when blood extends into the aneurysm sac outside of the stent, either by retrograde perfusion from an aortic arterial branch, leak from the proximal or distal end of the stent, or through the stent graft or where adjacent stent grafts overlap.[1] Serial post-treatment CT imaging should demonstrate gradual decrease in the size of the excluded aneurysm sac. In the presence of an endoleak, the sac will stay the same or enlarge.

When performing CT after endoluminal stent placement, a precontrast acquisition is necessary for distinguishing calcification or surgical material within the aneurysm sac from an endoleak, and improves specificity and positive predictive value in identifying endoleaks.[2,3] As shown in this case, high-attenuation calcification within an aneurysm sac can mimic an endoleak on post-contrast CT, but is definitively characterized as calcification by comparing to a non-contrast acquisition (Figure 67.1).

Importance

Calcification or surgical material within the aneurysm sac may mimic endoleak if only post-contrast images are obtained. Proper protocol design is an integral component to high-quality diagnostic interpretation. Knowledge of pitfalls such as this mandates use of a precontrast acquisition following endoluminal stent placement to serve as comparison for the post-contrast sequences. Endoleaks may be followed if small, but can require reintervention. If left untreated, an endoleak can eventually result in rupture of the aneurysm sac.[1]

Typical clinical scenario

Patients typically undergo lifelong serial follow-up imaging after the endovascular stent has been placed.[1] Approximately 25% develop an endoleak, most commonly type II.[1,4] Delayed endoleaks occur in 10% on average, with reports as high as 30%.[4]

Differential diagnosis

The primary differential consideration in the patient status post-endovascular stent placement is whether high density within the aneurysm sac reflects the presence of calcification or surgical material or is contrast extravasation reflecting the presence of an endoleak.

Teaching point

CT protocol optimization for endovascular stent follow-up requires use of a precontrast series, to serve as a comparison to post-contrast acquisitions and distinguish the potential etiologies for high density within the aneurysm sac.

REFERENCES

1. Stavropoulos SW, Charagundla SR. Imaging techniques for detection and management of endoleaks after endovascular aortic aneurysm repair. *Radiology* 2007;**243**:641–55.

2. Iezzi R, Cotroneo AR, Filippone A, Di Fabio F, Quinto F, Colosimo C, Bonomo L. Multidetector CT in abdominal aortic aneurysm treated with endovascular repair: are unenhanced and delayed-phase enhanced images effective for endoleak detection? *Radiology* 2006;**241**:915–21.

3. Rozenblit AM, Patlas M, Rosenbaum AT, Okhi T, Veith FJ, Laks MP, Ricci ZJ. Detection of endoleaks after endovascular repair of abdominal aortic aneurysm: value of unenhanced and delayed helical CT acquisitions. *Radiology* 2003;**227**:426–33.

4. Veith FJ, Baum RA, Ohki T, et al. Nature and significance of endoleaks and endotension: summary of opinions expressed at an international conference. *J Vasc Surg* 2002;**35**:1029–35.

Pearls and Pitfalls in Cardiovascular Imaging, ed. Stefan L. Zimmerman and Elliot K. Fishman. Published by Cambridge University Press. © Cambridge University Press 2015.

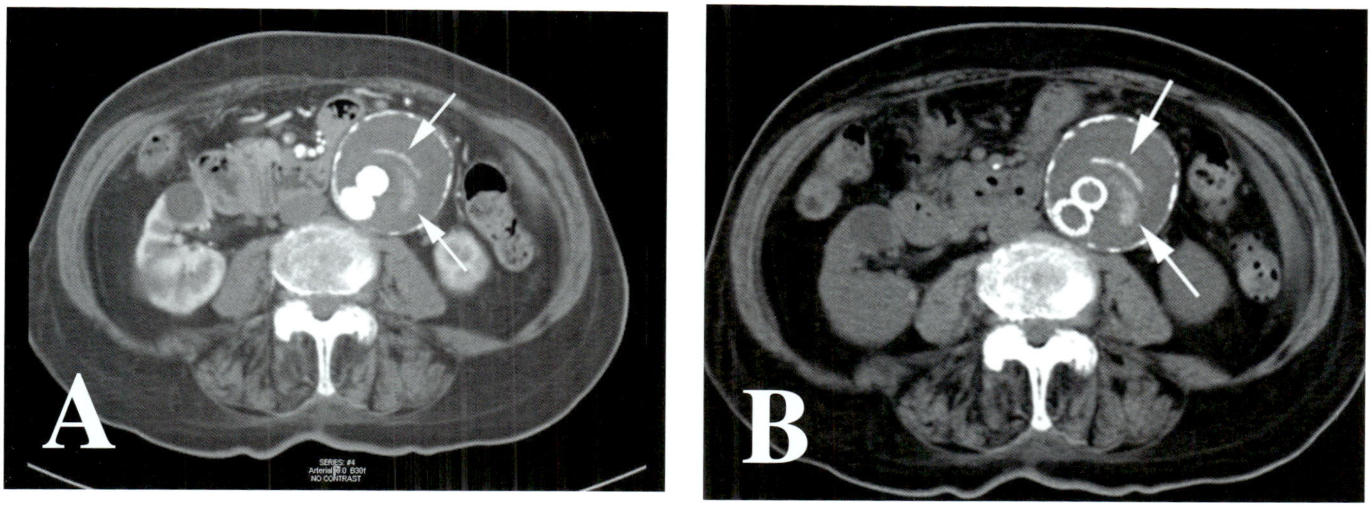

Figure 67.1 A 92-year-old woman status post-endovascular stent repair of infrarenal abdominal aortic aneurysm. High attenuation crescents within the aneurysm sac (arrows) could be mistaken for endoleak on the arterial phase post-contrast CT (**A**) but are confirmed as calcification on the precontrast acquisition (**B**). Reprinted with permission from Johnson P, Routine use of precontrast and delayed acquisitions in abdominal CT: time for change. *Abdom Imaging*. 2012; **38**.

CASE 68

Type II endoleak occult on arterial phase images

Pamela T. Johnson

Imaging description

Following endovascular stent repair of abdominal aortic aneurysms, the most common complication is a type II endoleak. Endoleaks occur when blood continues to flow into the aneurysm sac after the procedure, carrying the risk of continued aneurysm expansion. On CT, endoleaks are identified by the presence of intravenous contrast within the aneurysm sac around the stent, which should normally be completely thrombosed. Five subtypes of endoleaks exist, but only types I–III will show contrast in the aneurysm sac at CT. These endoleaks are classified by the source of blood flow. In type II endoleaks, there is reperfusion of the aneurysm sac by aortic branch vessels. These are typically the inferior mesenteric artery or a lumbar artery branch, and are located anterior or posterior in the aneurysm sac depending on the feeding vessel.[1]

Identification of a type II endoleak hinges on protocol optimization. The literature supports use of multiple acquisitions[2–5] and narrow reconstruction sections[6] to maximize likelihood of detecting an endoleak. With respect to the relative utility of different phases after contrast infusion, several studies have confirmed that use of delayed acquisition enables identification of more endoleaks than use of only an arterial phase acquisition. While many endoleaks are more conspicuous on the arterial phase, some will be more conspicuous or only visualized on the delayed phase (Figures 68.1and 68.2).[7]

Importance

Studies show that more than half of type II endoleaks will resolve spontaneously,[8–9] particularly those that do not result in enlargement of the aneurysm sac. However, the risk of a persistent endoleak is expansion of the aneurysm sac, which can result in rupture despite the presence of a stent. Arterial and delayed venous phase acquisitions are recommended for endovascular stent follow-up to avoid missing small type II endoleaks that may only be visible on the delayed phase.

Typical clinical scenario

Type II endoleaks occur in 19–24% of patients who undergo endovascular stent repair of an abdominal aortic aneurysm and account for 40% of endoleaks.[1,8,9] These can be identified on the first follow up CT examination, or develop later.

Differential diagnosis

The differential diagnosis of an endoleak is either calcification or surgical material within the aneurysm sac, which is distinguished by correlation with a precontrast acquisition.

Teaching point

Although type II endoleaks are the result of vascular reperfusion by an arterial branch, a small percentage of these are optimally visualized only on delayed acquisitions. Imaging protocols for post-stent evaluation should include precontrast, arterial, and delayed phases to avoid missing small type II endoleaks.

REFERENCES

1. Bashir MR, Ferral H, Jacobs C, McCarthy W, Goldin M. Endoleaks after endovascular abdominal aortic aneurysm repair: management strategies according to CT findings. *AJR Am J Roentgenol.* 2009; **192**: W178–186.

2. Golzarian J, Dussaussois L, Abada HT, Gevenois PA, Van Gansbeke D, Ferreira J, Struyven J. Helical CT of aorta after endoluminal stent-graft therapy: value of biphasic acquisition. *AJR Am J Roentgenol.* 1998; **171**:329–331.

3. Rozenblit AM, Patlas M, Rosenbaum AT, et al. Detection of endoleaks after endovascular repair of abdominal aortic aneurysm: value of unenhanced and delayed helical CT acquisitions. *Radiology.* 2003; **227**:426–433.

4. Iezzi R, Cotroneo AR, Filippone A, et al. Multidetector CT in abdominal aortic aneurysm treated with endovascular repair: are unenhanced and delayed phase enhanced images effective for endoleak detection? *Radiology.* 2006; **241**:915–921.

5. Iezzi R, Cotroneo AR, Filippone A, Santoro M, Basilico R, Storto ML. Multidetector-row computed tomography angiography in abdominal aortic aneurysm treated with endovascular repair: evaluation of optimal timing of delayed phase imaging for the detection of low-flow endoleaks. *J Comput Assist Tomogr.* 2008; **32**:609–615.

6. Iezzi R, Cotroneo AR, Filippone A, Di Fabio F, Santoro M, Storto ML. MDCT angiography in abdominal aortic aneurysm treated with endovascular repair: diagnostic impact of slice thickness on detection of endoleaks. *AJR Am J Roentgenol.* 2007; **189**:1414–1420.

7. Johnson PT, Fishman EK. Routine use of precontrast and delayed acquisitions in abdominal CT: time for change. *Abdom Imaging.* 2013; **38**:215–233.

8. Jones JE, Atkins MD, Brewster DC, Chung TK, Kwolek CJ, LaMuraglia GM, Hodgman TM, Cambria RP. Persistent type 2 endoleak after endovascular repair of abdominal aortic aneurysm is associated with adverse late outcomes. *J Vasc Surg.* 2007;**46**:1–8.

9. Tolia AJ, Landis R, Lamparello P, Rosen R, Macari M. Type II endoleaks after endovascular repair of abdominal aortic aneurysms: natural history. *Radiology.* 2005;**235**:683–686. Epub 2005 Mar 9.

Pearls and Pitfalls in Cardiovascular Imaging, ed. Stefan L. Zimmerman and Elliot K. Fishman. Published by Cambridge University Press. © Cambridge University Press 2015.

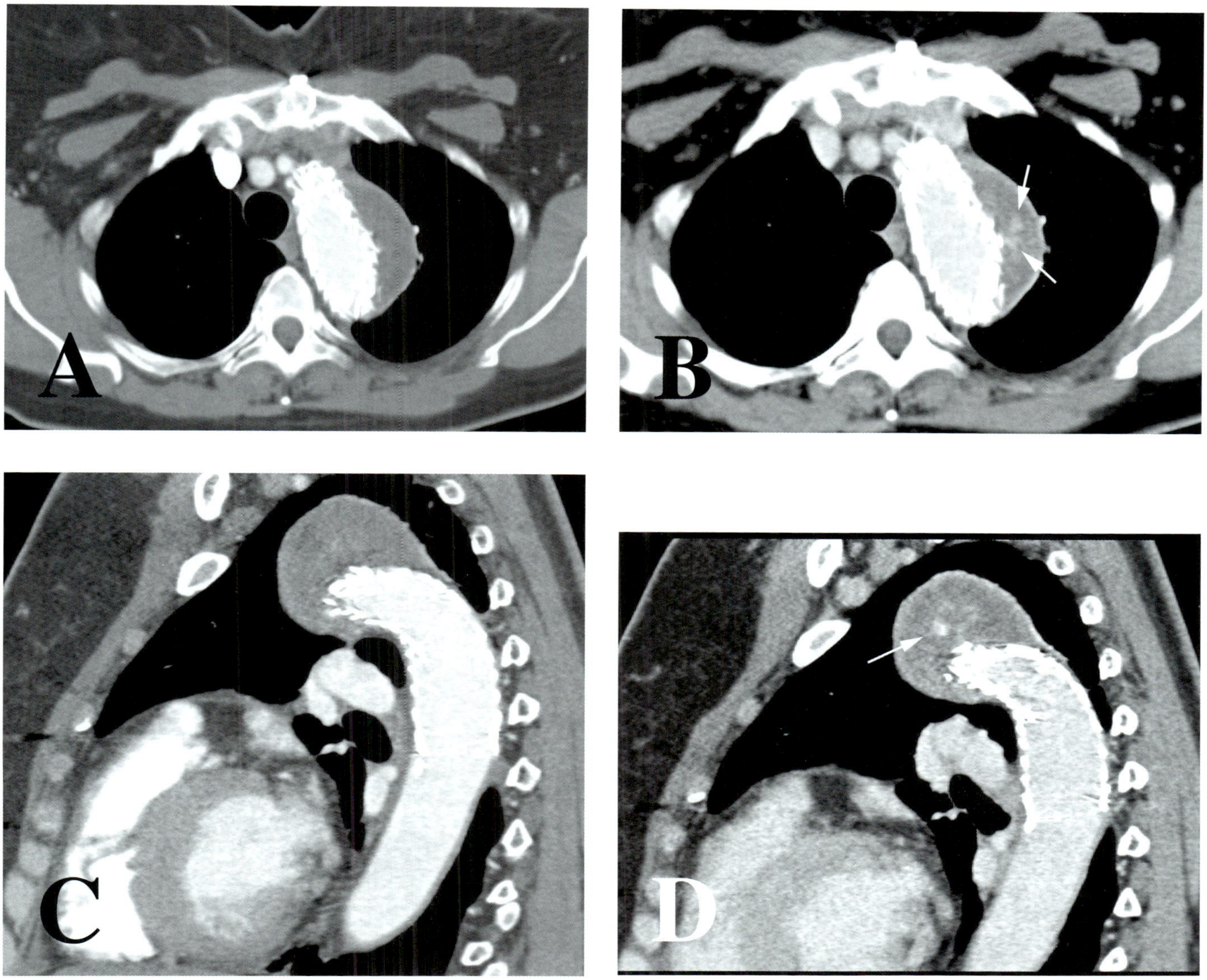

Figure 68.1 A 52-year-old woman status post-endoluminal stent grafting of the descending thoracic aorta for contained rupture. Axial arterial phase (A), axial venous phase (B), sagittal arterial phase (C), and sagittal venous phase (D) show an endoleak (arrow) that is only visualized on the venous acquisition. Reprinted with permission from Johnson P, Routine use of precontrast and delayed acquisitions in abdominal CT : time for change. *Abdom Imaging* 2012; **38**.

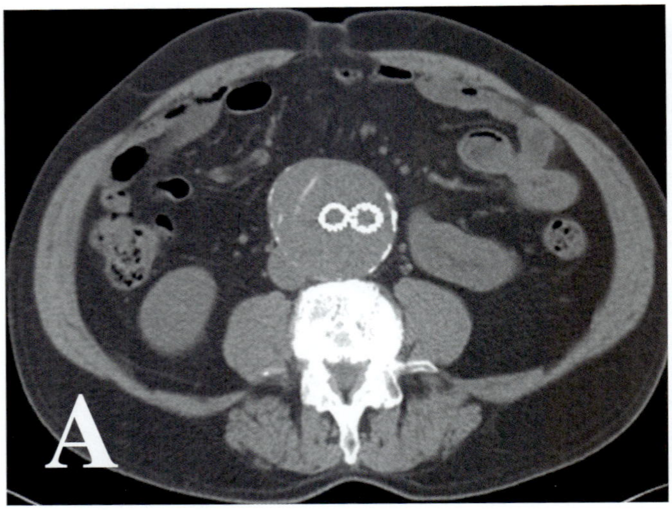

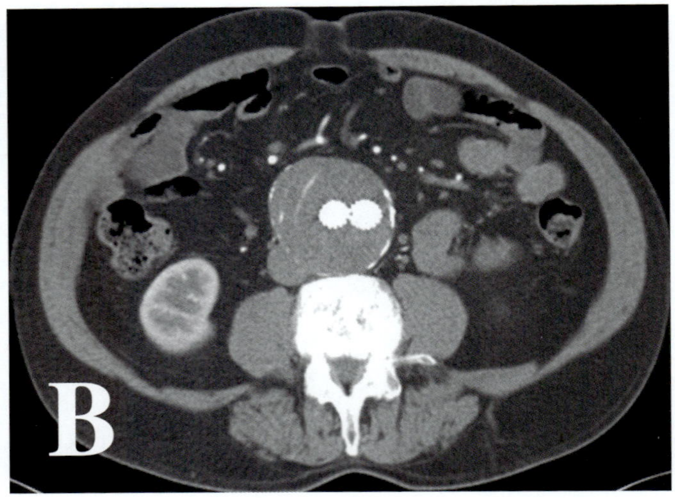

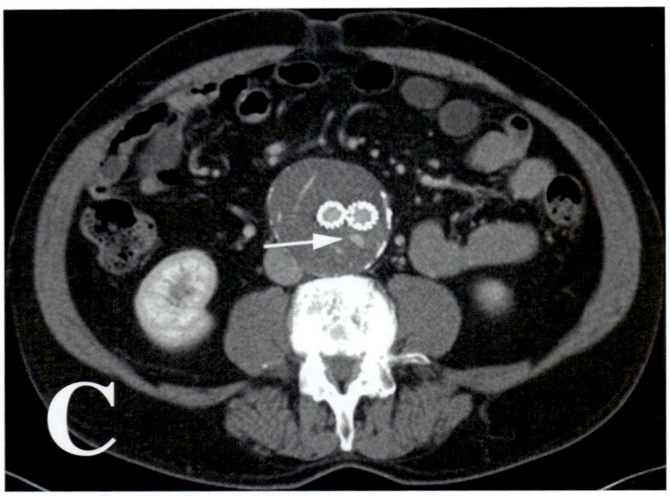

Figure 68.2 A 76-year-old male status post-endoluminal stent grafting of the abdominal aorta for a 7.1 cm aneurysm. Axial non-contrast (**A**), axial arterial phase (**B**), and axial venous phase show an endoleak (arrow) that is only visualized on the venous acquisition.

CASE 69

Elephant trunk graft mimicking aortic dissection

Pamela T. Johnson

Imaging description

Patients who require staged thoracic aneurysm surgery may have an "elephant trunk" prosthesis placed during the first surgery. The proximal graft is sutured into the aortic arch, while the distal edges of the graft are freely mobile within the lumen of the descending thoracic aorta (Figures 69.1 and 69.2). Owing to the configuration, the free edges of the distal end of the graft can simulate an intraluminal dissection on axial CT. Correlation with surgical history and review of 2D MPRs and 3D renderings enables the radiologist to make the correct interpretation of a normal elephant trunk prosthesis. The surgical procedure and typical imaging appearance have been described in detail in the literature.[1–4]

The free-floating graft serves to protect the descending thoracic aorta prior to the second surgery. It is then incorporated into either a surgical graft or endoluminal stent graft during repair of the descending aorta. Because the graft is positioned in the descending thoracic aorta, the second surgery can be performed at a distance from the first in unaltered anatomic planes; reoperating in the same location carries a high risk of hemorrhage. Patients may alternatively undergo endoluminal stent repair of the descending thoracic aorta. The elephant trunk graft has radiodense markers on the distal end (Figure 69.3), to enable localization during fluoroscopic endovascular stent placement.

It is important to distinguish the normal appearance from potential complications of this type of graft. These include graft entrapment in the patients with a residual dissection; the graft can migrate into one lumen and preferentially supply the blood flow to that lumen. Surgeons will excise the most cranial extent of the dissection to prevent this complication. Additionally, aneurysmal dilatation of the more distal aorta has been reported.[5] Ideally, this graft is a temporary structure that is incorporated into the final repair in a timely fashion to prevent such complication.

Importance

Misdiagnosis of the normal elephant trunk prosthesis as a dissection of the descending thoracic aorta can lead to unnecessary patient anxiety, additional imaging examinations, and potentially inappropriate interventions.

Typical clinical scenario

Patients with extensive aortic pathology (aneurysm, dissection) who require staged surgery are candidates for an elephant trunk prosthesis.

Differential diagnosis

The differential diagnosis for a linear intraluminal filling defect in the aorta of a patient with prior elephant trunk repair is either a graft or a dissection flap. Critical to correct interpretation in this case is an understanding of the CT appearance of the elephant trunk prosthesis in the descending thoracic aorta and knowledge of the surgical procedure performed.

Teaching point

Radiologists must be aware of the CT appearance of an elephant trunk prosthesis in a patient who has undergone the first of two-stage surgical procedures to repair extensive pathology of the thoracic aorta.

REFERENCES

1. Prescott-Focht JA, Martinez-Jimenez S, Hurwitz LM, Hoang JK, Christensen JD, Ghoshhajra BB, Abbara S. Ascending thoracic aorta: postoperative imaging evaluation. *Radiographics*. 2013; **33**:73–85.
2. Johnson PT, Corl FM, Black JH, Fishman EK. The elephant trunk procedure for aortic aneurysm repair: an illustrated guide to surgical technique with CT correlation. *AJR Am J Roentgenol*. 2011; **197**:W1052–1059.
3. Garrido JM, Miguelena J, Muñoz R, Prada P, Epeldegui A. Repair of multiple aneurysms of the thoracic aorta with a hybrid prosthesis. *J Card Surg*. 2011; **26**:197–200.
4. Jim J, Moon MR, Rubin BG, Sicard GA, Sanchez LA. Hybrid repair of distal arch aortic aneurysms: endovascular elephant trunk completion. *Ann Vasc Surg*. 2011; **25**:598–604.
5. Higuchi T, Takahashi T, Ishizaka T, Yoshioka D, Shirakawa Y, Kuratani T, Sawa Y. Rapid expansion of another downstream aortic aneurysm with the elephant trunk. *Gen Thorac Cardiovasc Surg*. 2010; **58**:617–619.

Pearls and Pitfalls in Cardiovascular Imaging, ed. Stefan L. Zimmerman and Elliot K. Fishman. Published by Cambridge University Press. © Cambridge University Press 2015.

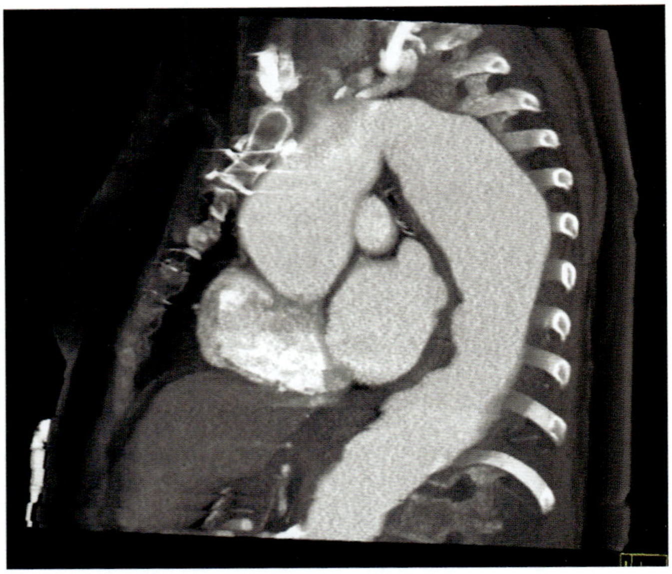

Figure 69.1 Preoperative sagittal oblique MPR from IV contrast-enhanced CT in an 81-year-old woman with extenstive thoracic aortic aneurysm involving ascending and descending thoracic aorta.

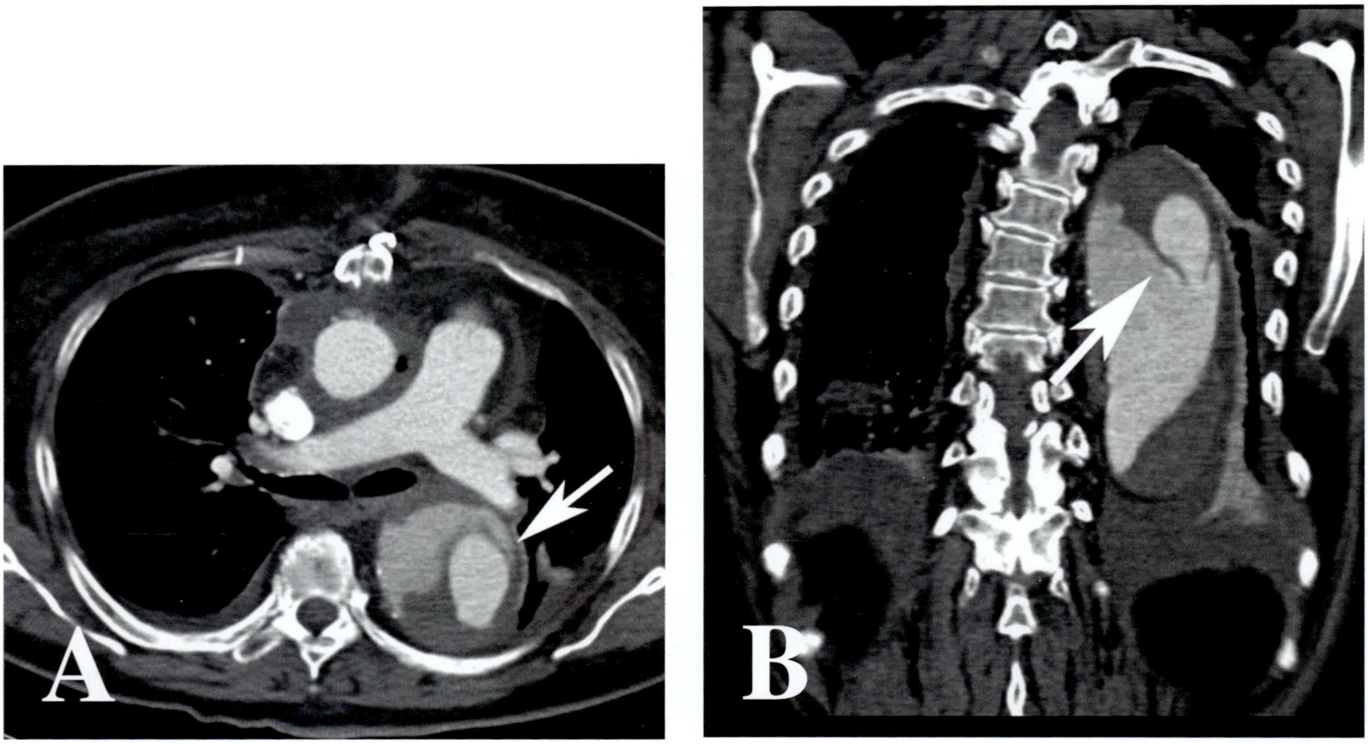

Figure 69.2 Post-operative CT in same patient as Figure 69.1. Axial section (**A**), coronal (**B**) and sagittal (**C**) MPRs from IV contrast-enhanced CT show the elephant trunk prosthesis (arrows) in the descending thoracic aorta. Cognizance of this normal post-operative appearance is critical to preventing misdiagnosis of post-operative aortic dissection.

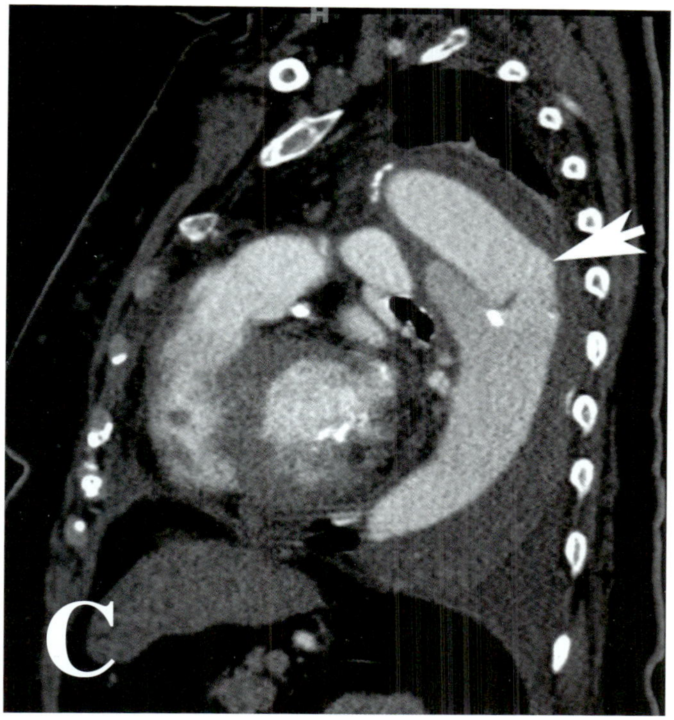

Figure 69.2 *(cont.)*

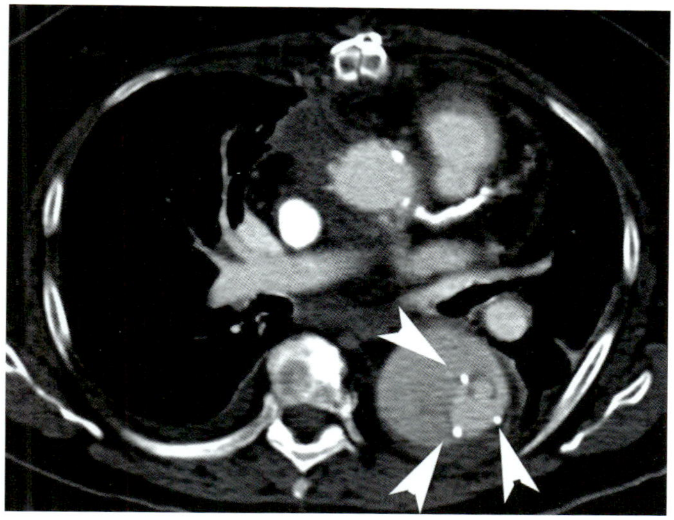

Figure 69.3 Same patient as Figure 69.1. Axial section through the lower edge of the elephant trunk graft shows radiodense markers (arrowheads), which can be used to localize the end of the graft during fluoroscopic endovascular stent repair of the descending thoracic aorta.

CASE 70

Pseudodissection due to aortic graft kinking

Stefan L. Zimmerman

Imaging description

Prosthetic aortic grafts often have areas of kinking where there is in-folding of the graft wall into the aortic lumen. This is a normal post-operative finding that is generally of no clinical consequence. On axial images, vertically oriented folds will have the appearance of an intraluminal flap and can mimic dissection (Figures 70.1 and 70.2).[1,2] Inspection of sagittal and coronal planes and volume-rendered images will allow visualization of the kinked segment and exclusion of dissection.

Importance

It is important to avoid misdiagnosis of aortic dissection as it may lead to unnecessary surgery or repeat imaging.

Typical clinical scenario

Kinking in the aortic graft is common in patients with prior open graft repair of the thoracic or abdominal aorta.

Differential diagnosis

Aortic graft kinking should be distinguished from a true aortic dissection. Careful inspection of multiplanar and 3D reformatted images should allow visualization of the kinking and prevent misdiagnosis. The location of abnormality can also be helpful as dissections do not occur within prosthetic aortic graft material. Dissections may, however, occur in the native aorta immediately adjacent to an anastomosis.

Teaching point

Kinking of aortic grafts after open aortic repair is common and can result in linear intraluminal filling defects that mimic dissection on axial images. The use of multiplanar reformatted and volume-rendered images will allow visualization of the kinked segment and help avoid misdiagnosis.

REFERENCES

1. J. K. Hoang, S. Martinez, L. M. Hurwitz. MDCT angiography after open thoracic aortic surgery: pearls and pitfalls. *AJR Am J Roentgenol* 2009; **192**: W20–7.
2. B. Sundaram, L. E. Quint, H. J. Patel, G. M. Deeb. CT findings following thoracic aortic surgery. *Radiographics* 2007; **27**: 1583–94.

Pearls and Pitfalls in Cardiovascular Imaging, ed. Stefan L. Zimmerman and Elliot K. Fishman. Published by Cambridge University Press. © Cambridge University Press 2015.

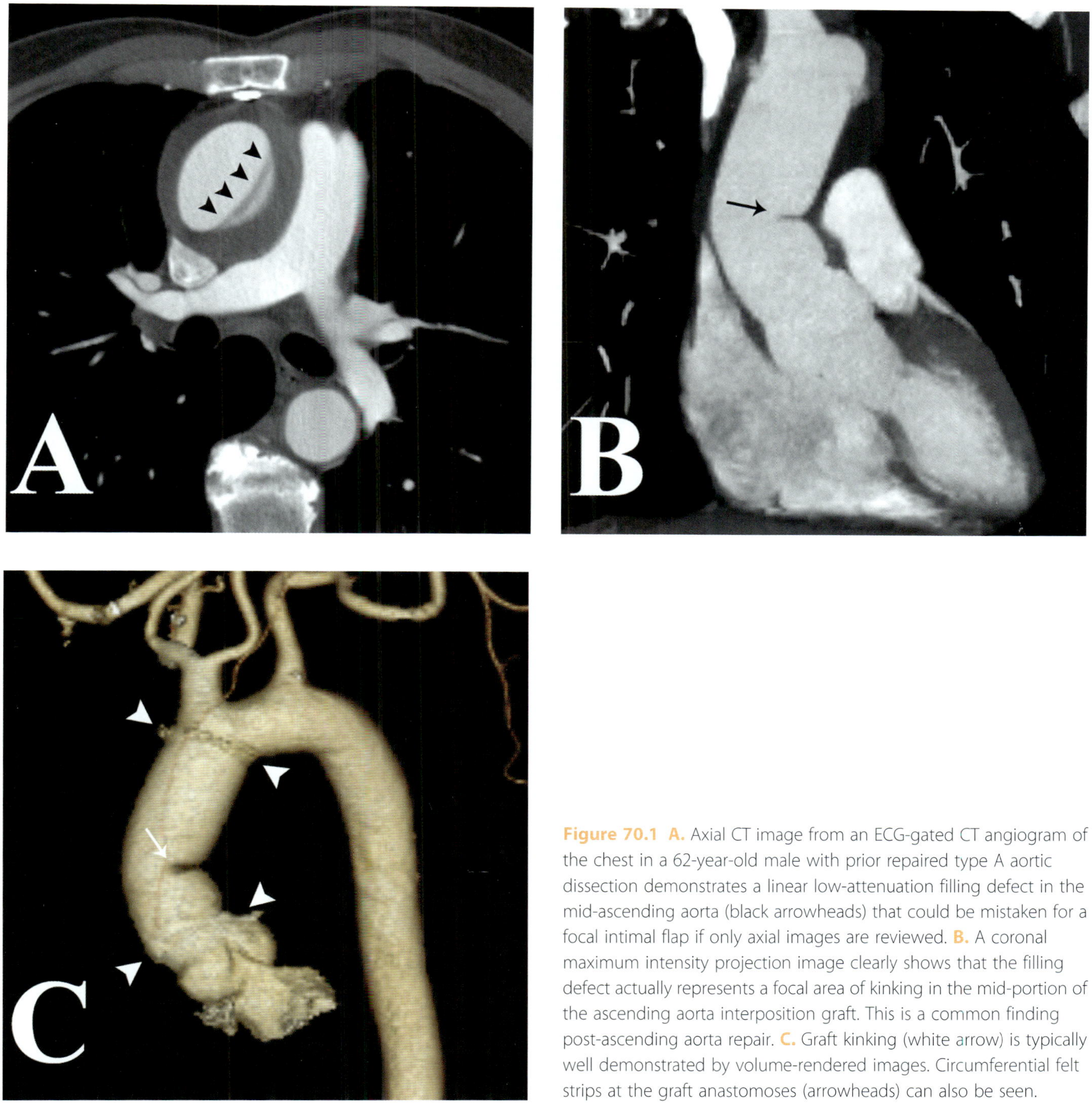

Figure 70.1 **A.** Axial CT image from an ECG-gated CT angiogram of the chest in a 62-year-old male with prior repaired type A aortic dissection demonstrates a linear low-attenuation filling defect in the mid-ascending aorta (black arrowheads) that could be mistaken for a focal intimal flap if only axial images are reviewed. **B.** A coronal maximum intensity projection image clearly shows that the filling defect actually represents a focal area of kinking in the mid-portion of the ascending aorta interposition graft. This is a common finding post-ascending aorta repair. **C.** Graft kinking (white arrow) is typically well demonstrated by volume-rendered images. Circumferential felt strips at the graft anastomoses (arrowheads) can also be seen.

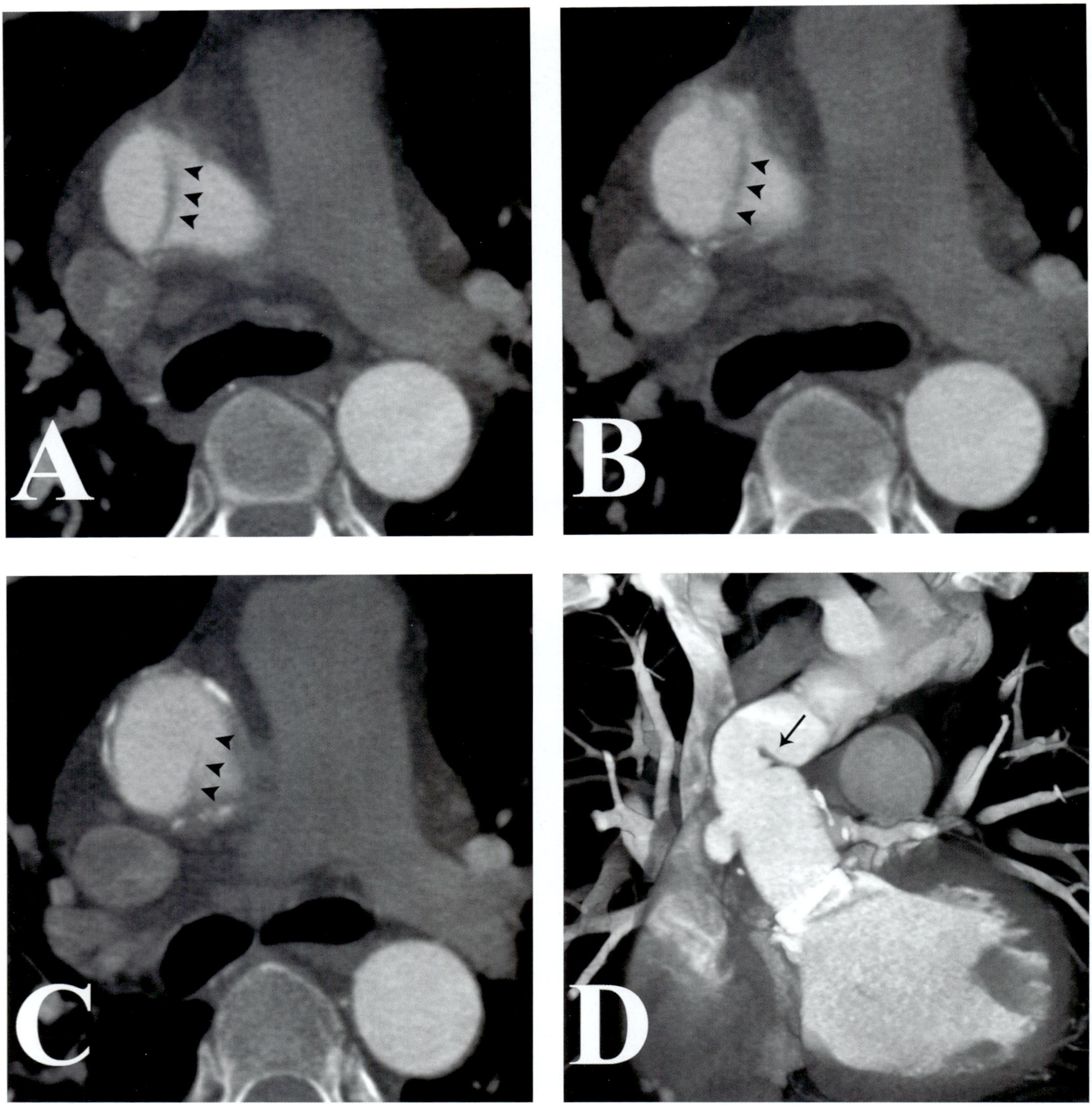

Figure 70.2 Three contiguous axial images (**A–C**) obtained from cranial (**A**) through caudal (**C**) in the region of the mid-ascending aorta in a 33-year-old male with a connective tissue disorder and prior aortic repair. There is a linear filling defect in the mid-ascending aorta that continues across several slices (black arrowheads), a finding that can be mistaken for a short dissection. However, on the coronal volume-rendered image (**D**), it is clear that this abnormality corresponds to a focal area of marked graft kinking (black arrow). This kinking is of no clinical significance but should not be mistaken for an acute aortic dissection or intimal injury.

CASE 71

Perigraft fluid collections

Stefan L. Zimmerman

Imaging description

Following ascending thoracic aorta surgery, it is common to identify fluid collections that surround the ascending aortic graft. These fluid collections are most often seen in the recent post-operative phase, are low in attenuation, and can range in thickness from millimeters to several centimeters (Figure 71.1).[1,2]

Importance

Perigraft fluid collections are important to distinguish from clinically significant causes of mediastinal fluid accumulation, namely post-operative mediastinal abscess or graft anastomotic dehissence.

Typical clinical scenario

Perigraft fluid collections are found in the majority of patients after graft repair of the ascending aorta and are generally of no clinical consequence.[1] These fluid collections will usually progressively decrease in size and resolve however, in some patients they may persist indefinitely (Figure 71.2).[1] The etiology of perigraft fluid collections is uncertain. In the immediate post-operative phase these collections have been postulated to represent evolving hematoma. Persistent collections may be due to an inflammatory response to graft material, something also noted in patients with prior open abdominal aneurysm repair.[3]

Post-operative perigraft fluid collections should be distinguished from infected fluid collections or anastomotic dehissence. Thickened, enhancing walls surrounding the collection, inflammatory changes in the mediastinal fat, gas, or extension of the fluid into the sternal wound are signs of infection. Increasing size of a perigraft fluid collection is an important finding that should raise suspicion for infection, anastomotic dehissence, or both. Extensive air can also be seen in the setting of an aortoesophageal fistula (Figure 71.3). The presence of new extraluminal contrast or pseudoaneurysm within the perigraft fluid is a definitive sign of anastomotic break down (Figure 71.3). In cases of slow or intermittent leaks, obvious signs of extraluminal contrast may be absent;[4] however, imaging will show a perigraft collection containing high-attenuation material due to hematoma.

Teaching point

Perigraft fluid collections are common following thoracic aortic surgery and usually insignificant. These collections should be closely inspected for evidence of enlargement, wall enhancement, gas, or new high-attenuation material that could be signs of infection or anastomotic dehissence.

REFERENCES

1. L. E. Quint, I. R. Francis, D. M. Williams, H. M. Monaghan, G. M. Deeb. Synthetic interposition grafts of the thoracic aorta: postoperative appearance on serial CT studies. *Radiology* 1999; **211**: 317–24.
2. B. Sundaram, L. E. Quint, S. Patel, H. J. Patel, G. M. Deeb. CT appearance of thoracic aortic graft complications. *AJR Am J Roentgenol* 2007; **188**: 1273–7.
3. A. K. Kadakol, T. J. Nypaver, J. C. Lin, et al. Frequency, risk factors, and management of perigraft seroma after open abdominal aortic aneurysm repair. *J Vasc Surg* 2011; **54**: 637–43.
4. B. Sundaram, L. E. Quint, H. J. Patel, G. M. Deeb. CT findings following thoracic aortic surgery. *Radiographics* 2007; **27**: 1583–94.

Pearls and Pitfalls in Cardiovascular Imaging, ed. Stefan L. Zimmerman and Elliot K. Fishman. Published by Cambridge University Press. © Cambridge University Press 2015.

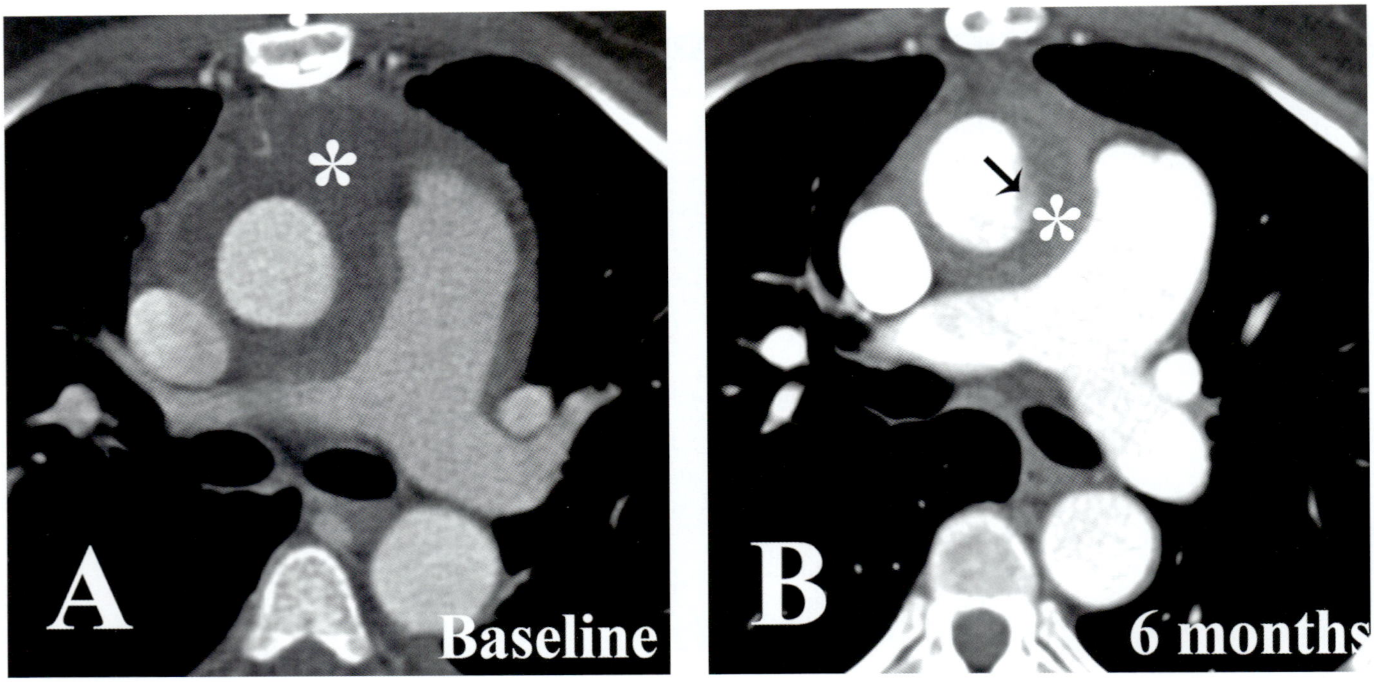

Figure 71.1 A. Axial contrast-enhanced CT image from a 42-year-old female post-operative from graft repair of the ascending aorta for acute type A intramural hematoma demonstrates a moderate-sized perigraft fluid collection (asterisk), not uncommon in the post-operative setting. **B.** Repeat CT of the chest obtained 6 months later shows decreased size of the perigraft fluid (asterisk), which will typically slowly resolve over time. Irregularity of the medial aortic graft wall is due to kinking of the graft material (black arrow).

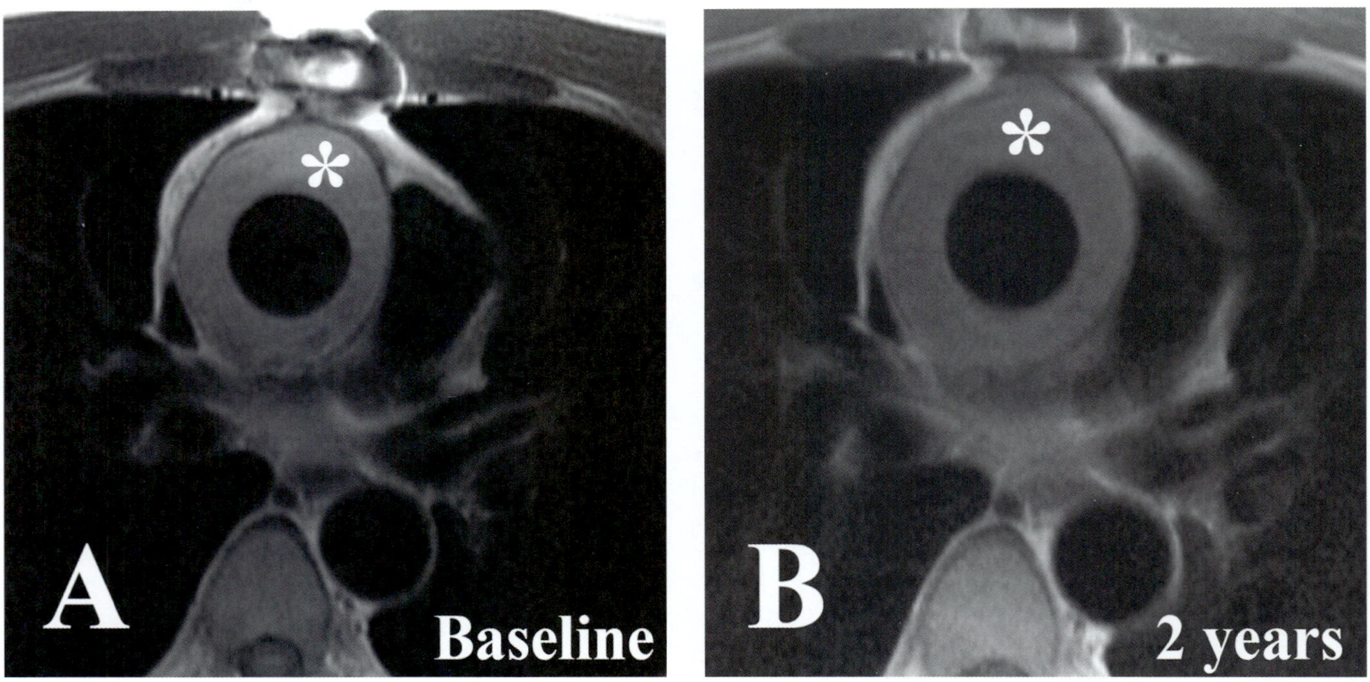

Figure 71.2 A. Axial dark blood spin echo image obtained from a thoracic MRI performed in a 47-year-old woman with recent graft repair of an ascending aortic aneurysm demonstrates an intermediate signal intensity perigraft fluid collection (asterisk). **B.** This fluid collection persists on subsequent follow-up MRI exam performed 2 years later with little change. **C.** On a follow-up contrast-enhanced CT of the chest performed 7 years later, there has been little change in the perigraft fluid collection. In some cases, perigraft fluid collections can remain stable indefinitely.

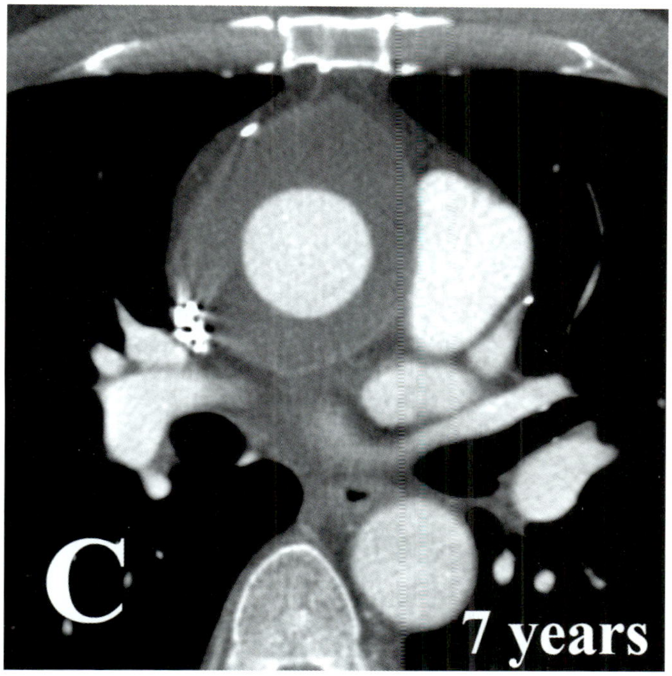

Figure 71.2 (*cont.*)

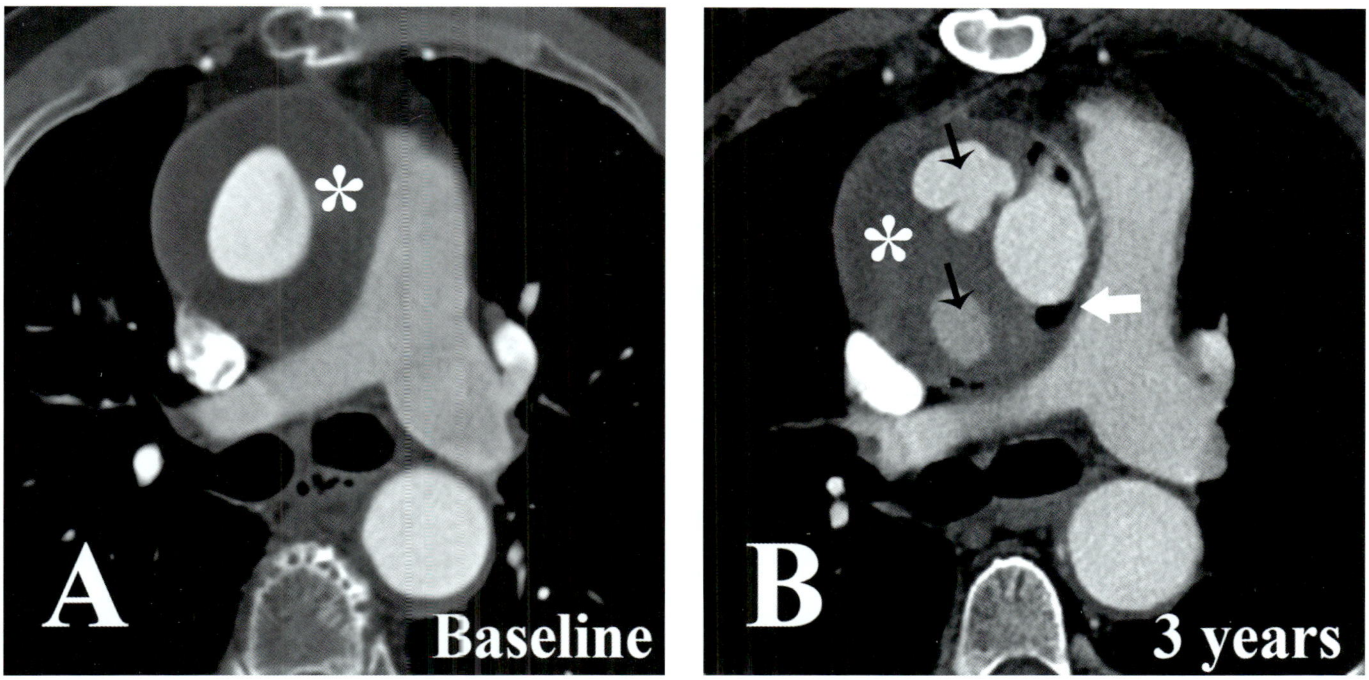

Figure 71.3 A. Axial contrast-enhanced CT examination of the chest obtained in a 75-year-old male with recent ascending aortic repair demonstrates a moderate-sized perigraft fluid collection (asterisk). B. On follow-up CT examination performed 3 years later for chest pain, the fluid collection (asterisk) has increased in size and now contains contrast (black arrows) and gas (white arrow). C. On a coronal image from the same examination, there is evidence of anastomotic dehissence (black arrow), with contrast leaking from the lumen, at the site of anastomosis, into the perigraft fluid. Extensive gas is also present in the perigraft collection (white arrow), which could be due to infection with gas-forming organisms or aortoesophageal fistula. This patient expired shortly after the CT scan due to massive gastrointestinal bleeding from an aortoesophageal fistula. Perigraft fluid collections that increase in size or demonstrate new contrast or gas should be viewed with suspicion for infection, dehissence, or both.

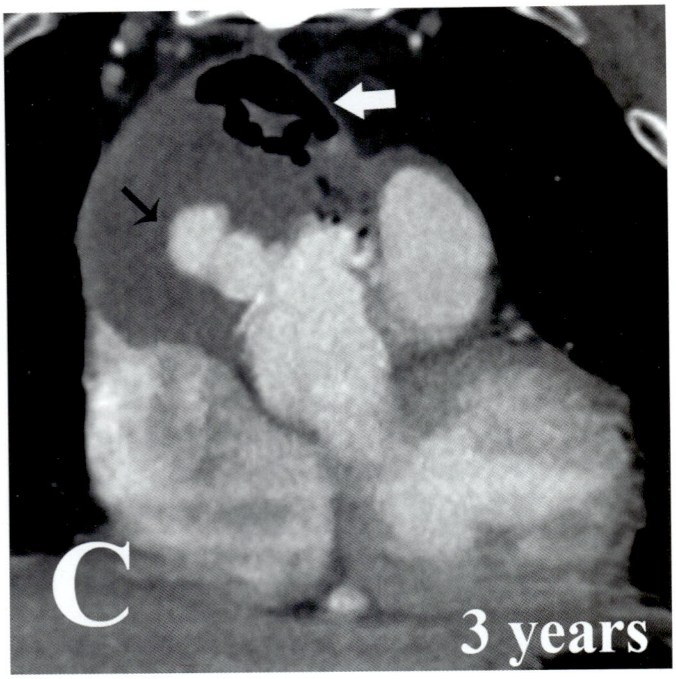

Figure 71.3 (cont.)

CASE 72

Post-operative air in the aorta: when is it of concern?

Saurabh Jha

Imaging description

The presence of air in the abdominal aorta[1] raises the possibility of recent surgery, instrumentation, infection (Figure 72.1) or aortoenteric fistula (AEF) (Figure 72.2).

Imaging features favoring post-surgical air include a fat plane between the aorta and bowel and no tethering of the bowel.[2] The presence of a fat plane essentially rules out AEF (Figure 72.3).

Importance

Air in the abdominal aorta may be a sign of important pathology or may be innocuous. Findings on imaging alone may not distinguish between the two. Specific inquiry should be made of the timing of intervention. Air is not atypical in the first 10 days after intervention.

Infection should be considered in a patient with fever and positive blood culture.

AEF is a surgical emergency and untreated can have a near-certain mortality. AEF can be clinically silent and imaging may provide the life-saving clues.

Typical clinical scenario

The patient is post-open or has a stent graft repair of abdominal aortic aneurysm. CT is obtained for surveillance or symptoms. Patients with AEF fistula may present with hematemesis, melena, sepsis, and abdominal pain. Air may be detected incidentally.

Differential diagnosis

The differential diagnosis for air in the aorta includes infection, aortoduodenal fistula, or instrumentation. Infection may lead to an aortoduodenal fistula and vice versa.

Teaching point

The presence of air in the abdominal aorta is both reflective of serious pathology and an expected finding post-intervention. Imagers should be aware of the bandwidth of possibilities and use findings on imaging and pertinent clinical information.

REFERENCES

1. Orton DF, LeVeen RF, Saigh JA, et al. Aortic prosthetic graft infections: radiologic manifestations and implications for management. *Radiographics* 2000; **20**: 977–993.
2. Vu QDM, Menias CO, Bhalla S, et al. Aortoenteric fistulas: CT features and potential mimics. *Radiographics* 2009; **29**: 197–209.

Pearls and Pitfalls in Cardiovascular Imaging, ed. Stefan L. Zimmerman and Elliot K. Fishman. Published by Cambridge University Press. © Cambridge University Press 2015.

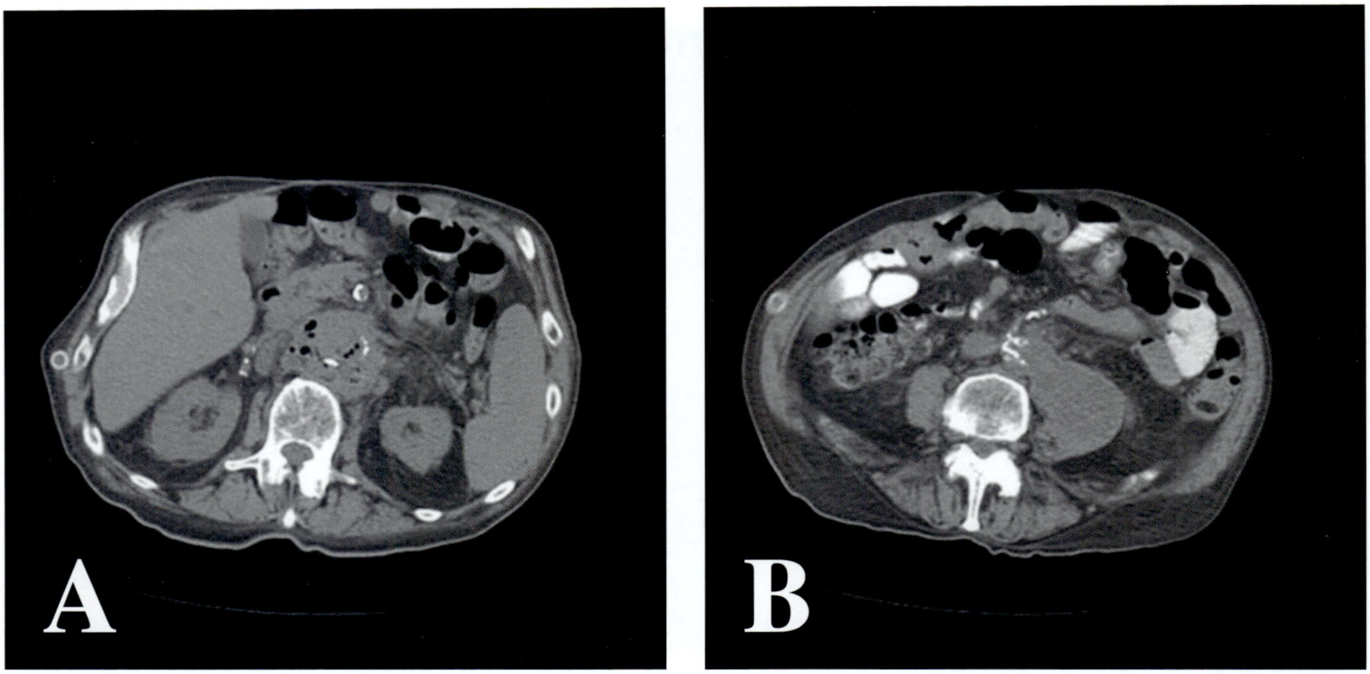

Figure 72.1 **A.** and **B.** A 68-year-old female with sepsis. Axial unenhanced CT shows extensive air in the abdominal aorta in a haphazard distribution. There was no antecedent history of instrumentation. The patient had an infected aortic aneurysm. The cultures showed streptococcus. Note also the presence of a left psoas abscess.

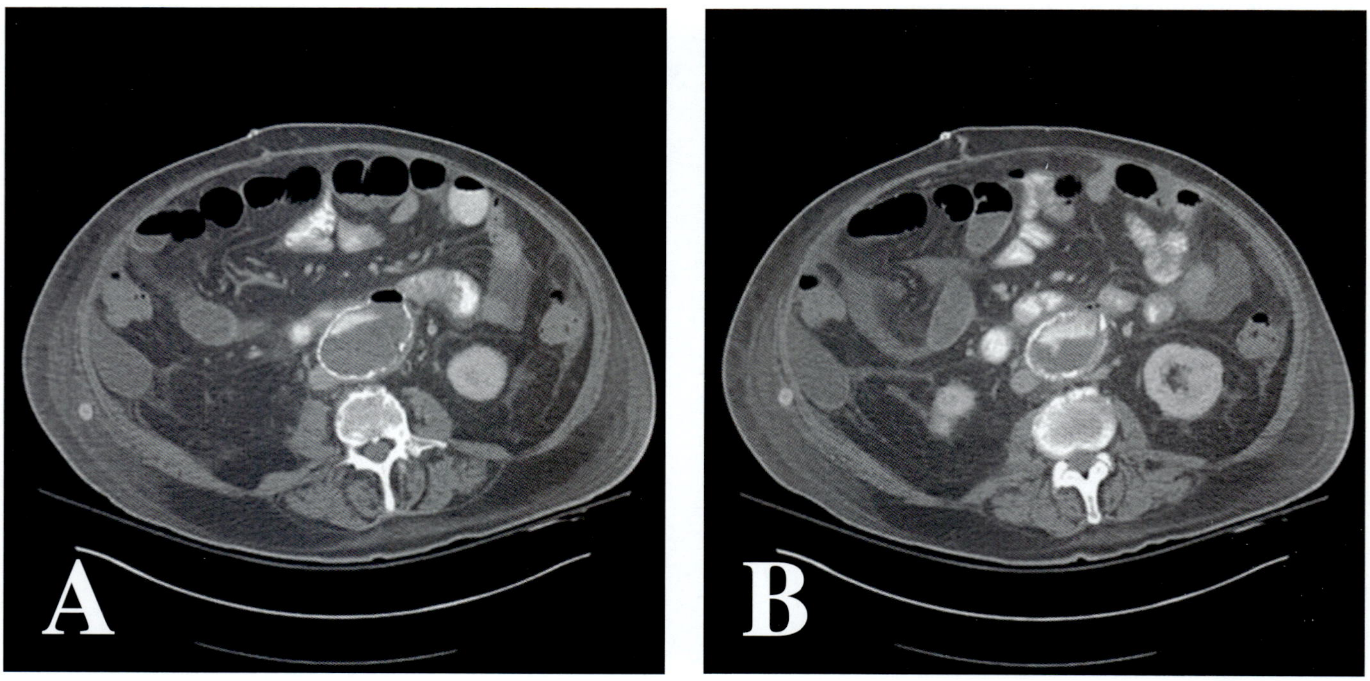

Figure 72.2 Primary aortoenteric fistula (AEF) in a 72-year-old female who presented with abdominal pain. Axial contrast-enhanced CT (**A–C**) shows the hallmarks of AEF including air in the most anterior aspect of the aorta and loss of the fat plane between the aorta and the transverse duodenum.

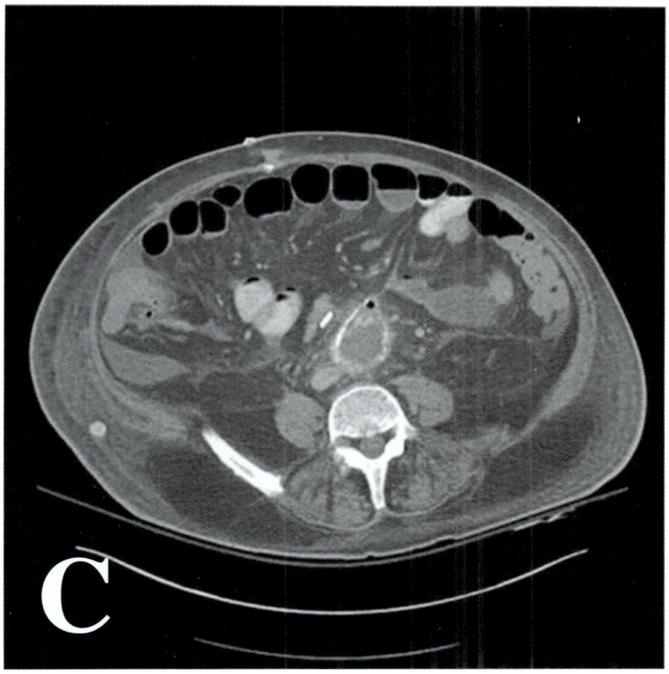

Figure 72.2 *(cont.)*

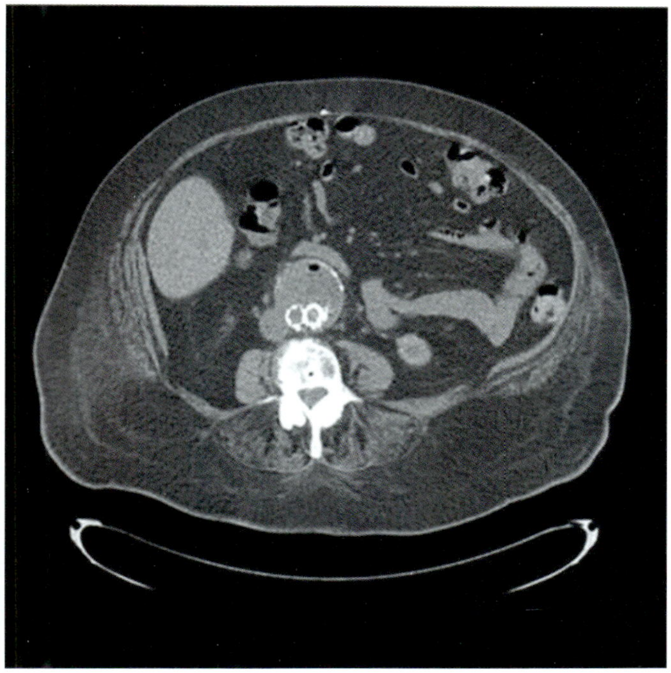

Figure 72.3 An 88-year-old male with post-stent graft repair of abdominal aortic aneurysm. Axial unenhanced CT shows air in the anterior aspect of the aorta. The presence of a fat plane between the aorta and the transverse duodenum rules out AEF. The stent graft was placed 8 days earlier.

CASE 73

Pseudostenosis of the common bile duct from crossing hepatic artery

Sumera Ali and Atif Zaheer

Imaging description

Psuedostenosis of the extrahepatic bile duct is a known diagnostic pitfall in magnetic resonance cholangiopancreatography (MRCP). The extrahepatic component of the biliary tree, which includes the common hepatic duct (CHD), left hepatic duct, and common bile duct (CBD), are crossed by the right hepatic artery (RHA) and the gastroduodenal artery (GDA). The pulsatile nature of the artery may result in non-pathologic obstruction of the extrahepatic bile duct, which appears as a focal signal loss on the multisection MIP reconstructed MRCP images.[1,2] It is most commonly seen where the RHA crosses the CHD just inferior to the confluence of the right and left ductal systems (Figures 73.1 and 73.2). The left hepatic duct compression is usually along the dorsal wall, while GDA may cross the middle segment of the CBD on its ventral wall. An apparent pseudostenosis at these levels can be further evaluated by identifying a normal biliary tree on the MRCP source images and identification of the crossing vessel on the coronal non-fat suppressed T2 or MR angiography images. Additional clues of a pseudostenosis include smooth- and short-segment narrowing ($< 1\,\text{cm}$) and lack of dilation upstream to the obstruction.[3]

Importance

A false positive diagnosis of a biliary stricture or hilar tumor could expose patients to risks of unnecessary invasive testing such as endoscopic retrograde cholangiopancreatography (ERCP) or biopsy.

Typical clinical scenario

Pathologic pseudostenosis of the extrahepatic biliary duct is a normal finding commonly seen at MRCP and has been reported in as many as 21% of patients.[3]

Differential diagnosis

Differential considerations include all the benign and malignant causes of biliary stricture. Benign conditions include post-surgical strictures, Mirizzi syndrome and those related to inflammation (e.g., chronic pancreatitis and sclerosing cholangitis). Malignant causes include strictures caused by pancreatic head carcinoma, cholangiocarcinoma, duodenal carcinoma, or metastasis. The length of obstruction can be helpful to distinguish these entities. In a study by Park et al. the mean length of strictures from malignant and benign causes were 30.0 mm ± 8.5 mm and 13.6 mm ± 9.1 mm, respectively;[4] while narrowing from pseudostenosis ranged in length from 4 to 11 mm (mean 7.9 mm).[3]

Teaching point

Crossing of the right hepatic artery behind the common hepatic duct or left hepatic duct and the gastroduodenal artery anterior to the mid-portion of the common bile duct can appear as a pseudostenosis on MRCP. These normal variants can be differentiated from pathological narrowing by their typical location, by the identification of a normal upstream biliary tree on the MRCP source images, and by finding a culprit crossing vessel on the coronal non-fat suppressed T2 or MR angiography images.

1. H. Irie, H. Honda, T. Kuroiwa, et al. Pitfalls in MR cholangiopancreatographic interpretation. *Radiographics* 2001; **21**: 23–37.
2. Y. Watanabe, M. Dohke, T. Ishimori, et al. Diagnostic pitfalls of MR cholangiopancreatography in the evaluation of the biliary tract and gallbladder. *Radiographics* 1999; **19**: 415–29.
3. H. Kondo, M. Kanematsu, Y. Shiratori, H. Moriwaki, H. Hoshi. Potential pitfall of MR cholangiopancreatography: right hepatic arterial impression of the common hepatic duct. *J Comput Assist Tomogr* 1999; **23**: 60–2.
4. M. S. Park, T. K. Kim, K. W. Kim, et al. Differentiation of extrahepatic bile duct cholangiocarcinoma from benign stricture: findings at MRCP versus ERCP. *Radiology* 2004; **233**: 234–40.

Pearls and Pitfalls in Cardiovascular Imaging, ed. Stefan L. Zimmerman and Elliot K. Fishman. Published by Cambridge University Press. © Cambridge University Press 2015.

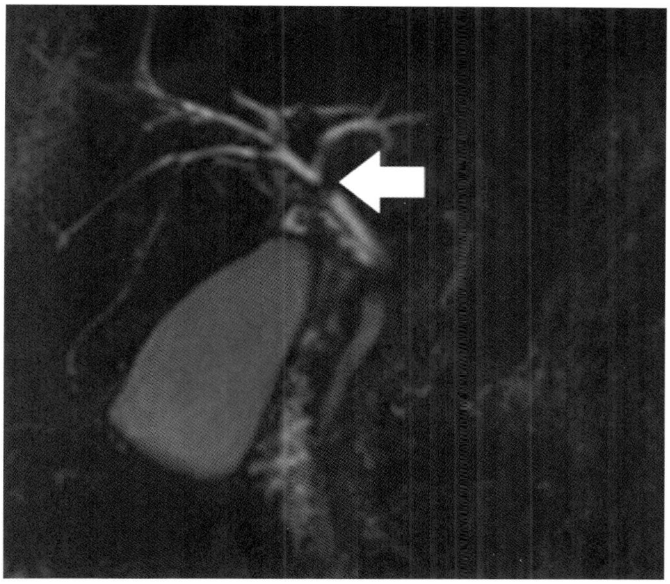

Figure 73.1 A 45-year-old female with abdominal pain. Coronal MIP reconstructed MRCP image demonstrates narrowing of the common hepatic duct (arrow) without evidence of intrahepatic biliary ductal dilatation.The finding of pseudostenosis is caused by crossing of the right hepatic artery.

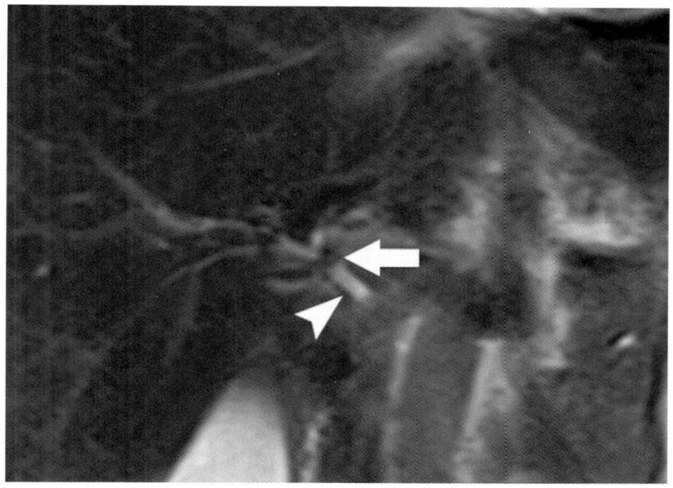

Figure 73.2 Common hepatic duct pseudostenosis caused by the right hepatic artery. Coronal T2-weighted MR image reveals the close anatomic relation between the common hepatic duct (arrowhead) and the right hepatic artery (arrow). The right hepatic artery appears as an area of signal void crosses the common hepatic duct just below the confluence of the right and left biliary ducts.

CASE 74

Pseudometastatic disease from hepatic arterioportal shunts

Atif Zaheer

Imaging description

Small nodular hepatic early enhancing areas on multiphasic contrast-enhanced CT or MRI imaging can mimic malignant pathology. These early enhancing lesions are typically located in the periphery of the liver, measure only a few millimeters and are visible predominantly on the arterial phase of contrast imaging fading to isodensity/intensity on the delayed-phase imaging (Figures 74.1 and 74.2).[1] Importantly, these lesions do not have a corresponding abnormality on the non-contrast T1- and T2-weighted MR imaging (Figure 74.3 and 74.4) and do not demonstrate restricted diffusion on diffusion-weighted imaging.[2]

Importance

An arterioportal shunt occurs as result of a direct connection between the hepatic arterial and the portal venous systems and is an important cause of transient hepatic attenuation/intensity difference (THAD/THID).[3] This tends to occur in the presence of diminished portal venous flow as in the case of cirrhosis or due to external factors such as trauma or percutaneous intervention.[4] These pseudolesions have to be differentiated from malignant ones to avoid unwarranted anxiety in patients and to avoid invasive testing such as biopsy or even surgical resection.

Typical clinical scenario

These lesions may be a source of concern in patients with cirrhosis or a known malignancy with hypervascular metastasis such as renal cell carcinoma or neuroendocrine tumors. Due to their small size biopsy is usually not an option and these lesions tend to disappear or remain stable on the follow-up examinations (Figure 74.5).

Differential diagnosis

A small flash-filling hemangioma is typically very bright on T2-weighted MR imaging and typically retains contrast on the more delayed-phase imaging. Hepatocellular carcinoma and even metastatic disease from cancers like renal cell, melanoma or neuroendocrine tumors tend to washout on the venous and delayed-phase imaging and appear as lower density/intensity than the liver. The absence of washout on delayed imaging, peripheral location, small size, and absence of abnormality on T1-, T2- and diffusion-weighted imaging along with long-term stability are features of a benign process such as an arterioportal shunt.

Teaching point

Small arterioportal shunts can mimic a malignant process. Typical imaging features on contrast-enhanced MRI may help with the diagnosis. Follow-up may be a reasonable option in high-risk patients.

REFERENCES

1. K. Ito, T. Fujita, A. Shimizu, et al. Multiarterial phase dynamic MRI of small early enhancing hepatic lesions in cirrhosis or chronic hepatitis: differentiating between hypervascular hepatocellular carcinomas and pseudolesions. *AJR Am J Roentgenol* 2004; **183**: 699–705.
2. U. Motosugi, T. Ichikawa, H. Sou, et al. Distinguishing hypervascular pseudolesions of the liver from hypervascular hepatocellular carcinomas with gadoxetic acid-enhanced MR imaging. *Radiology* 2010; **256**: 151–8.
3. J. J. Bookstein, K. J. Cho, G. B. Davis, D. Dail. Arterioportal communications: observations and hypotheses concerning transsinusoidal and transvasal types. *Radiology* 1982; **142**: 581–90.
4. J. H. Ahn, J. S. Yu, S. H. Hwang, J. J. Chung, J. H. Kim, K. W. Kim. Nontumorous arterioportal shunts in the liver: CT and MRI findings considering mechanisms and fate. *Eur Radiol* 2010; **20**: 385–94.

Pearls and Pitfalls in Cardiovascular Imaging, ed. Stefan L. Zimmerman and Elliot K. Fishman. Published by Cambridge University Press. © Cambridge University Press 2015.

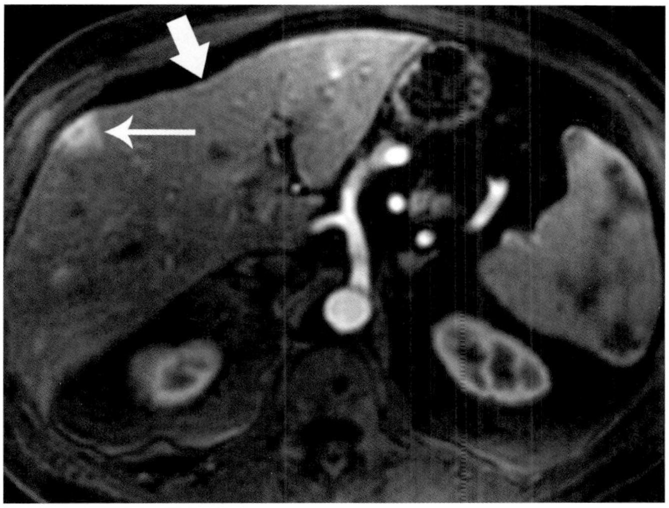

Figure 74.1 A 73-year old man with history of renal cell carcinoma and cirrhosis with a hepatic arteriovenous shunt. A small arterially enhancing wedge-shaped lesion is seen on axial contrast-enhanced T1-weighted image in a subcapsular location in the right lobe of the liver (thin arrow). Note the cirrhotic morphology of the liver with slight atrophy of the segment 4 (thick arrow).

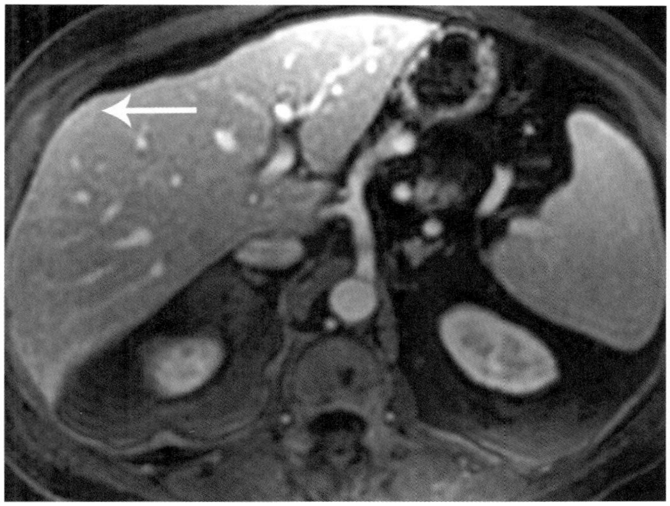

Figure 74.2 Axial contrast-enhanced venous phase T1-weighted image demonstrates blending in of the lesion with the adjacent liver parenchyma (arrow).

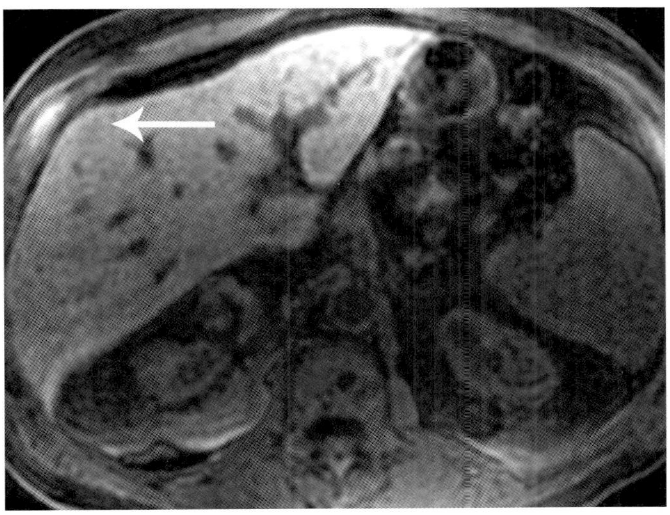

Figure 74.3 Axial precontrast T1-weighted image shows no abnormality in the area of the AV shunt (arrow).

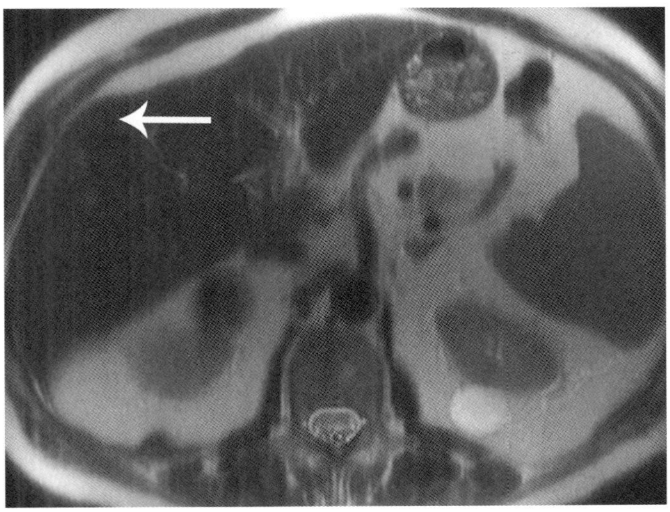

Figure 74.4 Axial T2-weighted image shows no abnormality in the area of the AV shunt (arrow).

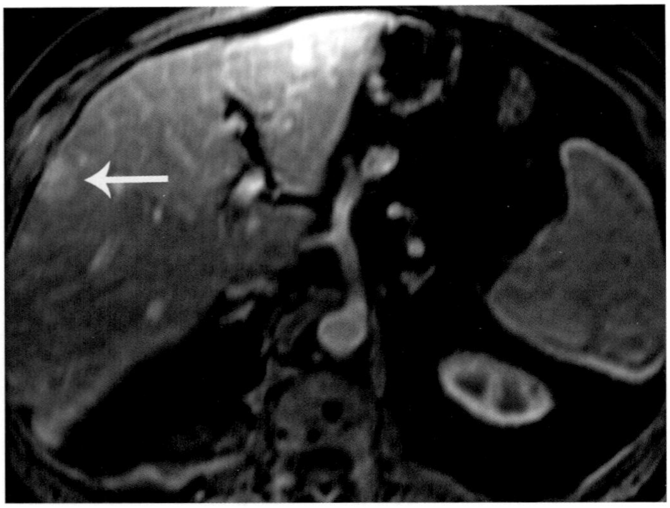

Figure 74.5 Axial contrast-enhanced arterial phase T1-weighted image obtained 5 years later shows stable appearance of the small arterially enhancing lesion in the same location (arrow). The imaging characteristics and the long-term stability confirmed the diagnosis of an AV shunt.

CASE 75

Pancreatic pseudomass due to thrombosed pseudoaneurysm

Vivek Halappa and Atif Zaheer

Imaging description

Pseudoaneurysm, also known as a false aneurysm, is a collection of flowing blood that is encapsulated and communicates with the ruptured arterial lumen contained only by the adventitia or surrounding soft tissue. After contrast administration, the sac may fill with contrast material if it is not completely thrombosed [1] and the enhancement follows that of the feeding artery (Figures 75.1 and 75.2). Thrombus within the sac may appear as high-attenuation filling defect on unenhanced CT or as high-signal-intensity defect on fat-suppressed T1-weighted MR images. Diagnostic specificity may be improved with 3D multidetector CT angiography (Figure 75.3).[2] Three-dimensional renderings are valuable for distinction from tortuous vessel or small, hyperattenuating islet cell tumor of the pancreas. Conventional angiography remains the standard of reference and provides the capability of endovascular management (Figure 75.4).

Importance

Pseudoaneurysms complicate 10% of cases of acute pancreatitis, most commonly affecting the splenic artery, although the hepatic, gastric, gastroduodenal, and pancreaticoduodenal arteries may also be involved due to erosion by pancreatic enzymes.[3] Early detection and management are paramount given the high mortality associated with rupture, which may be up to 90% if bleeding is left untreated.[4] Rupture can occur into the peritoneum, adjacent hollow organs, pseudocyst or pancreatic duct. Given enhancement characteristics, there is risk of mistaking pseudoaneurysms for a hypervascular pancreatic mass such as neuroendocrine tumor. Misdiagnosis leading to biopsy may have catastrophic consequences due to severe bleeding.

Typical clinical scenario

Pseudoaneurysm may be asymptomatic and could be detected incidentally during imaging patients with complicated pancreatitis and may be mistaken for a mass at routine imaging, especially if the lumen is completely thrombosed and fails to enhance on CT.[5] In case of hyperenhancement, it may also be mistaken for a hypervascular lesion such as a neuroendocrine tumor.

Differential diagnosis

Differential diagnoses for pseudoaneurysm include a hypervascular pancreatic mass such as a neuroendocrine tumor. Rarely, the second portion of the duodenum surrounded by annular pancreas may also mimic a pseudoaneursym, especially when filled with hyperdense oral contrast.

Teaching point

It is important to differentiate pancreatic pseudoaneurysms from pancreatic mass given the risks of misdiagnosis. Identification of increased attenuation/signal intensity on unenhanced CT and MRI scans, if thrombosed, and avid enhancement after contrast infusion similar to that of the feeding artery will help make the correct diagnosis.

REFERENCES

1. V. A. Sahni, K. J. Mortele. The bloody pancreas: MDCT and MRI features of hypervascular and hemorrhagic pancreatic conditions. *AJR Am J Roentgenol* 2009; **192**: 923–35.
2. K. M. Horton, E. K. Fishman. Volume-rendered 3D CT of the mesenteric vasculature: normal anatomy, anatomic variants, and pathologic conditions. *Radiographics* 2002; **22**: 161–72.
3. E. J. Balthazar. Complications of acute pancreatitis: clinical and CT evaluation. *Radiol Clin North Am* 2002; **40**: 1211–27.
4. C. N. Chong, K. F. Lee, K. T. Wong, W. W. Ng, J. Wong, P. B. Lai. Ruptured gastroduodenal artery pseudoaneurysm as the initial presentation of chronic pancreatitis. *Am J Surg* 2009; **197**: e38–40.
5. S. Murayama, Y. Shimoda. Completely thrombosed splenic artery aneurysm mimicking cystic pancreatic mass: computed tomographic findings. *Gastrointest Radiol* 1990; **15**: 205–6.

Pearls and Pitfalls in Cardiovascular Imaging, ed. Stefan L. Zimmerman and Elliot K. Fishman. Published by Cambridge University Press. © Cambridge University Press 2015.

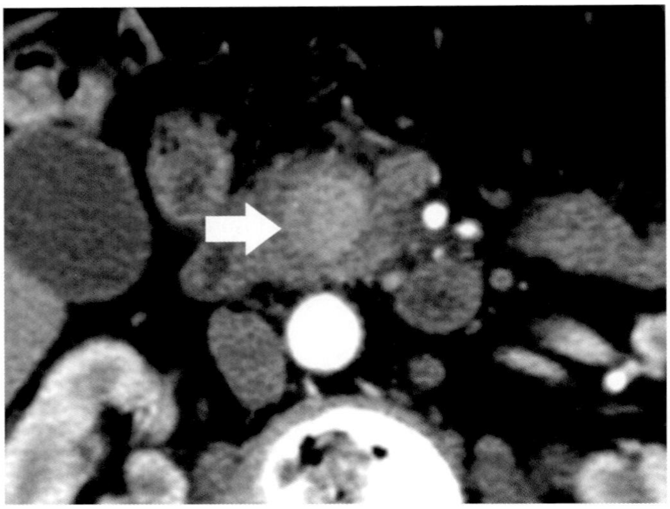

Figure 75.1 A 60-year-old man with history of acute pancreatitis. Axial MDCT through the level of the pancreas head in the arterial phase demonstrates a 2 cm hyperenhancing round mass-like lesion (arrow).

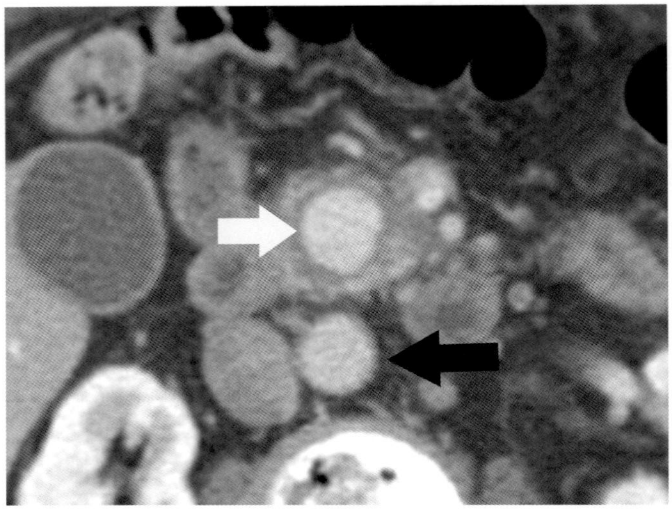

Figure 75.2 Axial MDCT through the level of the pancreas head in the venous phase demonstrates a pseudoaneurym (white arrow) with contrast enhancement similar to the aorta (black arrow).

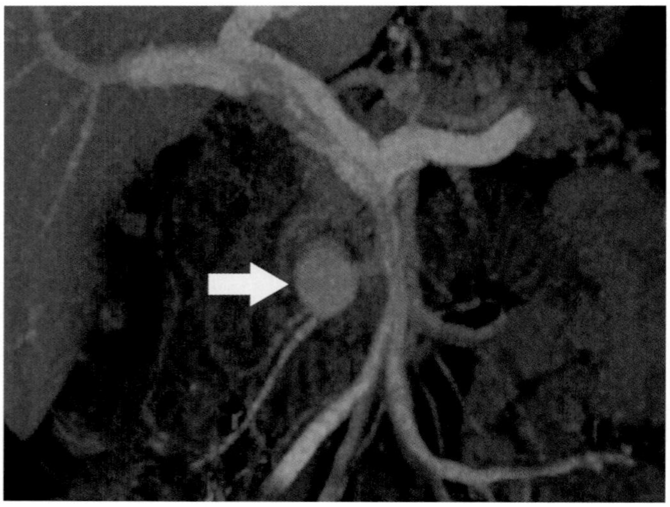

Figure 75.3 Coronal multiplanar reformat image in the venous phase demonstrates a pseudoaneurysm (arrow) with contrast enhancement similar to the adjacent vessels.

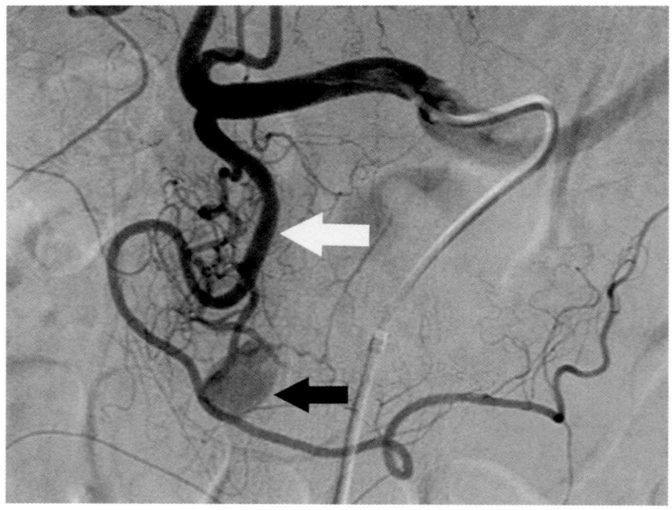

Figure 75.4 Digital subtraction angiogram of the gastroduodenal artery (white arrow) demonstrates a 2 cm gastroduodenal artery pseudoaneurysm (black arrow).

CASE 76

Splenic artery aneurysm mimicking pancreatic neuroendocrine tumor

Pamela T. Johnson

Imaging description

Pancreatic neuroendocrine tumors (PNETs) have variable CT appearances, but demonstrate a distinctive CT appearance when they present as small, hypervascular masses within the pancreatic parenchyma.[1] Unlike adenocarcinoma, which is typically hypovascular and most conspicuous on the venous phase, hypervascular PNETs are typically more vascular than the pancreatic parenchyma on the arterial and/or venous phase(s). This appearance can be mimicked by a splenic artery aneurysm that is partially or completely surrounded by pancreatic parenchyma (Figure 76.1). The distinction is made by demonstrating contiguity with the splenic artery on arterial-phase imaging, facilitated by use of 2D multiplanar reconstructions and 3D rendering.[2,3]

Importance

Distinction of a splenic artery aneurysm from a pancreatic neuroendocrine tumor is essential, for several reasons. Biopsy of a splenic artery aneurysm mistaken for a PNET could result in catastrophic hemorrhage. Resection based on a presumptive CT or MR diagnosis would subject the patient to an unnecessary surgical procedure with significant morbidity rates.

Typical clinical scenario

Splenic artery aneurysms are estimated to occur in 0.1 to 10.4% of the general population.[4] Splenic artery aneurysms have a strong female predominance, with a female to male ratio of 4:1.[4] Splenic artery aneurysms are defined by diameter greater than 1 cm. Splenic artery aneurysms may be mistaken for pancreatic neuroendocrine tumors when proper CT technique is not performed, including high spatial resolution, arterial and venous phase acquisitions, as well as 2D multiplanar reconstructions and 3D rendering. A single venous phase acquisition without narrow reconstruction sections can make the distinction of the two entities challenging.

Differential diagnosis

Differential diagnosis for a vascular lesion in the pancreas includes metastasis from renal cell carcinoma, gastrointestinal stromal tumor, peripancreatic paraganglioma, and intrapancreatic splenule.[1] The presence of calcification would be more common with either a PNET or a splenic artery aneurysm.

Teaching point

Splenic artery aneurysm should be considered when a highly vascular lesion, particularly with peripheral calcification, is identified in the pancreatic parenchyma. Protocol optimization with dual-phase imaging and dataset review with multiplanar processing tools will help avert misdiagnosing splenic artery aneurysm as pancreatic neuroendocrine tumor.

REFERENCES

1. Raman SP, Hruban RH, Cameron JL, Wolfgang CL, Fishman EK. Pancreatic imaging mimics: part 2, pancreatic neuroendocrine tumors and their mimics. *AJR* 2012 Aug; **199**:309–318.
2. Horton KM, Hruban RH, Yeo C, Fishman EK. Multi-detector row CT of pancreatic islet cell tumors. *Radiographics* 2006; **26**:453–464.
3. Agrawal GA, Johnson PT, Fishman EK. Splenic artery aneurysms and pseudoaneurysms: clinical distinctions and CT appearances. *AJR* 2007; **188**:992–999.
4. Al-Habbabi Y, Christophi C, Muralidharan V. Aneurysms of the splenic artery – a review. *The Surgeon* 2010; **8**:223–231.

Pearls and Pitfalls in Cardiovascular Imaging, ed. Stefan L. Zimmerman and Elliot K. Fishman. Published by Cambridge University Press. © Cambridge University Press 2015.

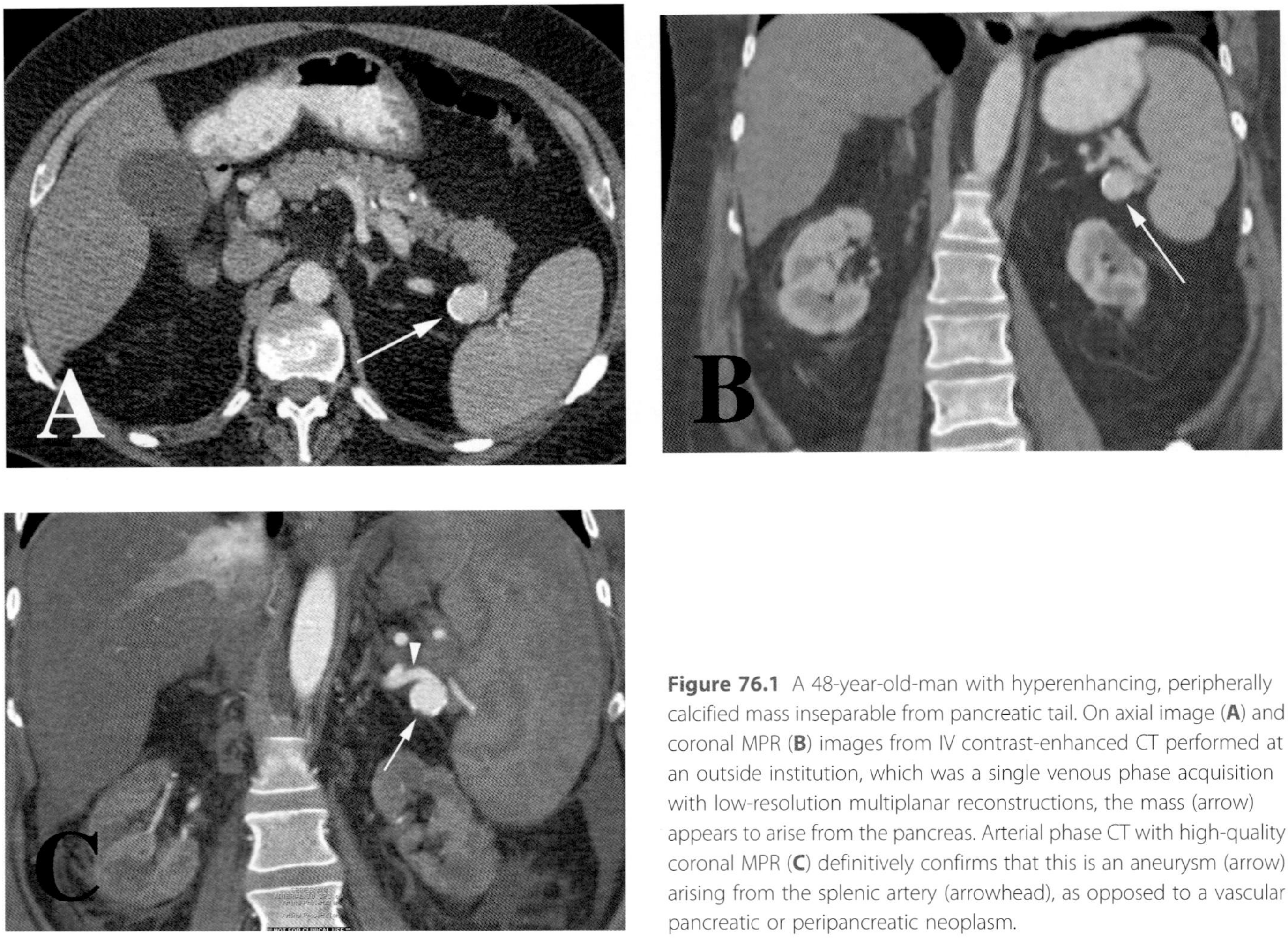

Figure 76.1 A 48-year-old-man with hyperenhancing, peripherally calcified mass inseparable from pancreatic tail. On axial image (**A**) and coronal MPR (**B**) images from IV contrast-enhanced CT performed at an outside institution, which was a single venous phase acquisition with low-resolution multiplanar reconstructions, the mass (arrow) appears to arise from the pancreas. Arterial phase CT with high-quality coronal MPR (**C**) definitively confirms that this is an aneurysm (arrow) arising from the splenic artery (arrowhead), as opposed to a vascular pancreatic or peripancreatic neoplasm.

CASE 77

Median arcuate ligament compression

Sumera Ali and Atif Zaheer

Imaging description

The acute angulation of the proximal celiac axis caused by a low inserting median arcuate ligament (MAL) and post-stenotic dilatation gives a characteristic appearance of a "hook" and can be demonstrated using multiplanar CT angiography (Figures 77.1 and 77.2).[1] Isolated expiratory compression of the celiac trunk may not be clinically significant and therefore images should be obtained at the end of maximum inspiration. Other associated findings include enlarged collateral vessels and gastroduodenal artery dilatation. Volume-rendered 3D images can assist in visualization of the severity of celiac axis compression and collateral vessels. The fibrous median arcuate ligament causing the compression can also be visualized on 3D reconstructions. Duplex ultrasound may be performed to study the severity of hemodynamic compromise. A peak systolic velocity greater than 200 cm/s is considered to be diagnostic of celiac artery stenosis.[2]

Importance

MAL is a fibrous band that connects the two cruras of the diaphragm across the aortic hiatus. It is normally located anterior to the aorta and superior to the origin of the celiac artery.[3] In about 10–24% of normal asymptomatic individuals, it is located anterioinferiorly to the celiac axis. In such cases, MAL may cause indentation and compression of the celiac artery, compromising blood flow and causing symptoms of celiac artery compression. MAL causing celiac artery compression can also be seen in asymptomatic people and therefore caution should be taken to attribute abdominal symptoms to compression based on imaging alone [4] and clinical correlation should be performed when incidentally noted on imaging.[5] The decision to intervene in established cases should be based on severity of clinical and imaging findings. Presence of post-stenotic dilation, collateral vessels and gastroduodenal artery dilatation suggests hemodynamic compromise, even in asymptomatic individuals, and early intervention should be considered.

Typical clinical scenario

Celiac artery compression is typically diagnosed in young to middle-aged patients presenting with symptoms similar to mesenteric ischemia (post-prandial pain and weight loss) but found to have patent mesenteric vessels. The presence of an epigastric bruit provides an important clue, but is rarely present.

Differential diagnosis

The main differential diagnosis is celiac artery stenosis secondary to atheromatous changes, which is typically seen in elderly patients and is associated with calcified and non-calcified plaque that is well visualized on CT.[1]

Teaching point

MAL compression of the celiac artery can be seen in normal asymptomatic individuals. However, in some patients, compression of the celiac axis can result in ischemic symptoms. Significant MAL compression can be diagnosed in symptomatic patients using CT angiography, which will demonstrate the characteristic "hook" like focal narrowing of the celiac artery that may be associated with enlarged collateral vessels depending on the duration and severity of compression.

REFERENCES

1. K. M. Horton, M. A. Talamini, E. K. Fishman. Median arcuate ligament syndrome: evaluation with CT angiography. *Radiographics* 2005; **25**: 1177–82.
2. A. Erden, M. Yurdakul, T. Cumhur. Marked increase in flow velocities during deep expiration: a duplex Doppler sign of celiac artery compression syndrome. *Cardiovasc Intervent Radiol* 1999; **22**: 331–2.
3. M. Loukas, J. Pinyard, S. Vaid, C. Kinsella, A. Tariq, R. S. Tubbs. Clinical anatomy of celiac artery compression syndrome: a review. *Clin Anat* 2007; **20**: 612–17.
4. R. M. Patten, D. M. Coldwell, Y. Ben-Menachem. Ligamentous compression of the celiac axis: CT findings in five patients. *AJR Am J Roentgenol* 1991; **156**: 1101–3.
5. N. E. Manghat, G. Mitchell, C. S. Hay, I. P. Wells. The median arcuate ligament syndrome revisited by CT angiography and the use of ECG gating – a single-centre case series and literature review. *Br J Radiol* 2008; **81**: 735–42.

Pearls and Pitfalls in Cardiovascular Imaging, ed. Stefan L. Zimmerman and Elliot K. Fishman. Published by Cambridge University Press. © Cambridge University Press 2015.

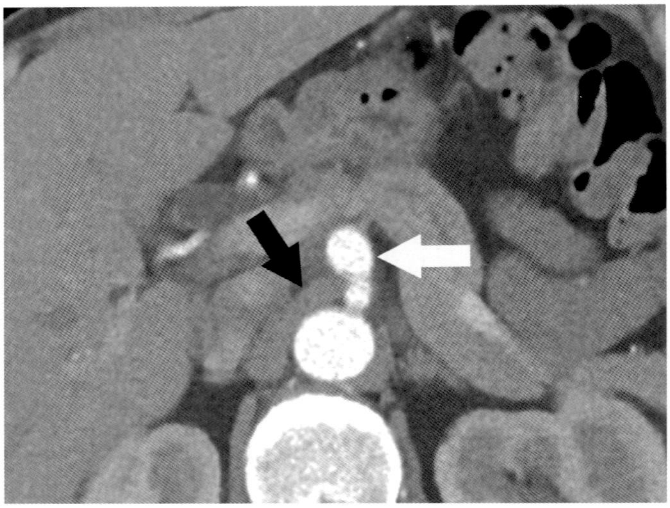

Figure 77.1 A 53-year-old man with epigastric abdominal pain. Axial contrast-enhanced MDCT arteriogram demonstrated narrowing of the celiac axis with post-stenotic dilatation (white arrow) due to a thickened MAL (black arrow). Note the absence of atherosclerotic disease.

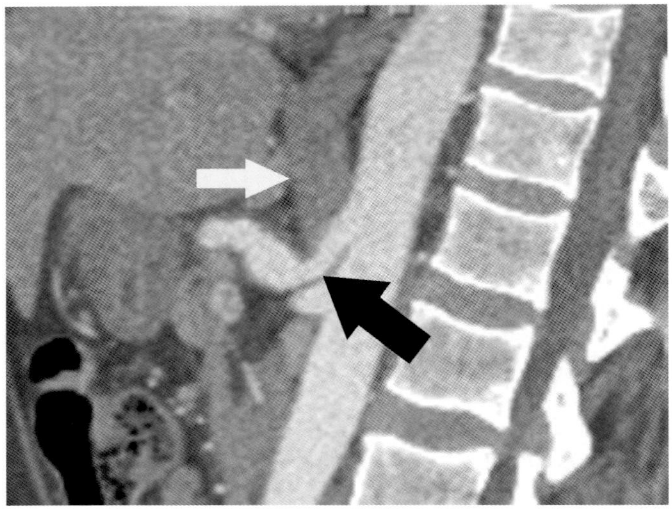

Figure 77.2 Sagittal multiplanar reformat image demonstrated acute angulation and narrowing of the proximal celiac axis (black arrow) due to thickened MAL (white arrow). The post-stenotic dilatation creates the characteristic "hooked" appearance.

CASE 78

Non-occlusive mesenteric ischemia

Atif Zaheer

Imaging description

Non-occlusive mesenteric ischemia (NOMI) is a condition in which bowel ischemia occurs secondary to slow flow in the mesenteric vessels in the absence of thrombosis. CT angiography demonstrates patent origin of the proximal vessels with poor visualization and pruning of the distal vasculature (Figures 78.1, 78.2, 78.3).[1] Delayed opacification of the mesenteric veins may be seen. Thickening of the bowel wall with or without pneumatosis may also be present (Figure 78.3). Selective angiography of mesenteric arteries serves as the gold standard in diagnosing NOMI.[2]

Importance

A low-flow state can be seen in conditions like hypovolemic shock, sepsis, heart failure, hypovolemia due to dehydration, and after dialysis in patients with chronic renal failure.[3],[4] NOMI constitutes about 25% of all cases of acute mesenteric ischemia with mortality as high as 70%.[5] The blood is shunted to maintain perfusion of the brain and heart, and an underlying cardiovascular disease may help precipitate the event. Although reversible, persistent ischemia may lead to bowel infarction. Superimposed infection may also occur. Accurate diagnosis is important as the treatment options differ from occlusive bowel ischemia and include correction of the underlying predisposing factor along with local or systemic vasodilators.

Typical clinical scenario

The typical scenario is of an older patient with underlying cardiovascular disease presenting with hypotension and decreased cardiac output followed by severe abdominal pain. Bowel sounds may be absent and gastrointestinal bleeding can also occur.

Differential diagnosis

Other causes of bowel ischemia such as arterial occlusion from atherosclerotic or thromboembolic disease and venous thrombosis of the mesenteric vasculature may be considered. In both cases filling defect in the effected vasculature may be seen (Figures 78.4 and 78.5).

Teaching point

NOMI is an important cause of ischemic bowel with high mortality and can be differentiated from other causes of bowel ischemia by the presence of narrowed mesenteric vasculature and absence of filling defects within the vessels.

REFERENCES

1. K. M. Horton, E. K. Fishman. Multidetector CT angiography in the diagnosis of mesenteric ischemia. *Radiol Clin North Am* 2007; **45**: 275–88.
2. M. Trompeter, T. Brazda, C. T. Remy, T. Vestring, P. Reimer. Non-occlusive mesenteric ischemia: etiology, diagnosis, and interventional therapy. *Eur Radiol* 2002; **12**: 1179–87.
3. T. S. Newman, T. H. Magnuson, S. A. Ahrendt, M. A. Smith-Meek, J. S. Bender. The changing face of mesenteric infarction. *Am Surg* 1998; **64**: 611–16.
4. S. M. Diamond, M. Emmett, W. L. Henrich. Bowel infarction as a cause of death in dialysis patients. *JAMA* 1986; **256**: 2545–7.
5. H. S. Bassiouny. Nonocclusive mesenteric ischemia. *Surg Clin North Am* 1997; **77**: 319–26.

Pearls and Pitfalls in Cardiovascular Imaging, ed. Stefan L. Zimmerman and Elliot K. Fishman. Published by Cambridge University Press. © Cambridge University Press 2015.

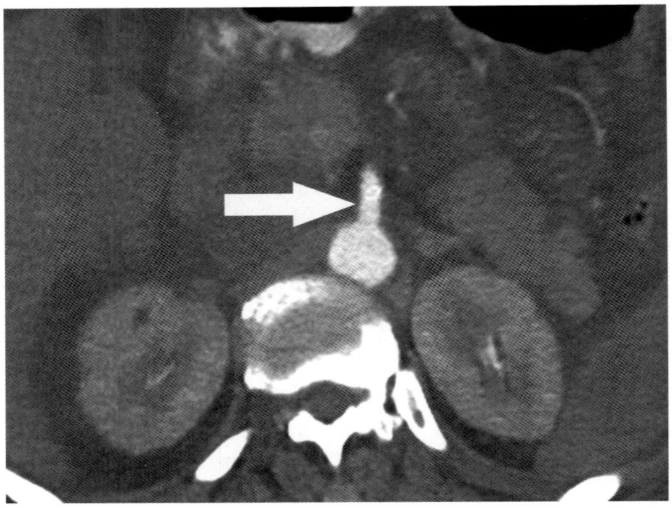

Figure 78.1 A 55-year-old man with end-stage renal disease on hemodialysis and ischemic cardiomyopathy presenting with abdominal pain. Axial contrast-enhanced arterial phase CT at the level of the kidneys demonstrates a patent origin of the SMA (arrow).

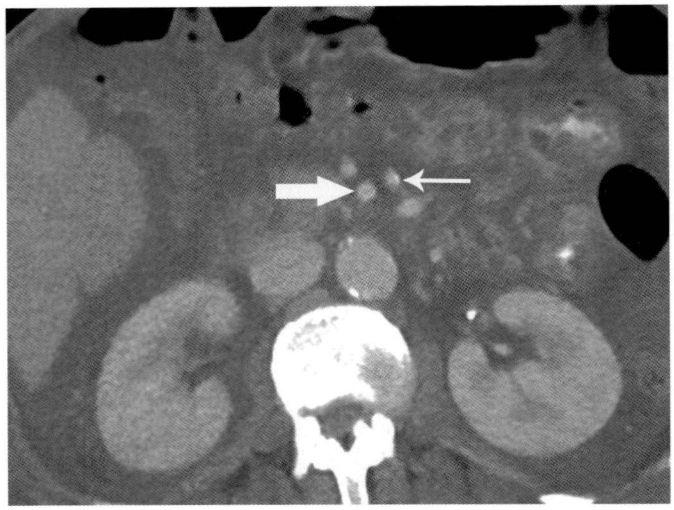

Figure 78.2 Axial contrast-enhanced arterial phase CT at a more caudal level demonstrates patent but diminutive SMA (thin arrow) and SMV (thick arrow).

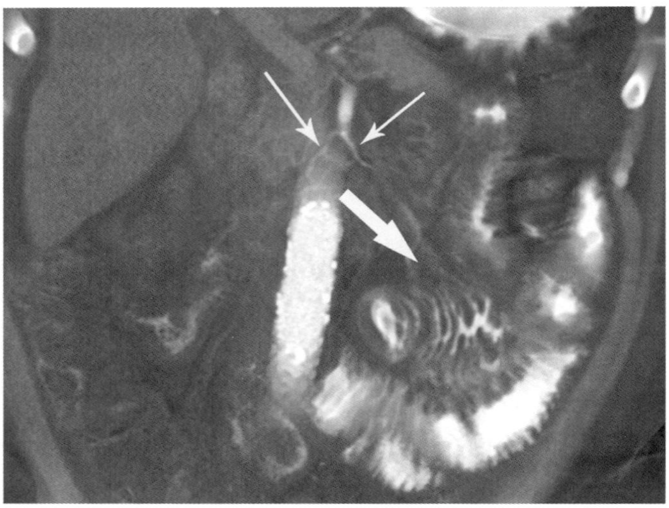

Figure 78.3 Coronal MIP image shows attenuated branches of the SMA (thin arrows). There is thickening of the bowel wall (thick arrow) secondary to non-occlusive small bowel ischemia.

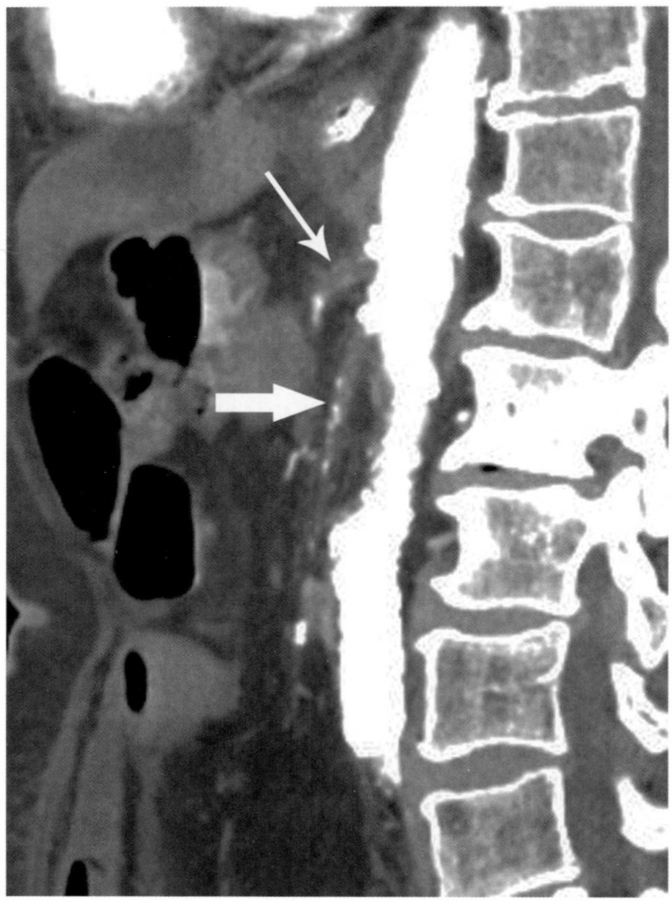

Figure 78.4 A 71-year-old woman presenting with abdominal pain. Sagittal contrast-enhanced arterial phase CT demonstrates lack of opacification of the celiac trunk (thin arrow) and the SMA (thick arrow) due to thrombosis.

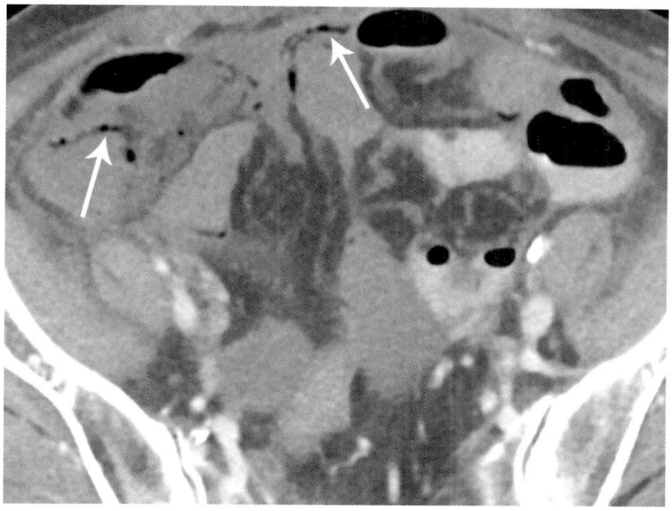

Figure 78.5 Axial contrast-enhanced image through the pelvis demonstrates pneumatosis of the small bowel (thin arrows) secondary to bowel ischemia from vascular thrombosis.

CASE **79**

Segmental arterial mediolysis

Atif Zaheer

Imaging description

CT angiography (CTA) provides a non-invasive method for the diagnosis of segmental arterial mediolysis (SAM), a rare non-atherosclerotic and non-inflammatory arterial disease. Smooth muscle degeneration of the outer layer of the media occurs primarily in the visceral branches of the abdominal aorta, leading to intramural hemorrhage and periadventitial fibrin deposition.[1] Contrast-enhanced arterial phase axial CT imaging in combination with multiplanar reconstructions and maximal intensity projections are useful imaging tools. Imaging findings include caliber irregularities of the splanchnic arteries including a "string of beads" appearance, aneurysm formation, or dissection (Figures 79.1, 79.2, 79.3 and 79.4).[2] Conventional angiography may be reserved for equivocal findings seen on CTA or MRA and for treatment.

Importance

Mortality related to SAM is about 26% and may be due to aneurysm rupture and subsequent hemorrhage.[3] Due to the lack of histopathologic confirmation of this disease in most cases, characteristic imaging findings may be the only way to diagnose this entity in patients with otherwise unexplained abdominal pain and gastrointestinal bleeding after excluding other possible etiologies. Axial and multiplanar CTA may help in the diagnosis while catheter angiography may be used for intervention.

Typical clinical scenario

SAM usually affects middle-aged patients[4] and presents with abdominal pain, gastrointestinal hemorrhage, retroperitoneal hemorrhage or intracranial bleeding.[5,6] Endovascular intervention has a high success rate while open surgical approach with vascular reconstruction may also be performed in select cases.[3]

Differential diagnosis

Fibromuscular dysplasia (FMD), although considered a variant of SAM given the similar imaging findings,[7] affects middle-aged women and involves primarily the renal and carotid arteries. Congenital conditions such as Ehlers–Danlos syndrome generally starts manifesting at a younger age while neurofibromatosis type 1 may cause vascular narrowing by mass effect from the surrounding neurofibromas easily seen on cross-sectional imaging. Mycotic aneurysms have a predilection for arterial bifurcations and will have surrounding inflammatory changes. Other differential considerations such as various types of vasculitis including polyarteritis nodosa, Takayasu's arteritis, Behçet's syndrome, and Henoch–Schönlein purpura[8] may have symptoms of systemic inflammation and detection of specific antibodies may help differentiate these entities from SAM.

Teaching point

Visceral branches of the abdominal aorta should be carefully scrutinized in patients undergoing CT for acute abdominal pain or gastrointestinal bleeding. CTA may be helpful in identifying abnormal vascular morphology, a bleeding source if present, and may be used for serial monitoring of these patients.

REFERENCES

1. R. E. Slavin, J. C. Gonzalez-Vitale. Segmental mediolytic arteritis: a clinical pathologic study. *Lab Invest* 1976; **35**: 23–9.

2. M. Michael, U. Widmer, S. Wildermuth, A. Barghorn, S. Duewell, T. Pfammatter. Segmental arterial mediolysis: CTA findings at presentation and follow-up. *AJR Am J Roentgenol* 2006; **187**: 1463–9.

3. M. Shenouda, C. Riga, Y. Naji, S. Renton. Segmental arterial mediolysis: a systematic review of 85 Cases. *Ann Vasc Surg* 2014; **28**: 269–77.

4. S. P. Kalva, B. Somarouthu, M. R. Jaff, S. Wicky. Segmental arterial mediolysis: clinical and imaging features at presentation and during follow-up. *J Vasc Interv Radiol* 2011; **22**: 1380–7.

5. C. K. Phillips, H. Lepor. Spontaneous retroperitoneal hemorrhage caused by segmental arterial mediolysis. *Rev Urol* 2006; **8**: 36–40.

6. A. Ro, N. Kageyama, A. Takatsu, T. Fukunaga. Segmental arterial mediolysis of varying phases affecting both the intra-abdominal and intracranial vertebral arteries: an autopsy case report. *Cardiovasc Pathol* 2010; **19**: 248–51.

7. J. T. Lie. Segmental mediolytic arteritis. Not an arteritis but a variant of arterial fibromuscular dysplasia. *Arch Pathol Lab Med* 1992; **116**: 238–41.

8. K. Geboes, I. Dalle. Vasculitis and the gastrointestinal tract. *Acta Gastroenterol Belg* 2002; **65**: 204–12.

Pearls and Pitfalls in Cardiovascular Imaging, ed. Stefan L. Zimmerman and Elliot K. Fishman. Published by Cambridge University Press. © Cambridge University Press 2015.

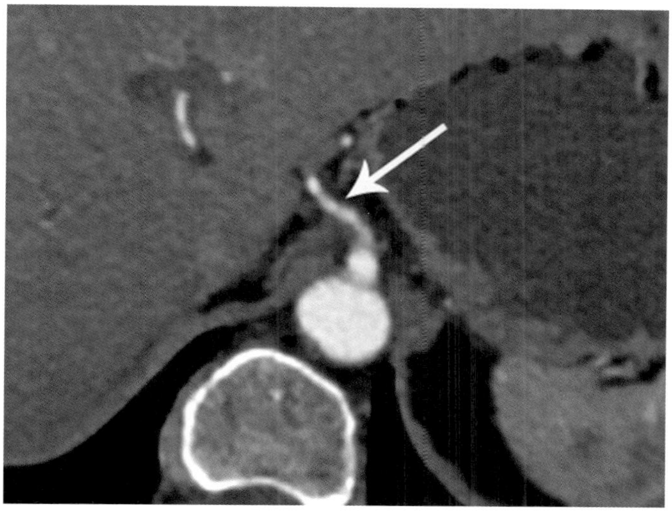

Figure 79.1 A 66-year-old woman with a right posterior inferior cerebral artery aneurysm. Imaging of the abdomen performed to evaluate for systemic disease. Axial contrast-enhanced arterial phase CT image demonstrates severe narrowing and beaded appearance of the celiac axis (arrow).

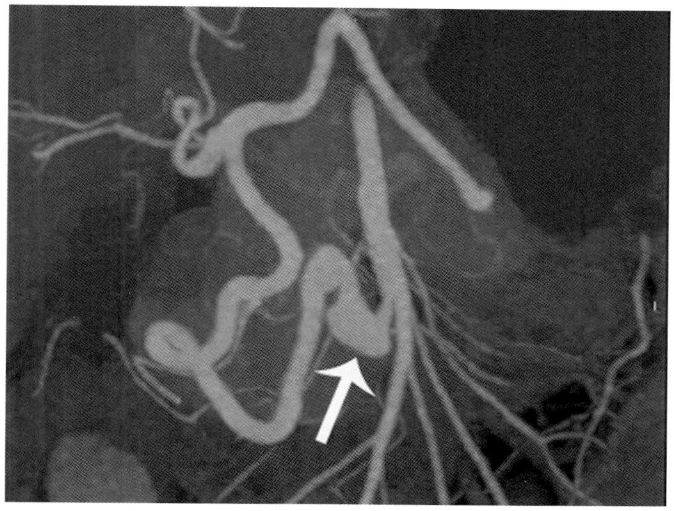

Figure 79.2 Coronal MIP CT image demonstrates a 1.5 cm aneurysm (arrow) of the inferior pancreaticoduodenal artery.

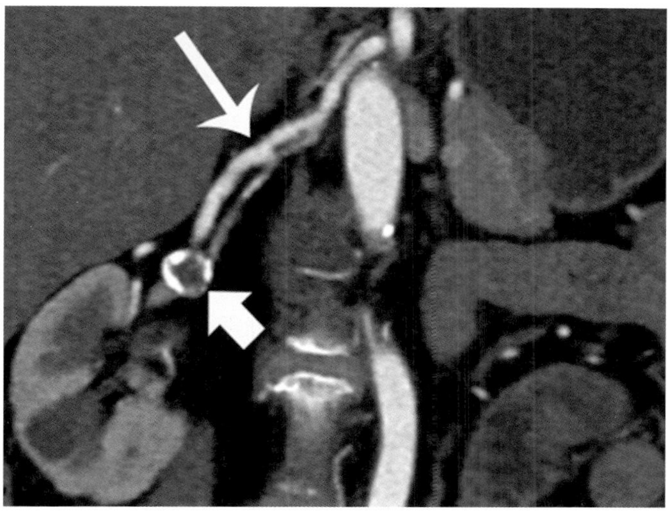

Figure 79.3 Coronal contrast-enhanced arterial phase CT images show a beaded and narrowed appearance of the right renal artery (thin arrow). Additionally, a small thrombosed aneurysm of the right renal artery is also seen (thick arrow).

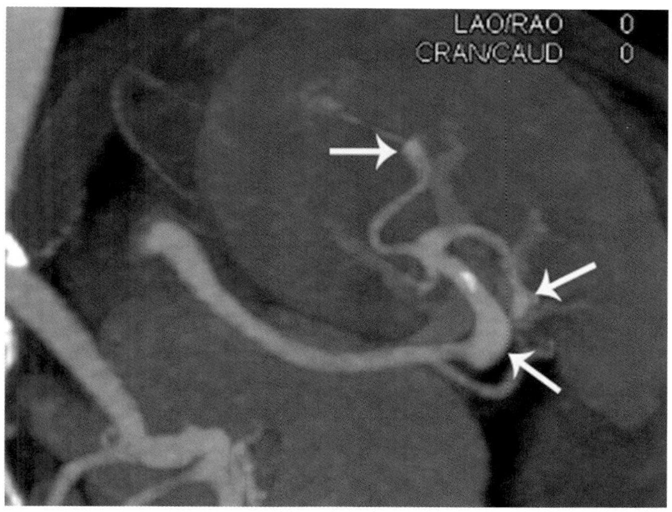

Figure 79.4 Coronal MIP CT image demonstrates multiple small aneurysms of the splenic artery (arrows). A presumptive diagnosis of segmental arterial mediolysis was made after excluding other potential etiologies by extensive laboratory work-up. These arterial abnormalities were followed up with CTA and remained unchanged over several years.

CASE 80

Superior mesenteric artery syndrome

Maera Haider and Atif Zaheer

Imaging description

Superior mesenteric artery syndrome is usually evaluated by contrast-enhanced CT or magnetic resonance angiography (MRA). The classic imaging finding is reduced space between the superior mesenteric artery and the anterior wall of the abdominal aorta that results in duodenal narrowing. The aortomesenteric angle, obtained from sagittal images, is significantly reduced from the normal range of 38–65°.[1] The combination of an aortomesenteric angle less than 22° and an aortomesenteric distance of less than 8–10 mm is considered by some authors to meet criteria for the diagnosis of SMA syndrome in the right clinical setting on CT (Figure 80.1).[2] Additional supportive findings include minimal intra-abdominal and retroperitoneal fat, duodenal compression between the aorta and SMA, dilation of the first and second portions of the duodenum, left renal vein enlargement, and enlargement of the left gonadal vein or other venous collaterals as a result of chronic renal vein compression (Figure 80.1).[2]

Importance

Young age and non-specific symptoms often lead to a delay in diagnosis, resulting in complications such as malnutrition, dehydration, and electrolyte abnormalities in patients with SMA syndrome.[3]

Typical clinical scenario

Superior mesenteric artery (SMA) syndrome is an atypical cause of high intestinal obstruction, with estimated incidence rates based on gastrointestinal barium series from 0.01% to 0.33%.[4] It occurs from an abnormally short distance between the aorta and SMA from loss of intra-abdominal fat, which normally separates them resulting in duodenal compression and is an important differential in patients with post-prandial abdominal pain, vomiting, and weight loss. The most common predisposing factors include severe weight loss and cachexia, surgical correction of spinal deformities, and congenital anomalies. Patients with recent bariatric surgery, cancer, or chronic immobilization are at risk.[5]

Common symptoms include intermittent epigastric pain, which is often post-prandial, early satiety, nausea, fullness, and voluminous vomiting, most frequently occurring in patients who have experienced rapid weight loss.[3] Anorexia may be resultant to these complaints. Most often, patients are adolescents or young adults. The symptoms are relieved when the patient lies in a left lateral decubitus, prone or knee-to-chest position.[1]

Differential diagnosis

During work-up for SMA syndrome, anorexia nervosa and bulimia should be considered. In addition, SMA syndrome should be differentiated from other disorders that could result in duodenal enlargement, such as diabetes mellitus, pancreatitis, peptic ulcer disease, or obstructing tumor.[6] Most importantly, SMA syndrome is not an imaging diagnosis alone and narrow aortomesenteric distance can be frequently seen in the normal population. Imaging must be interpreted in context of the proper clinical scenario.

Teaching point

SMA syndrome is a diagnosis of exclusion, and should be considered in patients with non-specific signs and symptoms of upper gastrointestinal tract obstruction. CT angiography findings of reduced aortomesenteric angle and distance supports the diagnosis in the correct clinical setting.[6]

REFERENCES

1. N. D. Merrett, R. B. Wilson, P. Cosman, A. V. Biankin. Superior mesenteric artery syndrome: diagnosis and treatment strategies. *J Gastrointest Surg* 2009; **13**: 287–92.
2. G. A. Agrawal, P. T. Johnson, E. K. Fishman. Multidetector row CT of superior mesenteric artery syndrome. *J Clin Gastroenterol* 2007; **41**: 62–5.
3. U. Baltazar, J. Dunn, C. Floresguerra, L. Schmidt, W. Browder. Superior mesenteric artery syndrome: an uncommon cause of intestinal obstruction. *South Med J* 2000; **93**: 606–8.
4. P. Ylinen, J. Kinnunen, K. Hockerstedt. Superior mesenteric artery syndrome. A follow-up study of 16 operated patients. *J Clin Gastroenterol* 1989; **11**: 386–91.
5. S. P. Raman, E. G. Neyman, K. M. Horton, F. E. Eckhauser, E. K. Fishman. Superior mesenteric artery syndrome: spectrum of CT findings with multiplanar reconstructions and 3-D imaging. *Abdom Imaging* 2012; **37**: 1079–88.
6. T. Welsch, M. W. Buchler, P. Kienle. Recalling superior mesenteric artery syndrome. *Dig Surg* 2007; **24**: 149–56.

Pearls and Pitfalls in Cardiovascular Imaging, ed. Stefan L. Zimmerman and Elliot K. Fishman. Published by Cambridge University Press. © Cambridge University Press 2015.

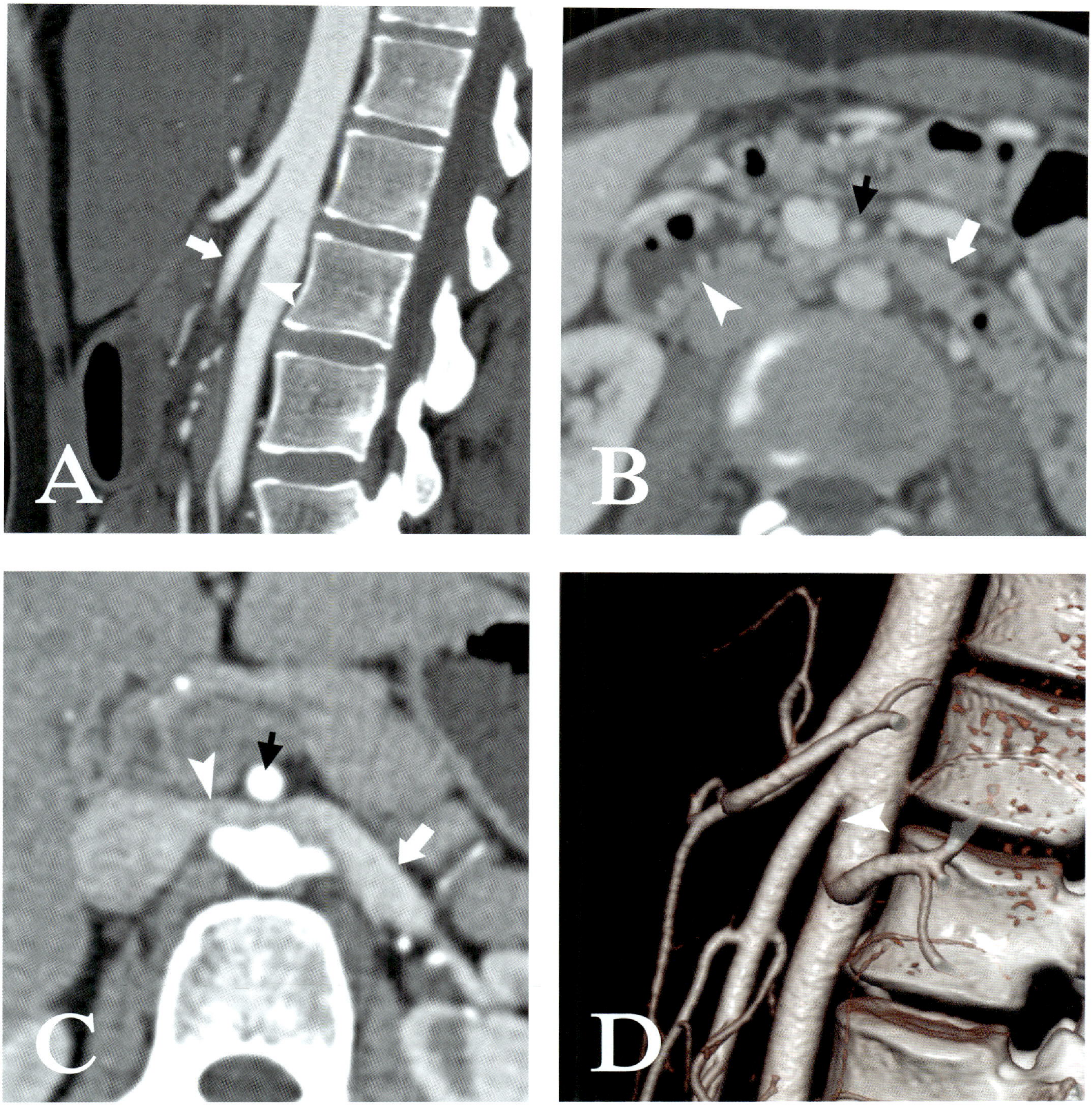

Figure 80.1 **A.** 32-year-old woman with recent weight loss and severe post-prandial abdominal pain. Sagittal contrast-enhanced CT images demonstrate severe narrowing of the aortomesenteric angle measuring 18°, with an aortomesenteric distance of 4 mm, and resultant compression of the duodenum (arrowhead) by the SMA (arrow). **B.** Axial CT image demonstrates a dilated duodenum (white arrowhead) proximal to the crossing of the SMA (short black arrow). The distal duodenum is normal in caliber (white arrow). **C.** Axial CT image demonstrates a dilated renal vein (white arrow) proximal to the crossing of the SMA (short black arrow). The distal renal vein toward the IVC is normal in caliber (white arrowhead). This is an ancillary finding of SMA syndrome. **D.** Volume-rendered image shows narrow aortomesenteric angle (white arrowhead).

CASE **81**

Renal fibromuscular dysplasia

Atif Zaheer

Imaging description

CT and MRI angiography provide a reliable and non-invasive method for diagnosis of renal fibromuscular dysplasia (FMD). The characteristic feature of renal FMD is a "string of beads" appearance of the mid- and distal renal artery due to the alternating stenosis and aneurysm formation (Figure 81.1). Axial imaging in combination with maximal intensity projection reconstructions are extremely helpful in making the diagnosis (Figure 81.2).[1] Contrast-enhanced 3D MRA can also be used as an alternate to CTA (Figure 81.3). Care should be taken not to misinterpret the stepladder image reconstruction artifact, resulting from faulty data reconstruction that produces a gap or overlap between sections or from source images that are too thick, as FMD (Figure 81.4). Conventional angiography, although considered gold standard, is not frequently used due to its invasive nature and may be reserved for equivocal findings seen on CTA or MRA and for treatment.

Importance

Fibromuscular dysplasia is the second most common cause of renovascular hypertension, after atherosclerotic disease, affecting mostly young or middle-aged women.[2,3] The disease is bilateral in two-thirds of the patients. It is classified according to the location of involvement within the vessel wall with medial fibroplasia accounting for 95% of cases. FMD is a non-inflammatory, non-atherosclerotic disease with presence of alternating areas of narrowing and small aneurysms causing the beaded appearance of the arteries. Vascular narrowing and dissections may occur.[4] FMD may also involve other visceral arteries such as the hepatic artery[5] as well as the carotid and vertebral arteries (Figure 81.5).[4] Accurate diagnosis is important as the treatment of FMD is distinct from other causes of renal artery stensosis such as atherosclerotic disease or vasculitis and can be treated with percutaneous transluminal angioplasty with a very high success rate.

Typical clinical scenario

Renal FMD may be incidentally found on imaging in a young potential renal donor or in a young or middle-aged woman with hypertension refractory to medical therapy. Contrast-enhanced CTA or MRA reveals a characteristic "string of beads" appearance of one or more renal arteries that can successfully be treated with percutaneous transluminal angioplasty.

Differential diagnosis

Renovascular hypertension from atherosclerotic disease affects older patients. Calcified or soft atherosclerotic narrowing typically develops in the proximal/ostial portion of the renal artery, as opposed to a beaded appearance of the renal arteries in the mid- or distal renal arteries seen in FMD. Other differential considerations include systemic vasculitis in conditions such as polyarteritis nodosa, Ehlers–Danlos syndrome, Alport's syndrome, pheochromocytoma, Marfan syndrome, and Takayasu's arteritis.[6]

Teaching point

Renal FMD is an important cause of renovascular hypertension affecting young and middle-aged women or may be incidentally found on contrast-enhanced CT or MRI. Contrast-enhanced CTA or MRA demonstrate a characteristic "string of beads" appearance.

REFERENCES

1. J. P. Beregi, S. Louvegny, C. Gautier, et al. Fibromuscular dysplasia of the renal arteries: comparison of helical CT angiography and arteriography. *AJR Am J Roentgenol* 1999; **172**: 27–34.
2. S. P. Youngberg, S. G. Sheps, C. G. Strong. Fibromuscular disease of the renal arteries. *Med Clin North Am* 1977; **61**: 623–41.
3. E. G. Harrison, Jr., J. C. Hunt, P. E. Bernatz. Morphology of fibromuscular dysplasia of the renal artery in renovascular hypertension. *Am J Med* 1967; **43**: 97–112.
4. J. W. Olin, J. Froehlich, X. Gu, et al. The United States Registry for Fibromuscular Dysplasia: results in the first 447 patients. *Circulation* 2012; **125**: 3182–90.
5. H. J. Jones, R. Staud, R. C. Williams, Jr. Rupture of a hepatic artery aneurysm and renal infarction: 2 complications of fibromuscular dysplasia that mimic vasculitis. *J Rheumatol* 1998; **25**: 2015–18.
6. C. Pontes Tde, G. P. Rufino, M. G. Gurgel, A. C. Medeiros, E. A. Freire. Fibromuscular dysplasia: a differential diagnosis of vasculitis. *Rev Bras Reumatol* 2012; **52**: 70–4.

Pearls and Pitfalls in Cardiovascular Imaging, ed. Stefan L. Zimmerman and Elliot K. Fishman. Published by Cambridge University Press. © Cambridge University Press 2015.

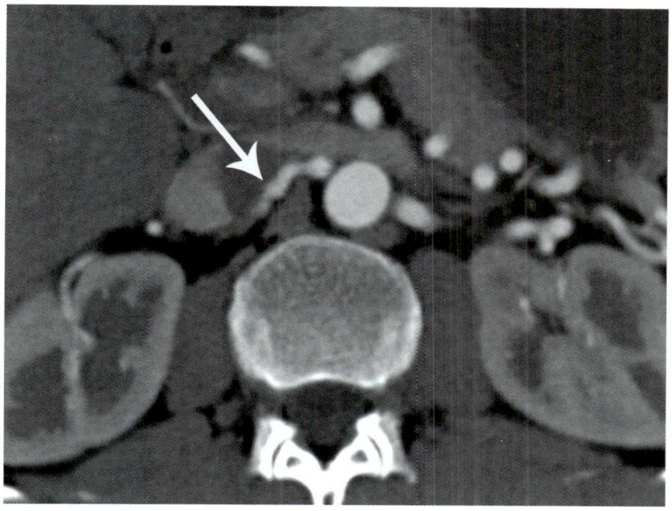

Figure 81.1 A 51-year-old man with renal fibromuscular dysplasia. Axial contrast-enhanced arterial phase CT at the level of the kidneys demonstrates a characteristic "string of beads" appearance of the mid-right renal artery (arrow).

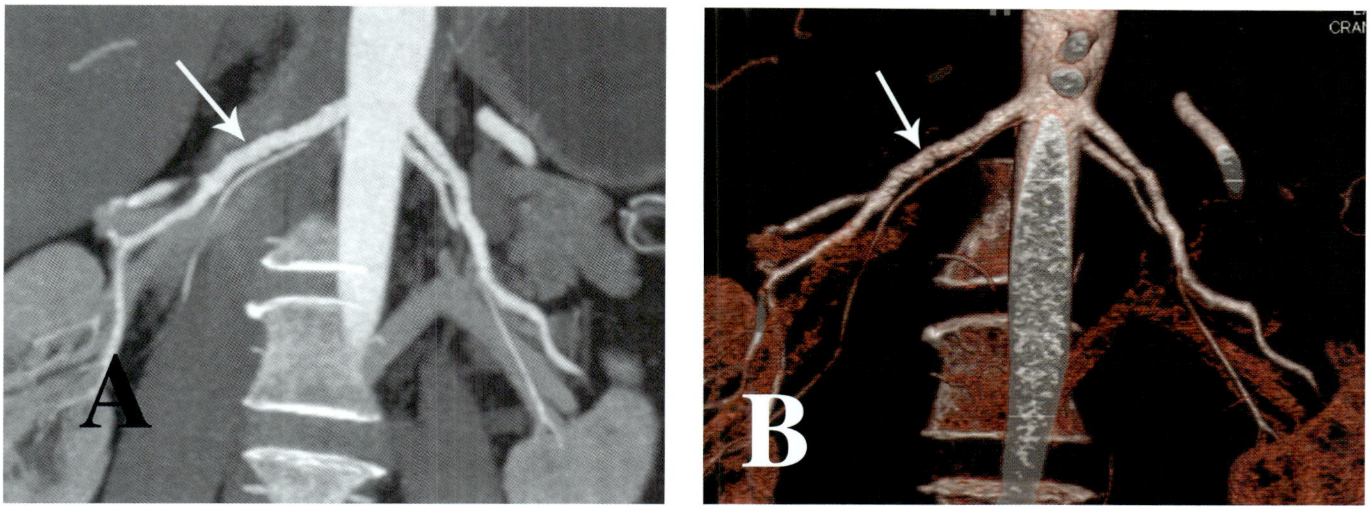

Figure 81.2 **A.** A 55-year-old potential renal donor woman with renal fibromuscular dysplasia incidentally found on a CT performed for evaluation of renal vascular anatomy. Coronal contrast-enhanced arterial phase CT maximal intensity projection image demonstrates beaded appearance of the mid-right renal artery (arrow). **B.** Anterior volume-rendered image demonstrates beaded appearance of the mid-right renal artery (arrow).

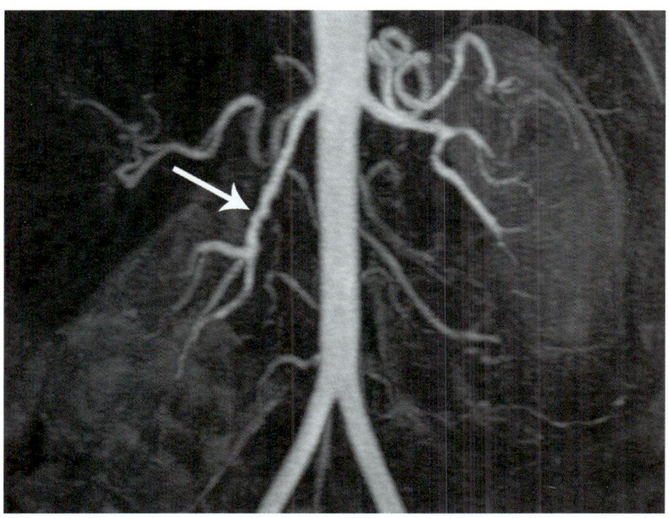

Figure 81.3 A 55-year-old woman with history of bilateral carotid artery dissections and presenting with hypertension. Coronal contrast-enhanced arterial phase MRA maximal intensity projection image demonstrates beaded appearance of the mid-right renal artery (arrow). Notice sparing of the proximal renal artery.

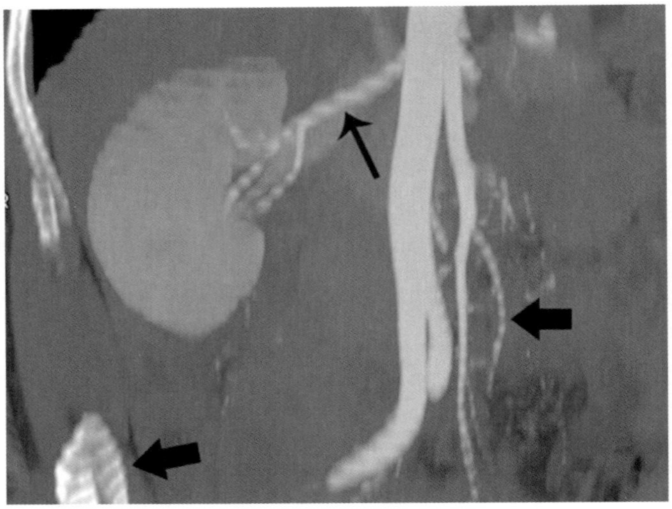

Figure 81.4 Coronal contrast-enhanced arterial phase MIP image demonstrating pseudo FMD from thick slab reconstruction with 5 mm axial slice thickness (thin arrow). Note that similar artifact is seen in other vasculature and the osseous structures (thick arrows).

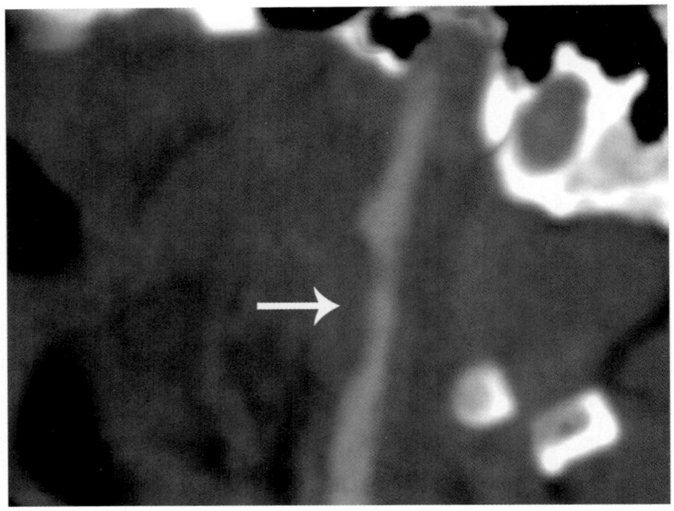

Figure 81.5 A 51-year-old man with aphasia and right leg numbness (same patient as in Figure 81.1). Contrast-enhanced arterial phase maximal intensity projection CT demonstrates dissection of the left internal carotid artery with luminal narrowing (arrow).

CASE 82

Reversal of superior mesenteric artery and vein in midgut volvulus

Vivek Halappa and Atif Zaheer

Imaging description

The misalignment of the superior mesenteric artery (SMA)–superior mesenteric vein (SMV) complex and malpositioning of bowel structures may be seen in an adult asymptomatic patient. Normally the SMV is to the right of the SMA; with malrotation, the SMV may occupy a position directly anterior or to the left of the SMA creating a distinctive "whirlpool" pattern (Figures 82.1A and 82.1B). This can be identified on cross-sectional imaging.[1] There is misplacement of the duodenojejunal junction to the right of the midline with the presence of the jejunal loops in the right abdomen and a left-sided-colon (Figure 82.1C). Associated pancreatic abnormalities may also be present such as aplasia of the uncinate process and short pancreas (Figure 82.1D).[2] Upper GI examination may also be performed to confirm the course of the duodenum and positioning of the ligament of Treitz (Figure 82.2).

Importance

Bowel malrotation occurs from shortening of the small bowel mesenteric root during embryologic development with less than 270° of counterclockwise rotation through the umbilicus between the fifth and tenth week of gestation. Midgut volvulus is a major complication and is the most common cause of bowel obstruction in adults with malrotation.[3] However, bowel malrotation mostly presents as chronic abdominal pain in adults. The symptoms may be due to acute or chronic intestinal obstruction caused by the presence of abnormal peritoneal bands (Ladd's bands) or a volvulus. There is also a high association with peptic ulcer disease, which may be caused by chronic partial gastric or duodenal outlet obstruction.[4]

Typical clinical scenario

Bowel malrotation is usually asymptomatic in adults and may present as vague chronic abdominal pain.[3] When complicated with midgut volvulus, symptoms of abdominal pain, bilious vomiting, and bloody stools may occur. Definitive treatment based upon the severity of symptoms is the Ladd procedure, which includes mobilization of the right colon and the duodenum, division of Ladd's bands and adhesions around the SMA, and appendectomy.[5]

Differential diagnosis

Abdominal pain associated with bowel malrotation in an adult patient presents as non-specific pain and differential considerations such as gallstone disease, chronic pancreatitis, inflammatory bowel disease etc. may be considered. When presenting with midgut volvulus, causes of bowel rotation such as bowel obstruction due to adhesions or internal hernia may be considered.

Teaching point

Bowel malrotation may be a cause of chronic abdominal pain in adults and can be identified as reversal of the SMA and SMV on cross-sectional imaging as well as misplacement of the duodenojejunal junction.

REFERENCES

1. D. M. Nichols, D. K. Li. Superior mesenteric vein rotation: a CT sign of midgut malrotation. *AJR Am J Roentgenol* 1983; **141**: 707–8.
2. R. Zissin, V. Rathaus, A. Oscadchy, E. Kots, G. Gayer, M. Shapiro-Feinberg. Intestinal malrotation as an incidental finding on CT in adults. *Abdom Imaging* 1999; **24**: 550–5.
3. A. K. Wanjari, A. J. Deshmukh, P. S. Tayde, Y. Lonkar. Midgut malrotation with chronic abdominal pain. *N Am J Med Sci* 2012; **4**: 196–8.
4. M. Pelucio, Y. Haywood. Midgut volvulus: an unusual case of adolescent abdominal pain. *Am J Emerg Med* 1994; **12**: 167–71.
5. L. R. Schultz, E. P. Lasher, A. H. Bill, Jr. Abnormalities of rotation of the bowel. *Am J Surg* 1961; **101**: 128–33.

Pearls and Pitfalls in Cardiovascular Imaging, ed. Stefan L. Zimmerman and Elliot K. Fishman. Published by Cambridge University Press. © Cambridge University Press 2015.

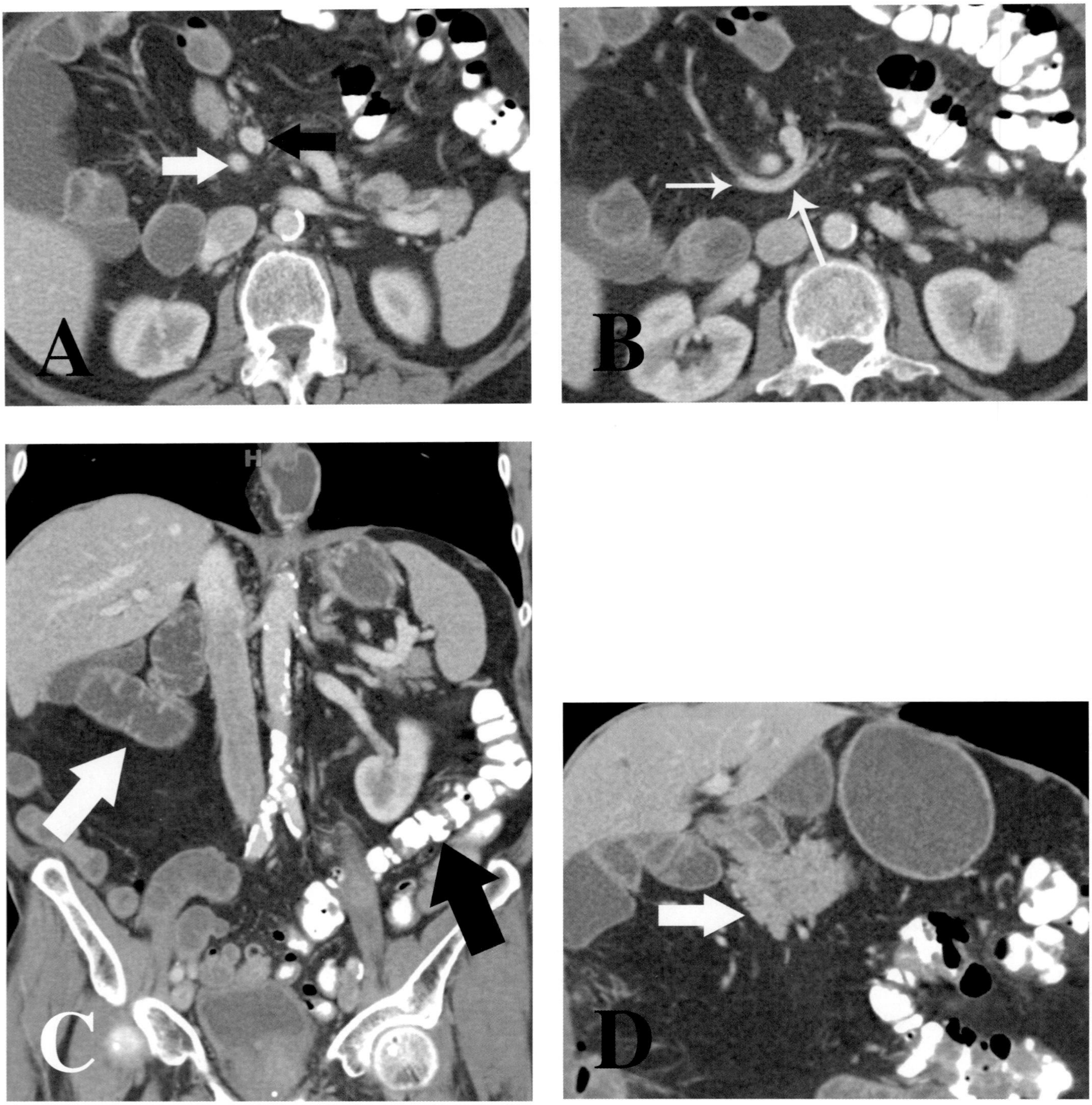

Figure 82.1 **A.** A 72-year old man with abdominal pain. Axial contrast-enhanced CT image demonstrates reversed SMA/SMV orientation with the SMV (black arrow) to the left of the SMA (white arrow). **B.** Axial contrast-enhanced CT image demonstrates going around, making a distinctive "whirlpool" pattern (arrows). **C.** Coronal contrast-enhanced CT image demonstrates jejunal loops in the right abdomen (white arrow) and the presence of large bowel in the left abdomen (black arrow). **D.** Coronal contrast-enhanced CT image demonstrates a short pancreas with aplasia of the uncinate process (white arrow).

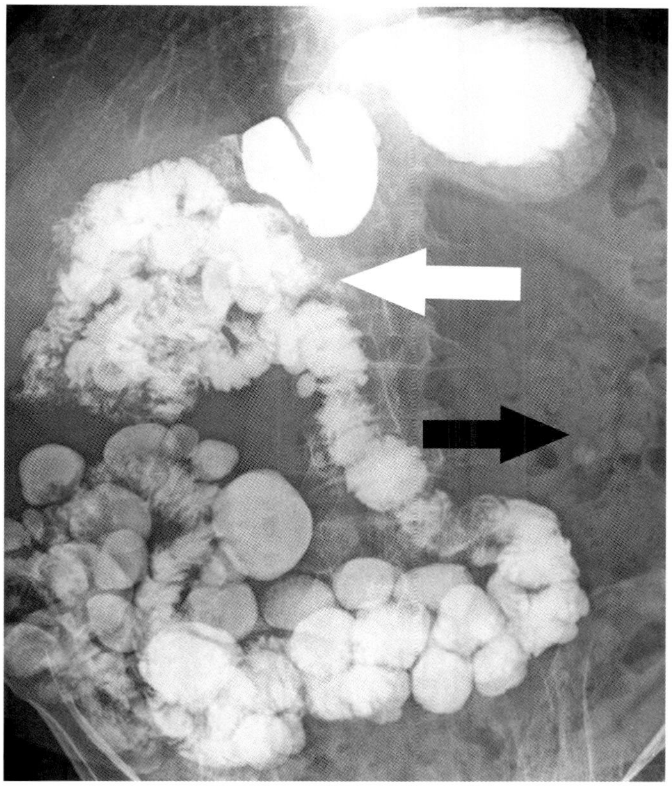

Figure 82.2 Small bowel follow-through in the same patient as above demonstrates the presence of jejuna loops in the left abdomen (white arrow). Stool can be seen present in the large bowel on the left (black arrow).

CASE **83**

Mesenteric artery collateral pathways

Atif Zaheer

Imaging description

The arc of Buhler is a persistent embryological communication between the proximal celiac axis and the superior mesenteric artery (SMA). It is short in length, arising from the proximal SMA and coursing vertically to anastomose with the proximal common hepatic artery. The arc of Buhler is a developmental variant, and can be present with or without associated celiac trunk stenosis. However, when present, it provides important collateral flow between the SMA and celiac trunk in the setting of celiac trunk occlusion or high-grade stenosis. Arterial phase CT angiography with the use of multiplanar reconstructions and three-dimensional volume rendered images will clearly demonstrate the anomalous vessel, which will be prominent in the setting of celiac artery disease (Figures 83.1 and 83.2).

Importance

Communication between the celiac axis, common hepatic artery, splenic artery, and the SMA known as the arc of Buhler represents a failure of embryologic regression of the ventral anastomosis between the celiac axis and the SMA. This persistent communication is seen in up to 4% of individuals.[1] The presence of this anastomotic variant leads to a change in the normal hemodynamics of the upper visceral circulation. The size of the arc of Buhler is usually less than 2.5 mm and may be considered significant when it preferentially fills the communicating visceral branches on diagnostic angiography.[2] The preoperative knowledge of this variant is essential for surgical planning in cases of liver transplantation, hepatic artery chemoembolization, and pancreaticoduodenal surgeries such as the Whipple procedure or total pancreatectomy, especially when the gastroduodenal artery needs to be ligated in the presence of celiac axis or SMA stenosis.[3,4]

Typical clinical scenario

This rare variant may be incidentally seen on routine angiography for the evaluation of gastrointestinal bleed or on CT angiography performed for liver or pancreas evaluation.

Differential diagnosis

A variant of the arc of Buhler is the Kirk's arcade, which is a communication of the splenic artery with the anterior and posterior pancreaticoduodenal arcades via the dorsal pancreatic artery.[4,5] Chronic celiac axis occlusion from vasculitis or atherosclerotic disease with prominent collateral vessels, typically the pancreaticoduodenal arcades, and gastroduodenal artery, may also be considered.

Teaching point

Arc of Buhler, an uncommon persistent embryologic communication between the celiac artery and the SMA, can be seen on CTA with or without associated celiac artery stenosis, and is important to identify prior to surgical or interventional procedures.

REFERENCES

1. E. Grabbe, E. Bucheler. [Buhler's anastomosis (author's transl.)]. *Rofo* 1980; **132**: 541–6.
2. W. E. Saad, M. G. Davies, L. Sahler, et al. Arc of Buhler: incidence and diameter in asymptomatic individuals. *Vasc Endovascular Surg* 2005; **39**: 347–9.
3. S. Y. Song, J. W. Chung, J. W. Kwon, et al. Collateral pathways in patients with celiac axis stenosis: angiographic-spiral CT correlation. *Radiographics* 2002; **22**: 881–93.
4. J. G. McNulty, N. Hickey, F. Khosa, P. O'Brien, J. P. O'Callaghan. Surgical and radiological significance of variants of Buhler's anastomotic artery: a report of three cases. *Surg Radiol Anat* 2001; **23**: 277–80.
5. H. Matsumura. The significance of the morphology of the dorsal pancreatic artery in determining the presence of the accessory right hepatic artery passing behind the portal vein. *Kaibogaku Zasshi* 1998; **73**: 517–27.

Pearls and Pitfalls in Cardiovascular Imaging, ed. Stefan L. Zimmerman and Elliot K. Fishman. Published by Cambridge University Press. © Cambridge University Press 2015.

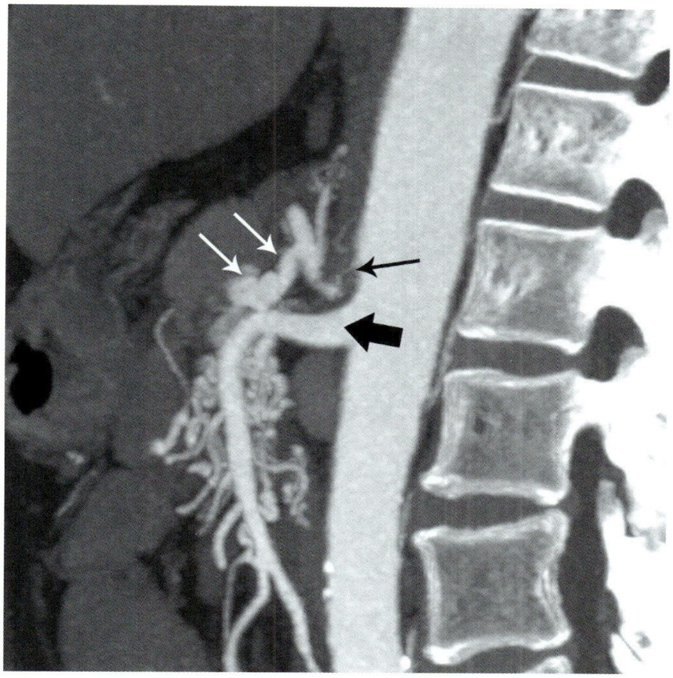

Figure 83.1 A 61-year-old woman with CTA performed for the evaluation of a pancreatic cyst. Contrast-enhanced arterial phase sagittal multiplanar reconstruction image of the aorta demonstrates an absent celiac artery (thin black arrow) and a patent SMA (thick arrow). A communication between the celiac axis and the SMA can be seen (thin white arrows).

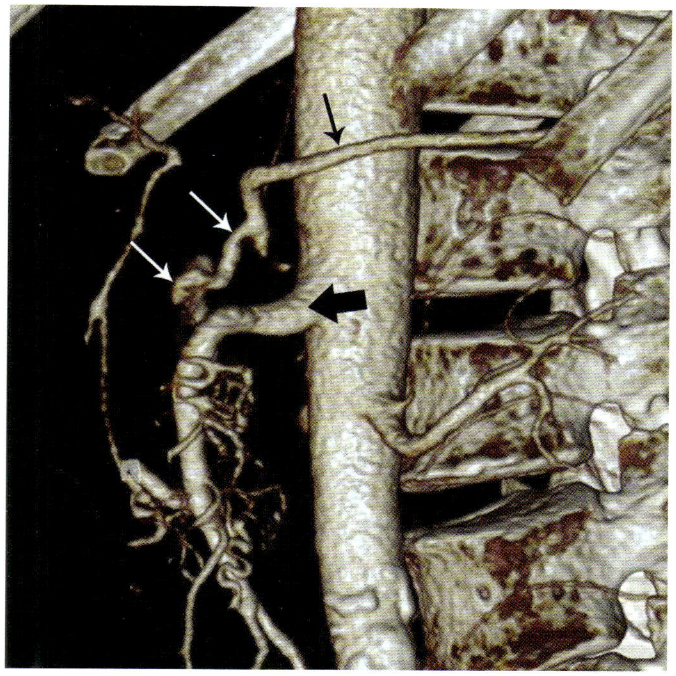

Figure 83.2 Contrast-enhanced arterial phase three-dimensional volume rendered image demonstrates a communication (thin white arrows) between the SMA and the splenic artery (thin black arrow). A patent SMA is also seen (thick black arrow).

CASE 84

Mesenteric artery anatomic variants

Satomi Kawamoto

Imaging description

In the classic anatomy, the common hepatic artery (CHA), left gastric artery (LGA) and splenic artery (SA) arise from the celiac axis (CA), and the superior mesenteric artery (SMA) arises from the aorta without an aberrant or accessory hepatic artery (61–76% of normal population[1–3]) (Figure 84.1). There are multiple types of variant anatomy of these vessels. The most common variations are a replaced or accessory left hepatic artery originating from the LGA (9.7–12.5%[3,4]), a replaced or accessory right hepatic artery originating from the SMA (7.5–10.6%[3,4]), or a combination of replaced or accessory right and left hepatic arteries (2.3–4.5%[3,4]) (Figure 84.2). Less commonly, the origin of the CHA arises from the SMA (1.5–3%[1,3,5]) (Figure 84.3) or directly from the aorta (0.2–2%[1,3,5]) (Figures 84.4 and 84.5). In these cases the splenic artery and left gastric artery often arise directly from the aorta (gastrosplenic, or lienogastric trunk) (Figures 84.3 and 84.5). Common origin of the CA and SMA (celiacomesenteric trunk) is seen in 0.7–1.1% of population (Figure 84.6).[2,5] Other uncommon variations include the splenic artery originating from SMA (splenomesenteric trunk) (0.24%[5]) (Figure 84.7), and the CHA originating from the left gastric artery (hepaticogastric trunk) (0.2–0.3%[2,5]) (Figure 84.7). Additional very rare patterns also have been described.

Typically, the common hepatic artery has a suprapancreatic, preportal course; however, there can be a variation in the pathway of CHA, such as a retrocaval course or passing through the pancreatic parenchyma, particularly when the CHA arises from the SMA (Figure 84.3).[2,5]

Importance

For preoperative planning of the abdominal surgery, it is important to understand the celiac axis, hepatic arterial, and mesenteric arterial anatomy to avoid or minimize serious ischemic complications. To perform interventional radiologic procedures such as intra-arterial hepatic tumor management and embolotherapy for hemorrhage, preprocedural evaluation of variant celiac axis and hepatic arterial anatomy is important for treatment planning.

Typical clinical scenario

Variant anatomy is usually an incidental finding of CT. It is best visualized on arterial phase, thin-slice images. Multiplanar reconstruction and 3D imaging created from thin slice reconstruction can demonstrate detailed anatomy and the spatial relationship of each vessel.

Differential diagnosis

Patients with a surgically created anastomosis may have findings that simulate variant anatomy, or potentially cause a confusing picture if the surgical history is uncertain.

Teaching point

A number of variants of the normal vascular anatomy of the celiac axis, hepatic artery, and SMA can be encountered. Accurate description is of critical importance for surgical planning of hepatic and other upper abdominal surgeries and interventional procedures. Thin-slice images acquired at arterial phase with multiplanar and 3D reconstruction are the most useful for demonstrating detailed vascular anatomy.

REFERENCES

1. Covey AM, Brody LA, Maluccio MA, Getrajdman GI, Brown KT. Variant hepatic arterial anatomy revisited: digital subtraction angiography performed in 600 patients. *Radiology* 2002;**224**:542–547.
2. Chen H, Yano R, Emura S, Shoumura S. Anatomic variation of the celiac trunk with special reference to hepatic artery patterns. *Annals of Anatomy = Anatomischer Anzeiger* 2009;**191**:399–407.
3. Hiatt JR, Gabbay J, Busuttil RW. Surgical anatomy of the hepatic arteries in 1000 cases. *Annals of Surgery* 1994;**220**:50–52.
4. Suzuki T, Nakayasu A, Kawabe K, Takeda H, Honjo I. Surgical significance of anatomic variations of the hepatic artery. *American Journal of Surgery* 1971;**122**:505–512.
5. Song SY, Chung JW, Yin YH, et al. Celiac axis and common hepatic artery variations in 5002 patients: systematic analysis with spiral CT and DSA. *Radiology* 2010;**255**:278–288.

Pearls and Pitfalls in Cardiovascular Imaging, ed. Stefan L. Zimmerman and Elliot K. Fishman. Published by Cambridge University Press. © Cambridge University Press 2015.

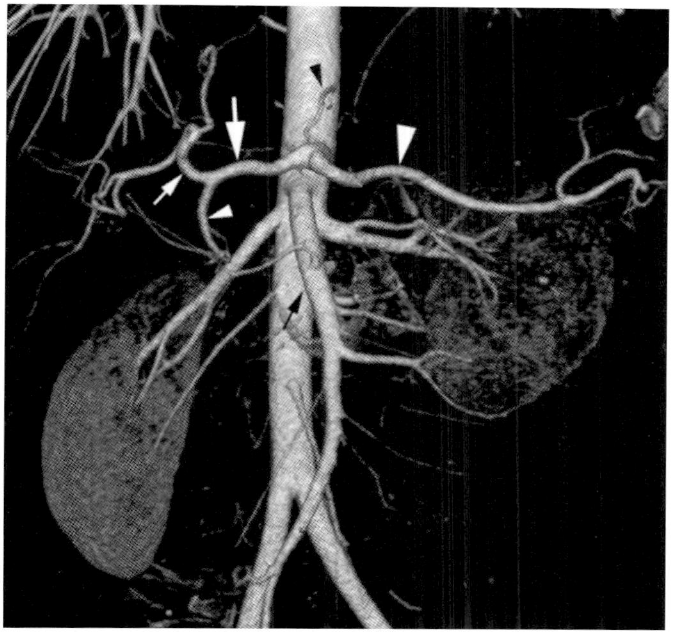

Figure 84.1 Classic anatomy of celiac axis and superior mesenteric artery. The common hepatic artery (large white arrow), left gastric artery (small black arrowhead) and splenic artery (large white arrowhead) arise from the celiac axis, and the superior mesenteric artery (small black arrow) arises from the aorta. Small white arrow: proper hepatic artery. Small white arrowhead: gastroduodenal artery.

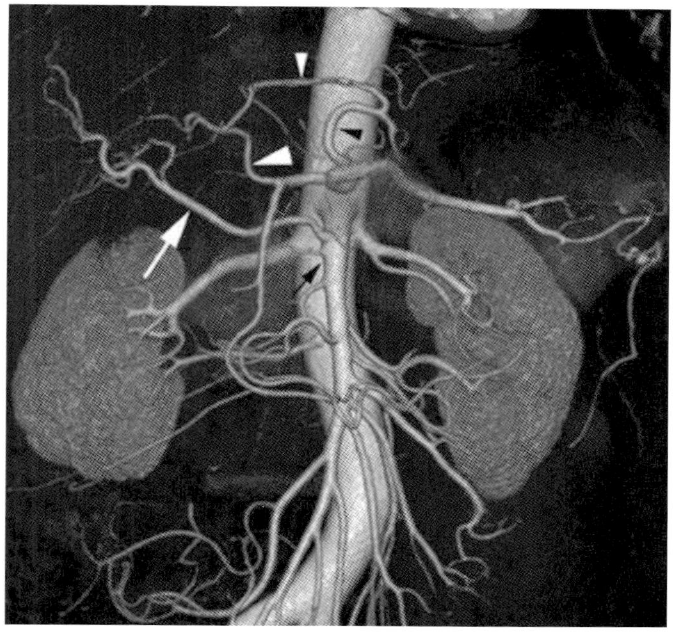

Figure 84.2 Accessory/replaced hepatic arteries. Replaced right hepatic artery (white arrow) arises from the superior mesenteric artery (black arrow). Accessory left hepatic artery (small white arrowhead) arises from the left gastric artery (black arrowhead). Large white arrowhead: left hepatic artery.

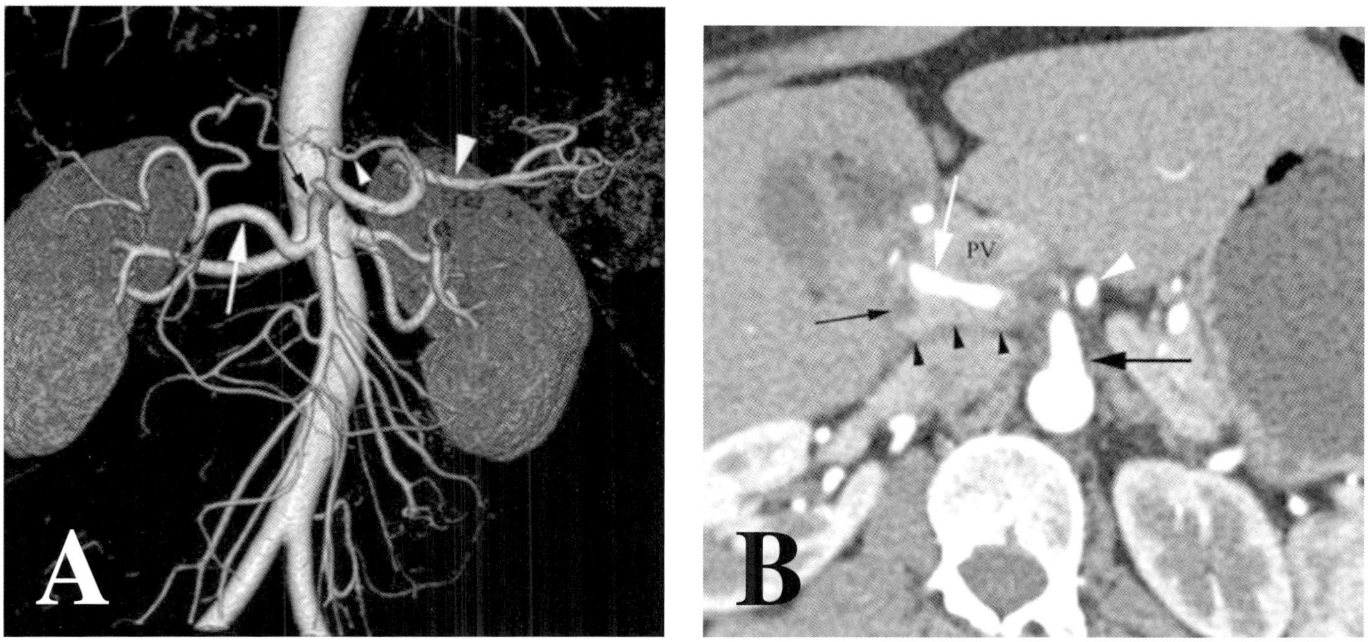

Figure 84.3 **A.** Hepaticomesenteric trunk and gastrosplenic trunk (2.6% [5]). The common hepatic artery (white arrow) arises from the superior mesenteric artery (black arrow). The left gastric artery (small white arrowhead) arises from the splenic artery (large white arrowhead). **B.** Hepaticomesenteric trunk and gastrosplenic trunk [5]. The common hepatic artery (white arrow) arising from the superior mesenteric artery (large black arrow) passes through the pancreatic parenchyma (black arrowheads). PV: portal vein. Small black arrow: common bile duct. White arrowhead: splenic artery.

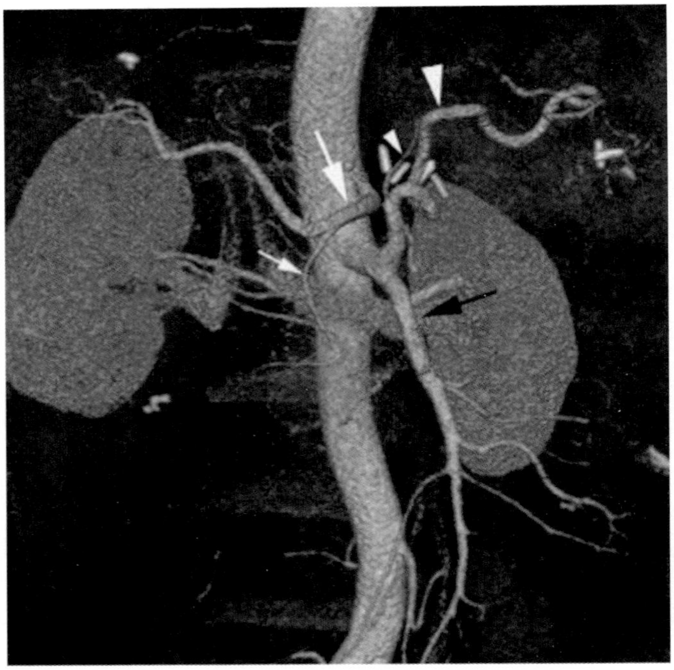

Figure 84.4 Common hepatic artery and gastrosplenomesenteric trunk (0.06% [5]). The common hepatic artery (large white arrow) arises from the aorta. The superior mesenteric artery (black arrow), splenic artery (large white arrowhead), and left gastric artery (small white arrowhead) arise from the common trunk. Small white arrow: gastroduodenal artery.

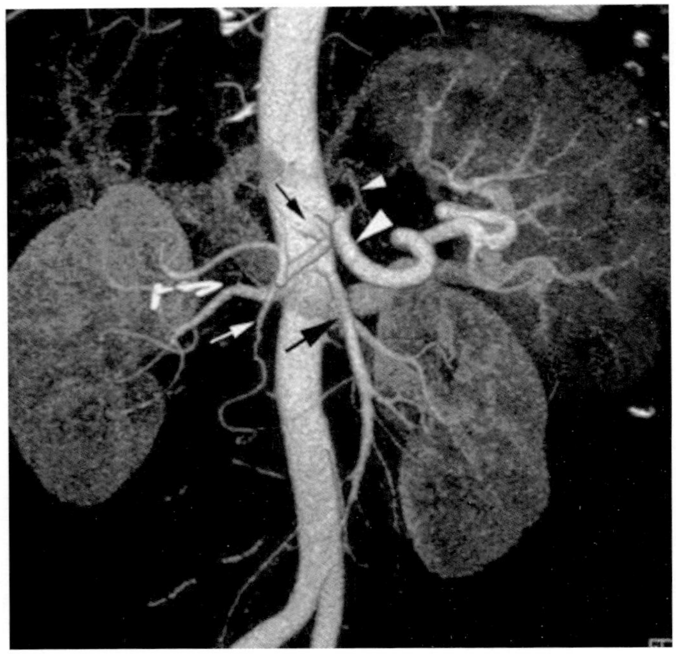

Figure 84.5 Common hepatic artery (small black arrow), gastrosplenic trunk, and superior mesenteric artery (large black arrow) (0.22% [5]). The left gastric artery (small white arrowhead) arises from the splenic artery (large white arrowhead). White arrow: gastroduodenal artery.

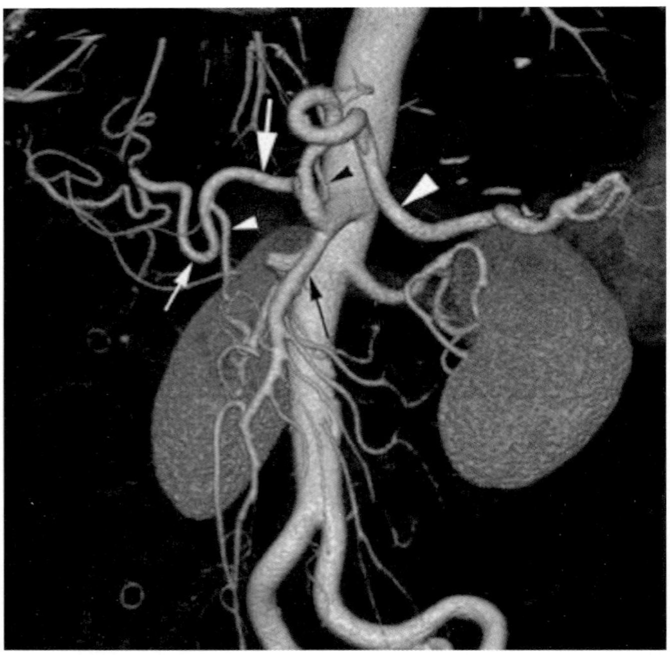

Figure 84.6 Celiacomesenteric trunk (1.1% [5]). The celiac axis and the superior mesenteric artery (black arrow) arise from a common trunk. Large white arrow: common hepatic artery, large white arrowhead: splenic artery, small black arrowhead: left gastric artery, small white arrowhead: gastroduodenal artery, small white arrow: proper hepatic artery.

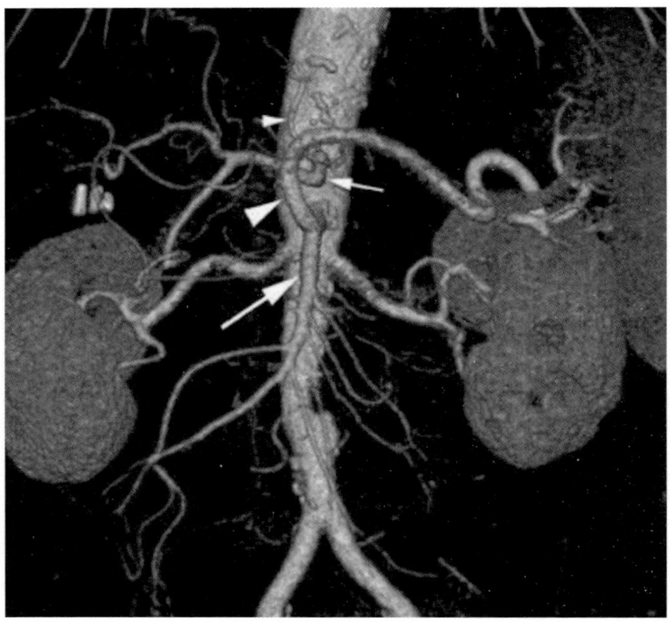

Figure 84.7 Hepatogastric trunk and splenomesenteric trunk (0.16% [5]). The splenic artery (large arrowhead) and superior mesenteric artery (large arrow) arise from a common trunk. The common hepatic artery (small arrow) and the left gastric artery (small arrowhead) arise from a common trunk.

CASE **85**

Superficial femoral artery occlusions

Stefan L. Zimmerman

Imaging description

Superficial femoral artery (SFA) occlusions may be missed in at least two scenarios at cross-sectional imaging. On standard abdominopelvic CT examinations, the SFAs are often only visualized on the last few slices obtained. In our experience, it is not uncommon for SFA occlusions to go unnoticed, particularly in patients with extensive atherosclerotic disease, given that they are an "edge of the film" finding and may not be included in the typical radiologist search pattern (Figure 85.1). The other scenario where SFA occlusions may be missed occurs with MRA examinations of the lower extremity. Symmetric bilateral occlusions may be difficult to appreciate on coronal maximum intensity projection (MIP) images of the lower extremities, given extensive collateral vascularity from the deep femoral arteries (Figures 85.2 and 85.3). In addition, SFA occlusions often begin at the origin of the vessel and continue for its entire length. In these cases, SFA occlusions must be recognized as the absence of a finding, i.e., the normal vessel, which can be challenging. The normal SFA should be recognized as a medially located vessel free from significant branches along its course through the thigh, unlike the deep femoral artery, which is located laterally and more posterior with numerous branches.

Importance

Occlusions of the SFA can be clinically important, potentially resulting in claudication symptoms, rest pain or, in extreme cases, tissue ischemia. SFA occlusions due to embolic phenomena are important to recognize as patients may require anticoagulation or thrombectomy and additional imaging studies may be necessary to identify the source of the embolus.

Typical clinical scenario

SFA occlusions may be encountered incidentally in patients with extensive atherosclerotic disease or may be the primary finding in patients being evaluated for suspected peripheral arterial disease (PAD). The prevalence of PAD is approximately 12% in older adults.[1]

Differential diagnosis

In patients with prior surgery for peripheral arterial disease, occlusions of grafts within the thigh may be mistaken for occlusion of the native vessel. Early acquisition after contrast injection with multidetector CT can result in the scanner outrunning the contrast bolus, resulting in SFAs that are unopacified with contrast. On MRA examinations, the presence of metal hardware, such as due to hip prostheses, may create susceptibility artifact that can result in signal voids in the SFA, simulating occlusion.[2]

Teaching point

Superficial femoral artery occlusions may be missed on routine CT examinations of the abdomen and pelvis and on MRA examinations of the lower extremity. Awareness of the typical imaging findings will help avoid misdiagnosis.

REFERENCES

1. M. H. Criqui, A. Fronek, E. Barrett-Connor, M. R. Klauber, S. Gabriel, D. Goodman. The prevalence of peripheral arterial disease in a defined population. *Circulation* 1985; **71**: 510–15.
2. H. Ersoy, H. Zhang, M. R. Prince. Peripheral MR angiography. *J Cardiovasc Magn Reson* 2006; **8**: 517–28.

Pearls and Pitfalls in Cardiovascular Imaging, ed. Stefan L. Zimmerman and Elliot K. Fishman. Published by Cambridge University Press. © Cambridge University Press 2015.

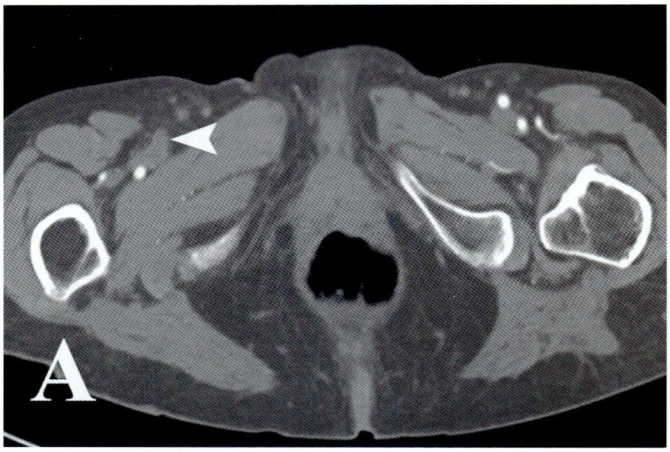

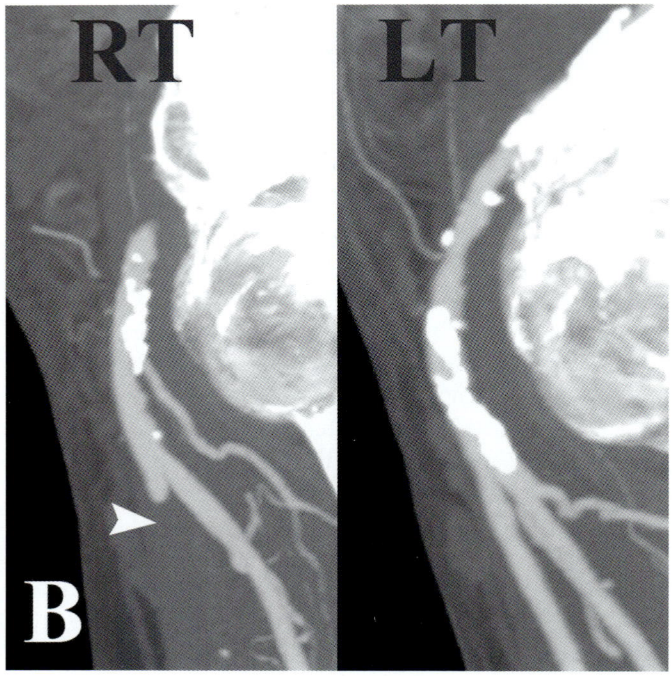

Figure 85.1 **A.** Axial image from a CT performed in an 84-year-old female with bladder cancer demonstrates right superficial femoral artery (SFA) occlusion (arrowhead) that had been missed on several previous examinations. SFA occlusions are not uncommonly missed on studies performed for non-vascular indications, given they are located at the edge of the film and outside of typical search patterns. **B.** SFA occlusion is confirmed on sagittal maximum intensity projection (MIP) images of the right (RT) and left (LT) femoral arteries. There is abrupt cutoff of the right SFA (arrowhead).

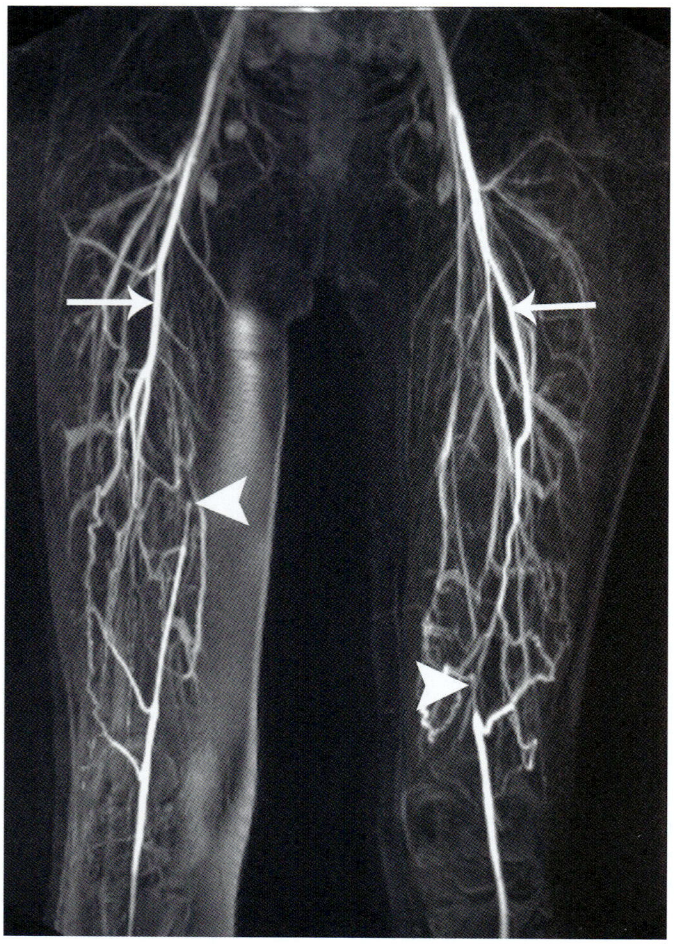

Figure 85.2 Coronal MIP from an MRA of the lower extremity performed in a 33-year-old female with Takayasu's arteritis demonstrates bilateral SFA occlusions. Reconstitution of the SFAs (arrowheads) is seen on the right side at mid-thigh level and on the left side just above the knee. There is extensive collateralization from the deep femoral arteries (thin arrows), which may distract the imager from identifying SFA occlusions. The deep femoral arteries can be recognized by the presence of multiple branches, whereas the SFA should have no significant branches in the thigh.

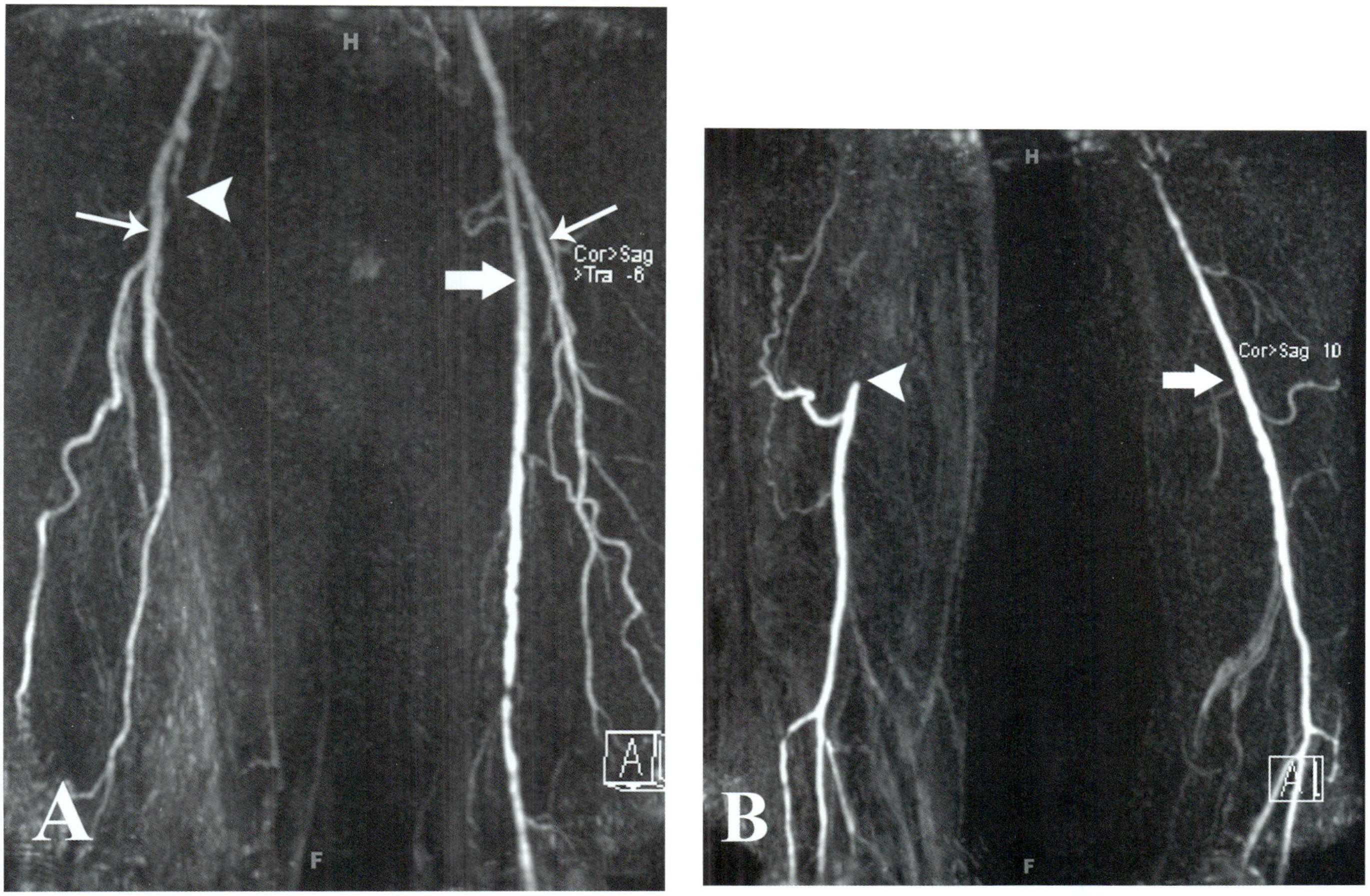

Figure 85.3 Coronal MIPs of the lower extremities from an MRA performed in a 73-year-old male with claudication. **A.** On the upper station, there is unilateral right-sided SFA occlusion (arrowhead). The deep femoral arteries are large with multiple prominent branches (thin arrows). The left-sided superficial femoral artery is patent and can be recognized by its medial location and lack of branches (thick arrow). **B.** On the middle station, reconstitution of right runoff at the popliteal is seen (arrowhead), via deep femoral collateral arteries. The left SFA and popliteal arteries are patent (arrow).

CASE 86 Popliteal artery entrapment

Vivek Halappa and Atif Zaheer

Imaging description

Popliteal artery entrapment is a developmental abnormality that results in compression of the popliteal artery due to abnormal relationships between the vessel and adjacent soft tissues within the popliteal fossa. Several types of developmental abnormalities that may result in entrapment have been identified.[1] In most cases, the popliteal artery is medially displaced. In some cases, this is due to an anomalous course of the vessel, which can wrap around the medial head of the gastrocnemius muscle. In other patients, the artery is deviated medially by anomalous muscular or fibrous bands or anomalous lateral insertion of the medial head of the gastrocnemius muscle. Finally, in some patients there are no anomalous structures but the artery is compressed by hypertrophied gastrocnemius muscles.

Conventional angiography in neutral, dorsi- and plantar flex maneuvers is the traditional gold standard for the diagnosis of popliteal entrapment as it can identify the site of arterial injury. However, it is not commonly used due to its invasiveness and inability to delineate surrounding anatomy. Color Doppler sonography demonstrates popliteal artery narrowing, changes in color flow, or increased peak systolic velocity on flexion maneuvers but may have a significant false positive rate.[2]

CT angiography with three separate intravenous injections in neutral, dorsi- and plantar flexion along with maximum intensity projection and volume-rendered images provide excellent contrast and spatial resolution of the surrounding abnormalities as well as the presence of occlusion and collateral formation.[3]

MR imaging and MR angiography with gadolinium is used to evaluate the anatomy of the popliteal fossa and the presence of any vascular compromise during compression maneuvers with superior capability of demonstrating surrounding soft tissue abnormality compared to CTA (Figure 86.1). Although MRI is comparable to conventional angiography, its main limitation is the underestimation of $< 50\%$ narrowing.[1]

Importance

Popliteal artery entrapment is an uncommon clinical syndrome seen in young adults, causing ischemic symptoms in the lower extremities. It occurs as a result of compression of the popliteal artery due to abnormal development resulting in abnormal anatomic relationship between the vessel and surrounding musculoskeletal structures.[4] Bilateral disease is present in 22–67% of patients.[5] Early diagnosis is very important since popliteal artery entrapment is a progressive condition and early treatment may prevent serious complications. Popliteal artery compression can cause chronic vascular microtrauma with arteriosclerosis and thrombus formation with distal ischemia. Stenosis and turbulent flow can lead to post-stenotic ectasia or aneurysm formation, which can result in aneurysmal dilatation, thrombosis or embolism and can potentially result in ischemia and threaten the viability of the limb. Treatment is surgical release of the entrapped vessel.

Typical clinical scenario

Mostly affecting young athletic men, popliteal artery entrapment patients present with progressive calf claudication and possibly with ischemia due to thrombosis in severe cases.

Differential diagnosis

Clinical correlation with symptoms is crucial given the presence of some degree of the narrowing of the vessel on stress maneuvers in as many as 50% of the general population.[6] Differential diagnosis in patients with popliteal artery entrapment include conditions causing intermittent claudication, namely cystic adventitial disease, arterial compression by bone lesions, fibromuscular dysplasia, Takayasu's arteritis, and Buerger's disease.

Teaching point

Diagnosis of popliteal artery entrapment involves identifying abnormalities in the affected artery as well as the abnormal anatomic structures responsible for the entrapment. MRI and MR angiography with stress maneuvers can demonstrate both the arterial findings and abnormal muscular or fibrous attachment necessary for diagnosis and further management.

REFERENCES

1. H. K. Kim, M. J. Shin, S. M. Kim, S. H. Lee, H. J. Hong. Popliteal artery entrapment syndrome: morphological classification utilizing MR imaging. *Skeletal Radiol* 2006; **35**: 648–58.
2. U. Hoffmann, J. Vetter, L. Rainoni, A. J. Leu, A. Bollinger. Popliteal artery compression and force of active plantar flexion in young healthy volunteers. *J Vasc Surg* 1997; **26**: 281–7.

Pearls and Pitfalls in Cardiovascular Imaging, ed. Stefan L. Zimmerman and Elliot K. Fishman. Published by Cambridge University Press. © Cambridge University Press 2015.

3. T. A. Macedo, C. M. Johnson, J. W. Hallett, Jr., J. F. Breen. Popliteal artery entrapment syndrome: role of imaging in the diagnosis. *AJR Am J Roentgenol* 2003; **181**: 1259–65.

4. N. M. Rich, G. J. Collins, Jr., P. T. McDonald, L. Kozloff, G. P. Clagett, J. T. Collins. Popliteal vascular entrapment. Its increasing interest. *Arch Surg* 1979; **114**: 1377–84.

5. P. S. Collins, P. T. McDonald, R. C. Lim. Popliteal artery entrapment: an evolving syndrome. *J Vasc Surg* 1989; **10**: 484–9; discussion 89–90.

6. L. S. Erdoes, J. J. Devine, V. M. Bernhard, M. R. Baker, S. S. Berman, G. C. Hunter. Popliteal vascular compression in a normal population. *J Vasc Surg* 1994; **20**: 978–86.

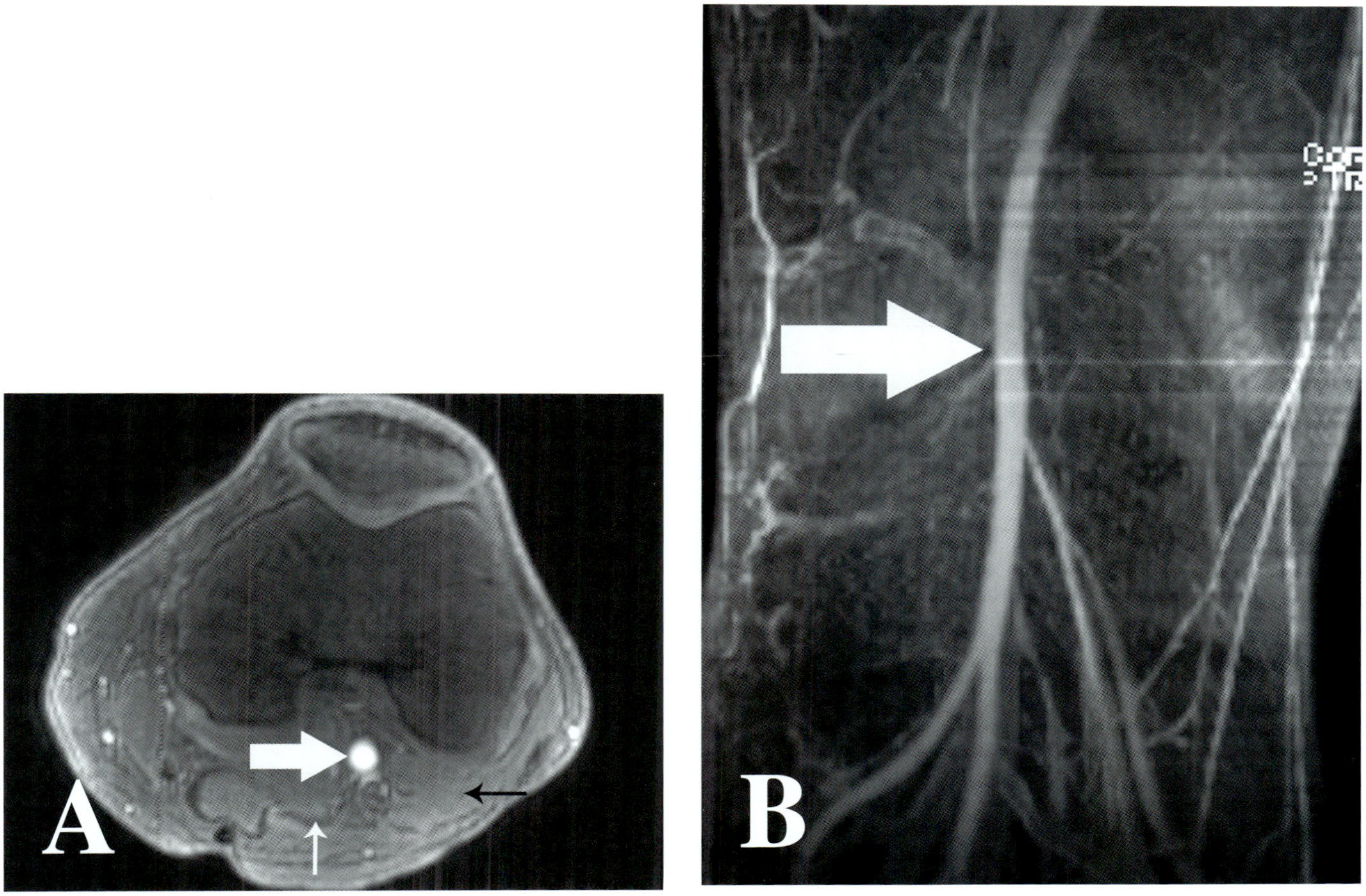

Figure 86.1 **A.** A 33-year old man with popliteal artery entrapment due to gastrocnemius muscle compression. Axial post-contrast T1-weighted image obtained in the neutral position demonstrates normal appearance of the popliteal artery (thick arrow) between the medial (thin white arrow) and the lateral (thin black arrow) heads of the gastrocnemius muscle. **B.** Maximal intensity projection image of the post-contrast MRA image obtained in the neutral position shows a normal popliteal artery (arrow). **C.** Axial post-contrast T1-weighted image obtained in the dorsiflexion position demonstrates >50% narrowing of the popliteal artery (arrow) between the 2 heads of the gastrocnemius muscle. **D.** Maximal intensity projection image of the post-contrast MRA image obtained in the dorsiflexion position shows a normal proximal popliteal artery (thick arrow) with severe narrowing in the popliteal fossa (thin arrows).

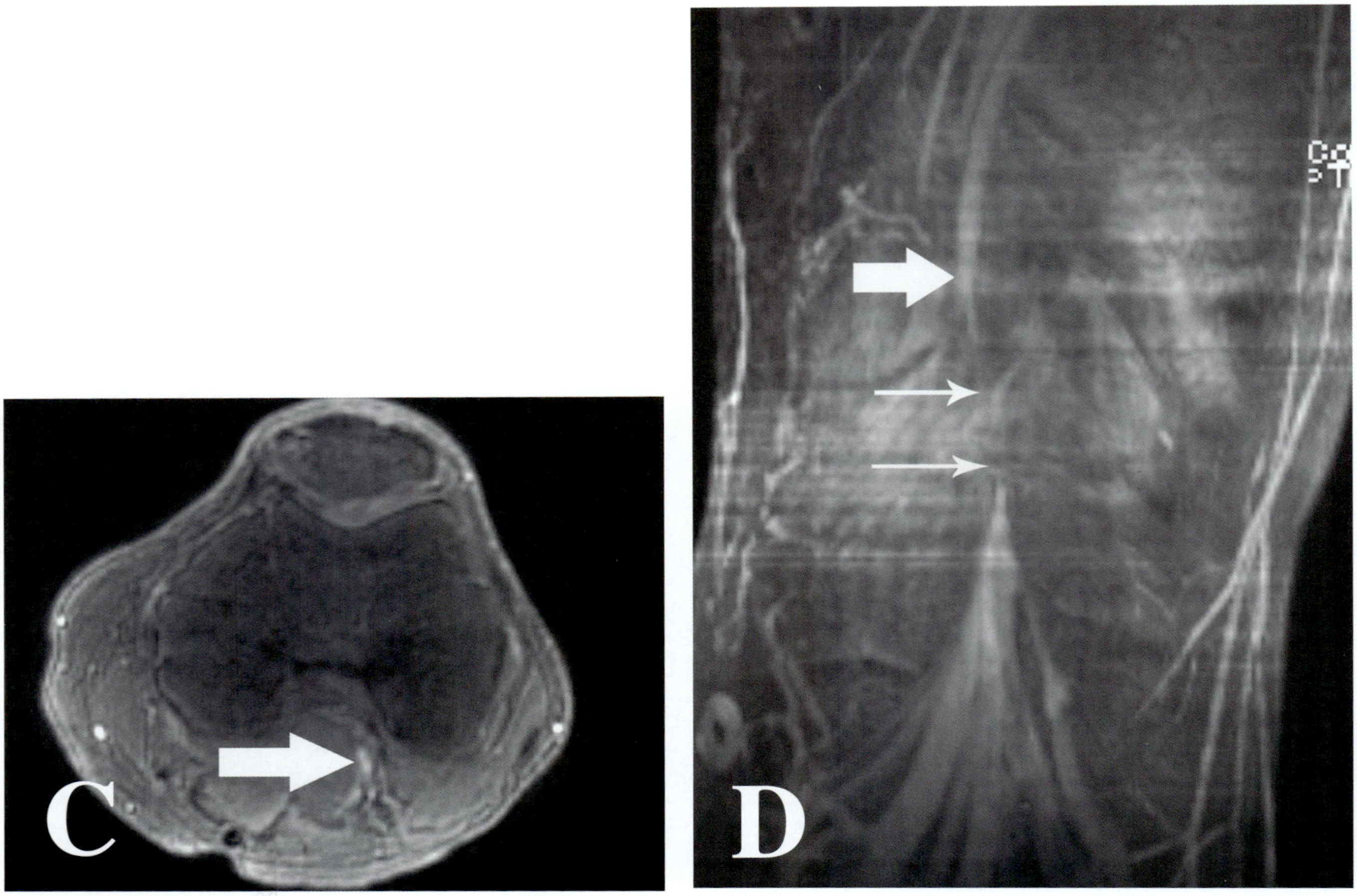

Figure 86.1 (*cont.*)

CASE 87

Suboptimal bolus timing in CT angiography of the extremities

Tessa S. Cook

Imaging description

Images with inadequate arterial opacification from suboptimal bolus timing demonstrate gradually decreasing opacification in the lower extremity arteries as they course distally. Often, the distal calf vessels are most severely affected, sometimes demonstrating a complete lack of opacification, which can simulate occlusion due to atherosclerotic or thrombotic disease. (Figures 87.1 and 87.2). However, immediate delayed images through the lower extremities will show complete opacification of the distal vessels, allowing for accurate characterization of vascular disease in the calf (Figure 87.3).

Importance

The use of multidetector CT for the evaluation of the abdominal aorta and lower extremity vasculature has become a routine clinical examination in multiple patient populations.[1] It is important to design protocols for these studies to avoid the common pitfall of suboptimal bolus timing. Disease in the aortoiliac or the femoropopliteal bed that results in sluggish downstream flow can be misinterpreted as occlusion in the calves if three-vessel runoff is not observed. Similarly, patients with very low cardiac output may require modifications to a standard protocol to account for the slow transit of contrast from the aorta to the feet. For this reason, it may be helpful to obtain immediate delayed images through the calves and feet, as the scanner may progress faster than the contrast bolus during the arterial phase of imaging. For dedicated lower extremity angiography, placement of the bolus tracker on the popliteal artery will also improve timing.

Typical clinical scenario

CT angiography of the abdominal aorta and lower extremities is performed for a variety of reasons. In the emergent setting, it is often required to assess for vascular injury in the setting of trauma or for acute vascular occlusion in a patient with a cold extremity. When ordered non-emergently, the goal is often to evaluate patients with peripheral vascular disease to determine if there is a need for surgical intervention. Regardless of the acuity, bolus timing is an important consideration. If there is stenosis proximally, distal vessels will demonstrate delayed opacification due to slower flow. However, if a study is obtained without proper timing, stenoses may erroneously be interpreted as occlusions.

Differential diagnosis

Asymmetric arterial opacification on a lower extremity CT angiogram can be due to arterial injury, vasospasm, atherosclerosis, popliteal entrapment or vasculitides affecting the extremities.

Teaching point

CT angiography of the lower extremities can be sensitive to bolus timing both in the setting of acute trauma as well as atherosclerotic disease. It can be helpful to obtain delayed images in the distal lower extremities to avoid incorrectly diagnosing vascular disease because of "outrunning the bolus."

REFERENCES

1. D. Fleischmann, R. L. Hallett, G. D. Rubin. CT angiography of peripheral arterial disease. *Journal of Vascular and Interventional Radiology* 2006; **17**: 3–26.

Pearls and Pitfalls in Cardiovascular Imaging, ed. Stefan L. Zimmerman and Elliot K. Fishman. Published by Cambridge University Press. © Cambridge University Press 2015.

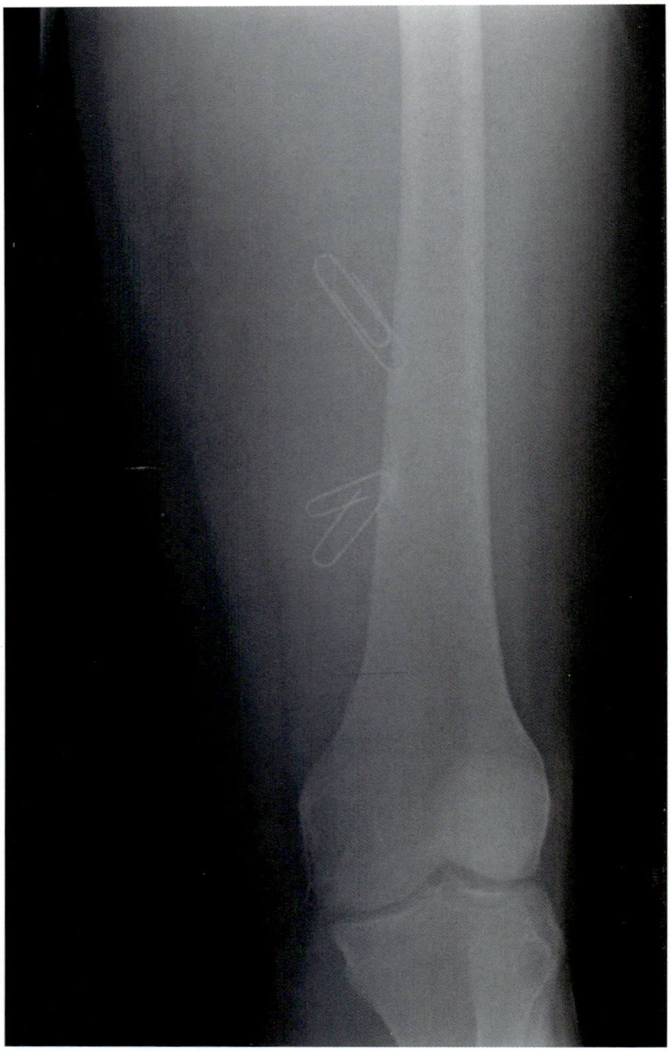

Figure 87.1 Coronal femur radiograph in a 24-year-old male status post-through-and-through gunshot wound demonstrates paper clips marking the entry and exit wounds but no visible bullet fragments in the thigh. A CT angiogram of the extremities was ordered to evaluate for vascular injury.

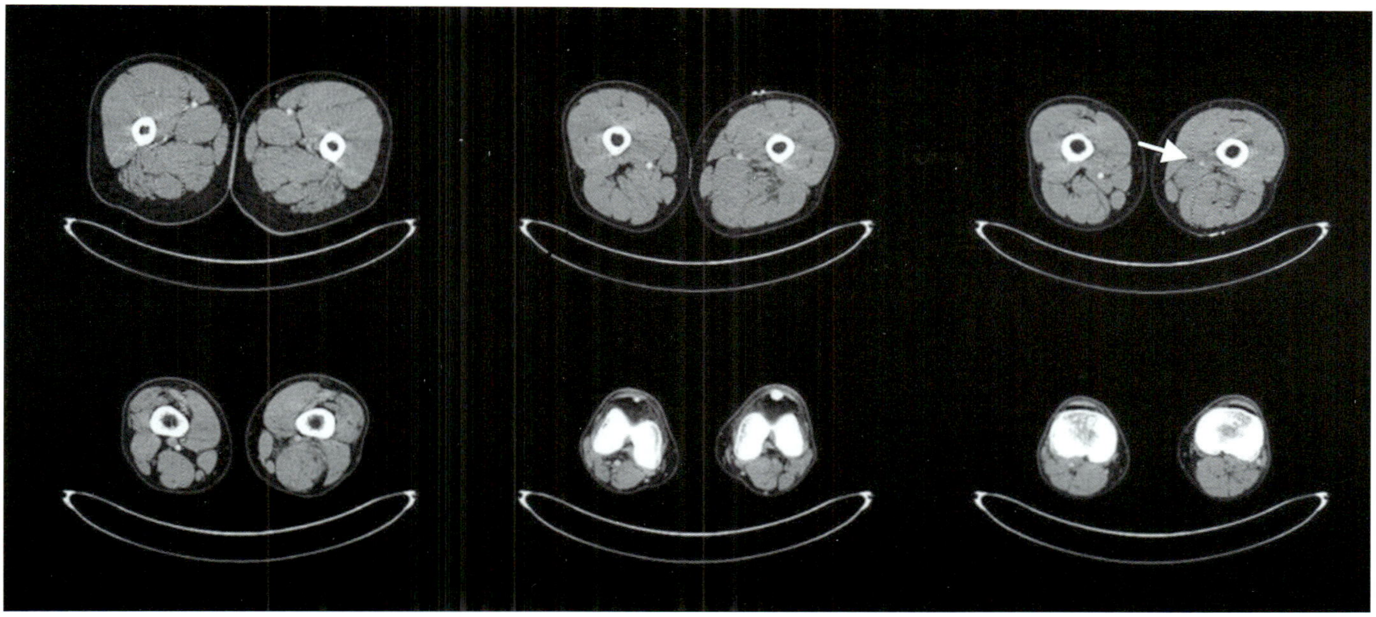

Figure 87.2 Axial images from a CT angiogram of the lower extremities during the arterial phase demonstrates gas in the left thigh in keeping with the recent gunshot wound, as well as asymmetric opacification of the superficial femoral arteries and progressively decreasing opacification of the left superficial femoral (arrow) and popliteal arteries. No active extravasation is seen in the thigh. In addition to the differential considerations associated with acute vascular injury, bolus timing should also be considered and delayed images obtained.

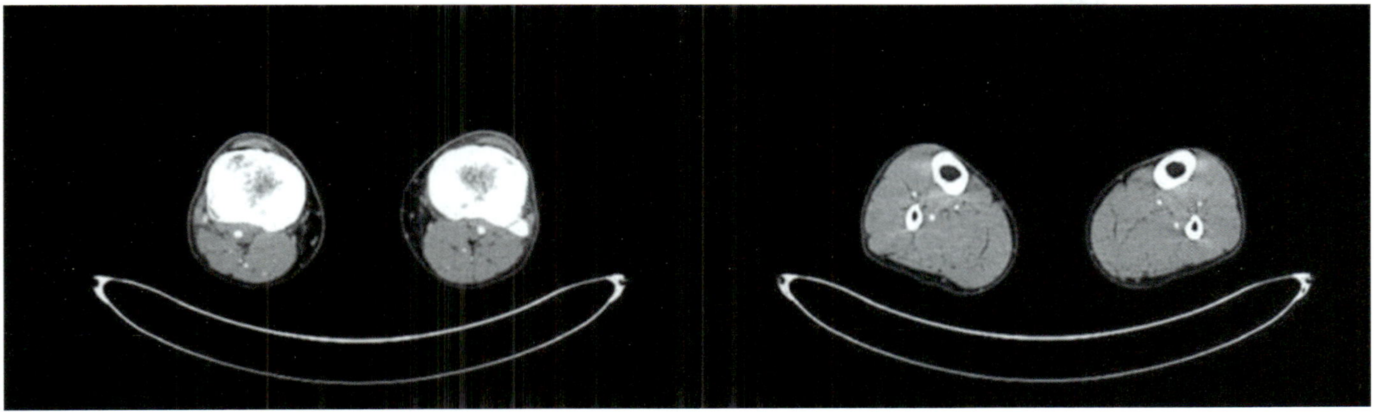

Figure 87.3 Axial images during the delayed phase of the CT angiogram demonstrate normal, symmetric opacification of the extremity arteries and three-vessel runoff bilaterally. Despite the suboptimal arterial opacification, there are no findings of vascular injury on the delayed phase.

CASE 88

Lower extremity arteriovenous fistula

Atif Zaheer

Imaging description

Multidetector computed tomographic angiography (CTA) is a fast non-invasive imaging technique with a sensitivity of 95% and a specificity of 99% for detection of arterial injuries in the extremities.[1] CTA is usually performed with 100–120 ml of contrast material injected at a rate of 4 ml/sec and images acquired at the time of maximal arterial enhancement (around 40 seconds). Bolus tracking may be used but is usually not necessary as most of the patients in the trauma setting are young adults. Evaluation is performed with axial images along with sagittal and coronal reconstructions and three-dimensional post-processing techniques such as volume rendering and MIP.[2] In the presence of an arteriovenous fistula (AVF) there is early filling of the involved vein on arterial phase imaging and lack of contrast opacification of the veins on the contralateral side (Figures 88.1 and 88.2).

Importance

AVFs are due to abnormal connections between the arterial and venous system bypassing the normal capillary beds. Acquired AVF usually occurs as a consequence of percutaneous vascular access but can also be secondary to penetrating injury to the lower extremity from stab wounds and gunshot injuries.[3] Accurate diagnosis is important as long-standing AVFs can cause edema, arterial aneurysm, ischemia, and even high-output cardiac failure.[4–6] There is excellent prognosis of AVFs after surgical or endovascular repair.[7]

Typical clinical scenario

Typically presentation would be a young person with history of lower extremity penetrating trauma presenting with limb edema. On examination machine-like murmur, bruit, or a pulsatile mass may be found.

Differential diagnosis

Inaccurate or mistiming of the bolus may cause opacification of the veins interfering with the evaluation of AVF. Absence of opacification of the contralateral veins helps differentiate mistiming of contrast bolus from an AVF. Intravenous contrast injection from the lower extremity causes opacification of the ipsilateral venous system; however, the contrast is usually denser than within the arteries (Figure 88.2). In the presence of central venous obstruction, early opacification of a peripheral vein can also occur due to the presence of collateral vessels (Figure 88.3).

Teaching point

Identification of an early draining vein in the setting of prior lower extremity trauma suggests the presence of an arteriovenous fistula. This should be differentiated from unilateral early venous opacification due to lower extremity contrast injection or collateral venous flow. Visualization of the site of arteriovenous communication with CT angiography will help confirm the diagnosis.

REFERENCES

1. J. A. Soto, F. Munera, C. Morales, et al. Focal arterial injuries of the proximal extremities: helical CT arteriography as the initial method of diagnosis. *Radiology* 2001; **218**: 188–94.
2. E. K. Fishman, K. M. Horton, P. T. Johnson. Multidetector CT and three-dimensional CT angiography for suspected vascular trauma of the extremities. *Radiographics* 2008; **28**: 653–65; discussion 665–6.
3. G. Lebreton, A. P. Uzel, J. Celerien, F. Roques, M. Deneuville. Popliteal arteriovenous fistula due to a gunshot injury. *Ann Vasc Surg* 2010; **24**: 952 e17–21.
4. Y. Sako, R. L. Varco. Arteriovenous fistula: results of management of congenital and acquired forms, blood flow measurements, and observations on proximal arterial degeneration. *Surgery* 1970; **67**: 40–61.
5. H. B. Shumacker, Jr. Aneurysm development and degenerative changes in dilated artery proximal to arteriovenous fistula. *Surg Gynecol Obstet* 1970; **130**: 636–40.
6. D. Kotelis, K. Klemm, H. von Tengg-Kobligk, J. R. Allenberg, D. Bockler. Intermittent claudication secondary to a traumatic arteriovenous fistula. *Vasa* 2007; **36**: 285–7.
7. D. C. Brewster, R. P. Cambria, A. C. Moncure, et al. Aortocaval and iliac arteriovenous fistulas: recognition and treatment. *J Vasc Surg* 1991; **13**: 253–64; discussion 264–5.

Pearls and Pitfalls in Cardiovascular Imaging, ed. Stefan L. Zimmerman and Elliot K. Fishman. Published by Cambridge University Press. © Cambridge University Press 2015.

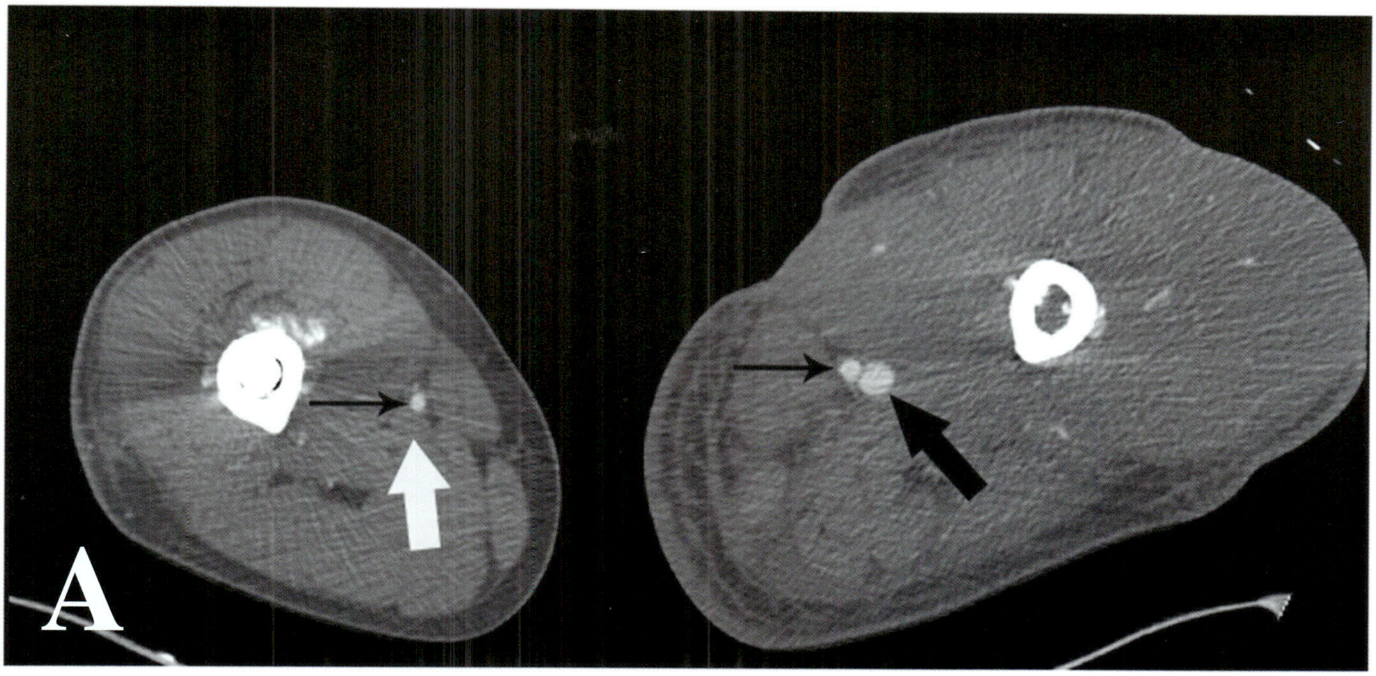

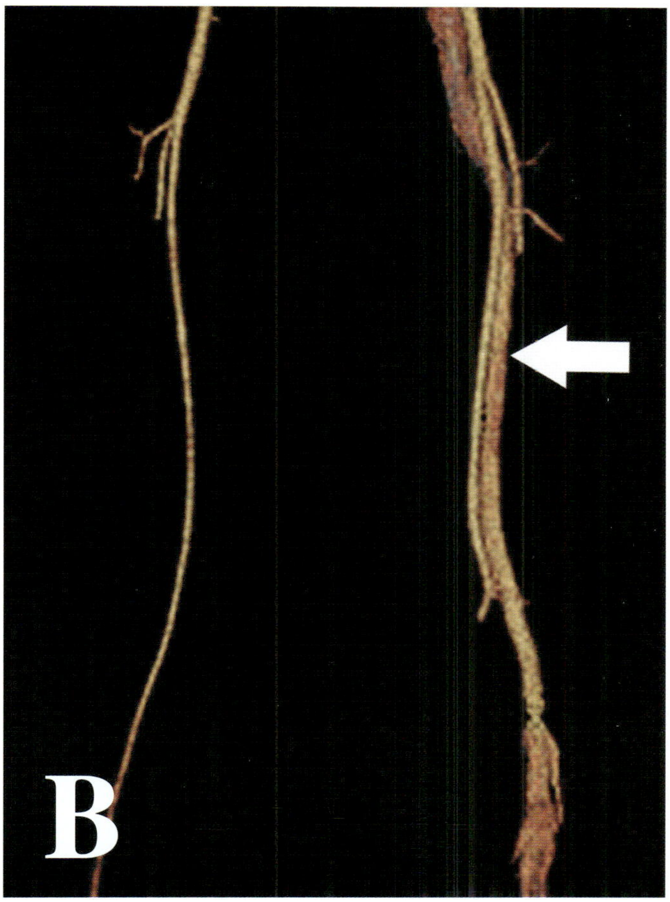

Figure 88.1 A. A 36-year old man with a history of penetrating trauma to the left lower extremity. Axial contrast-enhanced arterial phase CT at the level of the femur demonstrates contrast opacification of the femoral arteries (thin black arrows). There is abnormal filling of the left femoral vein on the arterial phase (thick black arrow). The right femoral vein is not opacified (thick white arrow). Note swelling of the left lower extremity. Findings are consistent with an AVF. **B.** Coronal post-contrast volume-rendered MIP image of the proximal lower extremity in the same patient as above demonstrates abnormal filling of the left femoral vein (white arrow) due to an AVF.

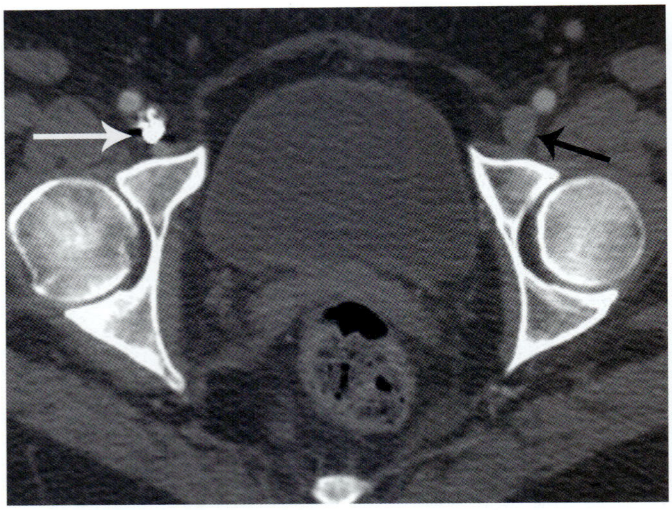

Figure 88.2 A 77-year-old woman with breast cancer and poor venous access. Axial contrast-enhanced arterial phase CT image shows a densely opacified right femoral vein (white arrow) secondary to a foot injection. Note lack of enhancement of the left femoral vein (black arrow).

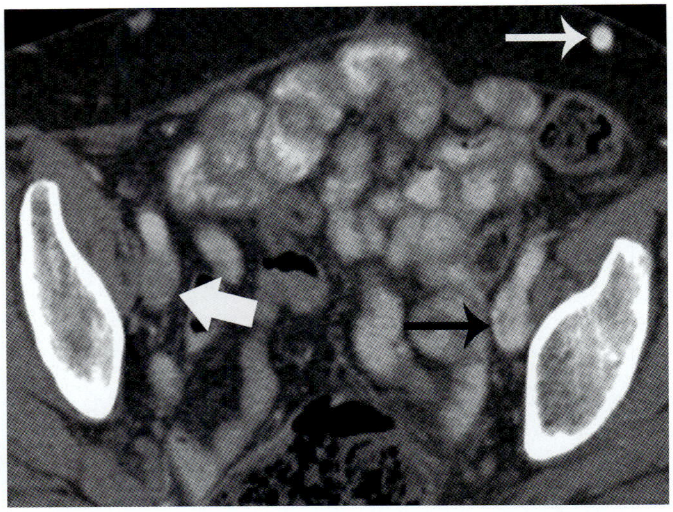

Figure 88.3 A 61-year-old woman with chronic SVC obstruction. Axial contrast-enhanced arterial phase CT image shows an opacified left external iliac vein (black arrow) and absence of filling of the right external iliac vein (thick white arrow). The early filling of the left external iliac vein is secondary to the collateral superficial thoracoabdominal venous route (thin white arrow) to bypass the SVC obstruction.

CASE 89

Persistent sciatic artery

Tessa S. Cook

Imaging description

A persistent sciatic artery can easily be identified using CT angiography of the pelvis and lower extremities. Sequential enhanced axial images through the pelvis demonstrate a vascular structure in the left hemipelvis that courses along the left acetabulum (Figure 89.1) before diving inferolaterally along the anterior aspect of the gluteus maximus into the left thigh (Figure 89.2). The vessel is of greater caliber than the ipsilateral external iliac, superficial femoral, and profunda femoris arteries. Its course is better appreciated on three-dimensional volume renderings (Figure 89.3), where the associated enlargement of the ipsilateral internal iliac artery can also be well appreciated. While this persistent left sciatic artery is mildly tortuous proximally, it is relatively uniform in caliber throughout its visualized course and does not contain any thrombus.

Importance

The persistent sciatic artery is a very rare vascular variant that can become clinically significant if complicated by aneurysm or thrombosis.[1,2] In such cases, patients often present with a pulsatile or enlarging gluteal mass or new onset of decreased pedal pulses, and surgical bypass (femoropopliteal or femorotibial) becomes necessary to restore blood flow to the leg.

Typical clinical scenario

The embryologic sciatic artery begins as a branch of the umbilical artery and perfuses the entire lower limb bud. By about the sixth week of gestation, the iliofemoral system begins to form and the sciatic artery begins to regress. Segments of the sciatic artery normally remain in the adult to form portions of the popliteal and peroneal arteries.[3]

In cases where the sciatic artery persists, it arises from the internal iliac artery and follows the course of the inferior gluteal artery. After passing through the sciatic foramen into the thigh, it may run adjacent to the posterior cutaneous or sciatic nerves.[4] This course can predispose patients to sciatic neuropathy if the vessel becomes enlarged due to aneurysm or thrombus. In cases where the superficial femoral artery is hypoplastic, patency of the sciatic artery becomes critical to preserve limb perfusion.

The incidence of a persistent sciatic artery is thought to be less than 0.04%.[1] It may be incidentally detected on CT or MR angiography performed for other reasons or discovered because the patient has symptoms related to thrombosis in the presence or absence of a persistent sciatic nerve aneurysm.

Differential diagnosis

The appearance of a vessel from the internal iliac artery perfusing the lower extremity is uncommon and there are no other differential considerations besides a persistent sciatic artery. However, a persistent sciatic artery is one of the differential considerations for multiple different clinical presentations, including a pulsatile gluteal mass, acute or chronic limb ischemia, and even sciatic neuropathy.[5]

Teaching point

A persistent sciatic artery is a very rare vascular anomaly that may be incidentally detected on CT or MR angiography of the pelvis and/or lower extremities. However, consideration of this entity is important in the setting of a pulsatile gluteal mass, acute or chronic limb ischemia or even sciatic neuropathy. Symptomatic patients may benefit from surgical intervention.

REFERENCES

1. V. Santaolalla, M. H. Bernabe, J. M. Hipola Ulecia, et al. Persistent sciatic artery. *Ann Vasc Surg* 2010; **24**: 691 e7–10.
2. G. L. McLellan, L. B. Morettin. Persistent sciatic artery: clinical, surgical, and angiographic aspects. *Arch Surg* 1982; **117**: 817–22.
3. V. S. Mandell, P. F. Jaques, D. J. Delany, V. Oberheu. Persistent sciatic artery: clinical, embryologic, and angiographic features. *AJR Am J Roentgenol* 1985; **144**: 245–9.
4. E. B. Bower, S. N. Smullens, W. W. Parke. Clinical aspects of persistent sciatic artery: report of two cases and review of the literature. *Surgery* 1977; **81**: 588–95.
5. M. Yamaguchi, S. Mii, T. Kai, H. Sakata, A. Mori. Intermittent claudication associated with persistent sciatic artery: report of two cases. *Surg Today* 1997; **27**: 863–7.

Pearls and Pitfalls in Cardiovascular Imaging, ed. Stefan L. Zimmerman and Elliot K. Fishman. Published by Cambridge University Press. © Cambridge University Press 2015.

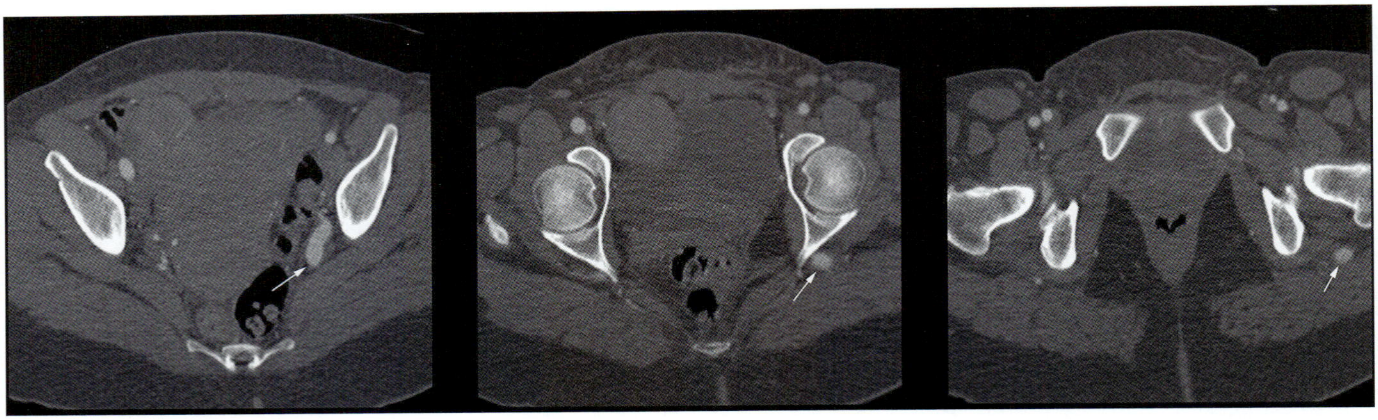

Figure 89.1 Images from a CT angiogram performed in a 47-year-old female, status post-repair of an ascending aortic aneurysm, who presented for follow-up of her aneurysm repair. Enhanced axial CT images (superior to inferior from left-to-right) through the pelvis demonstrate a mildly tortuous vessel (arrows), larger in caliber than the left external iliac artery, coursing posteriorly along the left acetabulum and anterior to the left gluteus maximus muscles, in keeping with an incidentally discovered persistent left sciatic artery. Note the caliber of the left superficial and deep femoral arteries, which are considerably smaller than the persistent sciatic artery.

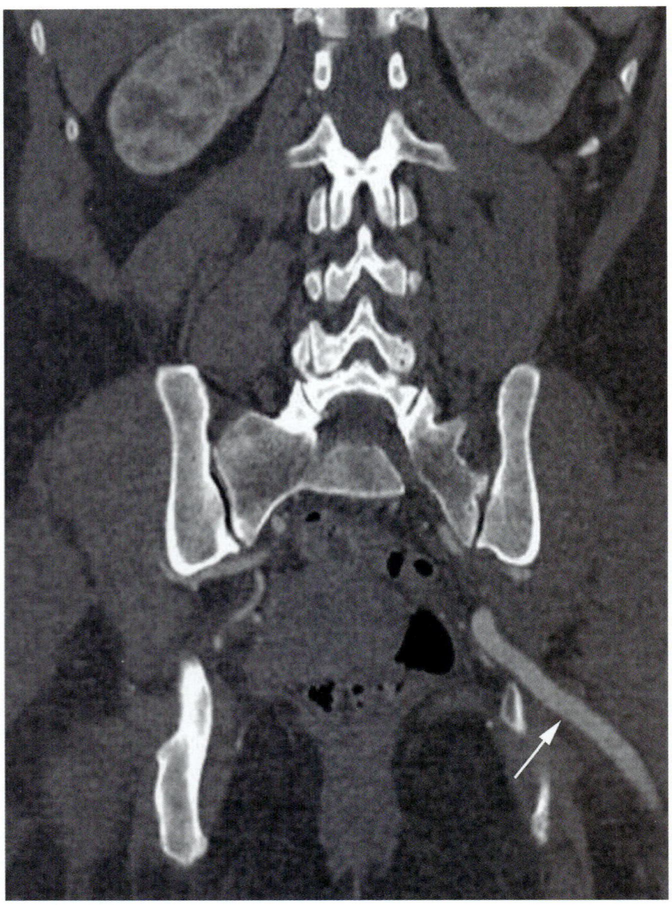

Figure 89.2 Coronal reformat from the same patient showing the persistent left sciatic artery (arrow) coursing posterolaterally, deep to the left gluteus maximus muscle.

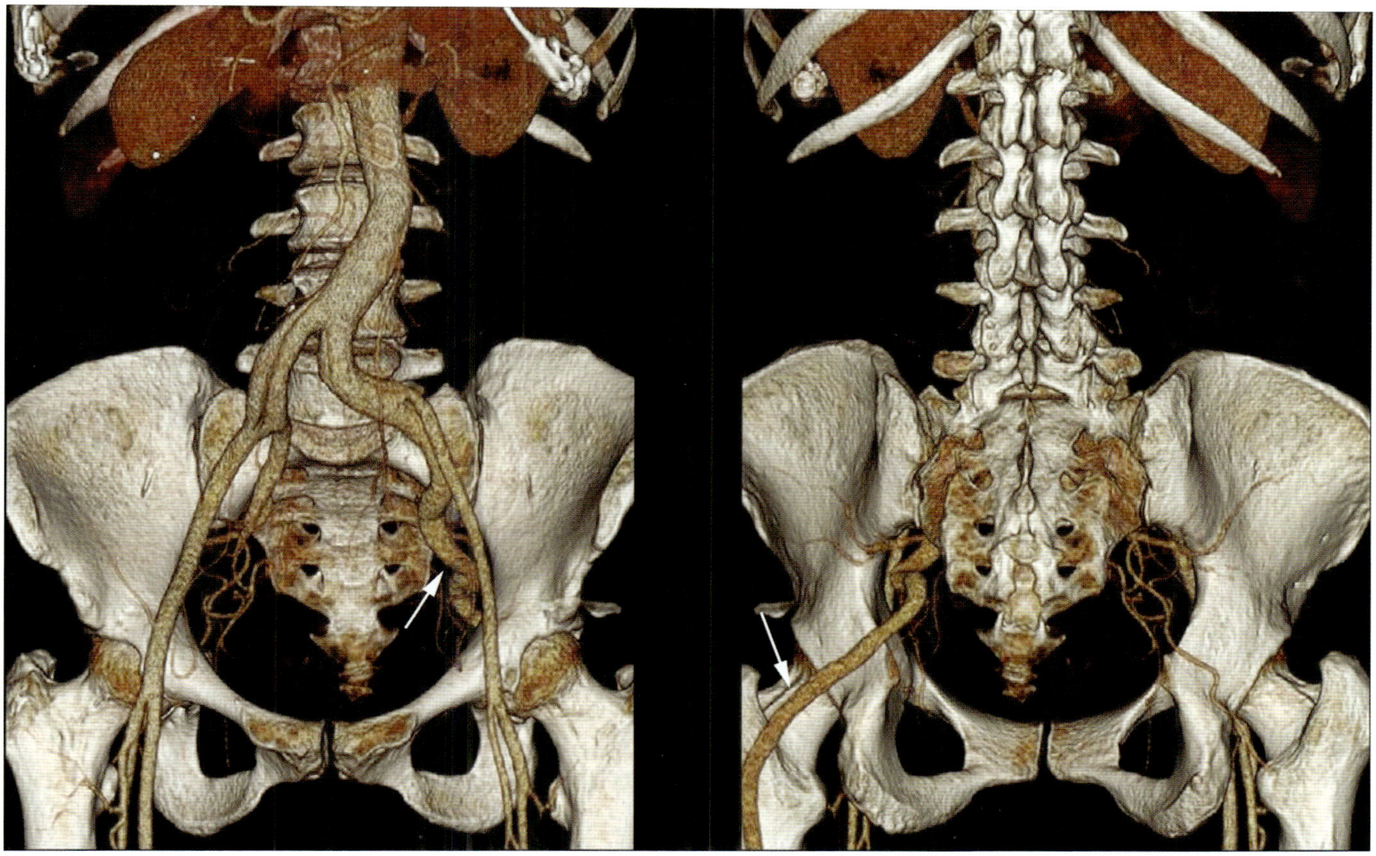

Figure 89.3 Anterior (left) and posterior (right) 3-D volume renderings from the same patient demonstrate the course of the persistent left sciatic artery (arrows), arising from the left internal iliac artery and coursing posterolaterally over the ischium and left femora neck.

CASE 90

Pseudolipoma of the inferior vena cava

Satomi Kawamoto

Imaging description

Localized fat collection adjacent to the intrahepatic inferior vena cava is an uncommon incidental benign finding on CT. It is usually seen as a round (Figure 90.1) or oval (Figure 90.2) fat collection on axial CT. It is located at or above the level of the confluence of the hepatic veins and the inferior vena cava,[1] and usually medial or anterior to the inferior vena cava,[1–3] but can be seen posterior to the inferior vena cava.[2,4] It demonstrates apparent fat attenuation on CT. On axial images, it may mimic a fat-containing lesion within the lumen of the inferior vena cava because of the acute angle of the fat collection with respect to the wall of the inferior vena cava. The right diaphragmatic crus forming a thin line medial to the fat collection may resemble the medial wall of the inferior vena cava on axial image (Figure 90.1).

Importance

Pericaval fat collection adjacent to the intrahepatic inferior vena cava represents a partial volume artifact of pericaval fat above the caudate lobe rather than true intraluminal lesion, and is usually of no clinical significance. However, it can be misdiagnosed as a mass in the inferior vena cava. Therefore, it is important not to misinterpret this finding as an abnormality of the inferior vena cava, such as thrombus or tumor.

Typical clinical scenario

The prevalence of pericaval fat collection near the intrahepatic inferior vena cava is considered rare, and this finding occurred in 0.5–0.55% in large CT studies.[1,5] In patients with chronic liver disease, it is more commonly seen. Gibo et al. reported that pericaval fat collection was seen in 16 (26.2%) of 61 patients with chronic liver disease.[4]

Pericaval fat collection near the intrahepatic inferior vena cava is related to anatomic variation of the subdiaphragmatic inferior vena cava, and chronic liver disease.[1,2,4] Han et al. reported that the rightward angulation and narrowing of the intrahepatic inferior vena cava caused the pericaval fat collections to appear within the lumen of the inferior vena cava on axial CT images (Figures 90.1 and 90.2).[2] In patients with chronic liver disease, a shrunken right lobe of the liver due to cirrhosis may provide a space between the inferior vena cava and diaphragm for pericaval fat to collect.[2] On coronal images, fat collection is contiguous to extracaval fat tissue (Figures 90.1 and 90.2).

Differential diagnosis

The differential diagnosis of pericaval fat collection includes fat containing tumor such as lipoma or fatty metamorphosis of hepatocellular carcinoma.[1] When attenuation of fat is not clearly demonstrated due to its small size or partial volume averaging, other filling defect such as thrombus, primary tumors of the IVC such as leiomyosarcoma, and secondary tumor extension, such as renal (Figure 90.3) or adrenal malignancy are considered as differential diagnoses. Thin-slice images should permit differentiation of fat and soft tissue density. Coronal reformatted images are helpful for identifying its extracaval origin (Figures 90.1 and 90.2).[2,4]

Teaching point

Localized fat collection adjacent to the intrahepatic inferior vena cava is an uncommon incidental benign finding. It should not be confused with intraluminal lesion such as thrombus or tumor. Fat attenuation and typical appearance and location help to differentiate localized fat collection from true intracaval lesion. Coronal reformatted images help to confirm the artificial nature of this finding.

REFERENCES

1. Miyake H, Suzuki K, Ueda S, Yamada Y, Takeda H, Mori H. Localized fat collection adjacent to the intrahepatic portion of the inferior vena cava: a normal variant on CT. *AJR American Journal of Roentgenology* 1992;**158**:423–425.
2. Han BK, Im JG, Jung JW, Chung MJ, Yeon KM. Pericaval fat collection that mimics thrombosis of the inferior vena cava: demonstration with use of multi-directional reformation CT. *Radiology* 1997;**203**:105–108.
3. Hines J, Katz DS, Goffner L, Rubin GD. Fat collection related to the intrahepatic inferior vena cava on CT. *AJR American Journal of Roentgenology* 1999;**172**:409–411.
4. Gibo M, Murata S, Kuroki S. Pericaval fat collection mimicking an intracaval lesion on CT in patients with chronic liver disease. *Abdominal Imaging* 2001;**26**:492–495.
5. Perry JN, Williams MP, Dubbins PA, Farrow R. Lipomata of the inferior vena cava: a normal variant? *Clinical Radiology* 1994;**49**:341–342.

Pearls and Pitfalls in Cardiovascular Imaging, ed. Stefan L. Zimmerman and Elliot K. Fishman. Published by Cambridge University Press. © Cambridge University Press 2015.

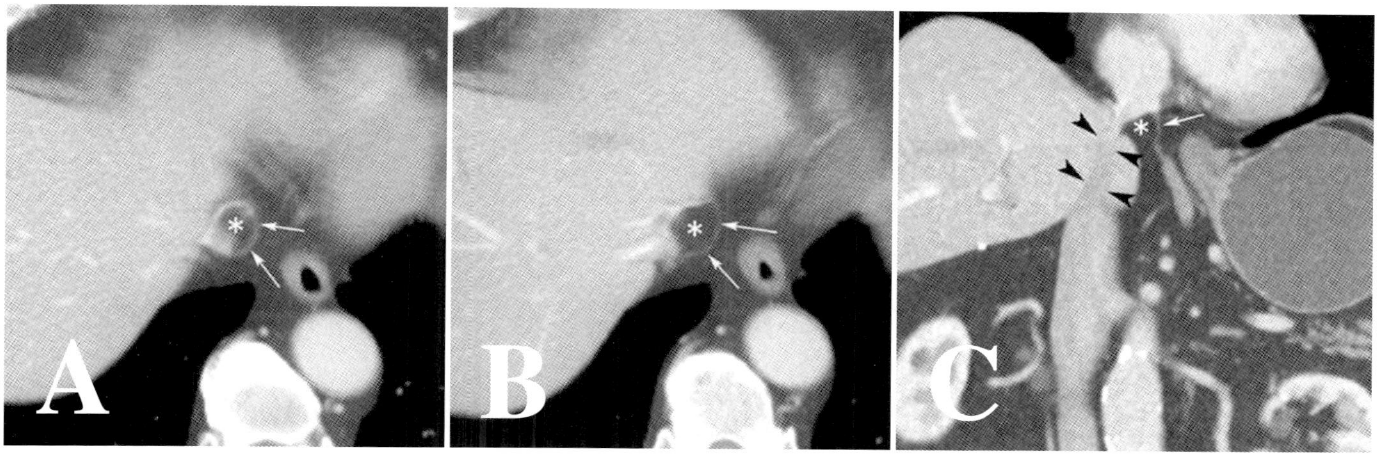

Figure 90.1 **A.** and **B.** Axial contrast-enhanced CT images incidentally show a round fat collection (asterisk) medial to the inferior vena cava immediately inferior to the diaphragm. The crus of the diaphragm (white arrows) simulates the medial wall of the inferior vena cava. **C.** Coronal reformatted CT shows rightward angulation and narrowing of the intrahepatic inferior vena cava (arrowheads), with pericaval fat (asterisk) extending above the caudate lobe of the liver. The medial wall of the inferior vena cava is contiguous to the diaphragmatic crus (white arrow).

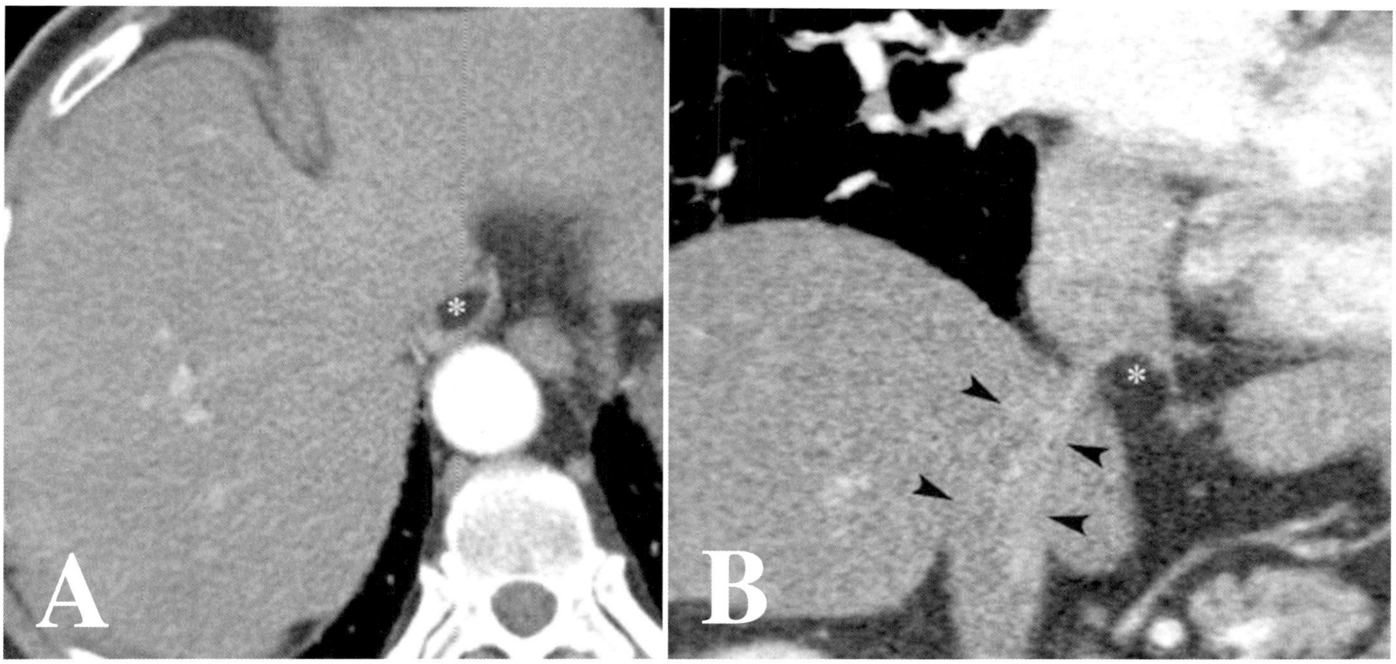

Figure 90.2 **A.** Axial contrast-enhanced CT performed to evaluate pulmonary embolism shows oval fat collection anterior to the inferior vena cava (asterisk) immediately inferior to the diaphragm. **B.** Oblique coronal reformatted CT image shows rightward angulation of the intrahepatic inferior vena cava (arrowheads), with pericaval fat (asterisk) extending above the caudate lobe of the liver.

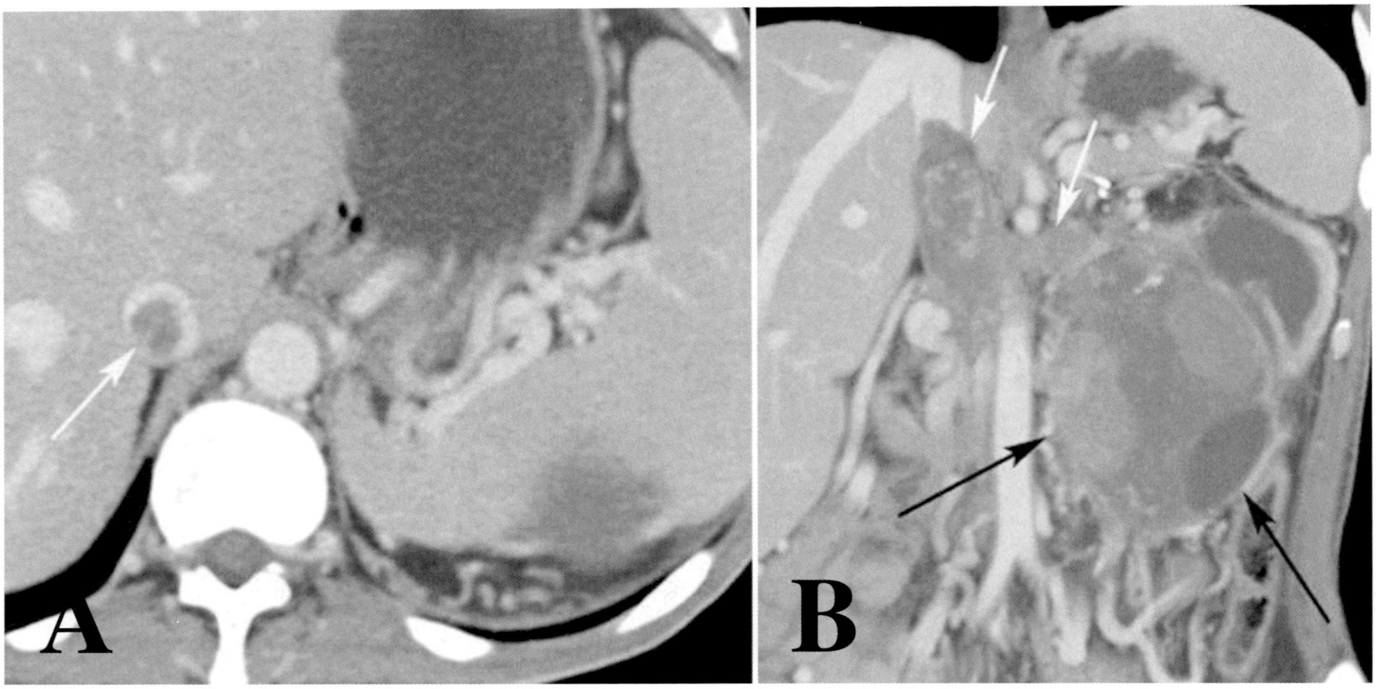

Figure 90.3 A. Axial contrast-enhanced CT shows soft tissue density filling defect (white arrow) within the intrahepatic inferior vena cava, representing tumor thrombus of renal cell carcinoma. Hypodense left renal mass is partially visualized posterior to the spleen. **B.** Coronal reformatted CT shows a large left renal mass (black arrows) extending into the left renal vein and IVC (white arrows).

CASE 91

Pseudomass from varicose veins

Satomi Kawamoto

Imaging description

Varicose veins may be seen as round or oval soft tissue density masses on CT, particularly when they are seen on a plane perpendicular to its course. Typically, varicose veins are easily diagnosed with intravenous contrast material, which helps to detect the continuity between varicose veins and other venous structures, and to determine the true vascular nature of the varicose veins. However, when contrast is not administered or enhancement of the vein is poor due to early arterial phase or thrombosis, it may be confused with lymphadenopathy or another mass (Figure 91.1).

Reformatted coronal or sagittal images along the course of the dilated vein will help to differentiate dilated veins from other pathologies. In patients with venous obstruction, knowledge of collateral pathways in chest, abdomen, and pelvis is essential to avoid misinterpretation.[1]

Importance

Varicose veins are commonly encountered at cross-sectional imaging of the thorax and abdomen. These vessels can be mistaken for adenopathy, which could lead to improper staging of patients with cancer or unnecessary work-up for malignancy. Erroneous biopsy of varicose veins may lead to profound hemorrhage.

Typical clinical scenario

Varicose veins are enlarged and tortuous venous channels, which are commonly caused by retrograde flow due to incompetency of valves or obstruction to flow.[2] Obstruction of the venous flow may be secondary to thrombus, external compression, or congenital.

In patients with occlusion of the superior vena cava and its tributaries, the collateral venous pathways are often categorized into four main pathways: lateral thoracic, internal mammary, azygos, and vertebral pathways (Figure 91.2).[1,3] In the abdomen, internal mammary pathways form anastomoses with the superficial epigastric veins, which may be seen in the anterior abdominal wall of patients with superior vena cava obstruction (Figure 91.3). When the inferior vena cava is obstructed, the ascending lumbar vein, which drains into the azygos–hemiazygos system, may be dilated.[4] Dilated azygos or hemiazygos veins can be confused with retroperitoneal, retrocrural, or paraspinal mass or adenopathy (Figure 91.4). In patients with portal hypertension, varicose veins may form in the esophagus or upper abdomen, and may simulate a mass or adenopathy (Figures 91.1 and 91.5).

A normal communicating vein between the left renal vein and the left ascending lumbar vein, or an azygos system have been reported in 69–91.5% of the autopsy studies.[2] Varicose dilatation of the communicating vein may be seen on CT in patients with backpressure changes in the renal vein or the lumbar vein/azygos system (Figure 91.6),[2] but is also commonly seen in the general population (Figure 91.7).[5] Yao et al. reported the communicating vein between the left renal vein and left ascending lumbar vein is visible in 35% of normal patients on CT.[5] The varicose communicating retroperitoneal venous channels have been confused with para-aortic adenopathy, adrenal masses, and renal artery aneurysms.[2]

Differential diagnosis

In patients with obstruction of major veins, collateral pathways may form, and may simulate mass or lymphadenopathy, particularly when contrast material is not used, or contrast enhancement of the vein is poor due to technical reasons or thrombosis.

Teaching point

Although varicose veins are usually easily diagnosed with contrast-enhanced CT, they may be confused with other pathologies such as lymphadenopathy or mass. The knowledge of typical collateral pathways associated with a specific location of central venous obstruction can help to prevent misinterpretation. The communicating vein between the left renal vein and left ascending lumbar vein is commonly visualized in the general population, and should not be mistaken for para-aortic lymphadenopathy.

REFERENCES

1. Kim HC, Chung JW, Yoon CJ, et al. Collateral pathways in thoracic central venous obstruction: three-dimensional display using direct spiral computed tomography venography. *Journal of Computer Assisted Tomography* 2004;**28**:24–33.
2. Jakhere SG, Yadav DA, Tuplondhe GR. Case report: Varicosity of the communicating vein between the left renal vein and the left ascending lumbar vein mimicking a renal artery aneurysm: Report of an unusual site of varicose veins and a novel hypothesis to explain its association with abdominal pain. *The Indian Journal of Radiology & Imaging* 2011;**21**:24–27.
3. Okay NH, Bryk D. Collateral pathways in occlusion of the superior vena cava and its tributaries. *Radiology* 1969;**92**:1493–1498.

Pearls and Pitfalls in Cardiovascular Imaging, ed. Stefan L. Zimmerman and Elliot K. Fishman. Published by Cambridge University Press. © Cambridge University Press 2015.

4. Kandpal H, Sharma R, Gamangatti S, Srivastava DN, Vashisht S. Imaging the inferior vena cava: a road less traveled. *Radiographics* 2008;**28**:669–689.

5. Yao Y, Okada Y, Yamato M, Ohtomo K. Communicating vein between the left renal vein and left ascending lumber vein: incidence and significance on abdominal CT. *Radiation Medicine* 2003;**21**:252–257.

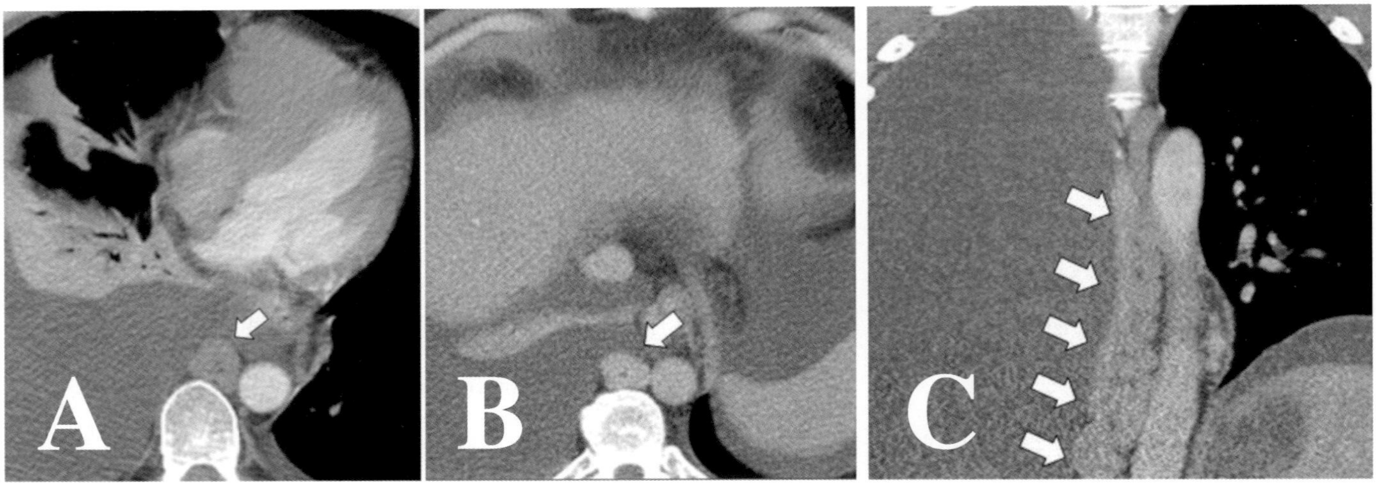

Figure 91.1 A. Arterial phase CT obtained in a patient with cirrhosis and hepatocellular carcinoma demonstrates a para-aortic soft tissue mass with central hypodensity, simulating an enlarged mediastinal lymph node with fatty hilum (arrow). **B.** Venous phase CT in the same patient demonstrates homogenous enhancement of this structure that matches the attenuation of blood pool in the inferior vena cava, suggesting it is venous in origin. **C.** Coronal reformatted venous phase image showing vertical course and tortuosity of the varicose veins (arrows).

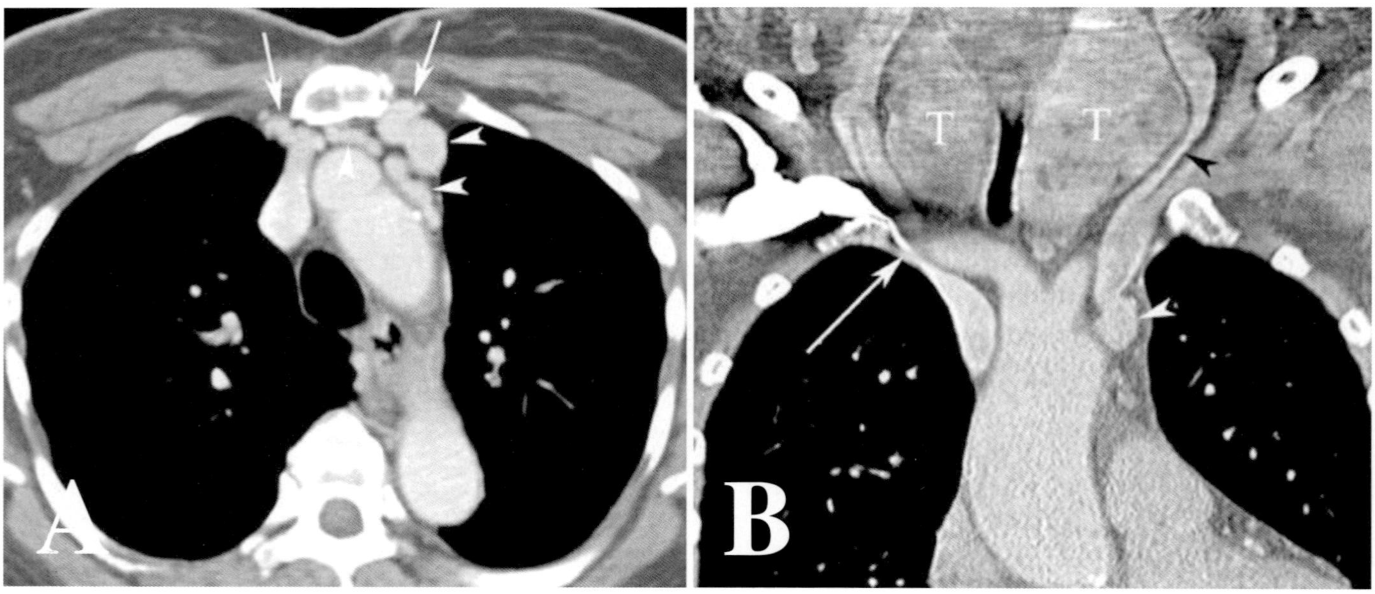

Figure 91.2 A. Contrast-enhanced CT shows multiple round and oval structures in prevascular space, representing dilated internal mammary veins (arrows) and collateral veins (arrowheads) simulating multiple lymph nodes. **B.** Contrast-enhanced coronal reformatted CT image shows markedly enlarged thyroid gland (T) exerting mass effect on the trachea, right innominate vein (white arrow) and left internal jugular vein (black arrowhead), with collateral vein (white arrowhead) in the mediastinum. The left innominate vein is also narrowed between the sternum and elongated aortic arch (not shown).

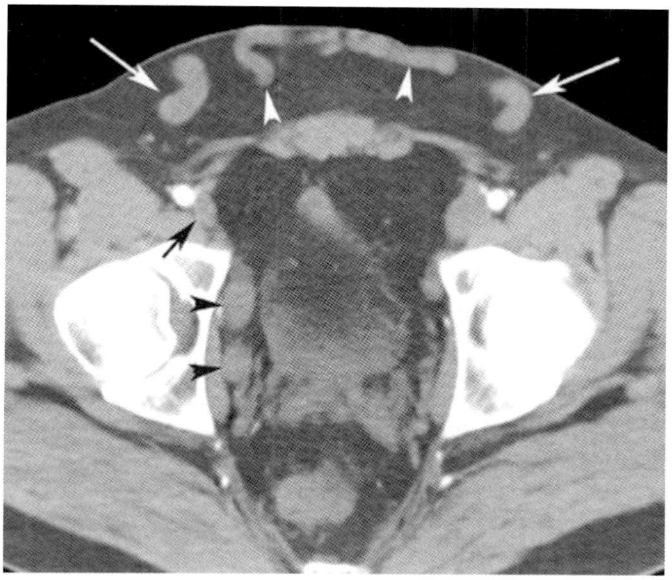

Figure 91.3 Arterial phase-contrast-enhanced CT incidentally shows bilateral varicose superficial epigastric veins (white arrows) communicating by collateral veins (white arrowheads). There is an asymmetrically small right external iliac vein (black arrow) and common femoral vein (not shown) with dilated right obturator veins (black arrowheads), suggesting chronic narrowing of the right external iliac and common femoral vein.

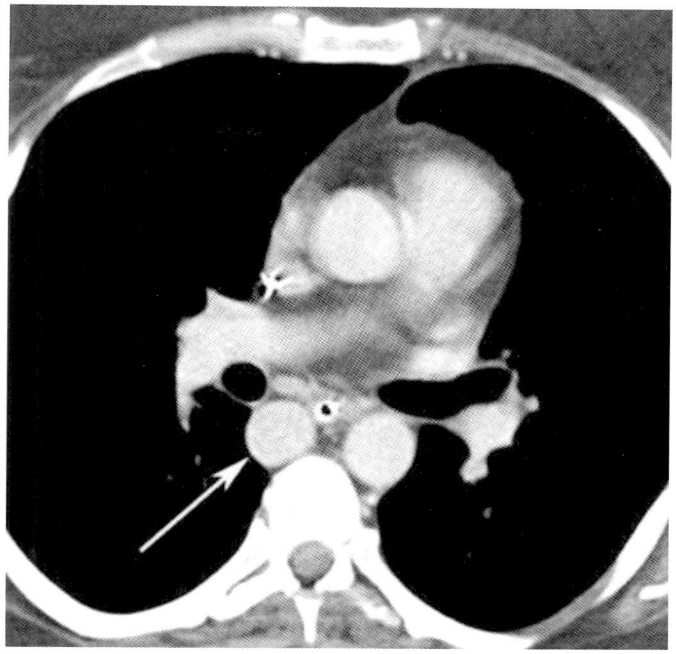

Figure 91.4 Contrast-enhanced CT shows dilated azygos vein (arrow) in a patient with congenital interruption of IVC and azygos continuation.

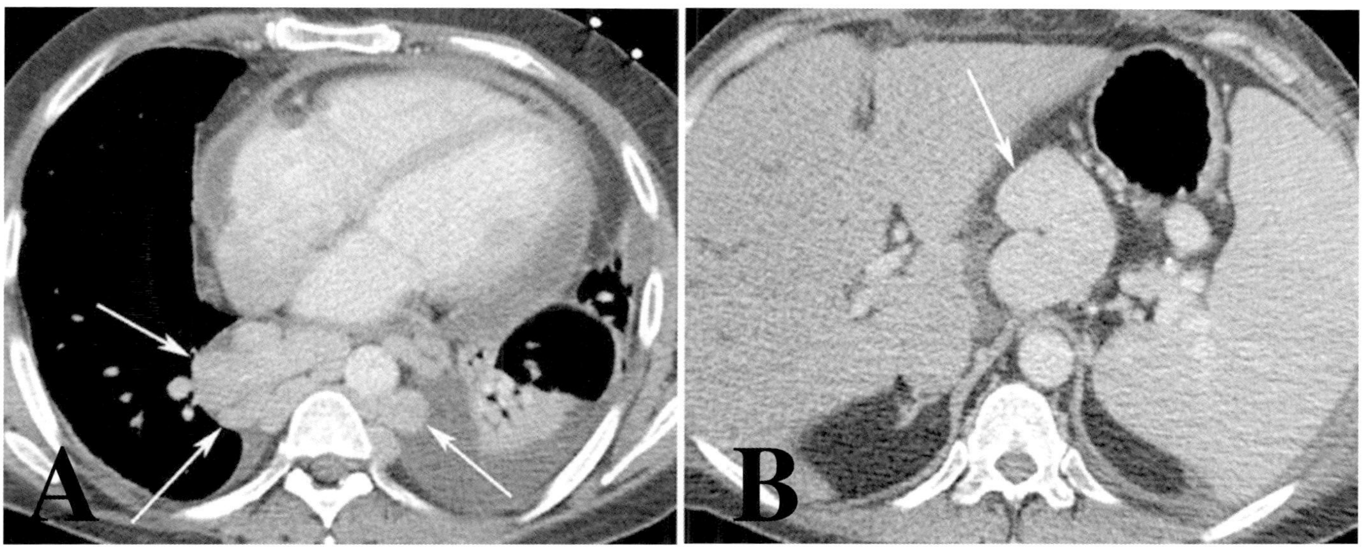

Figure 91.5 **A.** and **B.** Contrast-enhanced CT of a patient with an infected pericardial effusion and liver cirrhosis. Massive varices (arrows) are seen in the posterior mediastinum adjacent to the distal esophagus and near the gastroesophageal junction. Pericardial effusion and pericardial thickening, left pleural effusion, marked splenomegaly, and ascites are also seen.

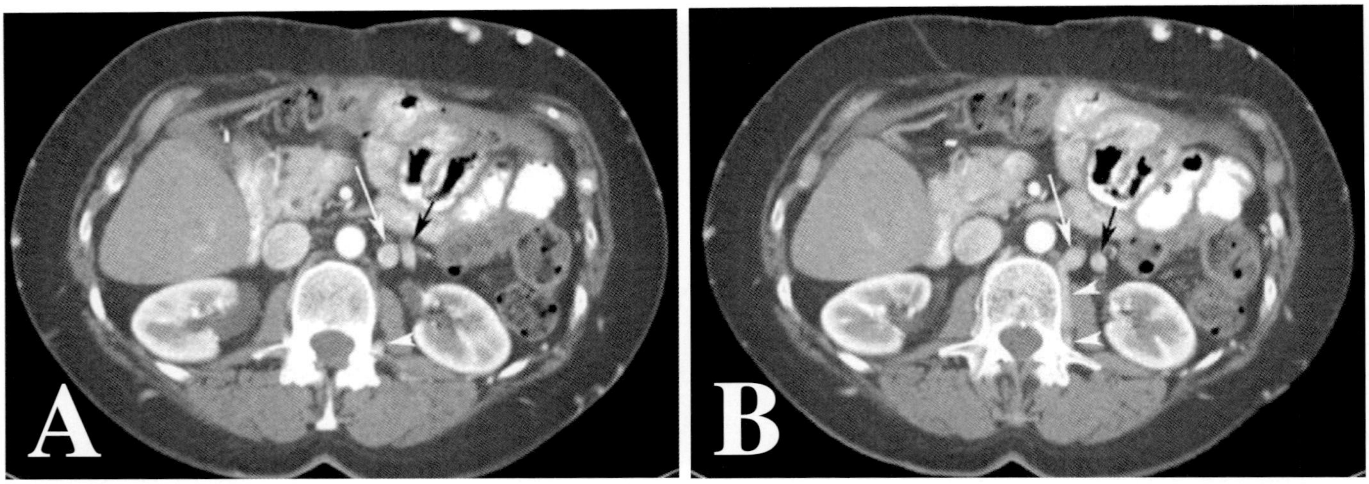

Figure 91.6 A. and **B.** Axial contrast-enhanced CT images show the communicating vein (white arrow) between the left renal vein (black arrow) and the ascending lumbar vein (white arrowheads). Note varicose dilatation of the communicating vein near the renal vein anastomosis. There are multiple collateral veins in the abdominal wall in this patient with chronic superior vena cava obstruction.

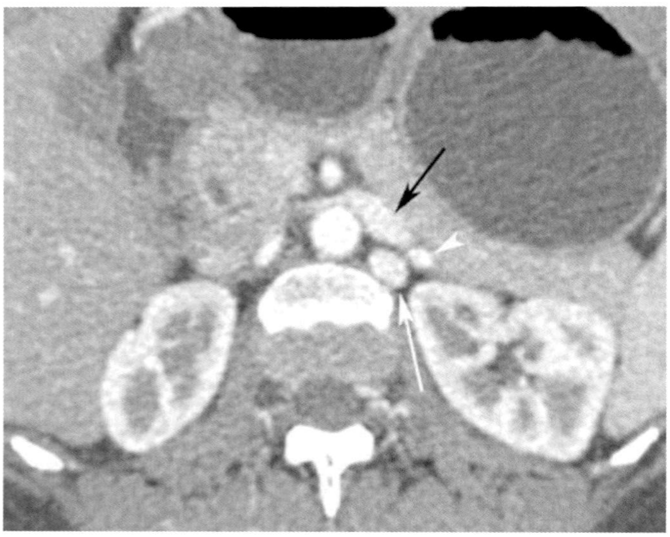

Figure 91.7 Contrast-enhanced CT in patient without pathology shows a varicose dilatation of the communicating vein (white arrow) between the left renal vein (black arrow) and the ascending lumbar vein. The left renal artery is indicated by the white arrowhead.

CASE 92

Catheter malpositions

Satomi Kawamoto

Imaging description

Catheter malpositions are found by identifying the tip of the venous or arterial catheter in the incorrect position, either within the incorrect vessel, or advanced too far or too short for acceptable use (Figures 92.1 to 92.4). Malpositions can occasionally be challenging to identify on radiographs due to overlying structures; however, they can typically be resolved with adjustments to brightness and contrast. Catheter malpositions are easily identified by cross-sectional imaging but are not uncommonly missed due to reader oversight.

Importance

Central venous catheterization is commonly used in modern medicine for various purposes; however, more than 15% of patients who receive these catheters have complications.[1] These complications include mechanical and chemical injury to the vessel wall with thrombus formation, development of a fibrin sheath, infection, and misplacement into other vessels.[2]

Malposition of central venous catheter placement may occur when advancing a catheter into an incorrect vein, or extending a catheter too far distally within a vessel.[3] Malposition of a central venous catheter can result in complications including thrombosis, and vascular perforation or even cardiac perforation and pericardial tamponade.[3] Positioning a catheter tip into the right atrium is thought to increase the likelihood of cardiac arrhythmias.[4] It is important to detect malposition of a central venous catheter on imaging studies.

Typical clinical scenario

There is controversy regarding the correct position for the tip of a central venous catheter. When a catheter is placed from the internal jugular vein or upper extremity veins, the traditional approach has been to place the tip of the central venous catheter within the superior vena cava; however, many believe that the performance and durability of the catheter will be improved by positioning the catheter tip within the upper right atrium.[4] Catheter malposition may occur in the azygos vein, hemiazygos vein, internal mammary vein, or contralateral innominate vein. Positioning of the catheter in an anomalous vein or a venous collateral may occur, including persistent left superior vena cava, dominant supreme intercostal vein, and pericardiophrenic vein. In patients with central vein occlusion due to thrombus or external compression, a central venous catheter may be advanced to an unintended position.

Although rare, catheters inserted from the left-sided upper extremity vein have been reported to have a higher incidence of vascular perforation.[4] The risk of azygos arch cannulation is also increased if catheters are inserted via left-sided veins. Bankier et al. reported azygos arch cannulation was observed in 16 of 1287 (1.2%) patients with central venous catheter placement, and 3 of 16 cases were complicated with venous perforations.[5]

Under normal circumstances, a femoral venous catheter tip is located in the common iliac vein or the inferior vena cava. Malposition of a femoral venous catheter may occur in the ascending lumbar vein.

Differential diagnosis

Usually, a central venous catheter is easily recognized on CT. When high concentration intravenous contrast material is present in the vein, a catheter may be obscured by contrast material, and may be better visualized on a wide window setting. Occasionally chronic thrombosis with linear calcification within a vein may simulate intravenous catheter.

Teaching point

Malposition of a central venous catheter can be related to complications including thrombosis, vascular perforation, and even cardiac perforation. It is important to recognize catheter malposition on imaging studies

REFERENCES

1. McGee DC, Gould MK. Preventing complications of central venous catheterization. *The New England Journal of Medicine* 2003;**348**:1123–1133.
2. Haygood TM, Brennan PC, Ryan J, et al. Central venous line placement in the superior vena cava and the azygos vein: differentiation on posteroanterior chest radiographs. *AJR American Journal of Roentgenology* 2011;**196**:783–787.
3. Patel RY, Friedman A, Shams JN, Silberzweig JE. Central venous catheter tip malposition. *Journal of Medical Imaging and Radiation Oncology* 2010;**54**:35–42.
4. Vesely TM. Central venous catheter tip position: a continuing controversy. *Journal of Vascular and Interventional Radiology : JVIR* 2003;**14**:527–534.
5. Bankier AA, Mallek R, Wiesmayr MN, et al. Azygos arch cannulation by central venous catheters: radiographic detection of malposition and subsequent complications. *Journal of Thoracic Imaging* 1997;**12**:64–69.

Pearls and Pitfalls in Cardiovascular Imaging, ed. Stefan L. Zimmerman and Elliot K. Fishman. Published by Cambridge University Press. © Cambridge University Press 2015.

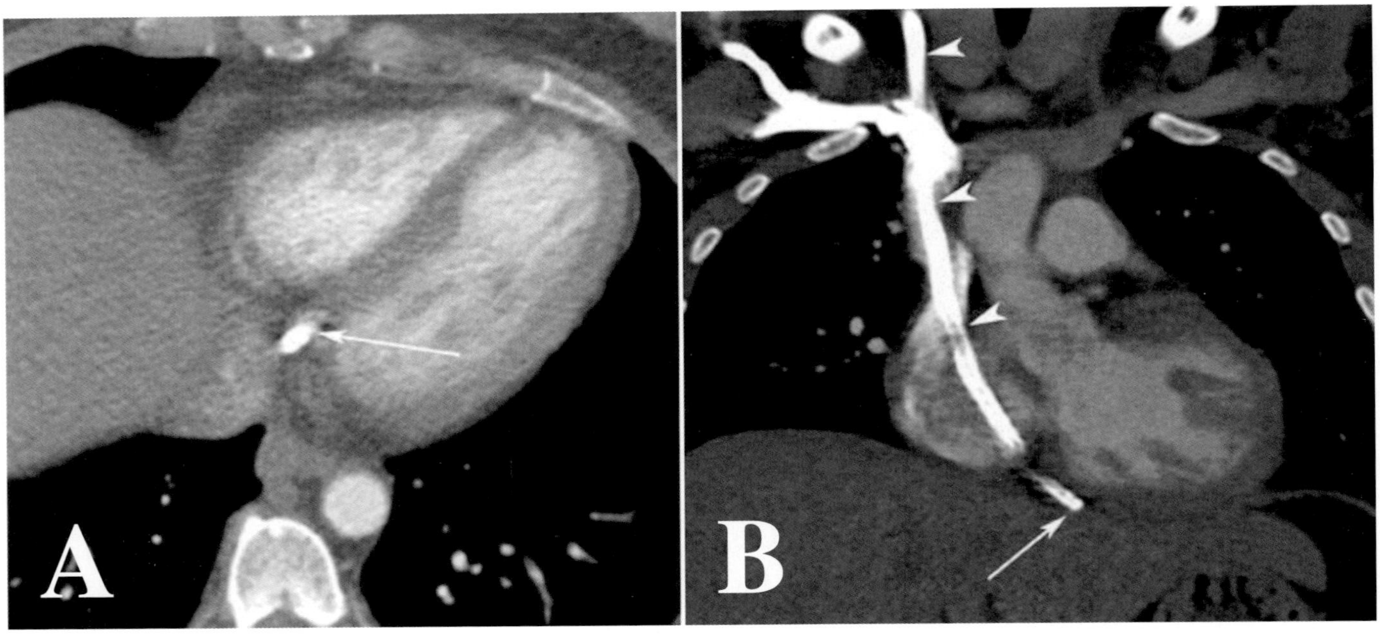

Figure 92.1 **A.** Contrast-enhanced axial and (**B**) coronal MPR CT, performed for evaluation of arrhythmia and shortness of breath, demonstrate a right-sided hemodialysis catheter (arrowheads) in the right atrium with the tip (arrow) in too low a position, which appears to be in the coronary vein at the base of the heart. Echocardiogram performed before catheter retraction showed that the catheter tip was within the right atrium. After catheter retraction, the patient did not have further episodes of palpitations.

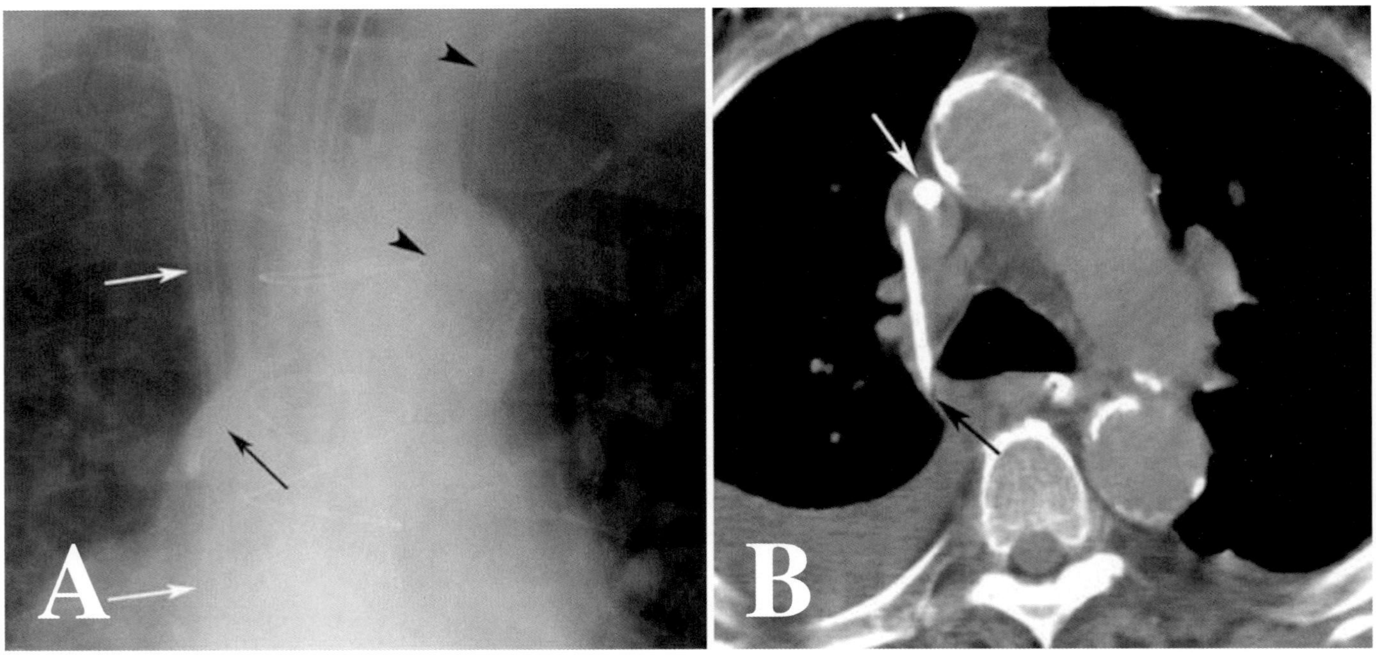

Figure 92.2 **A.** Portable AP chest radiograph shows left-sided central venous catheter (black arrowheads) with its tip (black arrow) arching upward and to the left in the region of the azygos arch, indicating catheter malposition in the azygos arch. The second large right-sided dialysis catheter is in the superior vena cava (white arrows). **B.** Axial non-contrast CT demonstrates the tip (black arrow) of the central venous catheter is located in the azygos arch. A large dialysis catheter is in the superior vena cava (white arrow). There is a small right pleural effusion and atherosclerosis of the thoracic aorta.

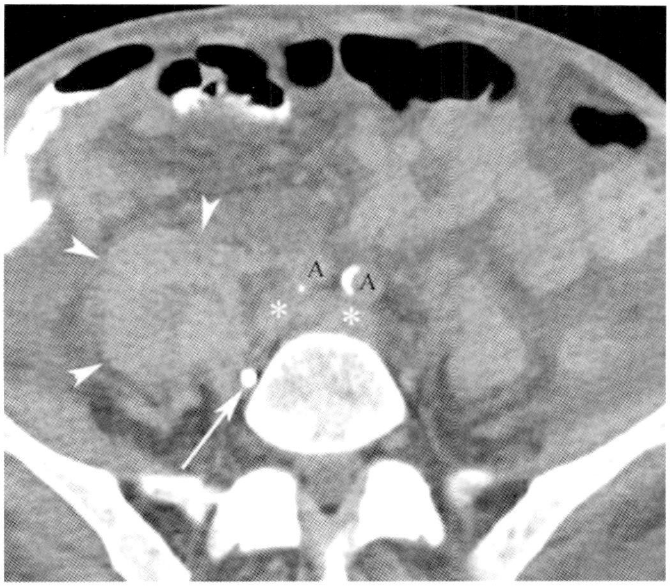

Figure 92.3 Non-contrast axial CT shows malposition of right femoral venous catheter with tip (arrow) in the ascending lumbar vein, which is located posterior to the common iliac veins (asterisk). There is a retroperitoneal hematoma surrounding the right psoas muscle (arrowheads). A small amount of ascites is present. (A: common iliac arteries.)

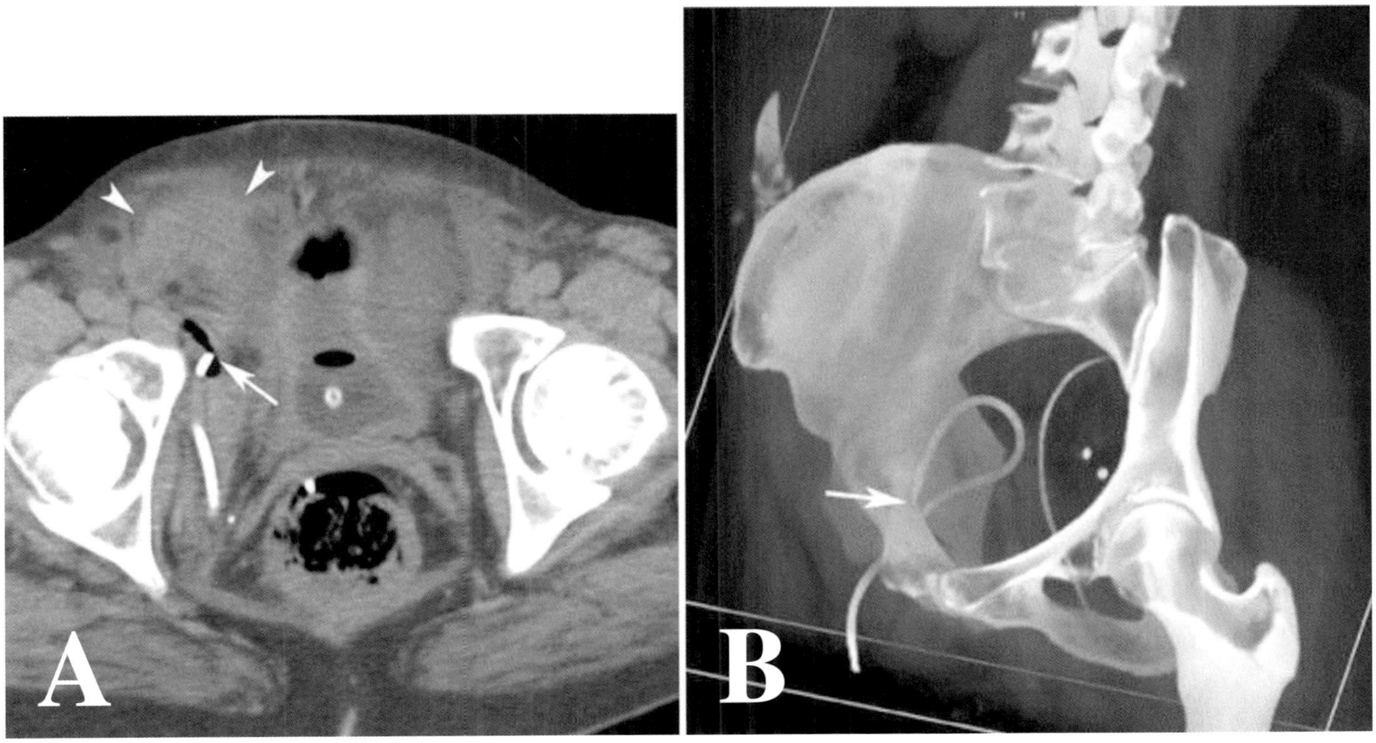

Figure 92.4 Non-contrast axial (**A**) and volume-rendered oblique sagittal (**B**) images show a right femoral venous catheter in an extravascular location in the right inferior pelvis through the right obturator foramen, with tip posterior to the right pectineal line (arrow). Air is seen near the tip of the catheter. There is a hematoma in the right anterior pelvis (arrowheads). A small amount of ascites is present. A Foley catheter and rectal probe are in place.

CASE **93**

Pseudothrombus in the inferior vena cava and other venous systems

Satomi Kawamoto

Imaging description

Filling defects within the inferior vena cava at CT or MRI may be a result of flow artifacts (Figures 93.1 and 93.4), bland thrombus (Figure 93.2) or tumor thrombus (Figure 93.3).[1] Within the inferior vena cava, the most common filling defect seen on CT is pseudothrombosis caused by laminar flow of enhanced blood from the renal veins streaming parallel to the column of unopacified blood returning from the lower body.[1] Its appearance is usually characteristic.[2] Coronal image may be helpful to show the characteristic pattern of a filling defect in relation to the renal veins (Figure 93.1). Artifactual filling defects may also result from poorly enhanced blood flowing into an opacified inferior vena cava, such as inflow from hepatic veins (Figure 93.4).

Artifactual filling defects can also be seen in other venous systems such as the internal jugular vein, portal vein, superior mesenteric vein (Figure 93.5), gonadal vein,[3] and iliofemoral vein.[4,5]

Importance

Artifactual filling defects seen in the venous system on CT and MRI can mimic true thrombus. Delayed imaging after administration of intravenous contrast material may be helpful for further characterization (Figure 93.5), and familiarity with anatomy and flow effects is important to distinguish between pseudo filling defects and true thrombus.[1]

Typical clinical scenario

Typically, pseudothrombosis is seen when enhanced and unenhanced blood flow is mixed related to normal anatomy (such as enhanced blood returning from renal veins mixed with unenhanced blood in the inferior vena cava from the lower body). Reflux of opacified blood mixed with unopacified blood may also cause pseudothrombosis;[1] for example, retrograde contrast enhancement of the inferior vena cava in patients with right-sided heart disease (such as tricuspid regurgitation, pulmonary hypertension, and right ventricular systolic dysfunction), or related to a higher injection rate (>3 ml/s) of contrast material.[6]

Asymmetric opacification of the venous system such as the gonadal veins and iliofemoral veins can also be a cause for pseudothrombosis. Asymmetric reflux of opacified blood into the left gonadal vein,[3] early venous return to the unilateral iliofemoral vein due to a portosystemic shunt,[5] abdominal wall collateral veins,[5] and renal transplant with renal vein and iliac vein anastomosis[4] have been described as causes for pseudothrombosis. In such situations, either the unopacified side or opacified side with mixing artifact can cause an appearance of pseudothrombosis.

Differential diagnosis

Bland thrombus and tumor thrombus should be differentiated from pseudothrombus. Pseudothrombus usually disappears on delayed images, but bland thrombus and tumor thrombus persist on delayed images. Malignant tumor thrombus extending into the inferior vena cava is typically seen in renal cell carcinoma (Figure 93.3), hepatocellular carcinoma, and adrenocortical carcinoma, and usually contiguous to the adjacent mass, and is associated with enhancement of the filling defect (Figure 93.3).[1]

Teaching point

Pseudothrombosis due to mixing artifact or asymmetric opacification is a time-dependent phenomenon that may be seen on early post-contrast CT and MRI,[5] and can mimic true thrombus in the inferior vena cava and other venous systems.

REFERENCES

1. Kaufman LB, Yeh BM, Breiman RS, Joe BN, Qayyum A, Coakley FV. Inferior vena cava filling defects on CT and MRI. *AJR American Journal of Roentgenology* 2005;**185**:717–726.
2. Zhang L, Yang G, Shen W, Qi J. Spectrum of the inferior vena cava: MDCT findings. *Abdominal Imaging* 2007;**32**:495–503.
3. Cranston PE, Hamrick-Turner J, Morano JU. Pseudothrombosis of the right ovarian vein. Pitfalls of abdominal spiral CT. *Clinical Imaging* 1995;**19**:176–179.
4. Gupta R, Rottenberg G, Taylor J. Pseudothrombosis of the iliac vein in patients following combined kidney and pancreas transplantation. *The British Journal of Radiology* 2002;**75**:692–694.
5. Desai G, Poder L, Wang ZJ, Yeh BM, Webb EM, Coakley FV. Computed tomography findings in pseudothrombosis of the iliofemoral vein. *Journal of Computer Assisted Tomography* 2010;**34**:146–148.
6. Kandpal H, Sharma R, Gamangatti S, Srivastava DN, Vashisht S. Imaging the inferior vena cava: a road less traveled. *Radiographics* 2008;**28**:669–689.

Pearls and Pitfalls in Cardiovascular Imaging, ed. Stefan L. Zimmerman and Elliot K. Fishman. Published by Cambridge University Press. © Cambridge University Press 2015.

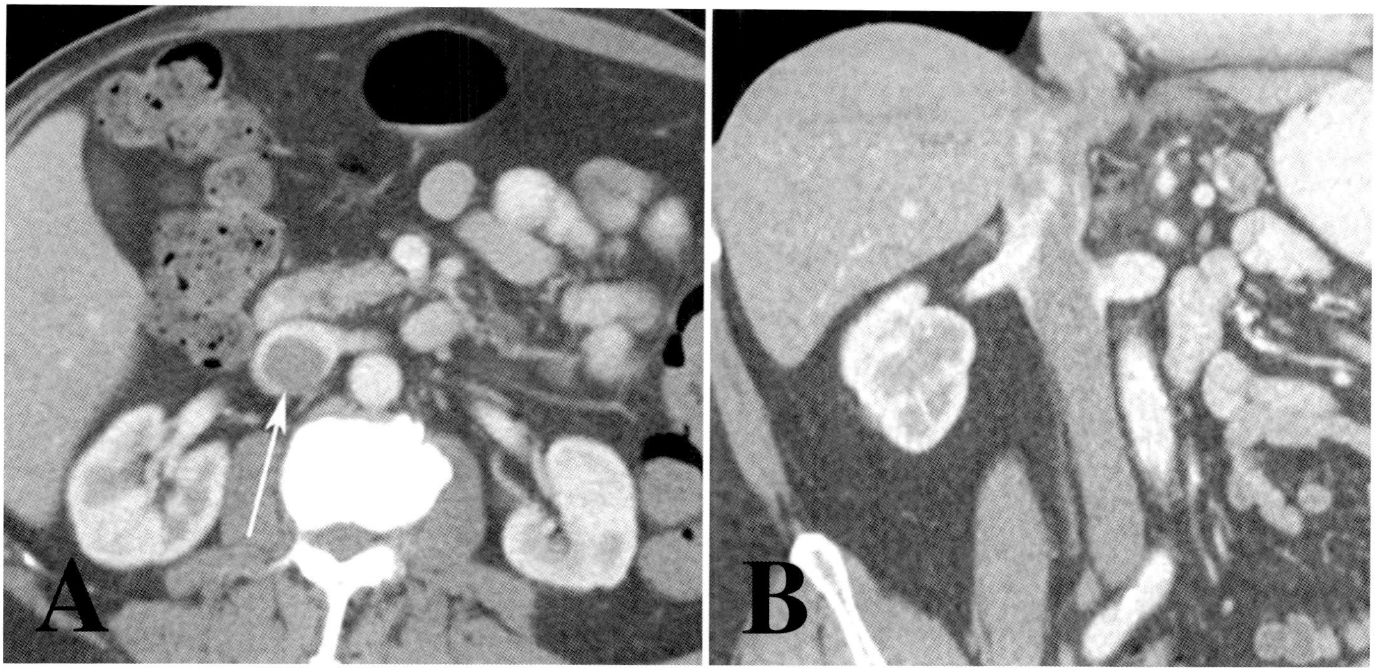

Figure 93.1 Pseudothrombus in the inferior vena cava. **A.** Axial contrast-enhanced CT shows a round filling defect (arrow) within the inferior vena cava. **B.** Coronal CT image shows the filling defect represents mixing artifact due to opacified blood from the renal veins and unopacified blood in the infrarenal vena cava from the lower body.

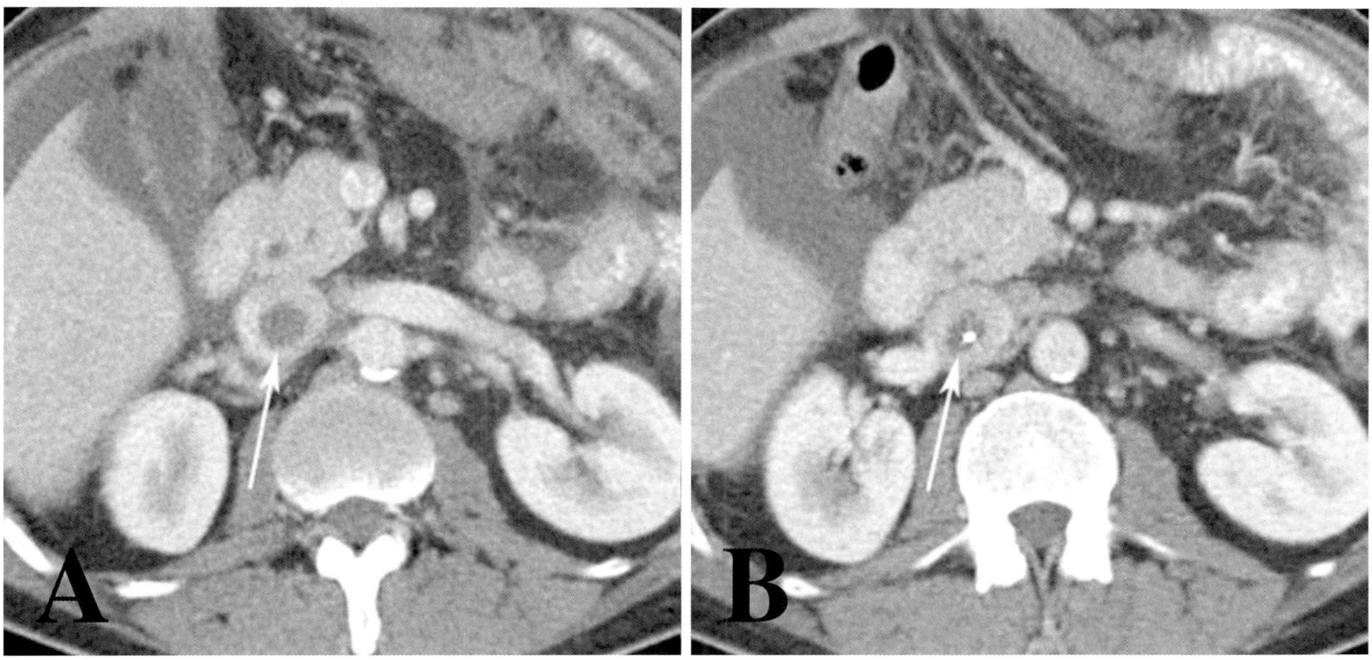

Figure 93.2 Bland thrombus in the inferior vena cava (IVC) attached to the IVC filter. **A.** and **B.** Axial contrast-enhanced CT images show a round filling defect (arrow) within the IVC attached to the IVC filter. **C.** Coronal image shows well-defined filling defect (arrows) attached to the IVC filter extending superiorly within the IVC representing bland thrombus.

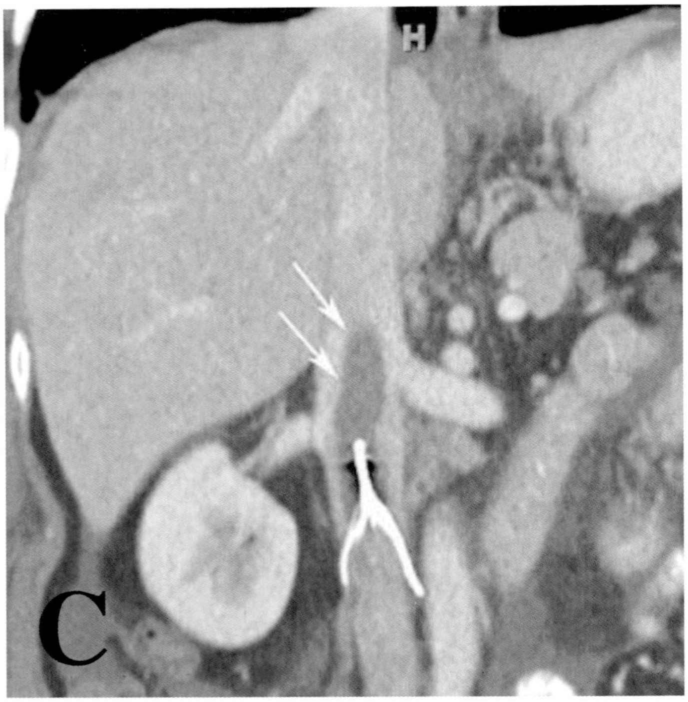

Figure 93.2 *(cont.)*

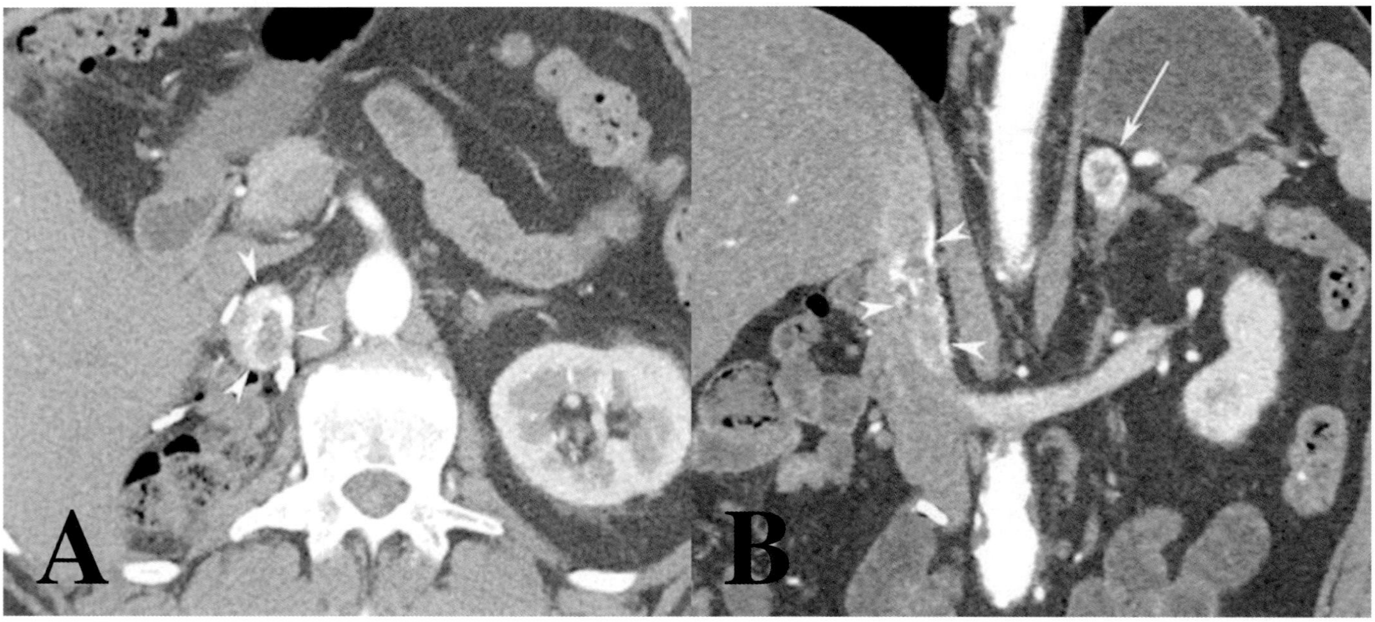

Figure 93.3 Tumor thrombus involving the inferior vena cava. Patient is status post-right nephrectomy for clear cell type renal cell carcinoma 4 years previously. Axial (**A**) and oblique (**B**) coronal arterial phase CT show intensely enhancing mass (arrowheads) in the inferior vena cava, representing tumor thrombus. There is also intensely enhancing left adrenal gland metastasis (arrow).

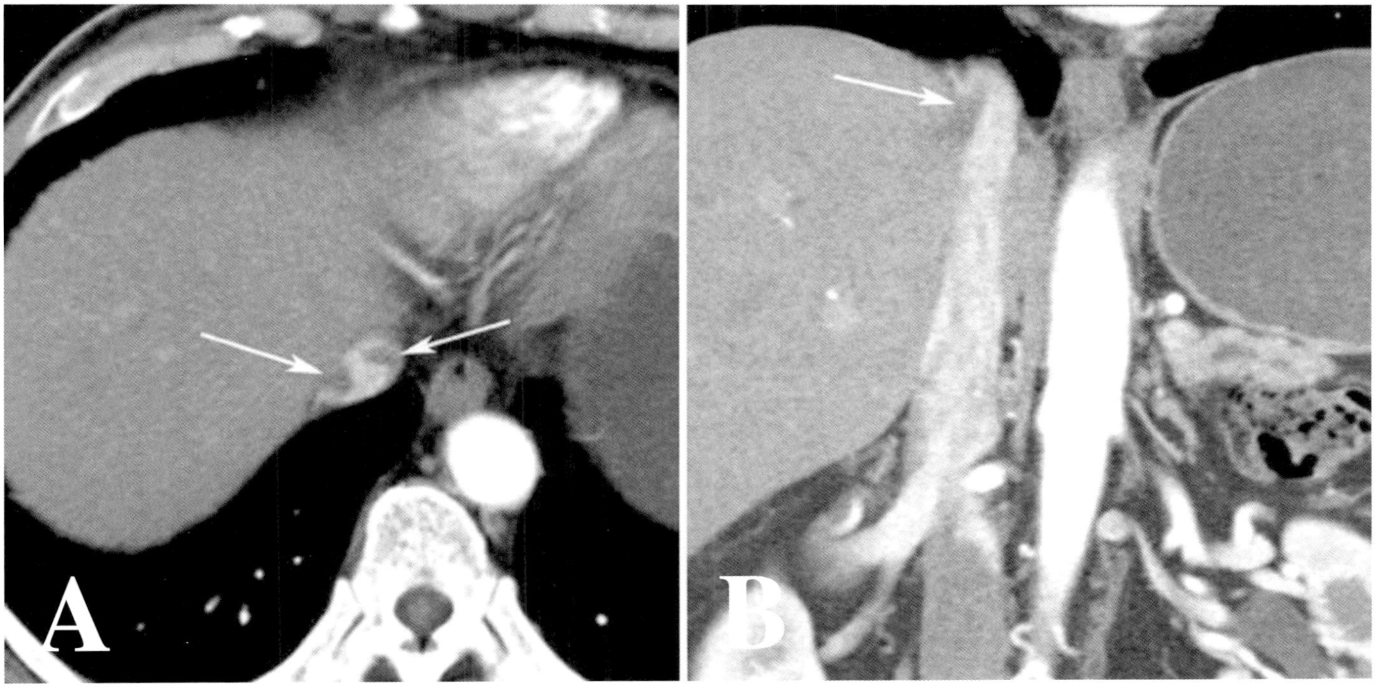

Figure 93.4 Pseudothrombus in the inferior vena cava. Axial (**A**) and coronal (**B**) contrast-enhanced CT show filling defects (arrows) within the hepatic portion of the inferior vena cava, due to mixing artifact from unopacified blood from the hepatic veins and opacified blood in the inferior vena cava.

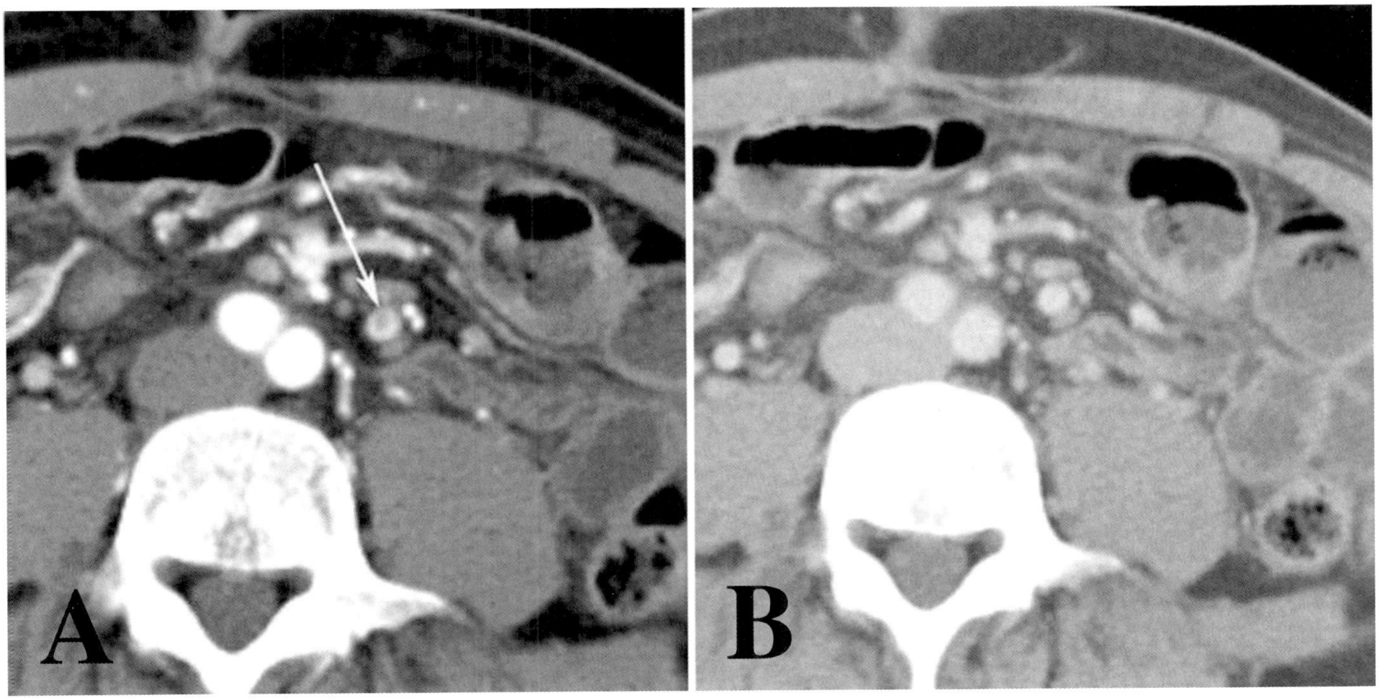

Figure 93.5 Pseudothrombus in the branch of the superior mesenteric vein. **A.** Arterial phase axial CT shows a small round filling defect within a branch of the superior mesenteric vein (arrow) representing mixing artifact from unopacified and opacified blood from the different branches of the superior mesenteric vein. **B.** Venous phase CT shows disappearance of the filling defect, confirming that it is mixing artifact.

CASE 94

Venous collateral pathways in caval obstruction

Sumera Ali and Atif Zaheer

Imaging description

Obstruction of the superior vena cava (SVC) may lead to the formation of portosystemic venous shunting leading to increased blood flow in the quadrate lobe (segment IV) of the liver as seen on contrast-enhanced CT (CECT) and also classically seen as the "hotquadrate lobe" sign on ^{99m}Tc–sulfur colloid scans of the liver.[1] Collateral flow from the subclavian vein goes to the superior epigastric vein via the internal mammary vein into the recanalized paraumbilical vein, which in turn drains into the left portal vein creating a characteristic wedge-shaped area of enhancement in the quadrate lobe during the arterial phase of the CT (Figures 94.1–94.5).[2,3] Blood is shunted to the IVC via the hepatic veins ultimately reaching the right atrium. The internal mammary vein also drains into inferior phrenic vein and subcapsular hepatic veins, which in turn drain into the intrahepatic portal tributaries. This pathway causes subdiaphragmatic focal enhancement near the bare area of the liver (Figures 94.4, 94.5, and 94.6). Additionally, the azygos and the hemiazygos veins may also become dilated and tortuous as a result of diversion of blood from the superior to the inferior vena cava (Figure 94.6).

Other collateral pathways for SVC obstruction include the lateral thoracic and superficial thoracoabdominal venous route, and the vertebral venous plexus route.[4]

Importance

Causes of obstruction of the SVC include compression by a mediastinal neoplasm, post-radiation fibrosis, mediastinitis, or thrombosis and stenosis due to presence of indwelling catheters. Cavoportal collaterals due to SVC obstruction may be seen as a hypervascular lesion on a contrast-enhanced CT and can be mistaken for a tumor. This could expose the patient to risks of unnecessary imaging and/or invasive testing such as a biopsy. Presence of collateral vessels seen on CT is a highly accurate predictor of SVC obstruction with a sensitivity of 96% and a specificity of 92%.[5]

Typical clinical scenario

SVC obstruction may be seen in patients with mediastinal masses, post-radiation fibrosis, or long-term indwelling catheters. A typical CT would show absence of contrast in the superior vena cava distal to the site of obstruction with luminal thrombus or stenosis, combined with enhancement of the collateral vessels.

Differential diagnosis

The differential for focally increased hepatic blood flow includes Budd–Chiari syndrome, hemangiomas, focal nodular hyperplasia, portocaval shunts associated with portal hypertension, and hepatocellular carcinoma.[1] Budd–Chiari syndrome can cause hyperenhancement in the caudate lobe while the other entities may occur in any hepatic segment.

Teaching point

The characteristic wedge-shaped enhancement in the quadrate lobe of the liver is a sign of SVC obstruction and should not be mistaken for a hypervascular liver mass. Detection of collateral pathways on contrast-enhanced CT carries a high sensitivity and specificity for the diagnosis of SVC obstruction.

REFERENCES

1. A. M. Dickson. The focal hepatic hot spot sign. *Radiology* 2005; **237**: 647–8.
2. H. Dahan, L. Arrive, L. Monnier-Cholley, P. Le Hir, M. Zins, J. M. Tubiana. Cavoportal collateral pathways in vena cava obstruction: imaging features. *AJR Am J Roentgenol* 1998; **171**: 1405–11.
3. S. Sheth, M. D. Ebert, E. K. Fishman. Superior vena cava obstruction evaluation with MDCT. *AJR Am J Roentgenol* 2010; **194**: W336–46.
4. B. Bashist, A. Parisi, D. H. Frager, B. Suster. Abdominal CT findings when the superior vena cava, brachiocephalic vein, or subclavian vein is obstructed. *AJR Am J Roentgenol* 1996; **167**: 1457–63.
5. H. J. Kim, H. S. Kim, S. H. Chung. CT diagnosis of superior vena cava syndrome: importance of collateral vessels. *AJR Am J Roentgenol* 1993; **161**: 539–42.

Pearls and Pitfalls in Cardiovascular Imaging, ed. Stefan L. Zimmerman and Elliot K. Fishman. Published by Cambridge University Press. © Cambridge University Press 2015.

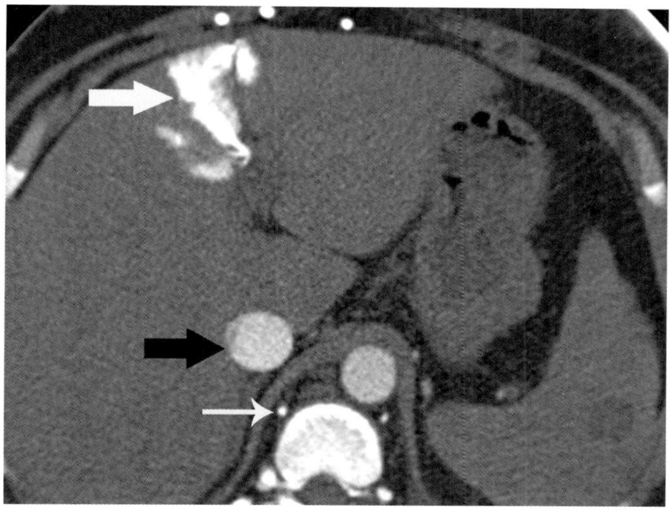

Figure 94.1 A 22-year-old woman with end-stage renal disease and chronic SVC thrombosis due to multiple central venous catheters used for hemodialysis. Axial contrast-enhanced arterial phase CT at the level of the liver demonstrates a triangular area of increased enhancement (thick white arrow). Early enhancement of the IVC (thick black arrow) and dense enhancement of the azygos vein is also seen (thin white arrow).

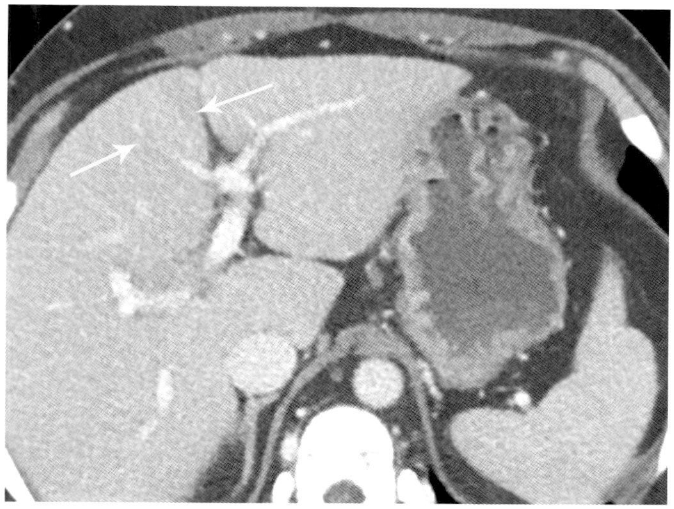

Figure 94.2 Axial venous phase from contrast-enhanced CT in the same patient demonstrates absence of the abnormality seen on the arterial phase (arrows).

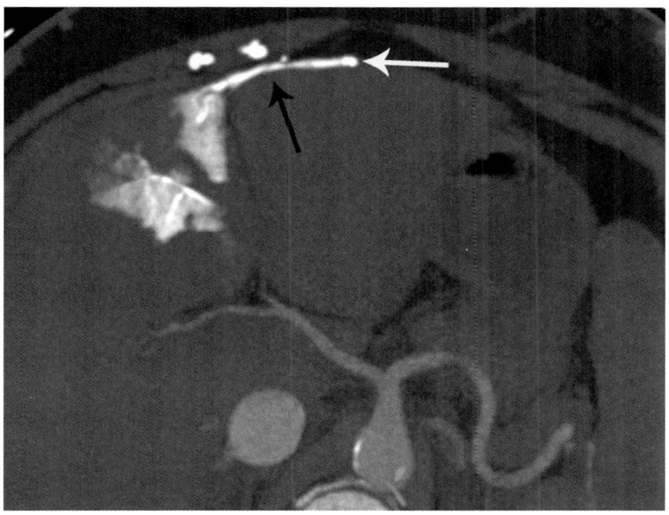

Figure 94.3 Axial contrast-enhanced arterial phase CT MIP image in the same patient shows a densely opacified right superior epigastric vein (white arrow) draining into a branch of the portal vein via the paraumbilical vein (black arrow).

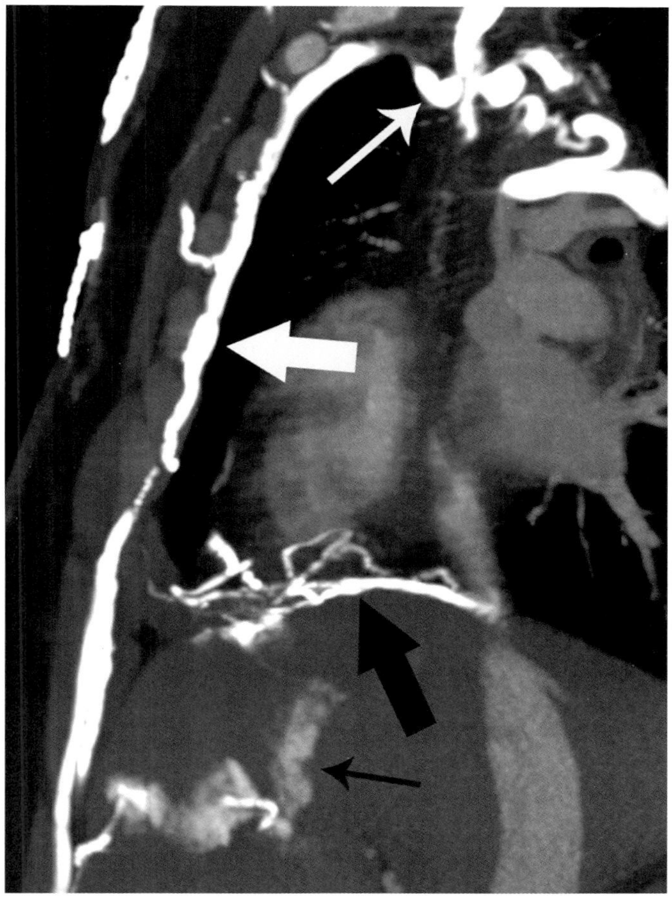

Figure 94.4 Sagittal MIP image in the same patient shows blood flow from the subclavian vein (thin white arrow) into the internal mammary vein (thick white arrow). Subdiaphragmatic focal enhancement near the bare area of the liver (thick black arrow) is due to the drainage of the internal mammary vein into inferior phrenic vein and subcapsular hepatic veins, and subsequently into the intrahepatic portal tributaries (thin black arrow).

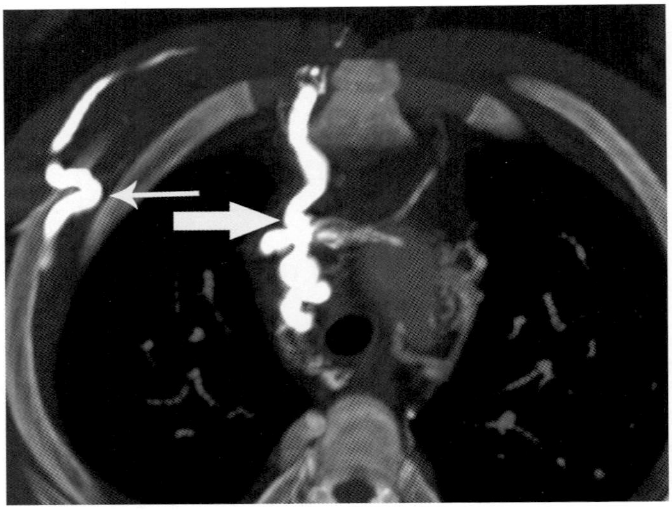

Figure 94.5 Axial contrast-enhanced arterial phase CT MIP image in the same patient shows densely opacified right internal mammary vein communicating with the right subclavian artery (thick white arrow). A dilated intercostal vein can also be seen (thin white arrow).

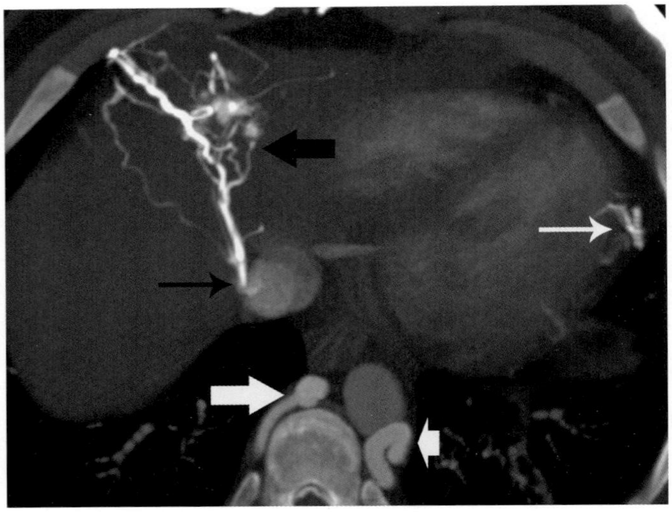

Figure 94.6 Axial contrast-enhanced arterial phase MIP image in the same patient demonstrates subdiaphragmatic focal enhancement near the bare area of the liver (thick black arrow) with drainage of internal mammary vein into inferior phrenic vein and subsequently into the IVC through subcapsular hepatic vein (thin black arrow). Dilated azygos (thick white arrow) and hemiazygos veins (short thick white arrow) as well as left pericardiophrenic vein (thin white arrow) are also seen.

CASE

95 Catheter-related thrombus and incidental small vein thrombosis

Satomi Kawamoto

Imaging description

Thrombosis within the relatively small veins such as the gonadal vein, inferior mesenteric vein, upper extremity veins, and thrombosis related to a central venous catheter may be symptomatic, but can also be an incidental finding on CT or MRI. Non-occlusive venous thrombosis is typically seen on contrast-enhanced CT as an intraluminal filling defect surrounded by contrast material (Figures 95.1 to 95.3). When the vein is occluded by thrombus, the venous lumen is not opacified. Central venous catheter-related thrombosis is seen as a filling defect within the vein around or attached to the catheter (Figure 95.3).

Importance

Thrombosis in relatively small veins can be easily overlooked on routine CT examination. Ovarian vein thrombosis has been considered rare, but recent data suggested that the diagnosis is more common than previously thought with the widespread use of cross-sectional imaging.[1] Anticoagulation is the mainstay of treatment for ovarian vein thrombosis.[2]

The clinical significance of central venous catheter-related thrombosis remains undefined, although all thromboses have the potential to embolize,[3] and patients often receive an anticoagulant therapy after detection of catheter-related thrombosis.[4]

Typical clinical scenario

Classically, ovarian vein thrombosis predominantly occurs in the postpartum period. It is also associated with pelvic inflammatory disease, gynecological malignancy, hypercoagulability, and surgery. Clinical presentation of ovarian vein thrombosis is variable. Patients may be asymptomatic, and thrombosis may be detected incidentally on CT, particularly after hysterectomy and salpingo-oophorectomy.[5] Other patients may present with fever and abdominal pain. Complications of ovarian vein thrombosis include extension of thrombus into the renal veins and the inferior vena cava, and pulmonary thromboembolism.[1] In asymptomatic patients, usually no perivascular stranding is seen on CT.[5] However, in patients with puerperal septic thrombophlebitis of the ovarian vein, tortuosity and perivascular edema are often associated.[6] Thrombosis of the ovarian vein is more commonly seen on the right side, likely related to long length of the right ovarian vein, lack of retrograde flow, and multiple incompetent valves.[5]

Septic thrombophlebitis of the inferior mesenteric vein can be associated with sigmoid diverticulitis. Thrombosis of the inferior mesenteric vein following total colectomy has also been reported.

Thrombosis is a known complication associated with central venous catheter. Catheter-related thrombosis can be small, and can be overlooked on CT. Catalano et al. reported 17 (3.5%) of 481 oncologic patients had a retrospective diagnosis of thrombosis related to central venous device on MDCT.[4] Eleven (65%) of these 17 cases of thrombosis were noticed retrospectively and not originally reported.[2] All of the 11 non-diagnosed cases were non-occlusive thrombi. They speculated the thrombus might be masked by the mix of unenhanced and enhanced blood coming from different veins, and beam hardening artifact from a catheter. Using appropriate window values is important in detecting catheter-associated thrombus.[2]

Differential diagnosis

When the veins are suboptimally opacified with contrast material, it may be difficult to differentiate true thrombus from artifactual filling defect related to mixing artifact. Delayed post-contrast image is helpful in distinguishing true thrombus from artifactual filling defect.

Teaching point

Thrombosis in the relatively small veins may be an incidental finding on CT, and can be easily overlooked. Central venous catheter-related thrombosis can be small and may be obscured by beam hardening artifact and mix of dense contrast material. Careful scrutiny of such veins may facilitate recognition of small thrombus. The use of appropriate window values is important in detecting catheter-related thrombus.

REFERENCES

1. Karaosmanoglu D, Karcaaltincaba M, Karcaaltincaba D, Akata D, Ozmen M. MDCT of the ovarian vein: normal anatomy and pathology. *AJR American Journal of Roentgenology* 2009;**192**:295–299.
2. Stafford M, Fleming T, Khalil A. Idiopathic ovarian vein thrombosis: a rare cause of pelvic pain – case report and review of literature. *The Australian & New Zealand Journal of Obstetrics & Gynaecology* 2010;**50**:299–301.
3. McGee DC, Gould MK. Preventing complications of central venous catheterization. *The New England Journal of Medicine* 2003;**348**:1123–1133.

Pearls and Pitfalls in Cardiovascular Imaging, ed. Stefan L. Zimmerman and Elliot K. Fishman. Published by Cambridge University Press. © Cambridge University Press 2015.

4. Catalano O, de Lutio di Castelguidone E, Sandomenico C, et al. Central venous device-related thrombosis as imaged with MDCT in oncologic patients: prevalence and findings. *Acta Radiologica* 2011;**52**:148–154.
5. Yassa NA, Ryst E. Ovarian vein thrombosis: a common incidental finding in patients who have undergone total abdominal hysterectomy and bilateral salpingo-oophorectomy with retroperitoneal lymph node dissection. *AJR American Journal of Roentgenology* 1999;**172**:45–47.
6. Twickler DM, Setiawan AT, Evans RS, et al. Imaging of puerperal septic thrombophlebitis: prospective comparison of MR imaging, CT, and sonography. *AJR American Journal of Roentgenology* 1997;**169**:1039–1043.

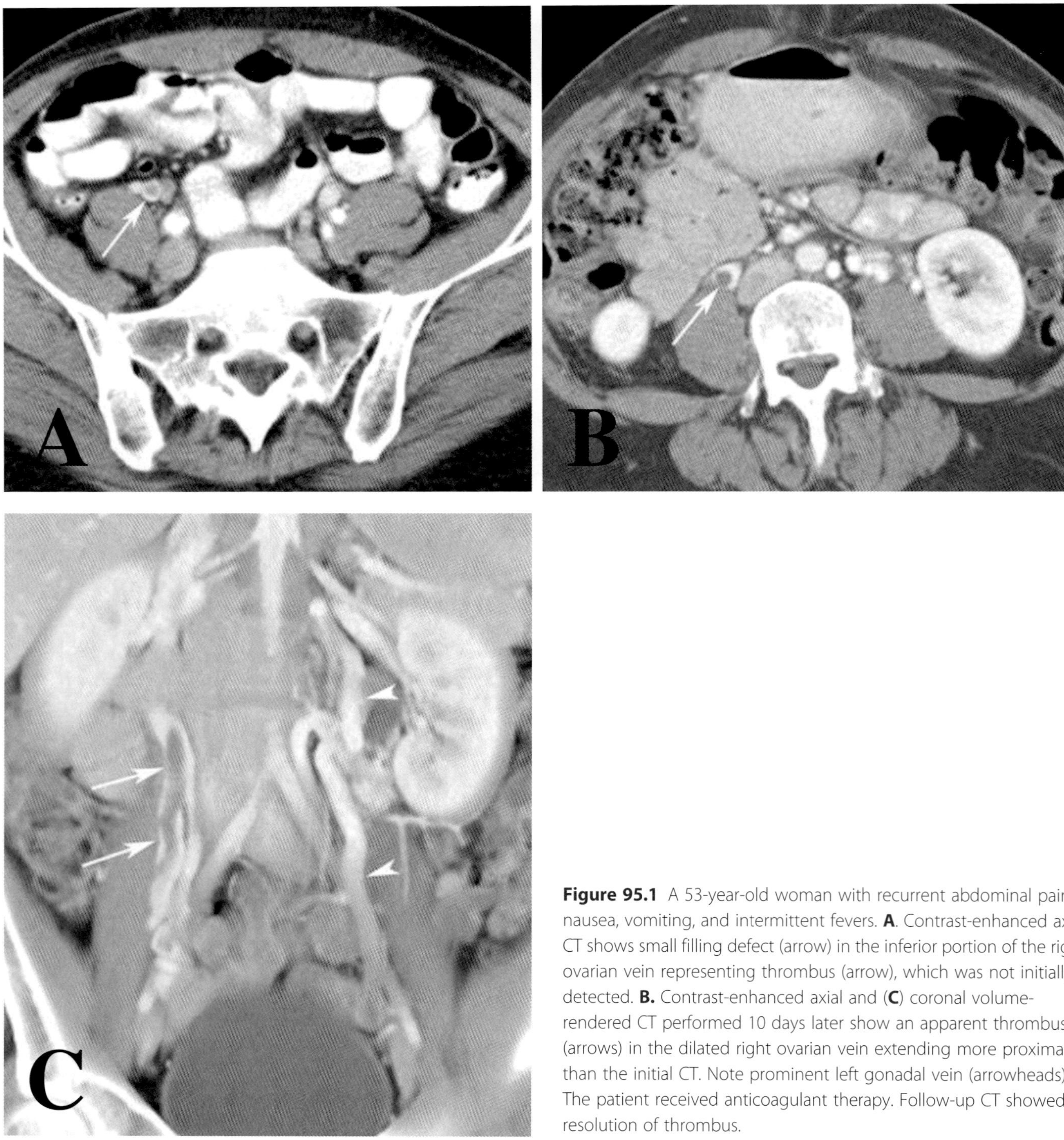

Figure 95.1 A 53-year-old woman with recurrent abdominal pain, nausea, vomiting, and intermittent fevers. **A**. Contrast-enhanced axial CT shows small filling defect (arrow) in the inferior portion of the right ovarian vein representing thrombus (arrow), which was not initially detected. **B.** Contrast-enhanced axial and (**C**) coronal volume-rendered CT performed 10 days later show an apparent thrombus (arrows) in the dilated right ovarian vein extending more proximally than the initial CT. Note prominent left gonadal vein (arrowheads). The patient received anticoagulant therapy. Follow-up CT showed resolution of thrombus.

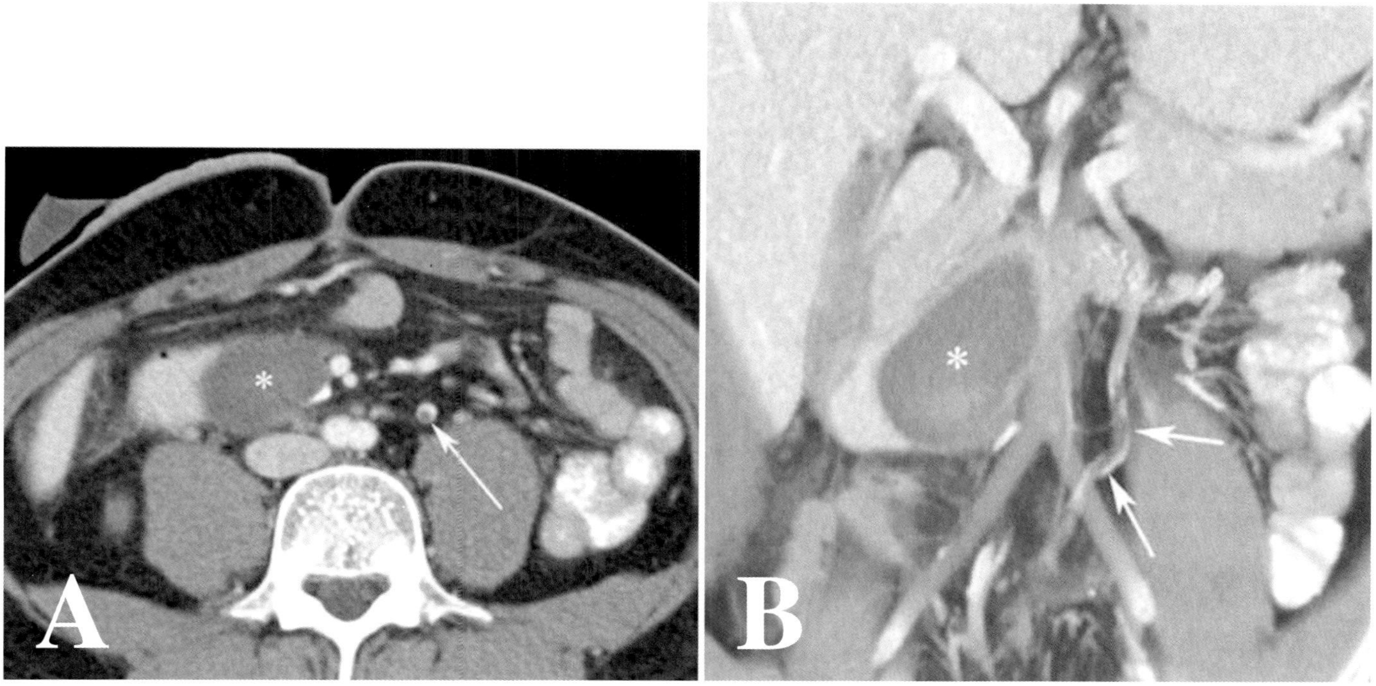

Figure 95.2 Contrast-enhanced axial (**A**) and coronal volume-rendered CT (**B**) show small filling defect in the inferior mesenteric vein (arrows) representing thrombus. The patient is status post-colectomy for ulcerative colitis. The patient later developed portal vein thrombosis, and received anticoagulant therapy. Subacute periduodenal hematoma (asterisk) is seen as a hypodense collection.

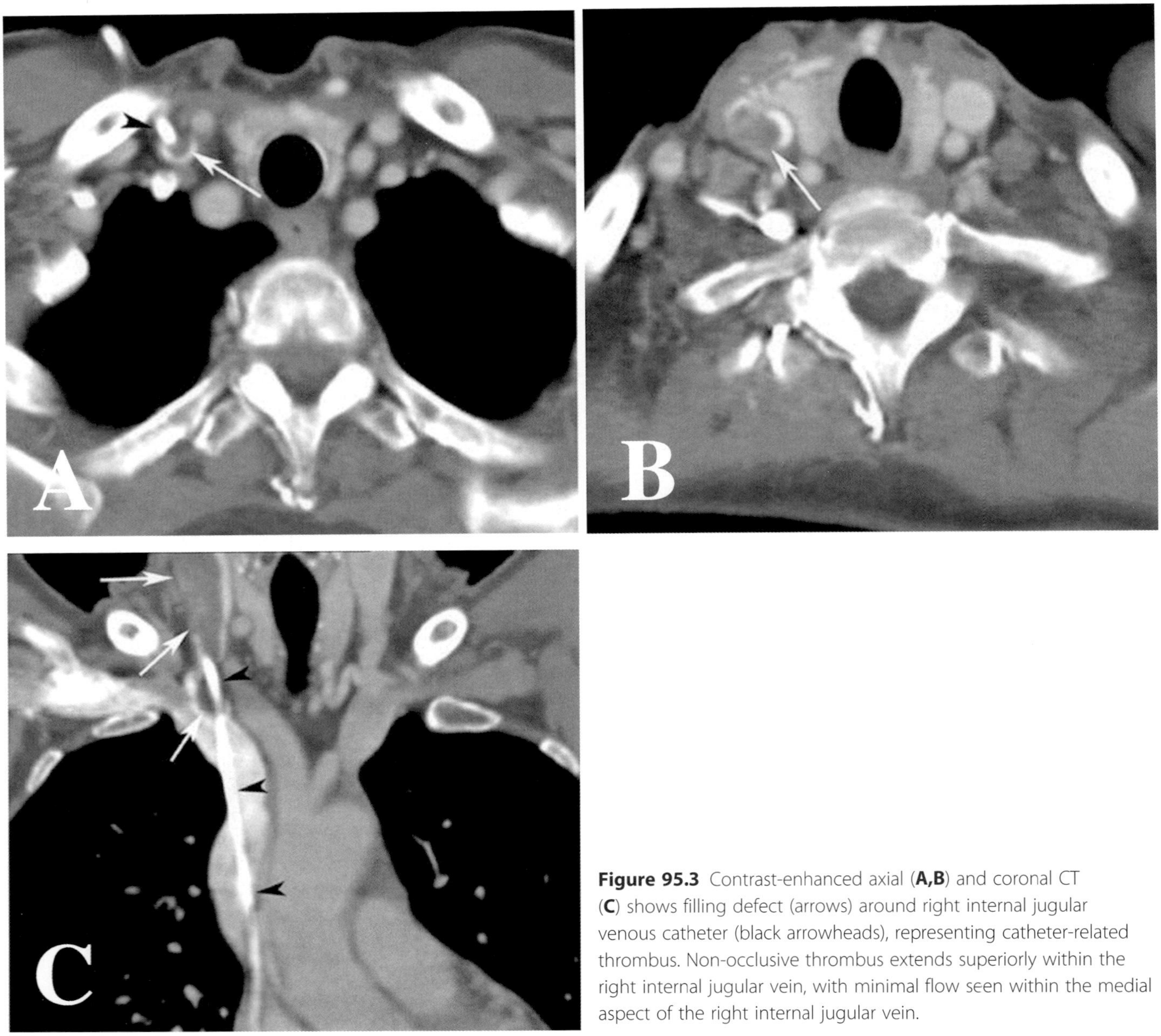

Figure 95.3 Contrast-enhanced axial (**A,B**) and coronal CT (**C**) shows filling defect (arrows) around right internal jugular venous catheter (black arrowheads), representing catheter-related thrombus. Non-occlusive thrombus extends superiorly within the right internal jugular vein, with minimal flow seen within the medial aspect of the right internal jugular vein.

CASE **96**

Nutcracker syndrome

Satomi Kawamoto

Imaging description

The nutcracker phenomenon, also known as left renal vein entrapment, refers to the compression of the left renal vein between the aorta and the superior mesenteric artery (Figures 96.1 and 96.2), with impeded outflow of the left renal vein.[1] Compression of the left renal vein can cause left renal-to-gonadal vein reflux resulting in pelvic congestion and varicocele. Patients may also have dilated, tortuous collateral veins around the left kidney, and left retroperitoneum (Figure 96.1). On sagittal images, an abnormally small angle between the abdominal aorta and superior mesenteric artery (normal: close to 90 degrees[2]) can be seen (Figures 96.1 and 96.2).[3] Asymmetric delayed cortical enhancement of the left kidney on the nephrographic phase of CT has been described.[3] On excretory phase CT, notching and displacement of the left renal collecting system and ureter due to dilated veins have also been described.[1]

Impeded outflow of the left renal vein has also been reported in association with a retroaortic course of the left renal vein. In this situation, the retroaortic left renal vein is compressed between the aorta and the vertebral column (Figure 96.1), which is called "posterior nutcracker."[2]

Importance

Symptoms of nutcracker syndrome are complex and include left flank and abdominal pain, macroscopic or microscopic hematuria, left renal-to-gonadal vein reflux resulting in pelvic congestion syndrome in females, varicoceles in males, orthostatic proteinuria, lower limb varices, and chronic fatigue symptoms.[1,4] The diagnosis of nutcracker syndrome is often difficult and is commonly delayed.[1] Differentiation should be made between asymptomatic dilatation of the left renal vein (nutcracker phenomenon) and symptomatic patients (nutcracker syndrome).

Typical clinical scenario

The exact prevalence of nutcracker syndrome is unknown but may be slightly higher in females.[1,4] Most symptomatic patients are in their second or third decade of life, and there may be a second peak in middle-aged women.[1,4] Spontaneous resolution of the nutcracker phenomenon has been described in children.[1]

Hematuria is the most commonly reported symptom.[1] Lopatkin et al. postulated that increased pressure in the venous system could rupture the thin-walled septum between the small veins and collecting system in the renal fornix resulting in hematuria.[5]

Diagnosis of nutcracker syndrome is based on history and physical examination, basic lab tests to exclude other causes of hematuria, and cystoscopy/ureteroscopy to confirm unilateral hematuria from the left side.[4] Cross-sectional imaging studies are used to demonstrate nutcracker anatomy and to exclude other causes for hematuria. Renal venography, combined with measurement of the pressure gradient between the left renal vein and the inferior vena cava, is the most reliable diagnostic tool for demonstrating renal vein hypertension.[4]

Differential diagnosis

Nutcracker anatomy is not always associated with clinical symptoms. The term "nutcracker syndrome" should be reserved for patients with characteristic clinical symptoms associated with demonstrable nutcracker morphologic features.[1] For patients with hematuria, the diagnosis of nutcracker syndrome is only made after exclusion of other causes of hematuria.

Teaching point

Nutcracker syndrome is characterized by impeded outflow from the left renal vein into the inferior vena cava due to extrinsic compression of the left renal vein, secondary to a narrow angle between the abdominal aorta and superior mesenteric artery. It is associated with complex symptoms including hematuria, abdominal/flank pain, varicoceles, and pelvic congestion. Cross-sectional imaging studies shows characteristic nutcracker anatomy.

REFERENCES

1. Kurklinsky AK, Rooke TW. Nutcracker phenomenon and nutcracker syndrome. *Mayo Clinic Proceedings* 2010;**85**:552–559.
2. Shokeir AA, el-Diasty TA, Ghoneim MA. The nutcracker syndrome: new methods of diagnosis and treatment. *British Journal of Urology* 1994;**74**:139–143.
3. Cho BS, Suh JS, Hahn WH, Kim SD, Lim JW. Multidetector computed tomography findings and correlations with proteinuria in nutcracker syndrome. *Pediatric Nephrology* 2010;**25**:469–475.
4. Ahmed K, Sampath R, Khan MS. Current trends in the diagnosis and management of renal nutcracker syndrome: a review. *European Journal of Vascular and Endovascular Surgery* 2006;**31**:410–416.
5. Lopatkin NA, Morozov AV, Lopatkina LN. Essential renal haemorrhages. *European Urology* 1978;**4**:115–119.

Pearls and Pitfalls in Cardiovascular Imaging, ed. Stefan L. Zimmerman and Elliot K. Fishman. Published by Cambridge University Press. © Cambridge University Press 2015.

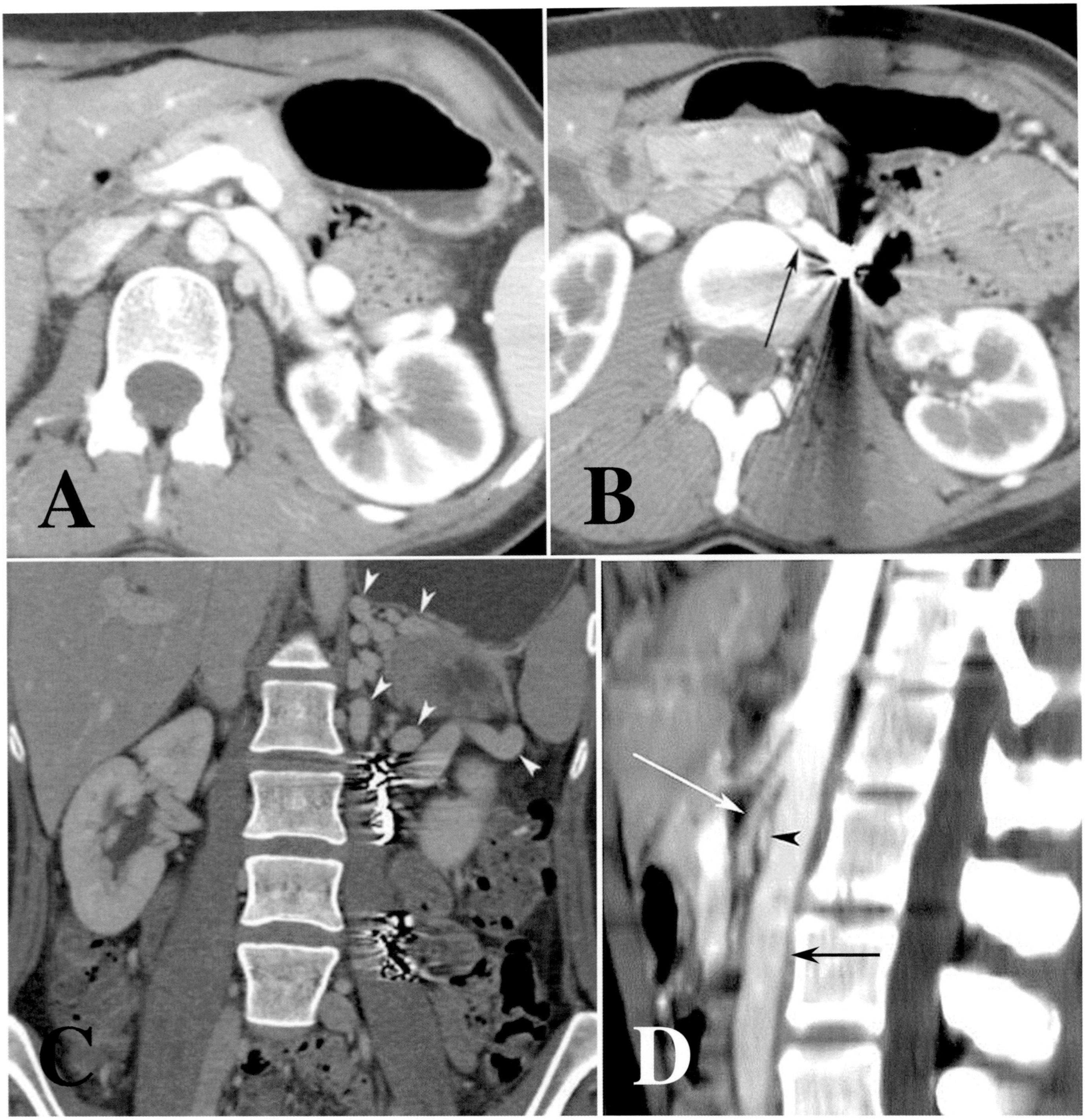

Figure 96.1 A 33-year-old woman with circumaortic left renal vein. History of left pelvic pain and left ovarian vein coil embolization. Worsening of left flank pain and left back pain. **A.** Axial contrast-enhanced CT shows compression of the left renal vein between the abdominal aorta and the superior mesenteric artery. **B.** Axial contrast-enhanced CT inferior to (**A**) shows compression of the retroaortic component of the left renal vein (arrow) between the abdominal aorta and the vertebral body. **C.** Coronal CT shows multiple collateral veins (arrowheads) around the left kidney. Multiple metallic densities from prior left ovarian vein coil embolization. **D.** Sagittal CT image shows small angle between the superior mesenteric artery (white arrow) and the aorta with compression of the left renal vein (black arrowhead). Retroaortic component of the left renal vein (black arrow) is also compressed between the abdominal aorta and the vertebral body.

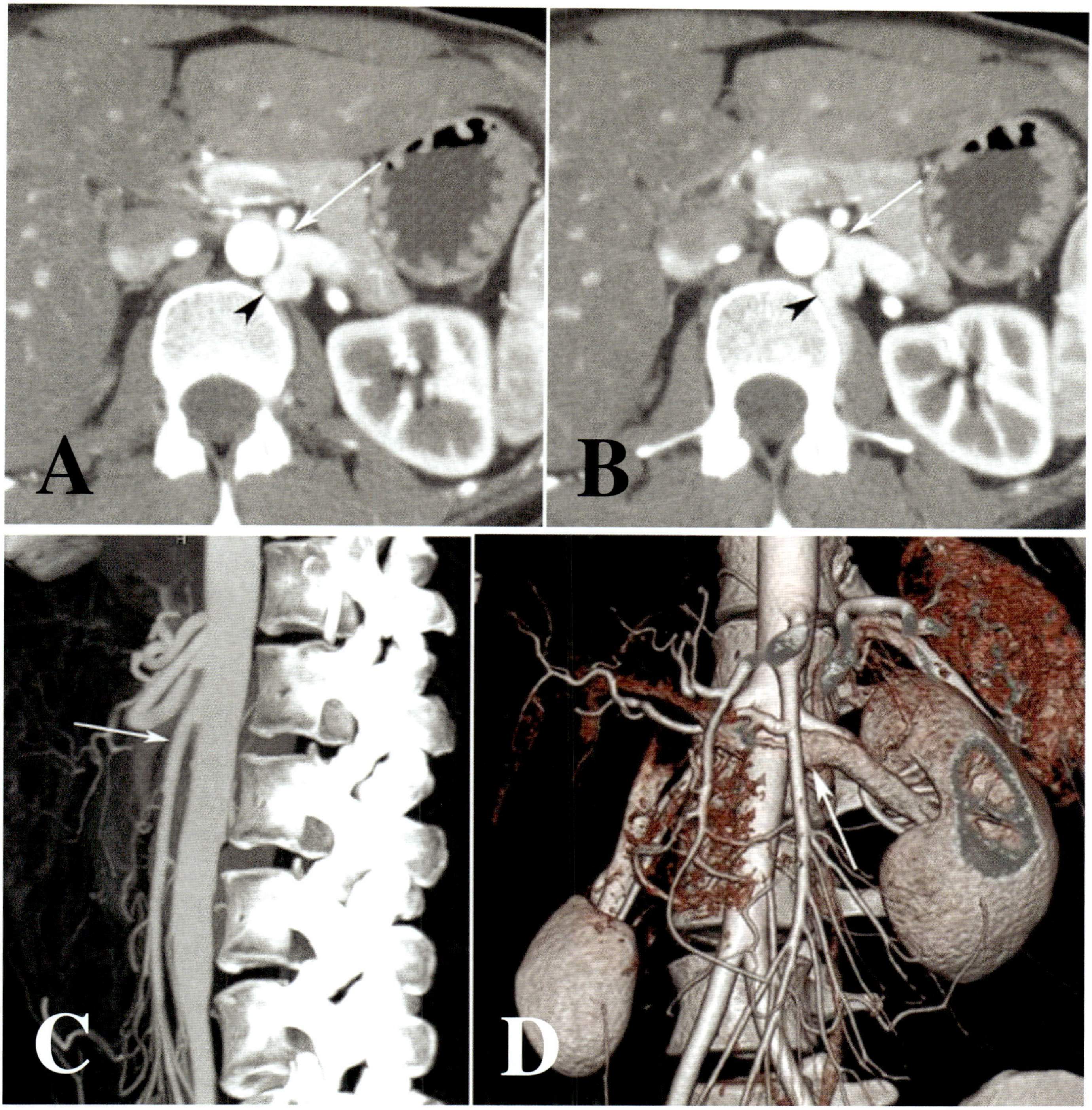

Figure 96.2 A 32-year-old woman with abdominal pain. CT was performed for suspected superior mesenteric artery syndrome. **A,B.** Contiguous axial contrast-enhanced CT images show compression of the left renal vein (arrow) between the abdominal aorta and the superior mesenteric artery. Dilated ascending left lumbar vein is also seen (arrowhead). **C.** Sagittal volume-rendered image shows small angle between the superior mesenteric artery (arrow) and the aorta. **D.** Anterior volume-rendered image shows compression of the left renal vein (arrow) between the abdominal aorta and the superior mesenteric artery.

CASE 97

May–Thurner syndrome

Satomi Kawamoto

Imaging description

May–Thurner syndrome, also known as iliac vein compression syndrome, or Crockett syndrome, is symptomatic compression of the left common iliac vein between the right common iliac artery and the lumbar vertebrae.[1] Axial CT images will show that the right common iliac artery compresses the left common iliac vein (Figures 97.1 and 97.2). Patients with May–Thurner syndrome have an asymmetrically small left common iliac vein, which measured an average of 3.5 mm in diameter in a study of 10 patients by Oguzkurt et al., which was significantly smaller than that in control subjects (11.5 mm). [1] The abnormality can be confirmed by iliac venography obtained via femoral access, which will demonstrate compression of the left common iliac vein in association with a pressure gradient (Figure 97.1). Patients with May–Thurner syndrome have a higher risk for acute or chronic deep venous thrombosis of the left-sided lower extremity (Figure 97.1). In patients with May–Thurner syndrome with chronic left common iliac venous occlusion, tortuous pelvic venous collaterals, which may connect to the contralateral veins, may be seen (Figure 97.2).

Importance

May–Thurner syndrome is important to recognize in patients with persistent left leg edema because relief of the mechanical compression of the left common iliac vein can prevent the development of deep venous thrombosis and venous insufficiency.[2] Endovascular treatment with angioplasty and stent placement has been shown to be a safe and effective means of treating May–Thurner syndrome.[3]

Typical clinical scenario

Patients with May–Thurner syndrome may present with acute or chronic left leg edema, limb pain, venous claudication, varicosities, deep venous thrombosis, chronic venous stasis, ulcers, phlegmasia cerulea dolens, or pulmonary embolism.[2,3] This condition has been estimated to occur in 2% to 5% of patients who undergo evaluation for lower extremity venous disorders.[2] It occurs predominantly in young to middle-aged women.[2]

Contrast-enhanced CT or MRI typically shows external compression of the left common iliac vein caused by the right common iliac artery. Monophasic flow without respiratory variation distal to the compression and a significant increase in flow velocity in the common iliac vein at the point of arterial compression has been described by Doppler ultrasound.[4] An iliac venogram remains the diagnostic test of choice by demonstrating venous compression, and pressure gradient.[2] A pressure gradient > 2 mmHg is abnormal across a stenosis in iliac veins.[4]

Differential diagnosis

Although compression of the left iliac vein by the right iliac artery against the lumbar vertebra has been thought to predispose to formation of deep venous thrombosis, this finding alone is commonly seen on CT in asymptomatic patients. The significance of this anatomic finding in asymptomatic patients has been the topic of debate for some time.[5] Kibbe et al. evaluated the CT of 50 asymptomatic patients: 24% of patients had greater than 50% compression and 66% had greater than 25% compression.[5] They proposed that some degree of compression of the left iliac vein may be a normal anatomic finding that by itself does not place the patient at increased risk for development of deep venous thrombosis.[5]

Teaching point

May–Thurner syndrome is symptomatic compression of the left common iliac vein between the right common iliac artery and the lumbar vertebrae. Cross-sectional imaging studies including CT show external compression of the left common iliac vein caused by the right common iliac artery against the vertebra. The diagnosis can be confirmed with venography, which will demonstrate compression of the left iliac vein and an abnormal pressure gradient across the stenosis.

REFERENCES

1. Oguzkurt L, Tercan F, Pourbagher MA, Kizilkilic O, Turkoz R, Boyvat F. Computed tomography findings in 10 cases of iliac vein compression (May–Thurner) syndrome. *European Journal of Radiology* 2005;**55**:421–425.
2. Cil BE, Akpinar E, Karcaaltincaba M, Akinci D. Case 76: May–Thurner syndrome. *Radiology* 2004;**233**:361–365.
3. O'Sullivan GJ, Semba CP, Bittner CA, et al. Endovascular management of iliac vein compression (May–Thurner) syndrome. *Journal of Vascular and Interventional Radiology: JVIR* 2000;**11**:823–836.
4. Oguzkurt L, Ozkan U, Tercan F, Koc Z. Ultrasonographic diagnosis of iliac vein compression (May–Thurner) syndrome. *Diagnostic and Interventional Radiology* 2007;**13**:152–155.
5. Kibbe MR, Ujiki M, Goodwin AL, Eskandari M, Yao J, Matsumura J. Iliac vein compression in an asymptomatic patient population. *Journal of Vascular Surgery* 2004;**39**:937–943.

Pearls and Pitfalls in Cardiovascular Imaging, ed. Stefan L. Zimmerman and Elliot K. Fishman. Published by Cambridge University Press. © Cambridge University Press 2015.

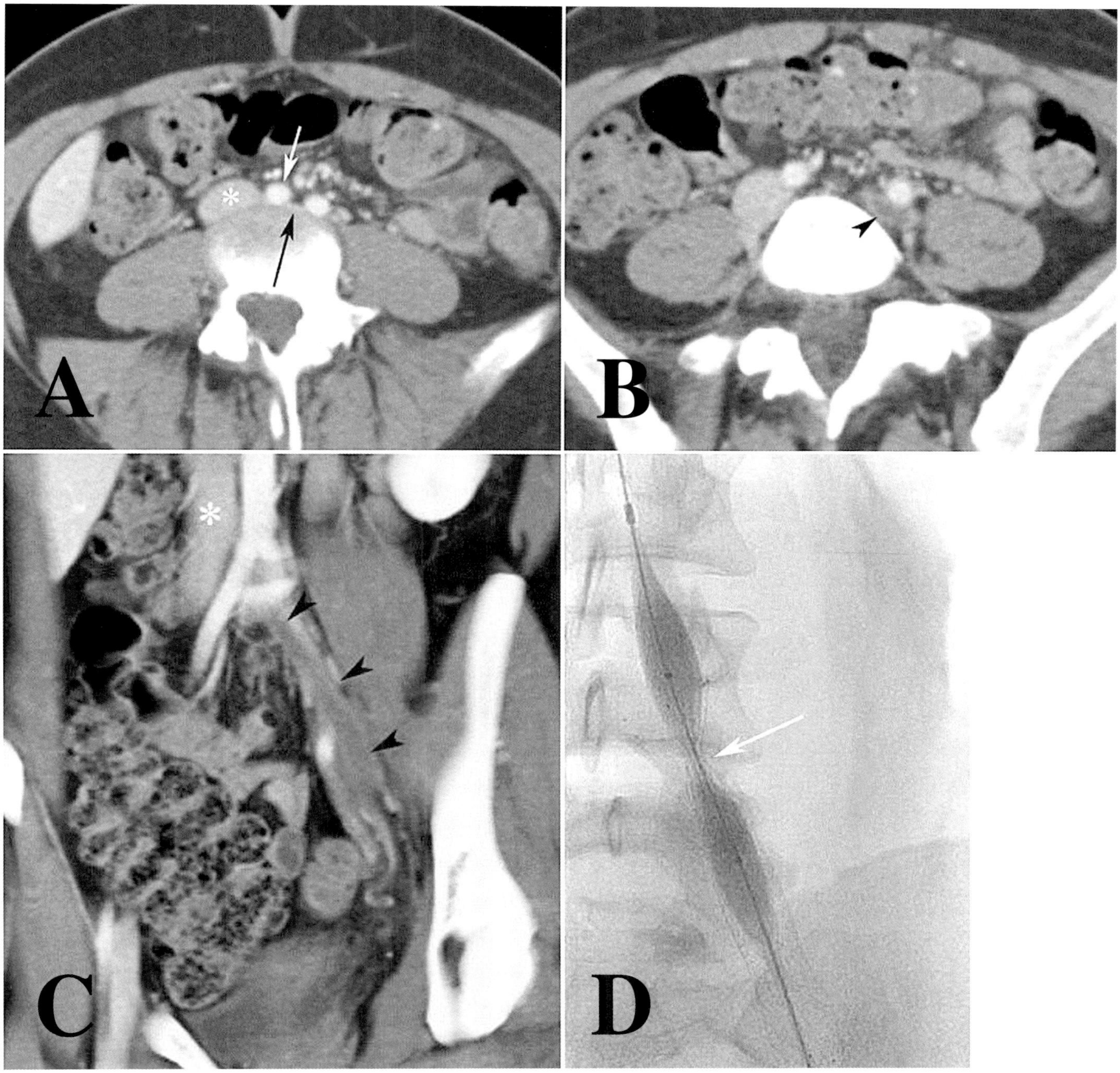

Figure 97.1 A 30-year-old woman with May–Thurner syndrome presented with acute deep venous thrombosis of the left lower extremity. **A.** Axial venous phase CT shows the left common iliac vein (black arrow) is compressed between the right common iliac artery (white arrow) and the vertebral body immediately below the level of the aortic bifurcation. Asterisk: inferior vena cava. **B.** Axial and (**C**) oblique coronal volume-rendered CT show acute thrombosis of the left common iliac vein and external iliac vein seen as hypodense filling defect (black arrowheads). Asterisk indicates the inferior vena cava. **D.** The patient underwent catheter-directed thrombolysis and angioplasty. A stent was placed over the short-segment stenosis at the origin of the left common iliac vein (arrow). Post-stent angioplasty was performed, and no residual stenosis was noted (image not shown).

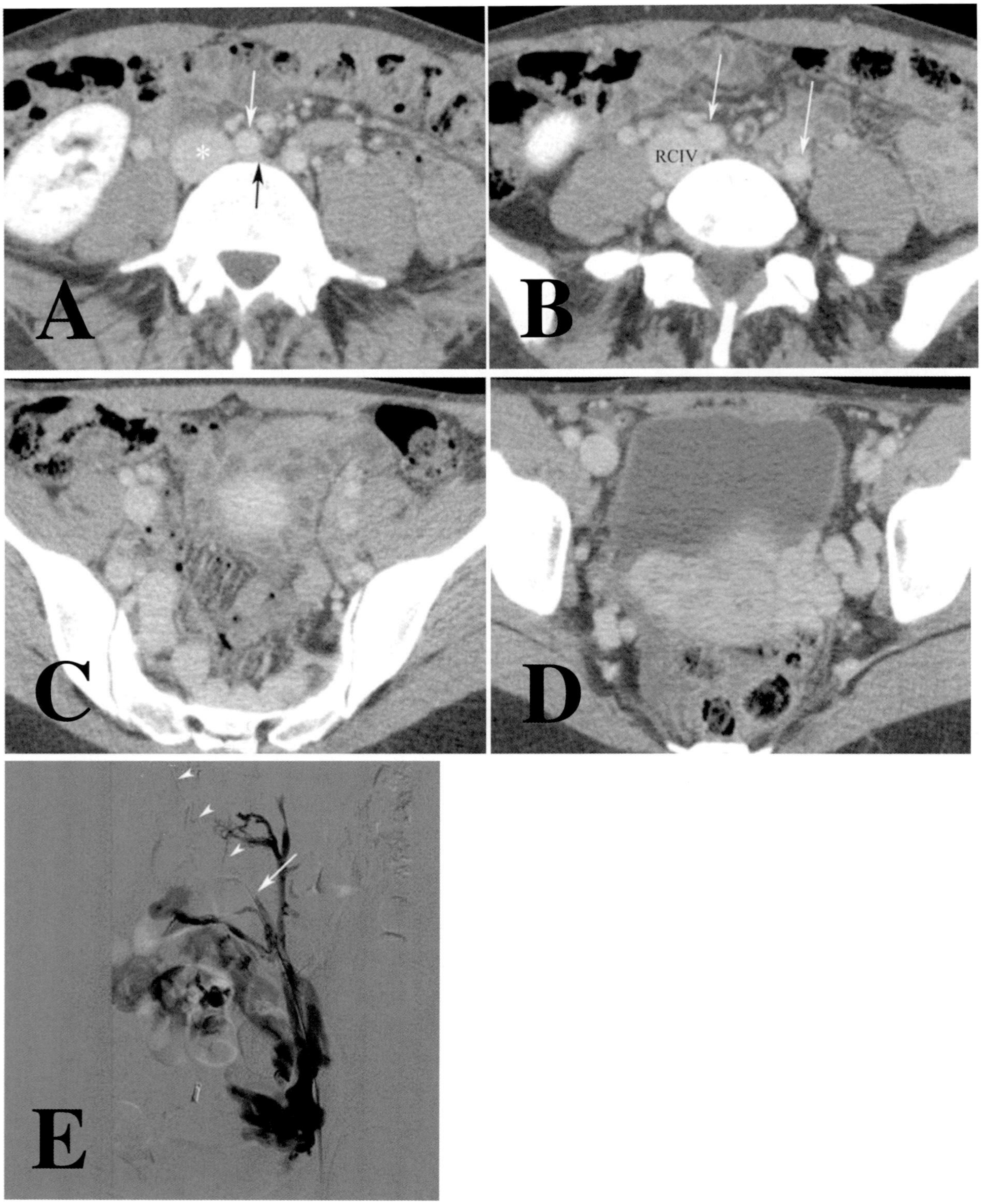

Figure 97.2 A 40-year-old woman with May–Thurner syndrome. Remote history of extensive deep venous thrombosis of the left lower extremity and chronic occlusion of the left common iliac vein resulting in pelvic congestion syndrome. **A.** Axial contrast-enhanced CT shows the left common iliac vein (black arrow) is compressed between the right common iliac artery (white arrow) and the vertebral body immediately below the level of the aortic bifurcation. Asterisk indicates inferior vena cava. **B–D.** Axial contrast-enhanced CT show non-visualized left common iliac vein due to chronic occlusion with marked pelvic venous collaterals. White arrows: right and left common iliac arteries. RCIV: right common iliac vein. **E.** Left iliac venogram shows chronic occlusion of the left common iliac vein (arrow) with venous drainage through an extensive complex of venous varices and via left lumbar/hemiazygos veins. The patient was treated with left common iliac vein reconstruction using venoplasty/stent. Arrowheads: wire in the left common iliac vein and inferior vena cava.

CASE 98 Pseudocarcinomatosis due to venous malformation

Atif Zaheer

Imaging description

Venous malformations are characterized by dilated venous spaces with normal arterial components.[1] They appear as soft tissue nodules on non-contrast computed tomography (CT) (Figure 98.1) and demonstrate slow, gradual nodular filling with contrast on delayed venous phase images with a prolonged contrast rise time of about 90 seconds (Figure 98.2).[2] If thrombosed, these show lack of enhancement on contrast-enhanced CT or MRI. Phleboliths are usually present and appear as calcified nodules on CT (Figure 98.1). On MRI, venous malformations are typically low-flow abnormalities characterized by decreased signal intensity on T1-weighted images and high signal on fat suppressed T2-weighted MR images (Figure 98.3).[1] High-signal intensity on T1-weighted images and internal fluid–fluid levels on T2-weighted images are indicative of the presence of hemorrhage or high protein content (Figure 98.3).[3] Delayed enhancement is often appreciated in the slow-flowing veins (Figure 98.4).[4] Furthermore, there is absence of arterial and early venous enhancement or arteriovenous shunting, distinguishing venous malformations from high-flow malformations or arteriovenous fistulas.[5] Phleboliths appear as small low signal intensity foci on all pulse sequences. Due to their nodular appearance, extensive venous malformations in the abdominal cavity can have an appearance similar to carcinomatosis (compare Figure 98.1 to Figure 98.5), particularly on non-contrast examinations.

Importance

Although present at birth, patients with venous malformations may become symptomatic in late childhood or early adulthood. Complications of venous malformations depend on the area of involvement and include rectal rectal bleeding, hematuria, epistaxis, deep vein thrombosis, pulmonary embolism, infection, and coagulopathy.[6] Misdiagnosis of venous malformations as carcinomatosis could lead to inappropriate biopsy with potentially disastrous consequences due to high bleeding risk.

Typical clinical scenario

Venous malformations may be seen in isolation or in combination with a variety of syndromes such as Klippel–Trenaunay–Weber, Sturge–Weber, and Proteus syndrome. Severe angiomatosis with extensive venous malformations seen in Klippel–Trenaunay–Weber is characterized by a triad of port-wine stain, venous varicosities and malformations, and osseous and soft tissue hypertrophy.[7,8] Although lower extremity is the site of involvement in about 95% of patients, venous malformations occur in both superficial and deep venous systems in the gastrointestinal and genitourinary tracts.

Differential diagnosis

The nodular densities on non-contrast CT can mimic soft tissue lesions. Peritoneal location can be mistaken for carcinomatosis and can be subject to needle biopsy (Figure 98.5A). The key differentiating feature is the presence of phleboliths which appear as calcified nodules on CT and the typical enhancement pattern on CT and MRI (Figure 98.5B). Differentiation between various syndromes associated with venous malformations is typically done on clinical grounds.

Teaching point

Venous malformation may be an isolated finding or seen in association with a wide variety of syndromes. Nodular lesions with phleboliths and delayed nodular filling on the venous phase are characteristic imaging findings that help differentiate venous malformations from mass lesions.

REFERENCES

1. T. Nozaki, S. Nosaka, O. Miyazaki, et al. Syndromes associated with vascular tumors and malformations: a pictorial review. *Radiographics* 2013; **33**: 175–95.

2. Y. Ohgiya, T. Hashimoto, T. Gokan, et al. Dynamic MRI for distinguishing high-flow from low-flow peripheral vascular malformations. *AJR Am J Roentgenol* 2005; **185**: 1131–7.

3. L. Flors, C. Leiva-Salinas, I. M. Maged, et al. MR imaging of soft-tissue vascular malformations: diagnosis, classification, and therapy follow-up. *Radiographics* 2011; **31**: 1321–40; discussion 1340–1.

4. H. Moukaddam, J. Pollak, A. H. Haims. MRI characteristics and classification of peripheral vascular malformations and tumors. *Skeletal Radiol* 2009; **38**: 535–47.

5. C. U. Herborn, M. Goyen, T. C. Lauenstein, J. F. Debatin, S. G. Ruehm, K. Kroger. Comprehensive time-resolved MRI of peripheral vascular malformations. *AJR Am J Roentgenol* 2003; **181**: 729–35.

6. S. A. Berry, C. Peterson, W. Mize, et al. Klippel-Trenaunay syndrome. *Am J Med Genet* 1998; **79**: 319–26.

7. T. P. Klippel M. Du noevus variqueux osteohypertrophiques. *Arch Gen Med* 1900; **3**: 641–72.

8. P. A. Baskerville, J. S. Ackroyd, M. Lea Thomas, N. L. Browse. The Klippel-Trenaunay syndrome: clinical, radiological and haemodynamic features and management. *Br J Surg* 1985; **72**: 232–6.

Pearls and Pitfalls in Cardiovascular Imaging, ed. Stefan L. Zimmerman and Elliot K. Fishman. Published by Cambridge University Press. © Cambridge University Press 2015.

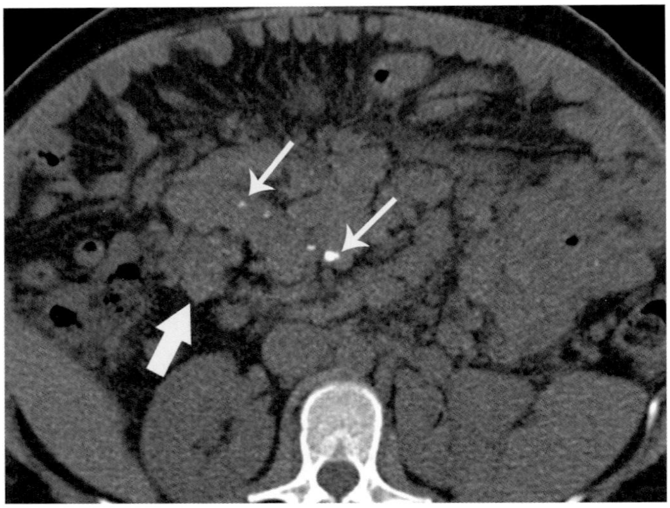

Figure 98.1 A 42-year-old woman with Klippel–Trenaunay–Weber syndrome. Axial non-contrast MDCT demonstrates multiple venous malformations in the mesentery, seen as multiple soft tissue nodules (thick white arrow). Multiple calcific foci are also seen, representing phleboliths (thin arrows).

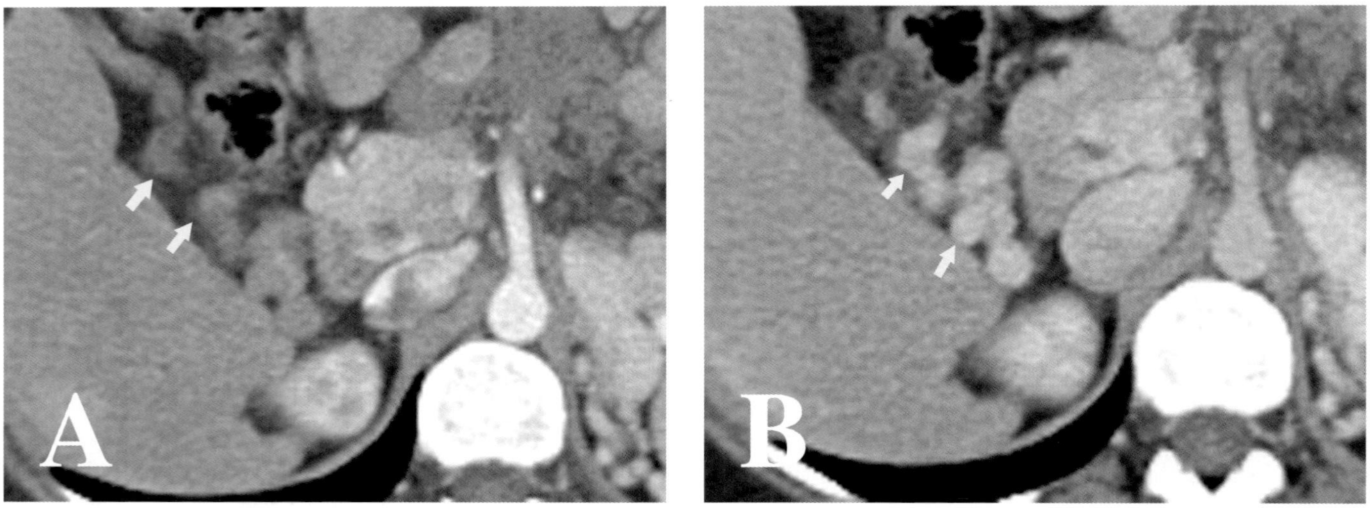

Figure 98.2 A. A 42-year-old woman with Klippel–Trenaunay–Weber syndrome. Axial contrast-enhanced arterial phase MDCT demonstrates venous malformation as serpiginous masses adjacent to the liver with minimal enhancement (arrows) in the arterial phase. **B.** Axial contrast-enhanced venous phase MDCT demonstrates venous enhancement (arrows) of the serpiginous masses, matching the enhancement of the inferior vena cava.

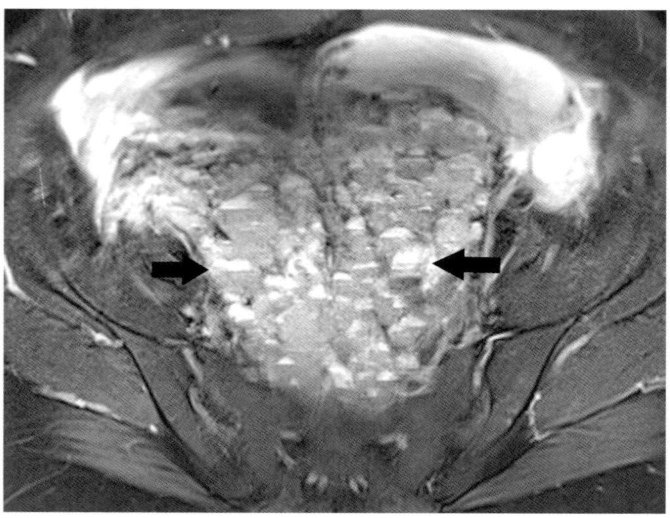

Figure 98.3 A 51-year-old woman with Klippel–Trenaunay–Weber syndrome. T2-weighted axial image demonstrates multiple venous malformations as areas of hyperintensity with internal areas of fluid–fluid levels (arrows) due to hemorrhage or high protein content.

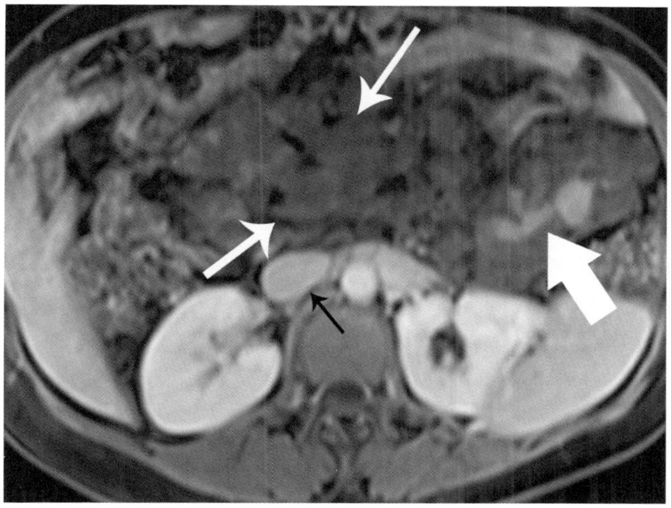

Figure 98.4 A 51-year-old woman with Klippel–Trenaunay–Weber syndrome. Axial post-contrast venous phase MR images demonstrate venous malformation as serpiginous lesions with venous enhancement (thick arrow), matching the enhancement of the inferior vena cava (thin black arrow). There is absence of enhancement in the thrombosed malformations (thin white arrows).

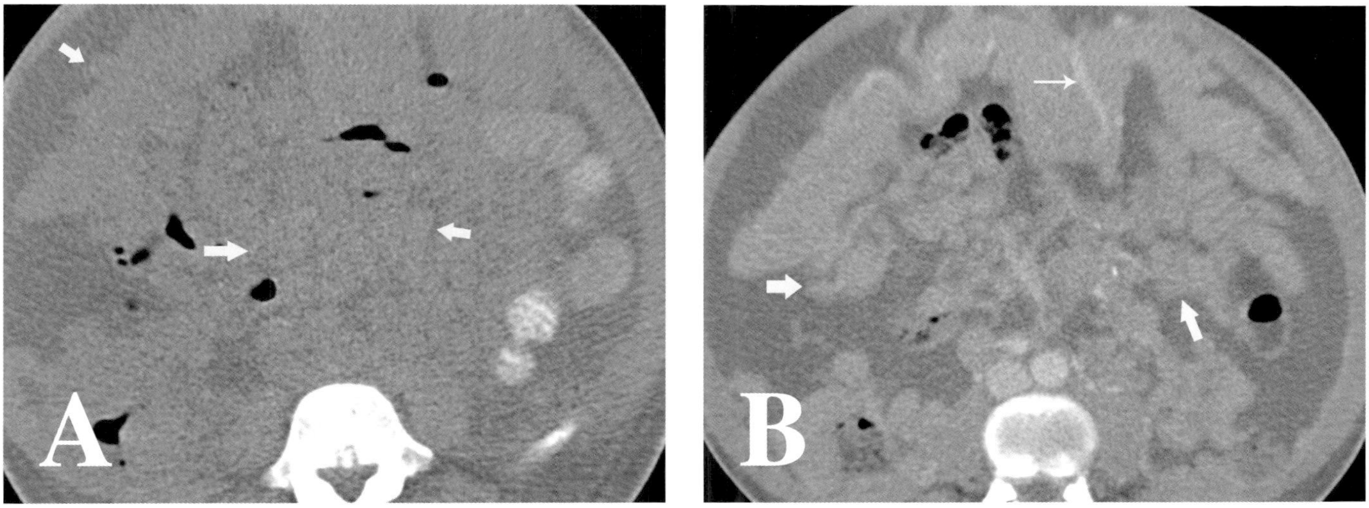

Figure 98.5 A. A 49-year-old man with metastatic ocular melanoma. Axial non-contrast-enhanced MDCT demonstrates multiple soft tissue nodules representing metastatic disease (arrows). **B.** Axial contrast-enhanced MDCT demonstrates multiple enhancing soft tissue nodules (thick arrows). An enhancing vein is seen, with a greater degree of enhancement than the adjacent nodular soft tissue, helping to distinguish this finding from a venous malformation (thin arrow). In venous malformations, the nodular soft tissue would be expected to enhance similar to adjacent veins and inferior vena cava.

CASE

99 Inferior vena cava anatomic variants

Satomi Kawamoto

Imaging description

Inferior vena cava (IVC) anomalies reflect an abnormal regression or persistence of the various embryonic veins,[1] and there are numerous variations.[2] In patients with double (right and left) IVC, two oval structures are seen on both sides of the abdominal aorta on axial images (Figures 99.1 and 99.2). There may be significant discrepancy in the size of the two veins.[3] Typically the right and left IVCs join to form a single right IVC at the level of the left renal vein (Figures 99.1 and 99.2). Different from dilated gonadal vein, the left IVC continues caudally to the left common iliac vein (Figure 99.1).

Retrocaval ureter is an anomaly related to the development of the inferior vena cava. The proximal right ureter is positioned posterior to the IVC, and then courses to the left of the IVC, and finally crosses anterior to the IVC (Figure 99.2).[4] Hydronephrosis due to ureteral obstruction may occur in patients with retrocaval ureter.

In patients with interruption of the IVC with azygos or hemiazygos continuation, the hepatic segment of IVC is absent (Figure 99.3), and the renal segment of IVC receives blood return from both kidneys and passes posterior to the diaphragmatic crus, and enters the thorax as the azygos or hemiazygos vein (Figure 99.3). The hepatic veins drain directly into the right atrium. In these patients, the azygos or hemiazygos vein is dilated (Figure 99.3), reflecting the increased flow through these vessels.

Importance

IVC anomalies usually are an incidental finding and do not have a clinical significance. However, it may simulate an abnormal structure such as lymphadenopathy or a mass. Before interventional or surgical procedures, such as IVC filter placement, anomalous anatomy of the IVC is important to be recognized. For example, in patients with double IVC, recurrent pulmonary embolism following placement of an IVC filter is possible.[4]

Other uncommon types of IVC anomaly include IVC agenesis,[5] right-sided double IVC, and left IVC with left retrocaval ureter. In patients with IVC agenesis, recurrent deep venous thrombosis may occur.[5]

Typical clinical scenario

Embryogenesis of the IVC is a complex process involving the formation of several anastomoses and regression of three paired embryonic veins (cardinal veins, subcardinal vein, and supracardinal veins).[1] A broad spectrum of congenital anomalies can affect the IVC.

The renal segment of the vena cava is formed by intersubcardinal and supracardinal anastomosis, and renal vein anomaly such as retroaortic renal vein and circumaortic left renal vein may occur at the time of development of this anastomosis. They are relatively common; the prevalence is 1.8–2.4% for retroaortic left renal vein, and 1.5–8.7% for circumaortic left renal vein.[1]

Anomalies of the IVC are present in 0.3–0.5% of otherwise healthy individuals, and in 0.6–2% of patients with other cardiovascular defects.[5] Left IVC has a prevalence of 0.2–0.5%. Usually, at the level of the renal vein, the left IVC passes in front of the aorta and runs to the right, assuming the normal position.[1] Double (right and left) IVC has 1–3% prevalence.[2,3] The left IVC typically crosses over to join the right IVC, usually anterior to the aorta at the level of the left renal vein.[1]

Retrocaval ureter is a rare congenital anomaly with a prevalence of 0.07%,[1]and usually occurs on the right side.[4] It is not an anomaly of ureteric development, but an anomaly related to the development of the IVC. It is one of the few congenital anomalies of the IVC that can be symptomatic.[3]

Interruption of the IVC with azygos or hemiazygos continuation results from failure to form the right subcardinal–hepatic anastomosis. Its prevalence is 0.6%.[1] Although these patients may be asymptomatic, this anomaly can be associated with congenital heart disease and asplenia or polysplenia syndrome (Figure 99.3).[4]

Differential diagnosis

Presence of the IVC in an unexpected location, or dilated azygos/hemiazygos vein may simulate retroperitoneal, retrocrural, or posterior mediastinal mass or adenopathy, especially when contrast material is not used, or the venous structures are not adequately opacified with contrast material related to technique or thrombus.

The left IVC may be mistaken for a large gonadal vein.[1] The left IVC continues caudally as the left common iliac vein, while a prominent gonadal vein courses toward the inguinal canal in males or the ovary in females.[1]

Pearls and Pitfalls in Cardiovascular Imaging, ed. Stefan L. Zimmerman and Elliot K. Fishman. Published by Cambridge University Press. © Cambridge University Press 2015.

Teaching point

IVC anomaly is often an incidental finding in asymptomatic patients. It is usually easily identified on contrast-enhanced CT. However, anomalies are important to recognize for better planning of interventional or surgical procedures. They should not be mistaken for a mass or lymphadenopathy.

REFERENCES

1. Kellman GM, Alpern MB, Sandler MA, Craig BM. Computed tomography of vena caval anomalies with embryologic correlation. *Radiographics* 1988;**8**:533–556.

2. Minniti S, Visentini S, Procacci C. Congenital anomalies of the venae cavae: embryological origin, imaging features and report of three new variants. *European Radiology* 2002;**12**:2040–2055.

3. Kandpal H, Sharma R, Gamangatti S, Srivastava DN, Vashisht S. Imaging the inferior vena cava: a road less traveled. *Radiographics* 2008;**28**:669–689.

4. Bass JE, Redwine MD, Kramer LA, Huynh PT, Harris JH, Jr. Spectrum of congenital anomalies of the inferior vena cava: cross-sectional imaging findings. *Radiographics* 2000;**20**:639–652.

5. Gil RJ, Perez AM, Arias JB, Pascual FB, Romero ES. Agenesis of the inferior vena cava associated with lower extremities and pelvic venous thrombosis. *Journal of Vascular Surgery* 2006;**44**:1114–1116.

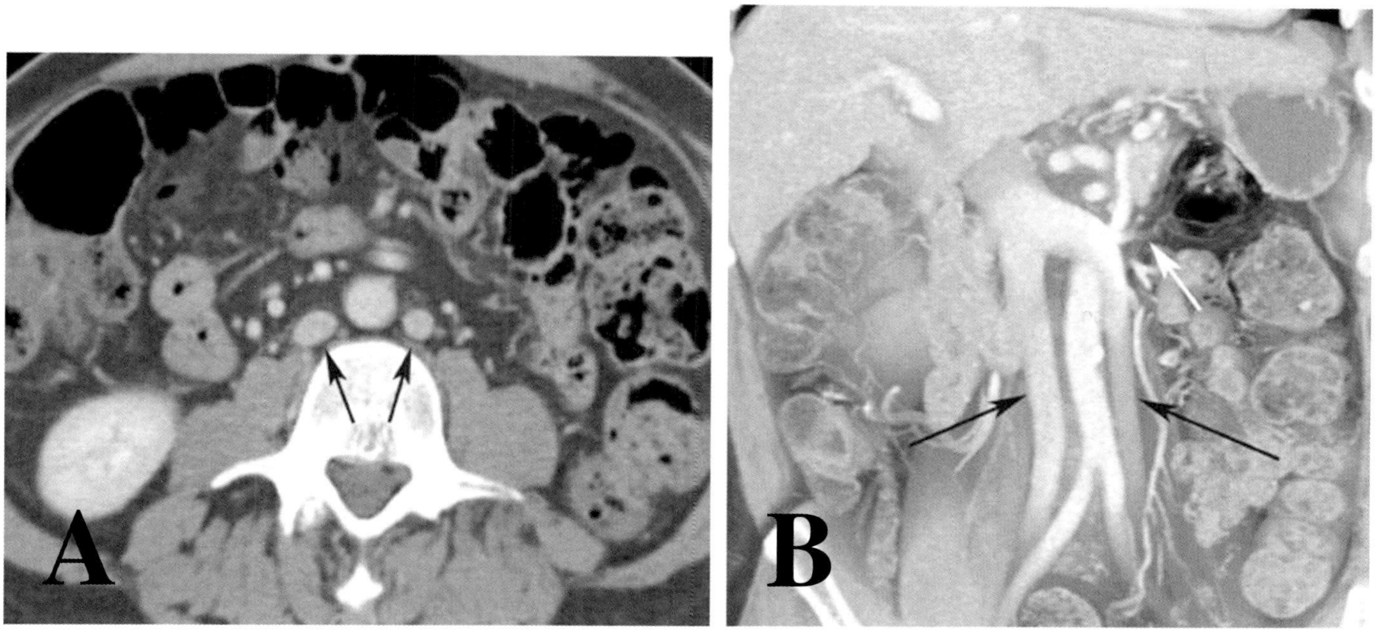

Figure 99.1 A. Contrast-enhanced axial and (**B**) coronal volume-rendered CT. Double IVC is incidentally demonstrated, seen on both sides of the abdominal aorta (black arrows). The right and left IVCs join to form a single right IVC at the level of the left renal vein (white arrow). The left renal vein is small in this patient with an atrophic left kidney (not shown). The left IVC continues caudally to the left common iliac vein.

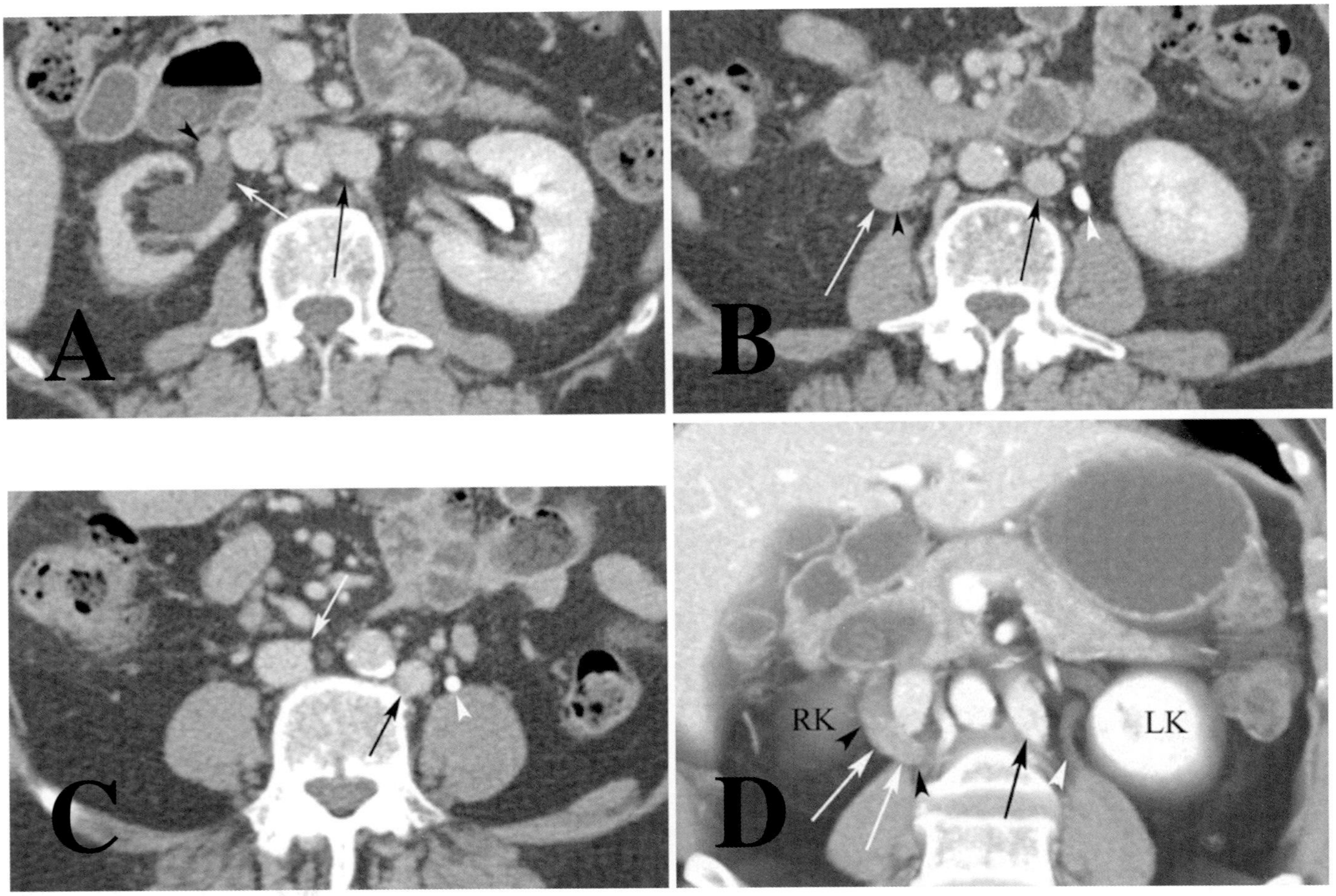

Figure 99.2 **A**.–**C**. Axial (excretory phase) and (**D**) oblique inferior volume-rendered (nephrographic phase) contrast-enhanced CT performed for evaluation of the patient's known bladder cancer demonstrate incidental double IVC and retrocaval right ureter. The proximal right ureter (white arrow) is positioned posterior to the right IVC, and then courses medially, and finally crosses anterior to the right IVC. Note normal course of the left ureter (white arrowhead). The proximal portion of the right ureter is filled with a soft tissue-density lesion (black arrowheads) thought to represent synchronous urothelial neoplasm. There is an atrophic right kidney with hydronephrosis (black arrow: left IVC; RK: right kidney; LK: left kidney).

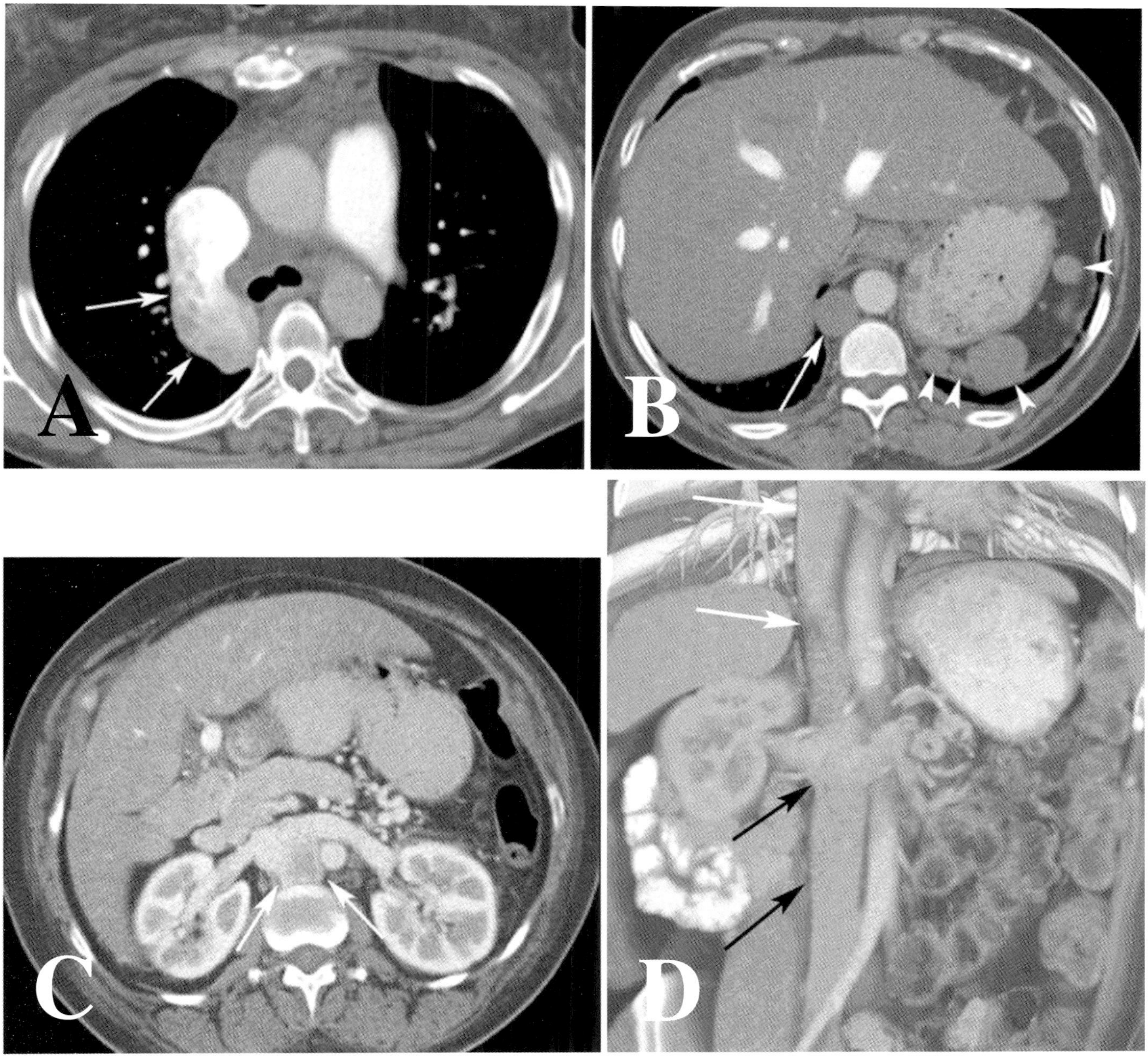

Figure 99.3. A.–C. Axial and (**D**) anterior volume-rendered contrast-enhanced CT performed for evaluation for pulmonary embolism and abdominal pain. **A.** There is dilatation of the azygos arch (white arrows). **B.** The hepatic veins are opacified with refluxed contrast material; however, the hepatic segment of IVC is absent. The dilated azygos vein is seen in the right retrocrural space (white arrow). Note multiple small spleens (white arrowheads), representing polysplenia. **C.** The renal segment of IVC drains posteriorly, connected to the dilated azygos vein (arrows). **D.** Right-sided renal and subrenal segments of the IVC (black arrows) drain to the dilated azygos vein (white arrows).

CASE 100

Superior vena cava anatomic variants

Pamela T. Johnson

Imaging description

Persistent left-sided superior vena cava (SVC) is the most common congenital venous anomaly of the chest. In this variant, the left-sided cava receives blood from the left subclavian and left jugular veins and courses inferiorly in the chest, lateral to the left aortic arch and hilum, and drains directly into the coronary sinus.[1] In the vast majority of cases, a separate right-sided SVC is also present.[2] These vessels communicate via a persistent bridging vein in 35% of patients.[2] On chest radiograph, left-sided SVC appears as superior mediastinal widening and a right-sided venous catheter will cross the mediastinum to enter the heart on the left side.[3] A CT will confirm the presence of left-sided SVC coursing lateral to the aortic arch and terminating in the coronary sinus (Figure 100.1). Duplicated inferior vena cava (IVC) and left-sided IVC are two congenital IVC anomalies where a left-sided IVC will be present in the left para-aortic region.[4,5]

Importance

Anomalous veins can be mistaken for lymphadenopathy or masses, particularly in studies performed without intravenous contrast. The presence of anomalous veins is also important for planning of central venous access.

Typical clinical scenario

Unless the patient has congenital heart disease, these anomalies are often identified incidentally during imaging. Persistent left-sided SVC is present in 0.3% of people, with a higher incidence (4.3%) in those who have congenital heart anomalies.[1,3]

Differential diagnosis

The differential diagnosis for a large venous structure coursing lateral to the ascending thoracic aorta is partial anomalous pulmonary venous return (Figure 100.2).[1] Unlike a persistent left SVC, which courses inferiorly into the coronary sinus (Figure 100.1), this venous structure courses into the left hilum and branches into the lung parenchyma, along with the left pulmonary arteries. A central line positioned in PAPVR (partial anomalous pulmonary venous return) will course away from the mediastinum at the level of the hilum (Figure 100.2), unlike one positioned in a duplicated SVC, which extends along the heart border into the coronary sinus (Figure 100.1).

Teaching point

Venous variants can be distinguished by their course and must not be mistaken for other pathology such as mediastinal or retroperitoneal adenopathy.

REFERENCES

1. L. P. Lawler, F. M. Corl, E. K. Fishman. Multi-detector row and volume-rendered CT of the normal and accessory flow pathways of the thoracic systemic and pulmonary veins. *Radiographics* 2002; **22** Spec No: S45–60.
2. G. M. Kellman, M. B. Alpern, M. A. Sandler, B. M. Craig. Computed tomography of vena caval anomalies with embryologic correlation. *Radiographics* 1988; **8**: 533–56.
3. T. J. Cole, D. A. Henry, H. Jolles, A. V. Proto. Normal and abnormal vascular structures that simulate neoplasms on chest radiographs: clues to the diagnosis. *Radiographics* 1995; **15**: 867–91.
4. C. S. Restrepo, A. Eraso, D. Ocazionez, J. Lemos, S. Martinez, D. F. Lemos. The diaphragmatic crura and retrocrural space: normal imaging appearance, variants, and pathologic conditions. *Radiographics* 2008; **28**: 1289–305.
5. J. E. Bass, M. D. Redwine, L. A. Kramer, P. T. Huynh, J. H. Harris, Jr. Spectrum of congenital anomalies of the inferior vena cava: cross-sectional imaging findings. *Radiographics* 2000; **20**: 639–52.

Pearls and Pitfalls in Cardiovascular Imaging, ed. Stefan L. Zimmerman and Elliot K. Fishman. Published by Cambridge University Press. © Cambridge University Press 2015.

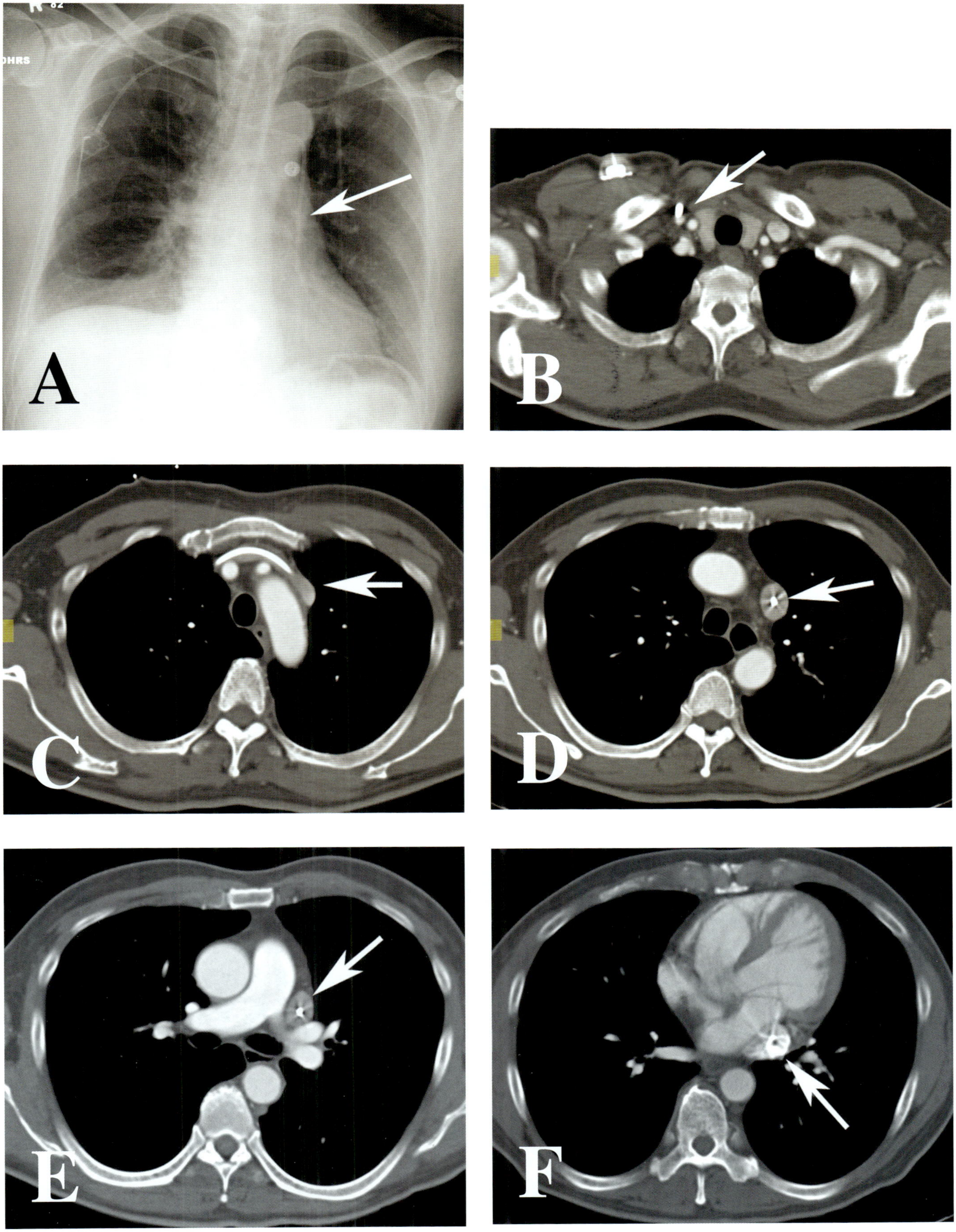

Figure 100.1 A 64-year-old man with a left-sided superior vena cava (SVC). **A.** Chest radiograph shows right subclavian venous catheter (arrow) coursing across the mediastinum and along the left heart border. **B–F.** Sequential axial images from IV contrast-enhanced chest CT demonstrate the catheter (arrow) coursing through the right internal jugular vein (**B**), then across the anterior mediastinum via the right innominate vein (**C**) to enter a left-sided SVC (**D,E**), which empties into the coronary sinus (**F**).

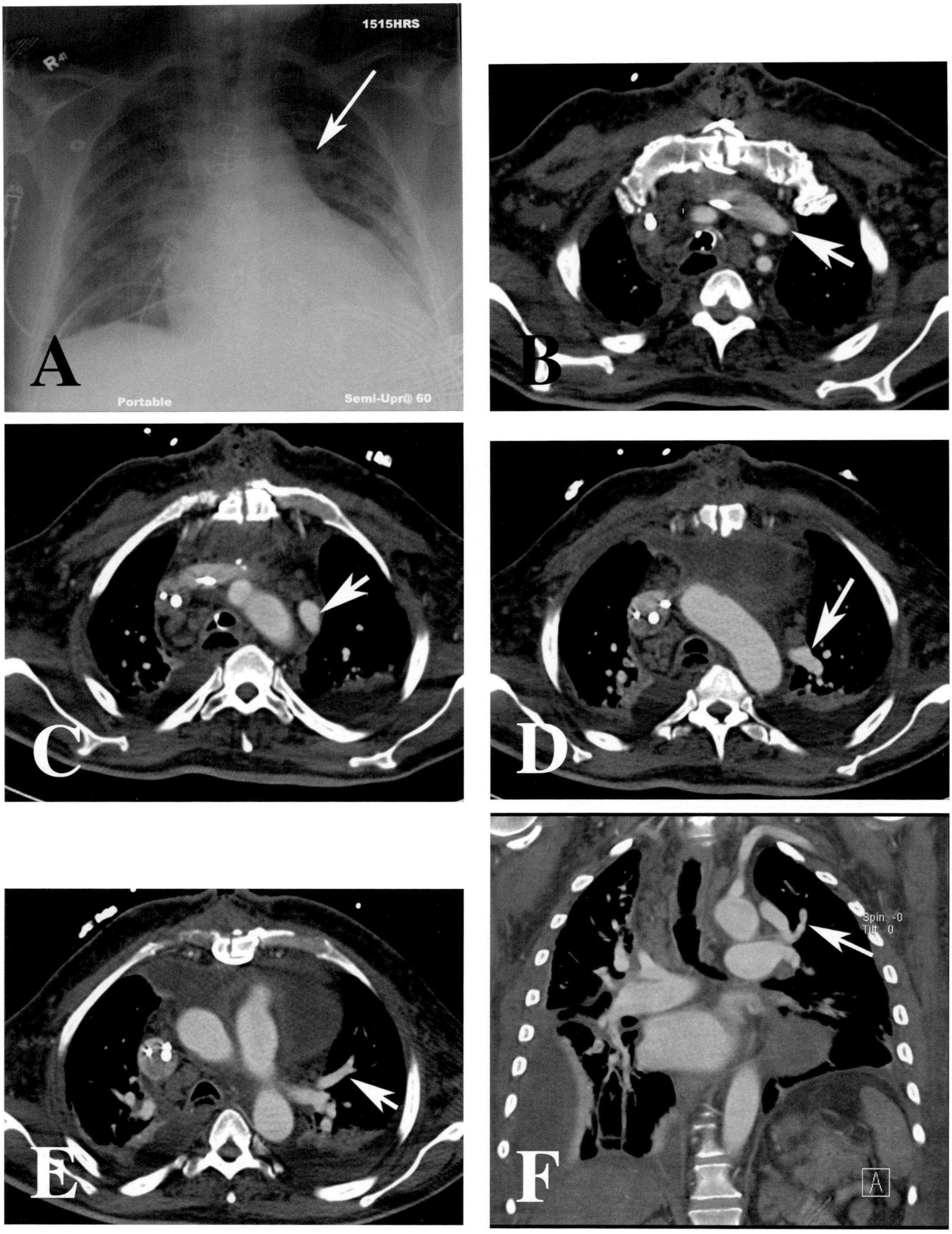

Figure 100.2 A 54-year-old man with partial anomalous pulmonary venous return (PAPVR). **A.** Chest radiograph shows a left-sided internal jugular venous catheter (arrow) coursing lateral to the mediastinum; the tip appears to be within the lung parenchyma. **B–E.** Sequential axial images from IV contrast-enhanced CT show this venous structure (arrow) coursing into the left hilum and into the lung parenchyma along with the left pulmonary arteries. **F.** Coronal MPR from IV contrast-enhanced CT shows the PAPVR (arrow) extending from left hilum into the lung parenchyma.

Index